MEASURING DISEASE

MEASURING DISEASE

A REVIEW OF
DISEASE-SPECIFIC
QUALITY OF LIFE
MEASUREMENT
SCALES

Ann Bowling

Open University Press
Buckingham · Philadelphia

Open University Press
Celtic Court
22 Ballmoor
Buckingham
MK18 1XW

and
1900 Frost Road, Suite 101
Bristol, PA 19007, USA

First Published 1995
Reprinted 1996, 1997

A catalogue record of this book is available from the
British Library

Library of Congress Cataloging-in-Publication Data
Bowling, Ann.
    Measuring disease: a review of disease-specific
quality of life measurement scales/Ann Bowling.
        p.   cm.
    Includes bibliographical references and index.
    ISBN 0-335-19226-2. – ISBN 0-335-19225-4 (pbk.)
    1. Health status indicators.   2. Quality of life.
I. Title.
RA407.B68 1994
613–dc20   94-28081
                                                CIP

Typeset by Type Study, Scarborough
Printed in Great Britain by St Edmundsbury Press Ltd,
Bury St Edmunds, Suffolk

CONTENTS

3 PSYCHIATRIC CONDITIONS AND PSYCHOLOGICAL MORBIDITY   61

4   RESPIRATORY CONDITIONS   149

5 NEUROLOGICAL CONDITIONS   175

6 RHEUMATOLOGICAL CONDITIONS

7 CARDIOVASCULAR DISEASES

8 OTHER DISEASE- AND CONDITION-SPECIFIC SCALES   259

9   COMMENTS ON MEASUREMENT ISSUES AND SOURCES OF INFORMATION   286

PREFACE

The aim of this volume is to review the most commonly used condition-specific measures of health-related quality of life. Although the title of this book includes the description 'disease', the scales reviewed here include both condition-specific and disease-specific instruments. The author accepts there is debate about the labelling of some conditions as diseases (e.g. mental health problems), and about where the dividing line is in the case of others, but the chapter headings are not meant to imply any statements about 'what is disease'. Most include the label 'condition' in order to reflect their broader content.

THE STRUCTURE OF THE CHAPTERS

Each chapter follows a similar, but not identical pattern, which is dependent upon the amount and type of research on health-related quality of life that has been carried out in that field. Investigators in psychiatry and cancer (oncology) have made the most progress with disease-specific quality of life measures in comparison with, for example, cardiovascular diseases, where there has been a greater reliance on generic measures of health-related quality of life.

Each chapter on condition- and disease-specific scales begins with an introduction to the methods of measuring quality of life in that area, and also references the commonly used generic and domain-specific (e.g. depression) health-related quality of life scales, before reviewing the disease- and condition-specific scales. The generic scales have already been reviewed by the author (Bowling 1991); interested readers are also referred to the source literature.

Disease- and condition-specific quality of life scales often require further supplementation with disease-specific symptom items, or other indicators of the presence of ill health (apart from clinical indicators). These range from self-reporting of symptoms and unwanted treatment effects, as in cancer, to assessments of grip strength among people with joint problems. This book would have been incomplete without some reference to these indicators, and so they are presented briefly before the disease- and condition-specific quality of life measures are reviewed. The speciality which has the most extensive literature on such self-report symptom instruments is psychiatry. A number of the most frequently used instruments are reviewed in the first part of Chapter 3. A smaller selection of commonly used screening instruments of depression can be found in Bowling (1991), with which there is a little overlap. Attempts have been made to minimize any duplication. The use of these instruments has been widespread in research across many medical specialities, thus Chapter 3 will be of relevance to most investigators. These screening instruments are also frequently used as indicators of quality of life in their own right, albeit narrow in scope. This is because, not only do they provide an index of psychological morbidity (a domain of quality of life), but they also include items on the impact of the condition on quality of life (e.g. on concentration, sleeping, energy levels, etc.).

The reader will also find some single-domain measures of need for care, behaviour, role functioning, adjustment and coping reviewed after the quality of life scales in Chapter 3. They are included because several of the broader scales overlap, almost indistinguishably, with quality of life scales. Some of them are popularly used with a range of physical and mental health problems.

Other major single-domain psychosocial scales, such as life satisfaction, social networks and support and self-esteem, have already been reviewed by the author (Bowling 1991), and only referenced in this volume. A fairly comprehensive range of scales of life satisfaction, morale and self-esteem can be found in reviews by Breytspraak and George (1982), Sauer and Warland (1982), Kane and Kane (1988), Andrews and Robinson (1991) and Blascovich and Tomaka (1991). A review of the measurement of social stress can be found in Kasl and Cooper (1987).

RECOMMENDATIONS

The strengths, weaknesses and coverage of each scale are presented in the text. Readers need to acquaint themselves with the range of available scales in their field of interest and select the ones which are most appropriate for the aims of their investigation. All scales have their good and bad points. Relatively few scales have been fully tested. Scale development is often ongoing, and promising but relatively untested scales today may be the scales of choice tomorrow. For this reason, no 'quasi-scientific' league table of 'best buys' has been attempted, although readers will find text comments, and a concluding section at the end of each chapter with some recommendations, which should help them to make up their own minds about whether a particular scale is appropriate for their study.

Finally, it is easier to criticize a scale than to construct one. Even scales that have insufficient evidence of reliability and validity will have involved its authors in a tremendous amount of work, and they are to be admired for their endeavours. Researchers are encouraged to use existing scales, or adapt them where necessary, rather than design them from scratch. Where scales have not been fully tested, users are encouraged to test further the reliability and validity of selected instruments when carrying out their research. In this way, a better body of knowledge will be developed.

COPYRIGHT

Many scales are only available for purchase commercially. This is particularly true of those developed in North America. In many cases, the purchase price simply covers administration costs and the cost of a manual and questionnaire; in others, the cost of the manual and scale can be several hundred pounds. Potential users are advised to contact the authors or distributors of scales for details of permission of use and, where applicable, purchase. The author would like to echo the plea of Wilkin *et al.* (1992): in view of the difficulty that can be experienced in obtaining scales, authors should be encouraged by publishers to either reproduce their questionnaire (if short) in a major article on the scale's psychometric properties, or publish the name and *address* of the scale distributor. This would save a great deal of unnecessary correspondence, searching for likely references and scanning of the catalogues of the different distributors.

ACKNOWLEDGEMENTS

I would like to thank Dr Robert Edelmann for his helpful and detailed comments on earlier drafts of the manuscript and ready assistance with scale location, Mr Robert Hall for the computer searches for relevant references at the UK Clearing House for Information on the Assessment of Health Outcomes, Dr Stephen Wright and Ms Sally Anne Francis for supplying relevant references and material on quality of life assessments. I am indebted to the librarians of St Bartholomew's Hospital, especially to the librarian of St Bartholomew's Hospital Medical College, Ms Rajalakshmi Gangadharam, for the many hours she spent helping me to track down and obtain references, and to Dr Richard Pearson and the library staff at the Royal Society of Medicine for helping me to access others. Thanks also to Doris Otomewo for her assistance with the merging and ordering of references and the compilation and printing of the final copy of the manuscript.

I would like to thank close friends and family, particularly John James Bowling, for their patience and good humour during a period when they must have questioned the quality of my life! Finally, I would like to take the opportunity to give thanks to Professor Lesley Southgate, Dr Bobbie Jacobson and Dr Jane Leaver for their support.

I am grateful to the Open University Press for permitting me to include a limited amount of the material on scales of functional ability and psychological well-being from *Measuring Health* (and also updated here), and to the many other publishers who gave me copyright permission to reproduce scale items. As always, any errors remain the responsibility of the author.

LIST OF
ABBREVIATIONS

ACSA	Amnestic comparative self-assessment
ADL	Activities of Daily Living
AHI	Arthritis Helplessness Index
AIDS	Acquired immune deficiency syndrome
AIMS	Arthritis Impact Measurement Scale
AMTS	Abbreviated Mental Test Score
APA	American Psychiatric Association
ARA	American Rheumatology Association
BCCQ	Breast Cancer Chemotherapy Questionnaire
BDI	Beck Depression Inventory
BPRS	Brief Psychiatric Rating Scale
BSC	Brief Symptom Checklist
BSI	Brief Symptoms Inventory
CABG	Coronary artery bypass graft
CAL	Chronic airflow limitation
CALGB	Cancer Leukaemia Group B Studies
CAPD	Continuous Ambulatory Peritoneal Dialysis
CARE	Comprehensive Assessment and Referral Evaluation
CARES	Cancer Rehabilitation Evaluation System
CES-D	Center for Epidemiologic Studies of Depression Scale
CHQ	(Guyatt's) Chronic Heart Failure Questionnaire
CINAHL	Cumulated Index for Nursing and Allied Health Literature
CIPS	Cancer Inventory of Problem Situations
CNS	Canadian Neurological Scale
COAD	Chronic obstructive airways disease
COPD	Chronic obstructive pulmonary disease
CRQ	(Guyatt's McMaster) Chronic Respiratory Questionnaire
CSQ	(Larsen's) Client Satisfaction Questionnaire
DIMS	Diabetes Impact Measurement Scales
DIS	Diagnostic Interview Schedule
DQOL	Diabetes Quality of Life Measure
DSM	Diagnostic and Statistical Manual
ECOG	Eastern Cooperative Oncology Group
EORTC	European Organization for Research on Treatment of Cancer
EURIDISS	European Research on Incapacitating Diseases and Social Support
FDA	US Food and Drugs Administration
FEV_1	Forced expiratory volume in one second
FLIC	Functional Living Index – Cancer
FLIE	Functional Living Index – EMESIS

FLP	Functional Limitations Profile	OECD	Organization for Economic Cooperation and Development
FSI	Functional Status Index		
FVC	Forced vital capacity	OMAC	Outcome Measures in Ambulatory Care
GAF	Global Assessment of Functioning Scale		
		OMAR	Office of Medical Applications of Research
GAIS	Global Adjustment to Illness Scale		
		OPCS	Office of Population Censuses and Surveys
GAS	Global Assessment Scale		
GHQ	General Health Questionnaire	PAIS	Psychosocial Adjustment to Illness Scale
GMS	Geriatric Mental State		
GWBS	(Psychological) General Well-Being Scale	POMS	Profile of Mood States
		PSE	Present State Examination
HAD	Hospital Anxiety and Depression Scale	QALY	Quality-adjusted life year
		QL/QoL	Quality of life
HAQ	(Stanford Arthritis Center) Health Assessment Questionnaire	Q-L Index	Spitzer's Quality of Life Index
		QLAF-C	European Neuroblastoma Study Group Quality of Life Assessment Form – Children
HIS	Health Insurance Study (Rand)		
HIV	Human immunodeficiency virus		
HOI	Health Outcomes Institute	QLI-MH	Quality of Life Index for Mental Health
HOPES	HIV Overview of Problems – Evaluation System		
		QLS	Quality of Life Scale
IBDQ	Inflammatory Bowel Disease Questionnaire	QLSC	Quality of Life Status and Change
		QWBS	Quality of Well-Being Scale
ICD	International Classification of Diseases	RA	Rheumatoid arthritis
		RCP	Royal College of Physicians
LASA	Linear Analogue Self-Assessment	RCT	Randomized controlled trial
LUSS	Leicester Uraemic Symptom Scale	RDC	Research Diagnostic Criteria
		REHAB	Rehabilitation evaluation
MACTAR	McMaster–Toronto Arthritis Patient Function Preference Questionnaire	RNL	Reintegration to Normal Living Index
		SADS	Schedule for Affective Disorders and Schizophrenia
MHIQ	McMaster Health Index Questionnaire		
		SAS-II	Social Adjustment Scale-II
MI	Myocardial infarction	SBAS	Social Behaviour Assessment Schedule
MMPI	Minnesota Multiphasic Personality Inventory		
		SBQOL	SmithKline Beecham Quality of Life Scale
MMSE	Mini-Mental State Examination		
MOS	Medical Outcomes Study (Rand)	SBS	Social Behaviour Schedule
		SCL	Hopkins Symptom Check-List
MPQ	McGill Pain Questionnaire	SCL-90	Symptom Check List-90
MQOLS-CA	Multidimensional Quality of Life Scale – Cancer	SEIQoL	Schedule for the Evaluation of Individual Quality of Life
MRC	Medical Research Council	SESS	Self-Evaluation and Social Support Schedule
MSQ	Mental Status Questionnaire		
NCI	National Cancer Institute	SF-36	Rand Medical Outcomes Study Short-Form 36-item health status questionnaire
NHP	Nottingham Health Profile		
OA	Osteoarthritis		
OAD	Obstructive airways disease	SGRQ	St George's Respiratory Questionnaire
OARS	Older Americans' Resources and Services Schedule		
		SIP	Sickness Impact Profile

SRPS	Social Role Performance Schedule	WAIS	Wechsler Adult Intelligence Scale
SRT	Symptom Rating Test	WHO	World Health Organization
SSIAM	Structured and Scaled Interview to Assess Maladjustment	WHODAS	World Health Organization Disability Assessment Schedule
STAI	State–Trait Anxiety Inventory	WHOQOL	World Health Organization Quality of Life Group
TAPS	Team for the Assessment of Psychiatric Services	WMS	Wechsler Memory Scale
TyPE	Technology of Patient Experience (TyPE) Specifications	WOMAC	Western Ontario and McMaster Universities Arthritis Index
VAS	Visual Analogue Scale		

1

HEALTH-RELATED QUALITY OF LIFE: A DISCUSSION OF THE CONCEPT, ITS USE AND MEASUREMENT

BACKGROUND: THE 'QUALITY OF LIFE'

Success in the West is usually determined by economic achievement and occupational status. In the developed world, with the emphasis on affluence and with the increasing longevity of populations, there is a general interest in how to achieve the 'goodness' of life, sometimes called life satisfaction or quality of life.

The following extract is taken from a dialogue between Serafin and Summerchild in Michael Frayn's (1991) novel, *A Landing on the Sun*, in which the plot centres on a government investigation of quality of life. It is used here, along with the discussion that follows it, to illustrate the ineffable nature and topicality of 'quality of life':

> . . . Now . . . To recapitulate: 'the quality of life', as you understand it, is some property which is in one way or another promoted or enhanced by washing machines . . . . (p. 81) . . . Does the class of things which to your mind promote(s) . . . the quality of life stretch far enough from the kitchen door to include the family television set? (p. 82) . . . Washing machines, and similar sorts of domestic machinery, are intended to save our

time and labour. Now no-one could claim that a television set saves time. On the contrary – it uses up the time we've saved with the dishwasher and the vacuum cleaner. And I think one might go on to argue that far from saving labour it creates it . . . (p. 83) . . . They enjoy watching it. Let's leap from the television to the central heating. Do they have central heating because they enjoy it? (p. 83) . . . Do you find the word 'motor car' on your list? (p. 85) . . . The list that you apparently keep inside your head of things that enhance the quality of life (p. 85).

> (Frayn 1991)[1]

Walter and Shannon (1990) described the current interest in 'quality of life' in the developed world, ranging from current concerns for the environment to the marketing of the products we buy, and to the evaluation of the benefit–burden ratio involved in medical treatments. More globally, quality of life as an outcome indicator has been added to social, as well as health, service programme development (DHSS 1989). It has also been added to the Worldwide Healthy Cities Programmes (e.g. The Quality of Life in Pasadena Project), and defined as spanning the visual arts, recreation, employment, transport, housing, environmental and conservation issues, health and other indicators of what has been labelled as 'the social temperature'. The Organization for Economic Cooperation and Development (OECD) has agreed on a list of quality

---

[1] Michael Frayn, *A Landing on the Sun*. Viking, 1991, pages 81, 82, 83, 85. Copyright © Michael Frayn 1991. Reproduced by permission of Penguin Books Ltd, Harmondsworth.

of life related social concerns of member states, including health, command over goods and services, employment and quality of working life (Andrews 1973). The salience of quality of life across disciplines has resulted in the recent emergence of generic quality of life questionnaires (Evans and Cope 1993), and quality of life questionnaires for use in health care evaluation (Chubon 1987; Patrick *et al*. 1988; Siegrist *et al*. 1993).

WHAT IS QUALITY OF LIFE AND HEALTH-RELATED QUALITY OF LIFE? A REVIEW OF THE CONCEPTS AND SOME ATTEMPTS AT MEASUREMENT

Quality of life research, then, spans a range of topics, from quality of life in the last year of life (Lawton *et al*. 1990) to quality of life in urban environments (Rogerson *et al*. 1989). As was illustrated earlier, quality of life is an amorphous concept, that has a usage across many disciplines – geography, literature, philosophy, health economics, advertising, health promotion and the medical and social sciences (e.g. sociology and psychology). It is a vague concept; it is multidimensional and theoretically incorporates all aspects of an individual's life. Quality of life has also been defined as the 'output' of the inputs of the physical and the spiritual (Liu 1974); as the degree to which a person accomplishes life goals (Cella and Cherin 1987); and even quantified crudely as a formula in which quality of life (QL) is a product of one's natural endowment (NE) and the effort made on one's behalf by the family (H) and society (S), such that $QL = NE \times H \times S$ (Shaw 1977). The meaning of the concept of quality of life is thus arguably dependent on the user of the term, his or her understanding of it, and his or her position and agenda in the social and political structure (Edlund and Tancredi 1985): 'Quality of life is a vague and ethereal entity, something that many people talk about, but which nobody very clearly knows what to do about' (Campbell *et al*. 1976). In view of its multitude of usages, it has been suggested that the term 'quality of life' is so misused that it should be banished from our lexicon (Annas 1990).

Health-related quality of life

Research on valued states of existence has reported

that health is the most valued state (Rokeach 1973; Kaplan 1993a), and there is a rapidly expanding literature on 'health-related quality of life'. Life expectancy at birth in the developed world has increased over the past 150 years, although most of the increase has taken place during the first half of this century. Expectation of life, and expectations of a morbidity-free life at older ages, has also increased and has led to international attempts to measure health expectancy (Bone 1992; Robine *et al*. 1992). Debate focuses on whether the extra years of life are spent in good or poor health, with one side arguing that chronic morbidity is being compressed into an increasingly shorter period before death, and the other arguing that there is an expansion of morbidity in old age. This interest in health expectancy, as opposed to simply analysing mortality rates, coincides with the more positive view of health measurement in relation to health-related quality of life, which is currently more fashionable than simply measuring mortality rates, disease and ill health. Similarly, purchasing debates in health care have been focusing on health care costs in relation to 'health gain' or benefit from the treatments and interventions that are contracted for (Øvretveit 1993; see also overview by Normand and Bowling in press).

In relation to health, health status is increasingly referred to as quality of life, and, so as to narrow down its operationalization in research studies, quality of life is increasingly referred to as health-related quality of life. Health-related quality of life, like subjective health status, is patient based, but focuses more on the impact of a perceived health state on the ability to live a fulfilling life (Bullinger *et al*. 1993). From a health (or disease) perspective, quality of life has been said to refer to the social, emotional and physical well-being of patients following treatment (Greer 1984), mirroring the World Health Organization's (WHO 1947, 1948) definition of health (see below), and as the impact of disease and treatment on disability and daily functioning (Kaplan 1985). It is a double-sided concept, incorporating positive as well as negative aspects of well-being and life, and it is multidimensional, incorporating social, psychological and physical health. It is also, ultimately, a personal and a dynamic concept for, as health status deteriorates, perspectives on life, roles, relationships and experiences change (Morris *et al*. 1986, Sherwood

1977). Grant *et al.* (1990) also define quality of life as 'a personal statement of the positivity or negativity of attributes that characterize one's life'. Taking these definitions into account, health-related quality of life is defined here as optimum levels of mental, physical, role (e.g. work, parent, carer, etc.) and social functioning, including relationships, and perceptions of health, fitness, life satisfaction and well-being. It should also include some assessment of the patient's level of satisfaction with treatment, outcome and health status and with future prospects. It is distinct from quality of life as a whole, which would also include adequacy of housing, income and perceptions of immediate environment.

The WHO definition

The theoretical framework of health-related quality of life, then, is largely based on a multidimensional perspective of health as physical, psychological and social functioning and well-being, along the lines of the WHO's (1947, 1948) definition of health: a 'state of complete physical, mental and social well-being and not merely the absence of disease or infirmity'. The WHO (1984) has since added 'autonomy' to this list. Ware (1987) has argued that five health concepts are inherent in this definition: physical health, mental health, social functioning, role functioning and general well-being. He restricts his definition because the goal of health care is to maximize the health component of quality of life. Health status may influence quality of life without determining it.

The WHO (1991) has a working party on quality of life under its umbrella, which is undertaking a ten-country study of health-related quality of life (Sartorius 1993). This is known as the World Health Organization Quality of Life Group (WHOQOL Group 1991, 1993a, 1993b, 1993c, 1994a). This group has provided a definition of quality of life which also takes individual perception and relationship to the environment into account:

> Quality of life is defined as an individual's perception of their position in life in the context of the culture and value systems in which they live and in relation to their goals, expectations, standards and concerns. It is a broad ranging concept affected in a complex way by the person's physical health, psychological state, level of independence, social relationships, and their relationships to salient features of their environment.
>
> (WHOQOL Group 1993b)

This definition underpins the current development of the WHOQOL, an instrument for measuring quality of life that can be used in a variety of cultural settings. The WHOQOL instrument is being developed as a core instrument, and editions are planned which will be specific to certain population groups (e.g. cancer patients, the elderly, etc.). The testing is ongoing.

Social science, social gerontology and the 'good life'

Psychologists, sociologists and social gerontologists in the USA carried out most of the early empirical social research on quality of life in studies which attempted to estimate well-being, satisfaction or happiness, and what people meant by 'the good life' (Gurin *et al.* 1960; Bradburn and Caplowitz 1965; Bradburn 1969). Lawton (1983) first proposed a theoretical model of quality of life as 'the good life', defined as psychological well-being, perceived quality of life, behavioural competence and the 'objective' environment. Andrews (1974) argued that quality of life is the extent to which pleasure and satisfaction have been obtained. Quality of life has been referred to as an affective response to one's role situation and values (Andrews and Withey 1976), as the discrepancy between desired and actual circumstances (Krupinski 1980), and well-being or 'ill-being' of people and/or their environment (Bubolz *et al.* 1980). The gerontological literature on the topics of 'successful ageing', 'positive ageing' and 'quality of older age' makes a similar point, focusing largely on life satisfaction and morale (Neugarten *et al.* 1961; Havighurst 1963; Williams and Wirths 1965; Bradburn 1969; Lawton 1975; Andrews and Withey 1976; Palmore 1979). There has been a rapid expansion of literature on correlates of life satisfaction as a proxy for quality of life (Bowling *et al.* 1991; Shahtahmasebi *et al.* 1992); and life satisfaction has become a key variable in analyses of health status and mortality in old age (Bowling and

Browne 1991; Bowling and Farquhar 1993; Bowling *et al.* 1994; Grundy *et al.* 1992). The work of social gerontologists has roots in philosophy. As long ago as 44 BC, Cicero (reprinted in 1979), argued that old age contains many opportunities for positive change and productive functioning, and should not be confused with illness.

In sum, quality of life research in gerontology overlaps with research on positive ageing and centres around feelings of control, social relationships and the quality of environmental settings (Day 1991), and on mental health, cognitive efficacy, social competence and productivity, personal control, life satisfaction and motivation (Baltes and Baltes 1990). Basically, quality of life is still taken to refer to the earlier conceptions of the 'goodness of life' (Zautra and Goodhart 1979). It can also be seen in terms of the difference between reality, or the perception of reality, and expectations (Calman 1984; Presant 1984). The question of what is quality of life ultimately remains philosophical.

Philosophical approaches

Overlapping with this research is the history of the exploration of happiness dating from the work of early Greek philosophers to present-day philosophy and social science (Morgan 1934; Barschak 1951; Tatarkiewicz 1975; Gallup 1976; Mason and Faulkenberry 1978; Andrews 1981; Parducci 1984; Veenhoven 1988, 1989, 1991). Bentham (1834/1983) introduced the dimension of well-being and its measurement which he defined as 'the difference in value between the sum of pleasures of all sorts and the sum of pains of all sorts which a man experienced in a given period of time'. Three alternative philosophical theories of 'the good life' are: (1) the hedonist, which takes the ultimate good for people to underlie certain conscious experiences; (2) preference satisfaction, which defines the good life as the satisfaction of people's desires or preferences; and (3) the ideal, which holds that part of a good life consists of the realization of specific, normative ideals (Brock 1993; Scanlon 1993).

Social indicators and human needs

Several commentators have pointed out that, in non-experiential social indicators research, quality of life encompasses all circumstances of life, for example housing, leisure activities, work, the environment, etc. (Campbell *et al.* 1976; Wingo and Evans 1978; Kaplan 1993a). Experiential social indicators research includes subjective well-being (see Elster and Roemer 1993). There are several meanings of the term 'quality of life' in social research, ranging from individual fulfilment to the ability to lead a 'normal' life (Edlund and Tancredi 1985; Fowlie and Berkeley 1987). Some have argued that human needs are the foundations for quality of life and that quality of life is the degree of satisfaction of those needs – for example, physical, psychological, social, activity, marital and structural (Hörnquist 1982). This is reminiscent of Maslow's (1954, 1962a, 1962b) hierarchy of need (physiological, safety and security, social and belonging, ego, status and self-esteem and self-actualization). There has been little attempt to examine these assumptions critically (Bauer 1966a; Ziller 1974).

Geography and societal approaches to measurement

Rogerson *et al.* (1989) reviewed the concept of quality of life, and pointed out that no definitive list of criteria of quality of life has yet been developed, and neither has an acceptable weighting system for the incorporation of subjective and objective indicators. Rogerson and co-workers' (1989) research in human geography was based on a national opinion survey of 1200 respondents in Britain. They were asked to rate 20 dimensions of quality of life in terms of their degree of importance in influencing their choice of where to live, on a scale of 5 (very important) to 1 (indicating minimal significance). The top five items were violent crime, non-violent crime, health provision, pollution levels, and cost of living. The bottom five related to travel to work time, leisure facilities, quality council housing, access to council housing and cost of private-rented housing. Thus, in research on quality of life in cities, health care ranks third in importance.

A postal survey based on a sample of adults in Leeds produced interesting results on quality of life domains and their importance to the public (Percy-Smith and Sanderson 1992). The survey was part of a community needs assessment exercise that involved data-gathering from numerous sources.

Some of the postal survey respondents were also interviewed in more detail and their responses were collated with those from interviews with community representatives, workers and with attenders at a public meeting. A list of 'needs' was drawn up, based on the literature, and respondents were asked to rate these according to the degree of importance they attached to each. Among the items rated as being of most importance were 'a good standard of health', 'access to health care', 'safe from acts of crime and violence', 'a decent standard of housing' and 'living in a pleasant, clean and peaceful area'. The lowest rankings were given to items such as 'having an influence on organizations which affect your life', 'having spare time for personal and leisure activities' and 'having access to social services'.

Individual meaning

Phenomenologists argue that quality of life is dependent upon the interpretation, and perceptions, of the individual (Ziller 1974). Cohen (1982) has also pointed out that the simple listing of quality of life domains is not a satisfactory way of measuring quality of life because it is unknown whether all important domains have been included. Researchers who construct health-related quality of life measurement scales are seldom philosophically sophisticated or concerned with competing accounts of 'the good life'. To some extent, the need to develop valid measures for use with large and varied samples of people necessitates compromises and the simplification of issues of philosophical importance (Brock 1993). Rosenberg (1992) has argued that the psychometric translation of quality of life into components such as emotional status, social interaction, economic status, health status and physical capacity, while incorporating the multidisciplinary nature of human beings, does not capture their subjectivity. He argued that hermeneutic thinking should be introduced into modern medicine, so that a naturalistic concept of mankind is presented along with a concept of the human being as a self-reflective individual responsible for his or her own actions. Ziller (1974) has also argued that the approach to quality of life is 'through the eye of the experiencer; that is, a phenomenological approach'. The health-related quality of life scales designed by Guyatt et al. (1987a, 1987c, 1989a, 1989d), O'Boyle et al. (1989, 1992), and Ruta (1992, 1994, in press), which take account of the individual's perspective, are exciting developments which are counteracting the trend towards the pre-definition of quality of life by the researcher.

Human judgement analysis

Promising research on health outcomes, which takes individual meaning into account, has involved the application of the techniques of human judgement analysis (Brehmer and Joyce 1988) to assess health-related quality of life (O'Boyle et al. 1989). With this technique respondents are asked to list the five areas of life ('cues') that they judge to be the most important to their overall quality of life (the technique is known as the Schedule for the Evaluation of Individual Quality of Life or SEIQoL). Open-ended questions are used to elicit the relevant cues. Then subjects rate their current status against a vertical visual analogue scale, labelled at the extremes 'as good as could possibly be' and 'as bad as could possibly be'. These ratings are recorded as bar charts. Respondents are then asked to rate their global quality of life on a similarly labelled horizontal visual analogue scale. Respondents use a disc to assess the relative importance of the individual dimensions to their overall quality of life rating, and a scoring procedure exists (O'Boyle et al. 1993). In research on hip replacement, social/leisure activities and family were nominated most frequently by both patients and controls; happiness, religion, independence and finances were also nominated. Health was nominated more frequently by controls than patients (O'Boyle et al. 1992). Among a healthy population, relationships, health, family and finances were the most frequently nominated domains (over 50 per cent of subjects), and among gastrointestinal clinic attenders, family, work, social and leisure and health were the most frequently nominated domains (McGee et al. 1991). The reliability of the scale was reported to be moderately high to high. A strong case could be made for the use of this scale as the core component of disease-specific measures, although more work is required on its acceptability.

Other research on individuals' judgements and ratings of health-related quality of life

Recent research on people's definitions of health-related quality of life includes work by Guyatt *et al.* (1987a, 1987c, 1989a, 1989d), Tugwell *et al.* (1987) O'Boyle *et al.* (1989, 1992, 1994), Partridge *et al.* (1991) Farquhar (1995) and Ruta *et al.* (1992, 1994a, 1994b). The research relating to specific diseases is described in later chapters, but as an example of some of this research, Ruta and co-workers' approach is outlined briefly here. This approach overlaps with that of O'Boyle *et al.* (1989, 1992) and Guyatt *et al.* (1987a, 1987c, 1989a, 1989d). Ruta *et al.* (1992, in press) asked patients (e.g. with back pain) about the five most important areas or activities of their life that were affected by their condition, and asked them to rate how badly affected each was on a scale of 0–100 (0 = worst they can imagine for themselves; 100 = exactly as they would like to be). A sixth category was provided for other areas of life affected by their medical condition not previously mentioned. They were finally asked to imagine that they could improve some or all of the chosen areas of their life, and were given 60 points which they could 'spend' across one or more areas. The points they allocated to each area were taken to represent the relative importance of potential improvements in that area. By multiplying each of the six ratings by the proportion of points allocated to that area, and summing, the authors generated an index between 0 and 100. The authors reported that the five most frequently mentioned areas of life were housework, gardening, sport, work and walking (these accounted for over 35 per cent of the areas mentioned).

Bowling (1993) carried out a study of the public's health service priorities in East London. This included a priority ranking exercise of six items in relation to perceived effect on health-related quality of life. Respondents ranked 'being free from pain or discomfort' as most important, 'being able to walk freely' as next important, 'being able to care for self (e.g. wash, feed)' third, 'being free from stress/nerves/anxiety/depression' fourth, 'being able to do main activity (e.g. work, study, housework)' fifth, and 'being able to pursue social and leisure activities' sixth (least important). While of interest, structured approaches using pre-coded questionnaires are less valuable than open-ended approaches, which attempt to measure people's conceptions of quality of life without being prompted, and hence biased, by researchers' definitions.

Delphi techniques

Dalkey (1972), after deriving lists of quality of life domains from graduate students, used the Delphi technique with a panel of people to rework the students' lists. The final list included: novelty (newness, surprise, variety), health (physical well-being, feeling good), dominance (superiority, power, control, aggression), self-respect (self-confidence, self-understanding), challenge (stimulation, competition, ambition), freedom (individuality, spontaneity, unconstrained), comfort (economic well-being, good things, relaxation), affection (love, caring, relating, understanding), security (peace of mind, stability, lack of conflict), achievement (sense of accomplishment, meaningful activity), status (prestige, social recognition, positive feedback) and involvement (participation, concern).

Valuations of health and ability

There have been several studies by health economists of valuations of health, although these are often narrow in focus (see later). One broader piece of research was reported by Berg *et al.* (1976), who carried out research on the valuation of states of health and ability (50 items) in a non-random sample of 150 health workers in the USA. They were asked to assign weights of between 0 and 10 in terms of their value to the quality and meaningfulness of life. The highest value was assigned to 'to be able to use your mental abilities' and the lowest was attached to 'to be able to go to a movie'. Other items with high values included 'to be able to see', 'to be able to think clearly', 'to be able to love and be loved in return', 'to be able to make decisions for yourself', 'to be able to live at home rather than in an institution', 'to be able to walk' and 'to be able to maintain contact with family and friends'. The results were consistent with previous research, and with Maslow's (1954) argument that once basic biological and survival needs have been met, emotional and social needs become more prominent. The authors concluded with reference to a statement by Lerner (1973): 'health is more than just a biomedical phenomenon; it involves a social human being functioning in a social environment with social roles he must fulfill'.

In summary, while the issue is complex, there is broad agreement that health-related quality of life includes physical, psychological and social health, and that each of these domains is multifaceted. A concept of health-related quality of life is clearly dependent on a concept of health and health status.

Unresolved questions

There are many vexing and unresolved questions in quality of life research. For example, as Schipper (1983) has asked: How can the quality of life of, say, a city and a country dweller be compared? Does their quality of life change in comparable ways in response to illness? Are some parameters of quality of life weighted differently by different groups of people, and in relation to different illnesses? The issue is not straightforward, and a multitude of additional questions are raised when attempting to consider the impact of an illness on an individual: What does the condition prevent the patient from doing? What do they miss doing as a result of the condition? What are their fears for the future? How do they cope with anger and frustration related to their condition? How does mood affect functioning and social relationships? Are there any positive consequences of the illness (e.g. bringing relatives closer together)? How do people spend their time, and how does this change when afflicted by certain illnesses (e.g. less time spent on leisure and domestic activities and social roles)? What is the impact of the condition on other family members? How have they adjusted, and have they been restricted? Rarely does one health status measure encompass any of these items, and researchers are forced to resort to lengthy, and sometimes impractical, batteries of several measurement scales.

A CONCEPT OF HEALTH

A measure of health status should be based on a concept of health. A medical conception of health is freedom from disease and abnormalities; a sociological view can be defined in terms of the possession of acceptable levels of mental and physical fitness in order to perform one's social role in society. As with the concept of quality of life, there is also a humanistic view of health in which optimal autonomy, personal strength and the positive meaning of life are central components (Heyrman and van Hoeck 1993).

The concept of positive health has been described elsewhere (Bowling 1991). Briefly, most health status instruments measure deviations away from a state of health and are really measuring ill health, or the absence of illness and disease. They rarely reflect the global definition of the WHO (1948), although this is the theoretical underpinning, explicit or implicit, in more recent attempts at scale development. There are multiple influences upon patient outcome, and these require a broad model of health. The non-biological factors which may affect recovery and outcome include patient psychology, motivation, coping, adherence to therapy, socio-economic status, availability of health care, social support networks, and individual cultural beliefs and health behaviours.

A negative conception and measure of health is more appropriate when measuring severely ill populations, but less appropriate in general population surveys. Negative definitions of, and measurements of, health status will tell us little about the health of the population. Positive health is therefore an increasingly popular concept, encompassing not just the absence of disease, but feelings of mental and physical well-being, full functioning, physical fitness, ability to cope, social support, adjustment and efficiency of mind and body. Collectively, these positive states have been referred to in the literature variously as positive health, social health and health-related quality of life. Even in disease-specific studies, where negative measures of health are appropriate, a more balanced scale including positive measures should also be used in order to assess outcome in relation to degrees of wellness as well as illness.

THE PUBLIC'S VIEW OF HEALTH

Dubos (1959) argued that health and disease cannot be defined merely in terms of anatomical, physiological or mental attributes, and that 'their real measure is the ability of the individual to function in a manner acceptable to himself and to the group of which he is part'. An absolute definition of health is not possible to construct and even the WHO (1947, 1948; WHOQOL Group 1993b) definitions can only be viewed as relative concepts (see above). People define their health variously, depending on sociodemographic factors and on their culture (d'Houtard and Field 1984; Currer and Stacey 1986). Their reported definitions include health as not being ill, absence of disease, as behaviour, as role functioning, physical fitness, energy and vitality, social relationships and emotional well-being. Wright (1990) has summarized lay definitions of health as health as *being*, health as *doing* and health as *having*. Wright (in press) also pointed to the debate about whether health is a 'state' or 'trait' (constructs which, he points out, are not mutually exclusive). He refers to the application of various constructs which he summarizes as 'dispositional resilience', such as 'hardiness', 'sense of coherence' and 'dispositional optimism' (Kobasa 1979; Scheier and Carver 1985; Antonovsky 1993). He argued that 'dispositional resilience' may influence health outcomes.

The concept of health is inevitably subject to cultural relativism (Heyrman and van Hoeck 1993), and while health may be a social goal common to all groups, the salience of health to individuals must be assessed relative to other goals. The place of health in one's value system will be reflected in one's definition of health. This has been amply demonstrated by the classic studies of Koos (1954) and Herzlich (1973), as well as by more recent research.

In a study of several thousand people attending health check-ups in Nancy in France, d'Houtard *et al.* (1990) reported that the most common and consistent definitions of health were 'hygiene, living conditions, to feel well in one's skin, to know oneself well, work, luck, to be at the top of one's form, personal unfolding and not to feel one's body'. These were comparable with findings from similar research carried out in Nijmegen in the Netherlands. D'Houtard and Field (1984) reported the results of a study of 4000 people from a health centre in Lorraine, France in more detail. When asked an open-ended question about what health meant to them, the most common replies were 'not to be sick', 'to be at the top of one's form' (more than 400 mentions), and 'good physical equilibrium', 'good mental equilibrium', 'joy of living' (300–400 mentions).

In the British National Health and Lifestyle Survey of 9003 adults living in randomly sampled households, Cox *et al.* (1987) reported that the concepts of health most often used for describing what health is in 'someone else' were, among female respondents in all age groups, 'never ill, no disease, never see a doctor', 'fit, strong, energetic, physically active', 'has healthy habits (e.g. not smoking, taking exercise, taking care of health)' and 'able to do a lot, work, socially active' (in order of frequency mentioned). Among male respondents in all age groups, the most common definitions were 'fit, strong, energetic, physically active', 'never ill, no disease, never see a doctor', 'has healthy habits (e.g. not smoking, taking exercise, taking care of health)' and 'able to do a lot, work, socially active' (in order of frequency mentioned). When asked about definitions of health used for describing 'what it is like to be healthy oneself', the most common response of more than half the males and females in all age groups was 'feel psychologically fit (e.g. good, happy, able to cope)', followed in order of frequency by 'fit, strong, energetic, physically active', 'able to do a lot, work, get out and about', and 'never ill, no disease, never see a doctor'. Respondents with A level education and above, particularly females, were more likely to mention 'physically fit, strong'.

Others have defined health in the context of interference with the performance of normal social roles and activities (Apple 1960), or ability to work (Twaddle 1969). The various lay definitions of health reported by Baumann (1961) pointed to three main orientations: a general feeling of well-being, the absence of illnesses and the ability to perform social roles. Definitions vary according to age, sex, level of education (Cox *et al.* 1987), cultural group (Bowling 1994b) and socioeconomic group, with those in the lower socioeconomic groups defining health more negatively (Blaxter and Patterson 1982) and more likely to perceive the causes of health as being outside their control (Blaxter 1983; Pill and Stott 1985, 1988; Coulter 1987; d'Houtard *et al.* 1990). On the other hand, Cox and co-workers' (1987) National Health and Lifestyle Survey in Britain reported that those in poor economic circumstances were not significantly more likely than those who were better off to associate poverty with ill health. They also reported that, while poverty and prosperity were seen generally as important determinants of health for society at large, it was rarely mentioned as a cause of ill health in the context of respondents' own lives. This pattern of responses was also found in relation to individual behaviours (diet, smoking, exercise). These beliefs and definitions are pertinent to measuring subjective health status, and have implications for the development of cross-cultural instruments.

These examples from the research literature on health beliefs illustrate that some groups of people do include social roles and social functioning in their definitions of health. However, for some decades there was much criticism of the previously described WHO (1947, 1948) definition of health as a complete state of mental, physical and social well-being. This was criticized as utopian and unrealistic, particularly given the many studies of community morbidity which imply that having unreported (to the doctor) symptoms is a normal condition of the population (Dunnell and Cartwright 1972). The lack of realism in the WHO definition, and the impossibility – even undesirability – of achieving 'perfect health' is emphasized by Dubos' view of health:

> Every manifestation of existence is a response to stimuli and challenges, each of which constitutes a threat if not adequately dealt with. The very process of living is a continual interplay between the individual and his environment, often taking the form of a struggle resulting in injury or disease. The more creative the individual the less he can hope to avoid danger, for the stuff of creation is made up of responses to the forces that impinge on his body and soul. Complete and lasting freedom from disease is but a dream remembered from imaginings of a Garden of Eden designed for the welfare of man.
>
> (Dubos 1959: 1–3)

Gradually, definitions of health, like health-related quality of life, have moved away from a total disease model to one which incorporates health and well-being. The most widely used measures of broader health status, or health-related quality of life, reflect this definition, and incorporate physical functioning, psychological well-being and social support and activity items. Also, in recognition of the emphasis on the positive as well

as the negative, evaluations of health and consequences of illness, Hyland and Kenyon (1992) have developed the Satisfaction with Illness Scale, and Argyle et al. (1989) have developed the Oxford Happiness Scale.

RECENT INTEREST AND DEVELOPMENTS IN MEASURING HEALTH-RELATED QUALITY OF LIFE

Quality of life was introduced by Medline as a heading in 1975, and accepted as a concept by Index Medicus in 1977; this was followed by acknowledgement and acceptance by various scientific bodies (Bech 1992). Since the 1970s, there has been an explosion of interest in the subject, with an increasing number of citations of quality of life in the medical literature. Both journal and review articles on quality of life now appear regularly in the medical literature (de Haes and van Knippenberg 1985, 1987; Cella and Tulsky 1990; Aaronson et al. 1991b). There has also been a proliferation of study groups, conferences and special journal issues (e.g. *Advances in Nursing Science* in 1985; *Journal of Chronic Diseases* in 1987; *Psychotherapy and Psychosomatics* in 1990; *Medical Care* in 1990; and *Social Science and Medicine* in 1995). In 1991, a journal entitled *Quality of Life Research* was published by Rapid Communications of Oxford devoted to the study of health-related quality of life. The February 1994 issue of *Quality of Life Research* was largely devoted to the publication of abstracts from the first meeting of the International Health-related Quality of Life Society, held in Brussels (3–4 February 1994). The focus of many of these was on the development of new disease-specific scales of quality of life.

Bardelli and Saracci (1978) reviewed all the clinical studies published in six major cancer journals between 1956 and 1976, and reported that in less than 5 per cent an attempt had been made to measure some aspect of quality of life. The situation changed from the late 1970s, and a comprehensive review of the literature by Fayers and Jones (1983) found over 200 papers published between 1978 and 1980 with the phrase 'quality of life' in the title. Aaronson et al. (1988) reported a review of clinical publications, using a Medline search between 1972 and 1987, and found that 3045 mentioned quality of life. Padilla *et al.* (1992b) reported that a search of the literature on quality of life in nursing journals, using the Cumulated Index for Nursing and Allied Health Literature (CINAHL), revealed over 1000 references about quality of life between January 1983 and December 1991. Literature reviews of two successive 5-year periods of the uses of quality of life measures in technology assessment were carried out by Najman and Levine (1981) and Hollandsworth (1988). Najman and Levine found 23 published studies between 1975 and 1979, and Hollandsworth found 69 studies between 1980 and 1984, a three-fold increase. It should be pointed out that not all of these studies included multidimensional measures of quality of life, and many were limited to fairly crude variables such as return to work and level of physical performance. Najman and Levine also reported that only one study in their search was based on a randomized controlled trial, and they criticized the measures of quality of life utilized in general, most of which were symptom checklists and scales of physical functioning. Almost half of the studies reviewed by Hollandsworth used only objective criteria. However, the use of subjective measures, which involve an evaluation by the patient, alongside objective measures, had markedly increased. Falotico-Taylor *et al.* (1989) have also criticized the methodology, as well as the measurements, used in most of these studies, and pointed out that few used control groups, few employed randomized controlled trials and few were longitudinal in design.

Today, a wide range of studies on the outcome of treatments and interventions include some form of quality of life measure, whether it be a limited assessment of symptoms and physical functioning, or a wider study including psychological well-being, life satisfaction, sexuality, social support and interaction, coping and adjustment, and self-concept and body image. The difference between the early outcomes research incorporating health-related quality of life and the research in the 1990s, is that the perspective is now broader and it is patient-based. The measurement of health care outcomes in the future is likely to demand disease-specific quality of life measurements, and health outcomes will increasingly be evaluated from the point of view of the patient.

THE NEED TO OPERATIONALIZE HEALTH-RELATED QUALITY OF LIFE

There has always been considerable debate among social scientists about 'operationalism', and the extent to which the gap between theory and empirical research can be bridged (for a discussion, see Blalock and Blalock 1971). However, for the concept of quality of life to have any value in descriptive or health outcome research, it must be decided what is to be measured and the agreed concepts need to be operationalized. This is essential if quality of life is to be researched in any coherent and logical way – and necessary before a quality of life scale can be said to be valid.

Scepticism has often greeted attempts to measure quality of life in clinical studies. This is unsurprising given that most investigators have not defined or operationalized their terms (Kaplan and Anderson 1990). Many assume that the concept refers to physical functioning, and/or psychological and mental status or symptom levels. Many scales purporting to be, or used as, quality of life scales are, in fact, simply health status scales, and they are also frequently single-domain scales (e.g. level of physical functioning or mental health).

The definition and measurement of health-related quality of life can, at a societal level, be limited to global indicators of mental and physical health and measurements can include, for example, the number of people who commit suicide, the number who are hospitalized, the numbers taking psychotropic medications, premature mortality and so on. Routine statistics can be used to provide the information, and these have been popularly used to estimate community mental health (Schneider 1976; Bloom 1978; Zautra and Goodhart 1979). Official rates always need careful interpretation in relation to their meaning.

In relation to disease-specific patient outcome, more thoughtful definitions and more sensitive measurements are required. The relevant domains of physical, social and psychological health require specification (e.g. pain, functioning, depression, social activity) and appropriate measurement scales need to be selected.

QUALITY OF LIFE ASSESSMENT AND RESEARCH ON HEALTH CARE OUTCOMES

Quality of life assessment as a supplement to more objective clinical indicators is becoming more topical in view of the increasing questioning of the effectiveness of many established medical treatments. The usually cited definition of health outcomes is that of Donabedian (1985), who defined health outcome as a change in patients' current and future health status that can be attributed to antecedent health care. Obviously, this definition is limited, as some interventions do not lead to such changes (i.e. some may stabilize conditions). Outcome indicators have traditionally included information on avoidable mortality, standardized mortality ratios, hospital re-admission or re-treatment rates (analysed in relation to cause), other service use indicators, laboratory investigations and other diagnostic tests, morbidity, case severity, adverse reactions, complications, the technical success of the treatment where quantifiable, symptom relief, pain and cost-effectiveness.

Some investigators are sceptical about patient-based indicators (e.g. self-reported health status and perceptions of well-being). However, it is important to include patient-based indicators in assessments of outcome *because* they do not necessarily correlate with objective measures of their level of physical functioning (Evans *et al.* 1985). There are many examples of studies which have reported low levels of agreement among doctors in relation to supposed objective clinical findings and variations in physicians' judgements (Wigton 1988). Subjective indicators (based on self-ratings) of quality of life, and health-related quality of life are increasingly popular due to the recognition of the importance of patient satisfaction and how individuals feel, rather than what statistics imply they ought to feel. Clinical indicators of outcome are no longer sufficient, particularly in view of the debate about whether to survive in a vegetative state is better or worse than death (see Jennett 1976).

The argument in favour of measuring quality of life as an outcome of clinical interventions has been neatly summed up by Ebbs *et al.* (1989). They argued that, in the case of chronic conditions with only partial or temporary amelioration of symptoms, a comprehensive evaluation is needed in order to determine the merits of treatment. Sullivan (1992) also pointed out that with incurable conditions, the realistic goal of care is to provide a life that is as comfortable, functional and as satisfying as possible. This argument can be extended to intervention for more acute conditions where the benefits of the treatment are complex and/or uncertain. The primary goals of medical treatment and care are to increase survival and to add quality to the survival. Quality of life as a measure of outcome redirects clinicians from limiting the measurement of outcome to post-intervention survival, complication rates and various physical or biochemical indicators towards consideration of the impact of the condition and the treatment on the patient's emotional and physical functioning and lifestyle. Quality of life indicators help to answer the question of whether the treatment leads to a life worth living, by providing a more patient-led baseline against which the effects of the intervention can be evaluated. The concept is not new to clinicians; many early health-related quality of life measures were developed by clinicians some decades ago, although they were often crude and limited to functioning (Karnofsky *et al.* 1948; Steinbrocker *et al.* 1949; Katz and Akpom 1976a, 1976b).

The measurement of health outcome of clinical interventions has become a cornerstone of health services research, and is also linked to the assessment of the appropriateness of health care interventions (Brook 1990). In Britain, health outcomes research has been given impetus by the division of health care into purchaser and provider organizations (Secretaries of State for Health 1989a, 1989b). Quality of life assessment as a supplement to the documentation of symptom rates, toxicity and adverse effects, and survival patterns is given more urgency in the light of information that some surgery is inappropriate or ineffective. For example, in the USA it has been estimated that only a third of operations for endarterectomy, a half of coronary artery bypass grafts and two-fifths of pacemaker implantations are carried out on patients likely to benefit from the procedure (Enthoven 1990, cited by Smith 1990). In an investigation of a random sample of 1302 Medicare patients in three areas of the USA who underwent carotid endarterectomy, Winslow *et al.* (1988) reported that just 35 per cent had the procedure for appropriate reasons, 32 per cent for equivocal reasons, and 32 per cent for inappropriate reasons. Quality of life assessment is also increasingly popular among pharmaceutical companies, with most reporting that they have used some type of quality of life instrument in their clinical trials of drugs (Luce *et al.* 1989). On the other hand, the US Food and Drugs Administration (FDA) considers that the state of the art of quality of life measurement is too immature to merit mandatory inclusion in clinical trials (Luce *et al.* 1989).

The health outcomes resulting from different methods of *delivering* care are also attracting increasing attention, as in the Rand evaluation of the outcome of different types of insurance plans in the USA (Brook *et al.* 1983, 1990). The increasing emphasis on health care provision as a scarce resource has given impetus to this trend. Health care is but one factor that influences the disease process, and this needs to be recognized. As Gulliford (1992) points out, health care outcome should be substituted for the ambiguous term 'outcome', and suitable disease-specific measures of health care outcome adopted and used in trials. In order to measure health care outcome, each potential indicator that might affect prognosis requires identification and measurement – from severity, age and treatment toxicity to sociopsychological factors (e.g. mental health, coping ability, adjustment and social support) and structural, non-service factors such as employment. Patient satisfaction is also arguably an outcome, rather than a process, indicator (Fitzpatrick 1990).

In sum, health care outcome measures must relate to the objectives and the known risks and benefits of the intervention or care. The Department of Health (1992) suggested the following should be incorporated in outcome assessment: survival rates, symptoms and complications, health status and quality of life, the experiences of patients and their carers, and the costs and use of resources. As their report continued: 'Many health technologies are intended to improve general health and the quality of life, so it is important to measure patients' subjective experiences of illness and the care they receive.' These dimensions have also been emphasized by Bardsley and Coles (1992) in relation to their Clinical Accountability, Service, Planning and Evaluation (CASPE) study. And as Frater (1992) also pointed out, the selection of an

outcome measure is also dependent on making the aims of health care explicit and agreed between all those involved.

UTILITY ASSESSMENTS AND QUALITY OF LIFE ASSESSMENT

Utility assessments

Health economists have concentrated on developing single-score scales of health-related quality of life. This is partly in response to the interest of health policy-makers in cost–benefit formulas for purchasing decisions. Their main focus in recent years has been on utility assessment. The researchers responsible for applying utility theory to the health care field include Kaplan, Bush and their colleagues in the USA (Kaplan and Bush 1982; Kaplan *et al.* 1984), Weinstein and his colleagues also in the USA (Weinstein *et al.* 1980), Williams in England (Kind *et al.* 1982) and Torrance and his colleagues in Canada (Torrance *et al.* 1972, 1982; Torrance 1986, 1987).

The QALY

Cost–utility studies need a common measurement of health outcome. With these cost–utility analyses, the cost of an intervention is related to the number of quality-adjusted life years (QALYs), a concept first introduced by Weinstein and Stason (1976). A QALY is a year of full life quality. Poor health may reduce the quality of a year (e.g. from 1 to 0.5). In QALYs, improvements in the length and quality of life are amalgamated into one single index. Each life year is quality-adjusted with a utility value, where 1 = full health. The utility value aims to reflect the health-related quality of life. Different types of medical interventions are then compared by calculations of costs per gained QALY (Williams 1985b). The Office of Health Economics (1989) compiled data analysed by Williams and presented a league table of costs and QALYs for selected interventions, ranging from advice from a general practitioner to stop smoking (extra cost per QALY gained: £170) to hospital haemodialysis (extra cost per QALY gained: £14,000).

QALYs are not really measures of quality of life

but measures of units of benefit from a medical intervention, combining life expectancy with an index of, for example, disability and distress. They are based on unvalidated value judgements. QALYs have been severely criticized (Carr-Hill 1989; Carr-Hill and Morris 1991) for their lack of validation. There are inadequate data on the conceptual basis, and on the validity of these types of scales, and the data on reliability and validity that do exist are based either on unrepresentative 'convenience' samples or random samples of the population with high rates of non-response, probably because people do not understand the exercise. The application of QALYs to health policy-making (i.e. purchasing) has led to ethical concerns, particularly given their crude state, over reliance on valuations by health professionals and non-representative groups of people (Grimley Evans 1992). There is no evidence that the judgements determining the QALY for a particular condition bear any relationship to real judgements faced by patients suffering from that condition.

Rosser Index of Disability

Williams (1985a) has pointed out that QALYs can be derived by several different methods. In the UK the basic measurement tool underlying the calculation of the QALY is the Rosser Index of Disability (Kind *et al.* 1982; Williams and Kind 1992), which was originally developed as an indicator of hospital performance (Rosser and Watts 1972; Rosser 1992). The Rosser Index is based on the concept of a health index, and subjects are graded into one of eight areas of disability, from none to unconscious, with each state being graded on four levels of distress, from none to severe. States are scored on a scale ranging from 0 at death to 1 = healthy (with negative values for states valued to be worse than death, such as vegetative states). The scaling and valuation of health state techniques of the scale have been clearly described and reviewed by Wilkin *et al.* (1992). Kind and Gudex (1991) have also developed a survey questionnaire – the Health Measurement Questionnaire – designed to collect self-reported information capable of being processed to yield Rosser disability/distress categories.

The approach of Kaplan and Bush

Kaplan and Bush (1982) and Kaplan *et al.* (1984) adopted a slightly different approach. They placed individuals with given health states into categories of mobility, physical activity and social activity, and then classified the symptoms and health problems that they had on a given day. Four hundred case descriptions were then compiled to illustrate the combinations of functional levels, symptoms or problems. The scale includes death. Random samples of the public gave preference ratings to the descriptions, and weights were derived for each level of mobility, physical activity, social activity, and symptom or problem. It is based on a measure of functional status. A utility value was assigned to each functional level, and questionnaire responses were used to assign subjects to one of a number of discrete function states. Kaplan's Index of Well-Being Scale is a single-score scale that has been developed out of this methodology, and has been used widely as a health status measure and methodological tool for health care decision-making (Kaplan *et al.* 1976; Bush 1984). The scale quantifies the health output of a treatment in terms of years of life, adjusted for the changes in quality, that it is responsible for.

Standard gamble, trade-off and rating scale techniques

In Canada, the McMaster group's approach was that QALYs should capture the subject's preferences concerning the length and quality of life, and proposed three approaches to the derivation of utility values (Torrance *et al.* 1972, 1982; Torrance 1986, 1987). The first is the standard gamble technique, in which subjects are asked to choose between their own health state and a gamble that they might die immediately or achieve full health status for the remainder of their lives (e.g. in relation to a specific treatment choice). The second is the time trade-off technique (Torrance *et al.* 1972), in which an individual is asked to consider a health state that is to last for a fixed period of time. A new procedure will give the individual normal health for a shorter period of time, but he or she will probably die or be severely disabled at the end of that time. The person is asked to 'trade-off' the time with reduced capacity for living with normal health for a shorter period of time. The time spent in normal health is varied until the point of indifference is found. Subjects may also be asked to evaluate the equivalences between the numbers of people helped by different treatments – how many people in state B must be helped to provide a benefit that is equivalent to helping one person in state A (see review by Kaplan *et al.* 1993a). The time trade-off technique has been reported to be more reliable and valid than the standard gamble technique (Dolan *et al.* 1993).

Third, Torrance *et al.* (1982) developed a rating scale approach, specifying six attributes that should be included in a health state: physical function, emotional function, sensory function, cognitive function, self-care and pain. Each of these attributes is given several levels of gradation, and the characteristics of a given health state would include a description of functioning, self-care and pain associated with that state. The descriptions can be shown on video or in written vignettes. The ratings assigned to the descriptions are placed on a visual analogue scale ranging from 0 (death/least desirable) to 100 (healthy/most desirable). Multiple Attribute Theory is then used to determine the value for each level of the attributes and the utility value of an associated health state.

Limitations

The disadvantages of all these methods are their cost, the requirements for skilled interviewers and complexity (leading to reliance on non-random or unrepresentative samples of the public). One of the main debates surrounding the use of these techniques is who should provide the utility values – the general public, health care providers and/or patients and their families themselves? While patients' assessments are undoubtedly important, proponents of obtaining utility values of the public and health professionals argue that patients' values may change over the course of an illness and thus their utility values would not be stable. The ethical concern is that the judgements of quality of life and utility assessments are poorly understood (Cohen 1990). A review by Kaplan *et al.* (1993a) has pointed to evidence from psychology experiments that suggest that methods commonly used for economic analysis do not represent underlying true preferences (Kahneman and Tversky 1983).

Health economists are now showing interest in a broader measure of health-related quality of life – the Euroqol. The aim of the Euroqol is to provide a standardized non-disease-specific survey instrument for describing health-related quality of life, and to generate a single index value for each health state (Euroqol Group 1990). It has suffered from very low response rates in a number of population surveys, and has relatively poor sensitivity (Brazier *et al.* 1993b) probably because of its crudity and lack of middle values for coding, and has accordingly been criticized (Carr-Hill 1992). It is also a highly skewed measure (Brazier *et al.* 1992, 1993a).

GENERIC, DOMAIN- AND DISEASE-SPECIFIC MEASUREMENT SCALES

Disease-specific

In choosing a measurement instrument, or set of measures, key questions to consider are whether a disease-specific and/or a generic measure is needed, and whether either requires supplementation with single-domain measures that are important to the study aims (e.g. depression). There is little point in utilizing a health status measure alone if it is unlikely to detect the effects of the treatment in question, or the symptoms specific to the condition. In addition, some measure of disease severity will also be required. Several severity and co-morbidity indexes have been developed (Kellerman and Hackman 1988; Parkerson *et al.* 1993a), although these are often fairly crude (Linn *et al.* 1968) and clinical investigators prefer to rely on biomedical indicators. Most health services researchers work closely with clinicians to ensure that the appropriate disease-specific outcome and severity indicators have been included in their batteries.

Clearly, criteria for assessing outcome of care will vary for different disease syndromes. A universal questionnaire to elicit the relevant information for a number of conditions would require a questionnaire of enormous length (Goligher 1987). Disease-specific quality of life scales are needed not simply for greater brevity, but to ensure sensitivity to sometimes small, but clinically significant changes in health status and levels of disease severity (for good illustrations of this point in relation to head and neck cancer, see Berg *et al.* 1976; Dhillon *et al.* 1982; Morris 1990). However, while different procedures require disease-specific quality of life outcome measures, there can still be a central core of quality of life questions common to a wide range of disease areas.

It is easy to assume that disease-specific measures *per se* will be more sensitive indicators of patient outcome than generic measures. However, a study of osteoarthritis patients by Kantz *et al.* (1992) reported that while knee-specific function measures and pain scales were more *specific* than the generic health status scale, the SF-36 (Ware *et al.* 1993), among patients with other co-morbid conditions, the SF-36 physical functioning sub-scale, plus knee-specific adaptations of that scale were just as specific as the disease-specific scales. Moreover, the disease-specific measures failed to distinguish between treated and untreated patients. A combined approach to outcome assessment, using both disease- (or condition-) specific and generic measures is preferable where a broad disease-specific quality of life instrument has not been satisfactorily developed. The generic measure of choice across many diseases is increasingly the SF-36. As Ware (1993) concluded, because the SF-36 is short, well tested and population norms exist, it may constitute a good generic core for use along with disease-specific outcome measures. The potential use of this scale as a generic core will be discussed more fully within the appropriate chapters of this book (see Chapter 8 for review).

Domain-specific scales

As the reviews of disease-specific indicators of quality of life will show, they can often be criticized for being too narrow in focus, while neglecting the measurement of important outcome and modifying variables (e.g. social support, adjustment, coping, life satisfaction, self-esteem, depression and other domains). Some investigators supplement their disease-specific scales with domain-specific measures. Generic and domain-specific measures have been reviewed by several authors (e.g. McDowell and Newell 1987; Bowling 1991; Wade 1992; Wilkin *et al.* 1992).

The domain-specific areas of interest will vary according to how the condition and its treatment affect the patient. Thus measures of psychiatric status will, for some diseases and conditions, necessitate the inclusion of a memory test, as well as a depression scale. The measurement of physical functioning may be restricted to global categories ranging from fully functioning to bedbound for more dramatic conditions and interventions where great changes are expected, but may need to be more refined and sensitive (i.e. at the 'less restrictive' end of the scale) in the case of more moderate cases.

Other domains of potential relevance may include occupational and social role functioning, including maintenance of social relationships and activities (Kaplan 1985; Bowling 1991, 1994a; Bowling *et al.* 1994). Psychological well-being can be important, and includes happiness/satisfaction, achievement of personal goals and aspirations, personal control, adjustment and coping ability (modifying variables), well-being, social support and interaction (outcome and modifying variables), self-concept and self-esteem, body image and somatic comfort (Lewis 1982, 1989; Young and Longman 1983; Schipper *et al.* 1984; Schipper and Levitt 1985, 1986; Ferrans and Ferrell 1990).

Some argue that a definition of quality of life should reflect the pre-illness situation of the patient; others argue that it reflects the attainment of an ideal quality (Calman 1984; Schipper and Levitt 1986). There is, of course, an individual judgement involved and people differ in their values. In medicine, the goal is to return patients to normal lives, rather than attain the ideal, and measurement scales should reflect this (Selby and Robertson 1987). Measures of quality of life should therefore reflect the range of normal activities that have been potentially affected by the condition and treatment. It is possible to obtain good response and completion rates with a comprehensive questionnaire (Sadura *et al.* 1992).

The specialized scales measuring specific domains are often long, and have to remain fairly lengthy in order to retain their sensitivity and psychometric properties. A caution must be made here in relation to the use of batteries of several scales, for example as a supplement to a brief disease-specific scale. Although disease- and condition-specific scales of quality of life are easy to criticize for their brevity, and their often narrow scope, no study can hope to measure every relevant domain, and most disease-specific scales are limited to the most essential. Domain-specific scales should be used when the area is of particular interest to the investigator, and the disease-specific (or generic) scale selected for use neglects that domain. They should not be included for the sake of having a comprehensive battery, without any theoretical or methodological justification. The danger is the production of a battery that contains too many and also overlapping items, which becomes tiresome to respondents, expensive to administer and analyse and produces an overwhelming amount of data which may not always be helpful.

Generic scales

Measures which implicitly or explicitly aim to tap health-related quality of life are usually referred to as broader measures of health status. They should encompass the dimensions of physical, mental and social health. Investigators have tended to supplement generic health status measures with specific disease items. They have used generic measures in order to make comparisons with other conditions, to broaden their outcome indicators, and because of the slow development of disease-specific questionnaires. On the other hand, generic instruments have an important constraint as they are unable to identify condition-specific aspects of a disease that are essential for the measurement of outcome (Hutchinson and Fowler 1992). Generic measures will always require supplementation with disease-specific measures in order to detect important clinical changes (Guyatt et al. 1986). McKenna (1993) has argued that the role of generic measures in health services and clinical research will diminish as more disease-specific measures are produced which can focus directly on the research issues. As McKenna points out, the use of disease-specific measures avoids asking irrelevant questions of respondents and maximizes the chance of detecting clinically significant changes, which is essential in clinical and policy-oriented research. However, it is unlikely that they will obviate the need for generic measures, or at least a generic core, as long as comparisons across disease groups within and between specialities are required.

The most popular generic measures include the Rand batteries, in particular the increasingly used SF-36 (Stewart and Ware 1992; Ware et al. 1993),

the Sickness Impact Profile (Bergner et al. 1981), the Nottingham Health Profile (Hunt et al. 1986) and the McMaster Health Index Questionnaire (Chambers et al. 1976). A popular and promising generic measure that is being developed for use in primary medical care is the Dartmouth Coop Function Charts (Nelson et al. 1987, 1990; McHorney et al. 1992; see review by Wilkin et al. 1992). However, while health-related quality of life measures are increasingly used in health services research, several reviews of clinical trials have indicated that they are still underused by clinicians (e.g. Guyatt et al. 1989b).

SATISFACTION WITH CARE AND OUTCOME

This domain is listed separately because it is an important and neglected component of disease-specific and generic scales or batteries of scales. A person's degree of satisfaction with his or her health status and outcome, and of fulfilment of expectations of the treatment, should be included. It is usually neglected because the detection of dissatisfaction has foiled all patient satisfaction questions and questionnaires. Reviews of the problems inherent in measuring patient satisfaction can be found in Roberts and Tugwell (1987), Ware and Hays (1988), Cartwright (1989), Fitzpatrick (1990), Wilkin et al. (1992) and van Campen et al. (1992). Davies and Ware (1991) have developed a promising Consumer Satisfaction Survey Questionnaire (including a 'Visit-specific satisfaction questionnaire') and user manual. The 'visit-specific' questions were developed from the Rand Medical Outcomes Study Questionnaires. Readers are referred to these sources where their measurement scales of choice do not address patient satisfaction issues.

WHO SHOULD RATE QUALITY OF LIFE?

Relatively few investigators have based their operational definitions and measurement decisions on what the public say are the relevant domains of quality of life. While some generic and disease-specific measures of health-related quality of life have included lay persons' perceptions of the effects of symptoms on their lives (e.g. Hunt *et al.* 1986), investigators have more commonly turned to the existing literature as their starting point. Some scales, particularly in mental health and oncology, bypass the patient's perspective altogether and base ratings on the perspective of a staff member or a 'significant other' (e.g. relative or friend).

In health care, the debate sometimes revolves around whether the quality of life assessment should be made by the patient or by a health professional (e.g. a doctor). Objections to physician ratings include the argument that while patients may judge their quality of life to be low, they may nevertheless value their lives as precious (Brock 1993). Some clinicians object to patients' ratings on the grounds of their subjectivity. This subjectivity, as it reflects the patient's point of view, should be viewed as their strength. There is now general recognition among health services researchers that measures of health outcome should incorporate the patient's perspective, not simply in terms of whether or not the treatment was a success, but more globally in relation to perceived mental and physical well-being as a consequence of an intervention. A person can feel ill without medical science being able to detect any apparent disease. A person's ill health is indicated by feelings of pain and discomfort, or perceptions of change in usual functioning and feeling. It has been known for many years that the utilization of health services is more closely associated with the perception of symptoms and people's feelings than with their actual medical condition (Mechanic 1962; Goldberg and Huxley 1980). Measures of health outcome need to take account of both the traditional disease model (pathological abnormality indicated by a set of symptoms and signs) and the patient's perspective.

The implication is that patients should complete a questionnaire about their quality of life themselves, or the questionnaire should be administered to them by a trained interviewer. 'Significant others' (e.g. relatives) and health care professionals should only complete ratings where their perspective is *also* required, and where the patient is too frail or ill to be questioned. However, a number of scales require a health professional to complete a questionnaire on behalf of the patient. These include Spitzer and co-workers' (1981)

Quality of Life Index, the rating scales of dependency, work and school performance, family and non-family relationships used by Horowitz and Cohen (1968), Taylor and Falconer (1968) and Rausch and Crandall (1982) in their studies of patients with temporal lobe seizures, and various other physical performance indicators, such as the Barthel Index (Mahoney and Barthel 1965) and the Karnofsky Performance Scale (Karnofsky *et al.* 1948).

On the other hand, although patient-based, self-report questionnaires are the ideal to be aimed for, it is not denied that there is also a practical need for supplementary, indirect measures of quality of life when the patient is too frail or ill to respond. The criticisms of these have arisen because some investigators have selected the latter rather than the former for routine use.

Discrepancies between doctors' and patients' assessments

Research suggests that there are wide discrepancies between patients' and doctors' ratings of outcome after specific therapies (Orth-Gomer *et al.* 1979; Thomas and Lyttle 1980; Jachuck *et al.* 1982; Slevin *et al.* 1988). The case against observer ratings of another person's quality of life, which is then taken as a proxy indicator, has been made by several empirical studies comparing doctors' and patients' ratings, and by the increasing literature on discrepancies in treatment preferences. This literature serves to indicate that the patient's feelings, values and opinions cannot be assumed. Jachuck *et al.* (1982) reported that, while all treating doctors in their study rated their patients' quality of life as having improved after they started antihypertensive treatment, three-quarters of the patients' relatives thought that it was worse; 8 per cent of the patients felt worse and 44 per cent felt the same (the remainder felt they had improved). Poor correlations between professionals' and patients' own self-assessments were also reported by Padilla *et al.* (1981). Large discrepancies in assessments between patients and doctors have been reported by Slevin *et al.* (1988), who compared their assessments using the Karnofsky Performance Scale, the Spitzer Quality of Life Index and the Linear Analogue Self-Assessment (LASA) scale.

Preference assessments and decision-making

On a related theme, there is increasing interest in assessing patients' preferences. These are generally known as 'preference assessments', and are defined as patient choice of intervention, based on the evidence. They are distinct from the preference assessments of different health states in the development of health status scales (Blischke *et al.* 1975). An example of a preference study is that by Wennberg *et al.* (1988) in relation to prostatic hypertrophy. As a result of their research, they recommended the development of procedures for objectively conveying information to patients about the options open to them in choosing a treatment. These developments have led some to caution that not all patients may want to exercise a choice, and not all patients who do make choices opt for the choice expected by clinicians (Wolberg *et al.* 1987; Wilson *et al.* 1988; Fallowfield and Hall 1991; Wolberg, 1991).

In relation to decision-making about quality *vs* quantity of survival, attitudes diverge within patient groups. Decision-making is never clear-cut, as a brief review of some of the literature by Byrne (1992) emphasizes. While research on patients across disease conditions has reported that people generally agree on what health states are worse than death (e.g. permanent coma, severe dementia, loss of essential functional ability such as being able to feed oneself; Pearlman *et al.* 1993), there is less agreement between clinicians and patients on the treatment of choice. For example, it was reported from one study of 104 patients with life-threatening illnesses, all of whom were estimated by their doctors to have less than a 50 per cent chance of surviving 5 years, that even the most seriously ill were more likely than their doctors anticipated to want cardiopulmonary resuscitation if their heart stopped beating. Doctors' preferences apparently corresponded more to their own personal preferences for what they would want in a similar situation, than to their patients' preferences (Schneiderman *et al.* 1993). Similarly, a study of 67 patients aged 70–96 years, due to be discharged from acute geriatric wards, reported that 73 per cent wished to be resuscitated if they had a cardiac arrest, and 70 per cent of their relatives also stated this, although few doctors had marked them for resuscitation should they have a cardiac arrest (Liddle *et al.* 1993).

Research in the USA has reported that some patients and proxy patients have expressed a preference to exchange survival for a shorter life of improved quality (McNeil *et al.* 1978, 1981). However, a study in the UK which asked patients with cancer, who were about to undergo chemotherapy to balance the price they were prepared to pay in terms of side-effects for a particular degree of benefit, showed that most patients would accept toxic chemotherapy for minimal benefit in terms of prolongation of life (Slevin *et al.* 1990). A study in the USA of women who had received adjuvant chemotherapy for early breast cancer, reported that 46 per cent thought that the inconvenience and toxicity of the treatment was worthwhile if they survived for as little as an extra 6 months; the results were similar when they were informed that the chances of survival were likely to be only slightly increased by the treatment (Coates and Simes 1992).

Mackillop *et al.* (1986, 1988, 1992) and Palmer *et al.* (1990) have conducted a series of studies comparing doctors' and non-medical laypersons' preferences for treatments. In one study of two clearly defined clinical trials in relation to lung cancer, they asked 400 lay people if they would participate in these trials if they had lung cancer. They compared their views with over 100 oncologists in Ontario. Fifty per cent of the lay sample said they would consent to a trial of lobectomy *vs* segmentectomy, compared with 64 per cent of the doctors, and 48 per cent of the lay sample would consent to the trial of five different forms of chemotherapy, compared with 19 per cent of doctors. Seventy-four per cent of the lay respondents believed that cancer specialists should be asked if they would be willing to participate in clinical trials before the trials were opened to patients. The authors concluded, on the basis of a series of similar studies, that patients cannot always be expected to recognize unacceptable experiments for themselves, and that many patients with non-small cell lung cancer are being asked to participate in trials that offer treatment options that many experts in the field would not be prepared to enter themselves because of their high risk–benefit ratios (Mackillop *et al.* 1986). The literature indicates moreover, that, despite the documented benefits of chemotherapy in specific cases (Coates *et al.* 1987; Rapp *et al.* 1988; Poon *et al.* 1989), it is still an aggressive therapy, with associated toxicity, and there is a great deal of variation among doctors in relation to treatment preferences (Mackillop *et al.* 1992).

In sum, the study method of choice is either subject self-completion scales or interviewer-administered scales. The latter method produces the best quality data with fewest ambiguities and missing data. Assessment of the patient's quality of life can also be made, with the patient's permission, by a close relative or friend; indeed, they are more likely than the patient to report adverse psychological changes (Jachuck *et al.* 1982). However, third party assessments are no substitute for the subject's own assessment. Other methodological and measurement issues are discussed briefly in the final chapter.

2

CANCERS

THE IMPORTANCE OF MEASURING THE QUALITY OF LIFE OF CANCER PATIENTS

After coronary heart disease, cancer is the most common cause of death in the Western world. The lifetime risk of developing cancer for a person in the West is 30 per cent, and there is a 20 per cent chance of dying from cancer (see Blackledge and Lawton 1992). When there is a reasonable prospect of cure for cancer, patients and doctors are likely to be willing to accept the associated risk of toxicity, with less concern for effects on quality of life. In cases where there is little or no chance of a cure, the aim of medical care is to prolong lives and to maintain the quality of those lives, which are at risk not only from the impact of the disease but also from the effects of the treatments. Biomedical advances in oncology have highlighted the potential trade-offs between the quality and length of life (Morrow et al. 1992). The measurement of quality of life can help clinicians – and patients – choose between chemotherapeutic agents when there is no clear survival advantage (Silberfarb et al. 1980; Selby and Robertson, 1987).

National oncology organizations and research grant bodies across the world are beginning to recommend the inclusion of quality of life measures in certain types of clinical trials of new technologies and drugs (Johnson and Temple 1985; Clinical Trials Cooperative Group Program 1988; Jones et al. 1988; Luce et al. 1989; Moinpour et al.

1989; Osoba 1992; Sadura et al. 1992). International workshops of quality of life assessment of cancer patients are now held on a more regular basis (see Ventafridda et al. 1986).

Probably the most extensive work on quality of life among cancer patients has been in relation to breast cancer (for reviews, see Fallowfield and Hall 1991; Kiébert et al. 1991; Lasry 1991). The precedent was set in this field probably because of concerns about the disfiguring nature of surgical treatment and the extensive rehabilitation needs associated with it, as well as changes in the treatment of choice away from radical mastectomy. Similar concerns are being expressed about other forms of cancer treatment, such as aggressive chemotherapy drugs. They can lead to cure or significantly longer survival, but they can also cause significantly greater treatment-related side-effects that may impair quality of life. Thus, in clinical practice, criteria other than survival period increasingly influence decision-making (Morrow et al. 1992).

WHAT HAS BEEN MEASURED IN STUDIES OF THE QUALITY OF LIFE OF CANCER PATIENTS?

Most studies of quality of life in oncology limit their definition and measurement to symptoms, physical functioning and psychological well-being, usually anxiety and depression (Morris 1990;

Gotay and Moore 1992). Of course, the traditional end-points in medicine are survival, recurrence or disease-free survival, various haematological and biochemical parameters, symptoms, toxicity, tumour response rate and duration of response (Buyse *et al.* 1984; Poon *et al.* 1989). Obviously, even small differences in such outcome indicators can be important in human terms (Early Breast Cancer Trialists' Collaborative Group 1992). Symptoms and toxicity of treatments can have severe effects on the quality of life of patients (Lindley *et al.* 1992).

In a review of 132 published clinical trials of cancer, Mosteller *et al.* (1980) noted that most studies reported outcome only in terms of survival or recurrence, while quality of life was mentioned but rarely measured. The concept has been slower to permeate into surgery (Ebbs *et al.* 1989); indeed, O'Young and McPeek (1987) found that only 3 per cent of trials reported in surgical journals mentioned quality of life. Most instruments reported to assess quality of life among cancer patients are weak or inadequate (van Knippenberg and de Haes 1988; Donovan *et al.* 1989).

There seems to be increasing agreement now that a quality of life instrument for use in oncology should be multidimensional (Aaronson *et al.* 1988). It should be cautioned, as in other chapters, that no one study can incorporate all relevant dimensions – the instrument or battery of measures would be too unwieldy and probably suffer from a high rate of non-response from patients. Investigators need to define clearly the aims of their investigations, and the domains of quality of life of interest, and focus on those aspects – in some cases, a disease-specific quality of life measure will suffice, and in others this will require supplementing with other batteries (e.g. of coping), depending on the aims of the study.

WHAT SHOULD BE MEASURED?

Maguire and Selby (1989), in their review of quality of life scales for the Medical Research Council, and Selby (1993) recommended that any quality of life assessment in patients with cancer should include physical well-being (symptoms and toxicities, such as pain, fatigue, nausea, physical activity and work, recreation and self-care activities), psychological well-being (body image, self-

esteem, emotional distress, anger, depression) and social well-being (effects on social activities, isolation, social support from family and friends, and sexual relationships).

In 1990, the National Cancer Institute and the Office of Medical Applications of Research (NCI/OMAR) in the USA co-sponsored a workshop on Quality of Life Assessment in Cancer Clinical Trials in order to agree on a definition of quality of life and the relevant dimensions of clinical decision-making to be measured. The quality of life issues that were identified were similar to those identified earlier by Maguire and Selby (1989), and included symptoms and toxicity of treatments, appetite and weight changes, pain, disfigurement, performance of activities of daily living (ADL), length of hospital stays, days off work, school attendance, social interaction and family life, intellectual, social and psychological functioning (Nayfield *et al.* 1992).

RECOMMENDED MEASUREMENT SCALES

The Southwest Oncology Group in the USA recommended that only instruments with established psychometric properties should be used in the assessment of quality of life (Moinpour *et al.* 1989, 1990). They recommended the use of self-completion questionnaires (by the patient), such as the short general health status measure from the Rand Medical Outcomes Study (MOS). Moinpour *et al.* recommended the 20-item version, although this has now been replaced in large part by the 36-item version – the Short Form-36 (SF-36) (Stewart and Ware 1992; Ware *et al.* 1993). They also suggested the quality of life 'uniscale' developed by Selby *et al.* (1984) and the Hospital Anxiety and Depression Scale (Zigmond and Snaith 1983). Non-disease-specific generic measures, such as the SF-36, do require supplementation with disease- (cancer-) specific items.

The scale of the European Organization for Research and Treatment of Cancer (EORTC), developed by Aaronson and co-workers' (1988, 1991a, 1993), is the main instrument promoted by the Quality of Life Committee of the National Cancer Institute of Canada Clinical Trials Group

(Osoba, 1992). This contains a disease-specific core section, with site-specific modules, and is undergoing an impressive level of testing.

NCI/OMAR suggested a number of instruments for which there was some evidence of reliability and validity: a generic measure such as the Short-Form (SF) 20- or 36-item versions (Stewart and Ware 1992); cancer-specific and site-specific instruments such as the Cancer Rehabilitation Evaluation System (Ganz et al. 1990; Schag and Heinrich 1988; 1990; Schag et al. 1991); the Breast Cancer Chemotherapy Questionnaire (Levine et al. 1988); the Functional Living with Cancer Index (Schipper et al. 1984; Schipper and Levitt 1985); or the previously mentioned EORTC (Aaronson et al. 1988, 1991a, 1993) and its site-specific modules. The latter is probably the best developed disease-specific quality of life scale to date. They also suggested the measurement of domain-specific areas such as adjustment and distress, using the Psychosocial Adjustment to Illness Scale – Self-Reported version, all conditions (PAIS-SR) (Derogatis and Lopez, 1983; Derogatis, 1986); the Symptom Distress Scale: Cancer (McCorkle and Young 1978; McCorkle and Quint-Benoliel 1983; Young and Longman 1983; McCorkle 1987; McCorkle et al. 1989); and the Rotterdam Symptom Checklist (RSCL) – Cancer (de Haes and Welvaart 1985; de Haes et al. 1986, 1987a, 1987b; de Haes and van Knippenberg 1987).

REVIEW ARTICLES ON QUALITY OF LIFE MEASUREMENT AND CANCER

A number of reviews have been published over the last decade which have identified and described commonly used health-related quality of life outcome measures for use with cancer patients. The list is long and, for the interested reader, includes: Kranth (1981), van Dam et al. (1984), de Haes and Welvaart (1985), Clark and Fallowfield (1986), Ventafridda et al. (1986), Cella and Cherin (1987), Fowlie and Berkeley (1987), Selby and Robertson (1987), van Knippenberg and de Haes (1988), Donovan et al. (1989), Maguire and Selby (1989), Moinpour et al. (1989), Fallowfield (1990), Aaronson et al. (1991b), Lindley (1992) and Saunders and Baum (1992). However, while there is some overlap between their scales of choice, there

are also several scales which are presented in one review but not in another, even in the more recent reviews.

THE DOMAINS OF MEASUREMENT

Symptoms and functioning

The symptoms associated with cancers are numerous and diverse, as are the treatments, which include chemotherapy, radiotherapy, radical or less invasive surgery. A disease-specific measure needs to be sensitive to the stage of cancer and the range and type of symptoms and treatment toxicities as they affect a person's quality of life. A common example of a symptom and toxicity (e.g. from chemotherapy) end-point in cancer research is nausea and vomiting (Edelstyn et al. 1979). Others include alopecia (hair loss), mood, appetite changes, headaches, stomatitis, diarrhoea, malaise or tiredness, shortness of breath, difficulty in falling asleep, lack of energy, lack of sexual interest, dry mouth, mouth ulcers, taste disturbances, indigestion, menstrual disturbances, cystitis, smell abnormalities, 'pins and needles', skin changes and various fungal and other infections. Pain is also commonly assessed and is experienced by about a third of all cancer patients (Bond 1979; Bonica 1985; Portenoy 1992). There are also numerous site-specific symptoms (see e.g. Burge et al. 1975), and specific symptoms associated with major surgery and chemotherapy, which are well documented in the literature (see e.g. Palmer et al. 1980, 1990; Vera 1981).

Saunders and Baum (1992) have described the disease-specific symptoms and the iatrogenic effects of treatment, particularly surgery, which lead to a decreased quality of life in cancer patients. They point out that, in the case of surgery, this can include mutilation, loss of self-esteem, changed body image, family rejection and physical handicap. The effects of radiation can include depression, nausea and vomiting, skin changes and tiredness. The effects of chemotherapy include nausea, vomiting, alopecia and tiredness. Hormone therapy can lead to menopause and hirsutism. They also point out that the disease-related threats to quality of life include the uncertainty of the prognosis, threat to survival, stigma of cancer, fear of pain and death, economic effects, sexual dysfunction and dissatisfaction with information.

Scales for monitoring toxicity related to treatment are used widely, as are classifications of physical functioning (Karnofsky *et al.* 1948; Zubrod *et al.* 1960; WHO 1979). Disease-specific performance tests have also been developed, such as the Carlens Vitagram, which is used widely (Carlens *et al.* 1970; Fergusson and Cull 1991). However, these are just part of the whole that constitutes health-related quality of life and its measurement.

Physical functioning and the effects of the condition or treatment on social roles and activities are important domains to measure. The most widely used scale of physical functioning is the Karnofsky Scale (Karnofsky *et al.* 1948) and adaptations of it (Zubrod *et al.* 1960), although this is a limited scale. It will be reviewed later.

Disease-specific measures of quality of life

The need for disease-specific measures to supplement generic quality of life scales in oncology is apparent from most studies. For example, an uncontrolled study by Dhillon *et al.* (1982) examined the impact of laryngectomy and the 'commando procedure' in 49 patients with cancer of the larynx. The results indicated that patients who had undergone a laryngectomy reported constant speech difficulties or an inability to speak, and problems with loss of taste, whereas the 'commando' patients reported severe eating difficulties (almost half had to rely on a fluid diet), dysphagia and severe dribbling. Because of the more visible nature of their problems, they were more likely to become social recluses, with experiences of depression. These problems were detected by disease-specific questions, and no standard quality of life instrument was used.

Different symptoms and unwanted treatment effects may be important in relation to different types of cancers and treatments, and it is not practical to include them all in any one scale. It is possible to overcome this problem by the use of modules within a questionnaire which alternate for different studies. Maguire and Selby (1989) and Selby (1993) recommended the development of scales using a core generic instrument for all studies, supplemented with disease-specific modules. This prevents the development of excessively long disease-specific instruments, and facilitates comparability between studies and disease sites. Selby *et al.* (1984), Warde *et al.* (1984) and Aaronson *et al.* (1991a, 1993) have been developing measures which incorporate core items of relevance for all studies, and alternative additional measures, or 'disease-specific modules for site-specific cancers (e.g. breast cancer, lung cancer and ovarian cancer).

While several quality of life scales for use with cancer patients have been developed, there are still many studies in which investigators have developed their own items of measurement due to the irrelevance of scale items to the research question. For example, some quality of life issues during recovery may be different to quality of life issues during treatment (Cella and Tross 1986; Fobair *et al.* 1986), leading researchers to design their own scales.

Generic measures of health-related quality of life

Few of the longer generic measures of health-related quality of life have been used with cancer patients. Because the range of physical experiences and treatment toxicities for cancer are so different from other conditions, investigators have either avoided generic measures or decided that disease- (site-) specific scales are more appropriate. Even the term 'cancer' itself covers over 100 different diseases (Ganz *et al.* 1992).

The Sickness Impact Profile (SIP) (Bergner *et al.* 1981), one of the most widely used and best tested scales, has on occasion been used with cancer patients. Its most well-known use in oncology is Selby and co-workers' (1984) attempt to construct a new scale incorporating a number of items from the SIP (see pp. 49–51). The SIP is a lengthy scale, with many repetitive items, and it is unlikely to be fully completed by people who are severely ill.

More promising is the Short Form-36, which was developed from the Rand Health Insurance Study (HIS) and Medical Outcomes Study (MOS) batteries (Ware *et al.* 1993). Several cancer organizations in the USA have recommended it for use, along with other scales (e.g. of anxiety and depression) and disease-specific items.

The use of batteries and scales

Domain-specific quality of life indicators are still popular among oncologists. For example, commonly used indicators of mood, body image, self-esteem and life satisfaction in oncology include the Profile of Mood States depression sub-scale, National Institute of Mental Health Center for Epidemiologic Studies (20-item) Depression Scale (Radloff 1975, 1977), Steinberg and co-workers' (1985) Body Image Scale (adapted by Lasry *et al.* 1987), Cantril's (1965) Ladder (9-item) Life Satisfaction scale and Rosenberg's (1965) Self-Esteem Scale.

In their pilot study, Morton *et al.* (1984) used a number of scales to assess the effects of treatment on the quality of life of 48 males aged 60 and over with buccopharyngeal cancer – hand grip; Karnofsky Performance Scale; functional disability; pain and discomfort; the Geriatric Mental State; Bradburn Affect–Balance Scale; and depression was classified according to DSM-III criteria. Differences in treatment groups were detected in relation to disability, well-being and depression.

The use of different groups of scales does not allow for comparison between studies. While a battery, or cluster, of scales is rewarding in terms of providing detailed information about the treatment of choice on the domains of interest, they can lead to lengthy administration times, and disease-specific measures will still be required in order to discover exactly what it is about the condition and/or the treatment that detracts from, or enhances, quality of life.

Domain-specific measures of quality of life

Psychological well-being

A person's ability to function physically and socially is influenced by their psychological well-being. It is important for psychological health to be incorporated into outcome end-points, and measured appropriately. Cancer is often associated with a decrease in psychosocial well-being and an increase in psychological morbidity (Maguire *et al.* 1980; McArdle *et al.* 1981; Fallowfield *et al.* 1986; Devlen 1987; Hopwood and Maguire 1992). Anxiety and depression are reported to be the most common psychological symptoms of cancer patients (Gottschalk 1983; Endicott 1984).

Affect and cognition

An important distinction for measurement purposes is that between affect and cognition (Campbell *et al.* 1976; Andrews and McKennell 1980; McKennell and Andrews 1980; Veenhoven 1984). *Affect* refers to an emotional phenomenon (e.g. positive/negative feeling) and *cognition* refers to rational appraisal (e.g. evaluation). The significance of this distinction in relation to the measurement of quality of life among cancer patients has been emphasized by de Haes *et al* (1987, 1992). Cognition may be more stable than the affective, and less sensitive to changes in life circumstances (Headey *et al.* 1984; de Haes *et al.* 1992). However, both are impaired in cancer patients (de Haes *et al.* 1992).

Anxiety, depression and mood

Several popular measures of mood, distress, anxiety and depression have been used with cancer patients, including the Profile of Mood States (POMS: McNair *et al.* 1971), the State–Trait Anxiety Inventory (STAI: Spielberger *et al.* 1983), the National Institute of Mental Health, Center for Epidemiological Studies – Depression Scale (CES-D: Radloff 1975, 1977), the Symptoms of Distress Scale (SADS: Endicott and Spitzer 1978), the General Health Questionnaire (GHQ: Goldberg 1972) and the Hospital Anxiety and Depression Scale (HAD: Zigmond and Snaith 1983). The short 10-item version of the Present State Examination (PSE: Wing *et al.* 1974) is also increasingly being used and regarded as suitable (Selby and Robertson 1987; Fallowfield *et al.* 1990), although others have adapted it (Pruyn *et al.* 1981).

General Health Questionnaire (GHQ)
Selby and Robertson (1987) suggested the General Health Questionnaire (GHQ: Goldberg 1972) as a method for assessing psychological morbidity (anxiety and depression) in oncology, although Maguire and Selby (1989), in their review of measures for the Medical Research Council, suggested that it does not work well with cancer patients. The GHQ is a general index of morbidity, measuring mainly anxiety and depression, although it contains a number of somatic and functional items which could artificially inflate the score for overall psychiatric morbidity.

Hospital Anxiety and Depression (HAD) Scale

Aaronson *et al.* (1988), Maguire and Selby (1989) and Selby (1992) have recommended the HAD (Zigmond and Snaith 1983), because it is short and does not contain any somatic items. It has been used successfully with cancer patients (Achard and Zittoun 1993; Cody *et al.* 1993), and reported to be acceptable to patients (Clark and Fallowfield 1986). However, not all reports of the use of the HAD with cancer patients are reassuring.

Slevin *et al.* (1988) compared the performance of the HAD with other LASA scales measuring quality of life, anxiety and depression in 108 patients with advanced malignant disease. The HAD correlated relatively poorly with the other scale items measuring anxiety and depression ($r = 0.39–0.60$). The authors concluded that in cancer patients the elements of the HAD scale are not the major contributors to anxiety and depression. They found that one of the anxiety items in the HAD ('worrying thoughts') contributed 70 per cent of the total variation in relation to the anxiety sub-scale, and one depression item ('the extent to which the patient looked forward') contributed 64 per cent of the variation in relation to the depression sub-scale. The authors suggest that this problem arose because cancer patients are anxious and worry about the future.

Profile of Mood States (POMS)

A popular mood scale in oncology, and in other specialities, is the Profile of Mood States (POMS: McNair *et al.* 1971). Reliability, validity and sensitivity have been tested and norms provided for cancer patients (McNair *et al.* 1971; McCorkle and Quint-Benoliel 1983; Cella *et al.* 1987, 1989; Cassileth *et al.* 1985). Cella *et al.* (1989) tested it on 923 recently diagnosed cancer patients. The POMS scores were significantly different for the cancer patients in comparison with norms for other population groups, and the authors advised other investigators to use their norms for making comparisons with cancer patients. Levy *et al.* (1989) reported that the POMS was sensitive to treatment type among breast cancer patients, and Cassileth *et al.* (1992) reported that it was sensitive to improvements in condition at 3 months follow-up.

Cognitive impairment

Intelligence and memory are often assessed in relation to children, in view of the uncertain effects of treatment (as well as time taken off school for treatments) on their functioning. The Wechsler Memory and Intelligence Tests are the instruments generally used (Wechsler 1945, 1958, 1981a, 1981b; Wechsler and Stone 1973).

Adjustment and coping

Quality of life may also be partly determined by the way in which a patient copes with illness (Weisman 1979). The ability to cope can be a modifying factor in relation to outcome. An equally essential concept in this process is adjustment to the condition. The importance of these psychological factors was demonstrated by de Haes *et al.* (1992), who reported that patients able to adjust are best able to maintain their quality of life.

Schedules often used in oncology in relation to coping and adjustment include: the Ways of Coping Scale (Folkman and Lazarus 1980); the Structured and Scaled Interview to Assess Maladjustment (Gurland *et al.* 1972a, 1972b); the Global Adjustment to Illness Scale, which was developed from interviews with cancer patients by five site collaborators from the Psychosocial Collaborative Oncology Group (Morrow *et al.* 1981); the Psychosocial Adjustment to Illness Scale (Morrow *et al.* 1978), which was recommended for use with cancer patients by Selby and Robertson (1987); and the Reintegration to Normal Living Index (Wood-Dauphinee and Williams 1987).

Self-concept, self-esteem and body image

Self-esteem is the overall affective evaluation of one's self-worth. It has long been viewed as a relevant variable in the study of adjustment to chronic illness (Moos and Tsu 1977; Turk 1979), including cancer (Foltz 1987; Curbow *et al.* 1990).

The self-concept has been defined as the 'sum total of all that a person feels about himself/herself' (Schain, 1980). It is akin to what the psychological literature terms 'self-esteem', which is the affective component of the self-concept: it describes an attitude, feeling or evaluation of the self (Greenwald *et al.* 1988). It is measured, in a global sense, by standard instruments such as Rosenberg's (1965) Self-Esteem Scale; it can also be reduced to compartments (e.g. feelings about body image following an amputation, colectomy, or mastectomy). In a review of 36 studies of self-concept in relation to neoplasms (cancer) Curbow *et al.* (1990), stressed the importance of definitions of terms – that the self-concept is best viewed as a collection of self-representations, and that self-esteem is a component of this group of representations.

The most popular scales are Rosenberg's (1965) Self-Esteem Scale and Fitts' (1965) Tennessee Self-Concept Scale, and the most common type of cancer studied in relation to self-esteem and self-concept is breast cancer (Curbow *et al.* 1990). Several other esteem scales are used in social science research on health outcomes (e.g. the Self-Esteem Questionnaire: Hoffmeister 1976). Readers are referred to McCarthy (1985).

The lack of disease-specific self-concept scales poses problems for researchers, and has led several to design their own scales. For example, in a study of 123 breast cancer patients undergoing a range of treatments from total or partial mastectomy to radiation therapy, Lasry *et al.* (1987) designed a series of ten questions about the impact of breast cancer on body image. Following analyses of reliability, three questions were excluded, and the remaining seven items had high internal consistency (Cronbach's alpha = 0.81). Their seven items related to body image and included: satisfaction with breast appearance; satisfaction with breast texture, satisfaction with body appearance, attractiveness according to others, change in attractiveness due to operation, description of scar (scale of 'revolting' to 'beautiful'); and fear of not being sexually attractive. The convergent validity of the index was confirmed by the findings which supported the investigators' hypothesis, that more positive body image was significantly associated with breast-conserving surgery, and body image was negatively affected by the more extensive surgery.

Life satisfaction

Most scales used in oncology generally cover the negative aspects of quality of life in cancer patients. The assumption underlying this practice is apparently that there is little that is positive in cancer patients' lives, although this was not borne out in the research undertaken by Hörnquist *et al.* (1992).

The most commonly used measures of life satisfaction and morale, across all disease groups, include the scales by Neugarten *et al.* (1961), Lawton (1972, 1975), Andrews and Withey (1976), and Bradburn (1969). An example of their use in oncology is Vinokur and co-workers' (1989, 1990) study of the life satisfaction of breast cancer patients which used items from Andrews and Withey's (1976) life satisfaction scale and Bradburn's (1969) Affect–Balance Scale. A popular life satisfaction item is Cantril's (1965) Ladder scale.

Social support

Social well-being includes feelings of intimacy, of belonging and the experience of social acceptance and approval, as well as being able to depend on people for instrumental help. It depends on having a social network, which may be enhanced or maintained by involvement in social activities. Scales have been developed to measure perceived support, network structure and/or participation in social activities. There is some evidence to support the buffering effects of social support in the face of a crisis. Social support is also an outcome variable – illness can impair the ability to maintain social relationships and activities. Support also includes the openness of communication and relationships with professionals, and its measurement should take account of satisfaction with medical and nursing care (Slevin 1984; Andersen 1985; Aaronson 1986; Fobair 1987). In some cases, the measurement of the quality/strain of the social relationship with key family members might also be important (Wellisch *et al.* 1983a; Wellisch 1987).

The social support literature and scales have been reviewed by Bowling (1991, 1994a). One popular scale because of its brevity is Berkman and Breslow's (1983) Social Network Index, which is based largely on dichotomized responses to questions about activities: attendance at church/religious services, clubs/voluntary organizations, talking on the telephone to family, friends or neighbours and frequency of contact with family, friends and neighbours. This has also been used with oncology patients. Vinokur *et al.* (1989), for example, used it with patients with breast cancer. However crude it may be, it was sensitive to health outcomes and mortality. It is relatively short and easy to administer, hence its appeal in clinical studies.

Vinokur *et al*. (1989) also used a number of supplementary support scales, including seven questions to assess satisfaction with marital relationships (Spanier 1976), such as: 'How often do you feel satisfied with this relationship?', 'How often are things between the two of you going well?' The responses form a 6-point scale ranging from 1 = never to 6 = all of the time/more than once a day. Vinokur *et al*. reported the alpha coefficient of this scale to be 0.82. They also used Caplan and co-workers' (1984) questions on social functioning, which provided an assessment of how respondents felt they had handled their roles, interpersonal relationships and emotions. Fourteen questions were included, for example: 'How well have you done in handling responsibilities and daily demands?. . . getting along with others . . . acting in a relaxed manner? . . . staying level headed?' Little testing of these questions has been conducted, but the value of the topics they cover is evident. A better subjective scale of perceived support is the scale developed for the Rand Medical Outcomes Study (Sherbourne and Stewart 1991), which asks respondents about the perceived availability of persons when they need help with, or support over, various aspects of life and when they are ill.

Patient satisfaction

Items on patient satisfaction and expectations should also be included. These have not been well-developed for disease-specific studies, and measurement of dissatisfaction is difficult. Relevant references were included in Chapter 1.

THE MEASUREMENT SCALES

SCALES MEASURING PHYSICAL FUNCTIONING, PAIN AND SYMPTOMS

Functional status scales used with cancer patients

Most existing functional status scales are not totally appropriate for use with cancer patients. Many

were developed for use in rheumatology and neurology, and are insufficiently sensitive to the particular problems of cancer patients. Despite this, the Karnofsky Scale (Karnofsky *et al*. 1948) is a popular scale among oncologists, although it is extremely crude. A condensed version of the Karnofsky scale was developed for use with cancer patients and is known as the Zubrod Scale (Zubrod *et al*. 1960). This is the most widely used scale of physical functioning, or performance, in oncology. Other scales of functioning which have been used in oncology include the Katz Activities of Daily Living Scale (Katz and Akpom 1976a, 1976b), the Barthel Index (Mahoney and Barthel 1965) and the Quality of Well-Being Index (Kaplan *et al*. 1976). The Karnofsky Scale will be reviewed below as its use is so widespread. The other scales mentioned are reviewed in Bowling (1991). While the Karnofsky Scale is still very popular, it is unlikely that it will survive, as increasing effort is being put into developing disease-specific quality of life scales for international use, which also include physical functioning as a major domain.

A literature review of the frequency of measurement of quality of life in clinical trials of outcome of care in six international cancer journals showed that only 6 per cent attempted to measure it, and of these most used the original performance criteria of Karnofsky (Bardelli and Saracci 1978). This is despite the many critical reviews of the scale which do not recommend its use (e.g. Donovan *et al*. 1989). Frequency of use is no necessary hallmark of a reliable and valid scale. Moreover, while it measures physical performance, it does not measure other dimensions of quality of life, despite users' claims to have conducted a quality of life study.

THE KARNOFSKY PERFORMANCE INDEX

Originally developed as a measure of nursing workload, the Karnofsky Index has been in use longer than any other measure of functional status, and remains popular among clinicians as a prognostic indicator, despite its poor performance in tests of reliability. It was not designed as a quality of life measure, but is frequently used as such. The Karnofsky Index emphasizes physical performance and dependency. It was originally designed for use with lung cancer patients in relation to assessing palliative treatments (Karnofsky *et al.* 1948; Karnofsky and Burchenal 1949), but is popular among clinicians for use with patients with other types of cancer, including breast cancer (Buchanan *et al.* 1986).

Content

The scale is heavily weighted towards the physical dimensions of quality of life, rather than social and psychological dimensions. Patients are assigned to categories by a clinician or other health care professional. It takes no account of the patient's feelings. It is widely used in the USA and Europe.

Administration and scoring

The classifications are made by health professionals. The 11 descriptions on the scale relate to rank-ordered decile points from 0 (dead) to 100 (normal) per cent. The patient is assigned a score after the most appropriate criteria are selected. Scores are summed to produce an overall score. The scoring procedure has not been assessed for validity. Various categorizations exist. It takes a few minutes to complete.

Examples from the Karnofsky Index

Criteria: Normal, no complaints, no evidence of disease (index: 100)
Criteria: Requires occasional assistance from others but able to care for most needs (index: 70)
Criteria: Disabled, requires special care and assistance (index: 40)
Criteria: Moribund (index: 10)
Criteria: Dead (index: 0)

Validity

The results for construct and concurrent validity (in relation to physical functioning) are generally good. Mor *et al.* (1984), in their national hospice evaluation, reported that the construct validity of the scale was adequately achieved: it was strongly related to two other independent measures of patient functioning (Katz's ADL Scale and another quality of life assessment). It was also able to predict longevity (0.30) in the population of terminally ill cancer patients, which indicates that it

has predictive validity. The Karnofsky Scale is a crude, although successful, predictor of survival. Mor (1987), again in a study of cancer patients ($n = 2046$), reported a moderate correlation between the Karnofsky Scale and the Spitzer Quality of Life scale; the correlation was probably moderate because the latter is multidimensional. One of its recent well-known applications has been in the US National Heart Transplantation Study (Evans *et al.* 1984). Results from this study showed a marked shift in the distribution of Karnofsky scores before and after transplantation. Ganz *et al.* (1988b) reported that the scale correlated well with the Functional Living Index. Other studies with lung cancer patients have reported inconsistent results in correlations between treatment response and the Karnofsky Index (Bakker *et al.* 1986; Harvey *et al.* 1987; Splinter 1990). The Karnofsky Performance Index has been reported to be a significant predictor of broader quality of life (measured with CARES) in three regression models relating to survivors of cancer of the lung, colon and prostate (Schag *et al.* 1994). The authors concluded that functional status is impaired when a variety of other factors relating to quality of life are also affected.

A major disadvantage of the Karnofsky Scale, apart from its crude and limited content, is that it involves categorization of patients by another person. This is a fundamental flaw given the evidence of discrepancies between patient and physician ratings of functioning and quality of life. In Evans and co-workers' (1984) study, for example, there were wide discrepancies between patients' self-assessments, based on the Sickness Impact Profile, and physicians' assessments, based on the Karnofsky Index, with the latter rating patients as being less impaired than the former.

Levine *et al.* (1988) reported that the Karnofsky Index was able to discriminate between women with stage II breast cancer who had completed treatment and those who were still undergoing treatment. It has not always been regarded as a sensitive scale to differences in patients' level of functioning, especially when they are mobile. For example, in a study of 81 patients with cancer of the bladder and colorectal cancer patients attending hospital clinics, Hurny *et al.* (1987) reported that the Karnofsky Performance Status scores of most patients were good, with only mild to moderate problems being recorded for most of them.

Yates *et al.* (1980) carried out the first objective validation of the scale with patients with advanced cancer – more than 30 years after its publication! They pointed out that the index is not appropriately scaled and that scale values may bear no relation to clinical significance. This criticism has been upheld in research by Schipper and his colleagues (Schipper *et al.* 1984; Schipper and Levitt 1986).

The fuller psychometric properties of the index have only recently begun to be seriously examined (Hutchinson *et al.* 1979). The scale's 'numeric' status has not been seriously challenged, and it has generally been uncritically accepted and applied in a large number of clinical settings (Schag *et al.* 1984). A basic problem is that the different conceptual elements do not appear on all scale points so that interpretations are liable to vary.

There are conceptual problems with the scoring method, particularly with the assumption that a patient with a low score due to immobility necessarily has a poorer quality of life than a patient with a higher score, and vice versa. For example, a patient with a poor score may have better social support than a patient with a good score and thus, despite his or her immobility, may have a better quality of life. Moreover, the Karnofsky ratings are often reported as a mean score, yet there is no evidence that the intervals between the ten categories represent the same degree of dysfunction (O'Brien 1988).

Reliability

Various studies have reported poor inter-rater agreement (Hutchinson *et al.* 1979), although the Karnofsky Index is still shown to be correlated with survival in cancer patients (Hyde *et al.* 1973; Stanley 1980). Slevin *et al.* (1988) reported a study involving 108 cancer patients, in which two groups of patients filled in the same collection of instruments, including the Karnofsky Index, on a single day, and then daily for five consecutive days. Although the Karnofsky Index was more robust than the other measures tested (Spitzer's Quality of Life Index, the Hospital Anxiety and Depression Scale and LASA visual analogue scales), the same score was achieved on only 54 per cent of

occasions, despite the fact that only the five top points on the Karnofsky Index were covered.

A study of 100 French cancer patients by Mercier *et al.* (1992b) reported that there was perfect agreement between doctor and patient using the Karnofsky Index in just 25 per cent of patient–doctor pairs. Mercier *et al.* (1992b) reported moderate agreement (62 per cent) by doctors and patients using the Karnofsky Index with cancer patients. In another study, inter-rater reliability was reported to be as low as 29–43 per cent with Cohen's kappa coefficient (Hutchinson *et al.* 1979). However, Yates *et al.* (1980) reported higher correlations using Pearson's coefficient of correlation (0.66–0.69). Mor *et al.* (1984), on the basis of a national hospice evaluation, reported that the inter-rater reliability coefficient of the 47 interviewers employed at test–retest at 4-month intervals was 0.97. Attempts have been made recently to improve the objectivity of the scale by the provision of a structured interview format, guidelines for examination of chart data, and input from significant others to arrive at a reliable rating. This can increase inter-rater reliability to 0.90+ (Grieco and Long 1984).

The index covers a very narrow dimension of quality of life (physical functioning), and requires supplementation with one of the many more recently developed psychosocial scales and symptom scales. It is included here because it is commonly used in oncology as a quality of life instrument, and it is frequently the only quality of life outcome indicator used, despite its narrow focus. Although it is most commonly used in studies of lung cancer (Minet *et al.* 1987; Fergusson and Cull 1991), it has been used in settings where its applicability has been questioned due to a lack of psychometric testing, for example bone marrow transplantation in children (Hinterberger *et al.* 1987).

Despite its limitations, the Karnofsky Scale has been used widely among cancer patients and has been popular with oncologists, partly because it has been shown to be a reasonable predictor of treatment outcome in a number of disease sites (Cella and Cherin 1987). The major flaw has been the assumption by clinicians that it measures global quality of life.

Two other versions of the scale have been developed, but with no obvious improvements in effectiveness over the original version (Zubrod *et al*. 1960; Nou and Aberg 1980). The World Health Organization (1979) has also developed a simpler alternative.

OTHER VERSIONS OF THE KARNOFSKY SCALE

THE WORLD HEALTH ORGANIZATION FUNCTIONAL SCALE

The World Health Organization (WHO 1979) has recommended an alternative 5-point performance scale which is simpler to use, but it still awaits an acceptable level of testing for reliability and validity, and it is also a narrow, physician-completed scale.

Examples from the WHO Functional Scale

0 = Able to carry out all normal activity without restriction

2 = Ambulatory and capable of all self-care but unable to carry out any work; up and about more than 50 per cent of waking hours

4 = Completely disabled, cannot carry on any self-care; totally confined to bed or chair

---

THE ZUBROD SCALE (OR, THE EASTERN COOPERATIVE ONCOLOGY GROUP PERFORMANCE SCALE: ECOG)

This scale, referred to variously as the Zubrod Scale, the ECOGP or the ECOG Scale, is really a condensed version of the Karnofsky Performance Index, from which it was developed. Work on its development in relation to disease-specific modules is ongoing (Zubrod *et al*. 1960; Skeel 1989). It is a measure of performance. It is valuable, like the Karnofsky Scale, as a predictor of the functional outcome of tumour treatment in certain sites. And, also like the Karnofsky Index, it is a limited scale in that it does not encompass any psychosocial indices of quality of life.

Content

The scale was designed as part of a battery of clinical measures of outcome in patients with cancer of the breast, lung, malignant melanoma and a lymphoma (Hodgkin's disease). It is an observer rating scale of 'patient reaction'. Scores range from 0 to 4 for performance. It also includes three single items on pain (rated 0 = none to 3 = severe), food intake (3 = poor and 1 = good) and nausea (0 = none to 2 = marked).

Administration and scoring

It is an observer-rated scale of ability, not performance (despite being called a performance scale). Observers are instructed to record the performance that a patient is capable of rather than what they actually choose to do. The range of scores is from 0 (*no impairment*) to 4 (*bedridden*). It provides a 5-point scale of performance. It is simple to use but is narrow in its coverage (i.e. it is limited to a single domain of quality of life – ability and mobility).

Performance scale of the ECOGP

0 = Normal activity

1 = Symptoms, but nearly fully ambulatory

2 = Some bed time, but needs to be in bed less than 50 per cent of normal daytime

3 = Needs to be in bed greater than 50 per cent of normal daytime

4 = Unable to get out of bed

Validity

It was not subjected to rigorous, systematic testing for reliability and validity by its author, although some studies have reported on some of its psychometric properties. It correlated well with a linear analogue self-assessment of quality of life (general well-being, mood, pain, nausea, vomiting, appetite, breathlessness, physical activity) (Coates *et al*. 1983). A study by Verger *et al*. (1992) compared the performance of the Karnofsky Scale with that of the ECOG Scale in 150 cancer patients. They reported that both scales were highly correlated, but a wide spread was observed in the lower performance status ranges, which should lead to some caution in the use of either scale. It does not always correlate well with scales of socio-psychological domains of quality of life (see Cella and Cherin 1987).

Reliability

Inter-observer correlations have been reported to be good (0.914) (Roila *et al.* 1991). However, a study of treatment for breast cancer by Guyatt *et al.* (1989c) and Levine *et al.* (1989) reported that the scale lacked clinical sensitivity as a measure of subjective health status.

Despite these fundamental weaknesses, the ECOG is the *performance* status measure of choice within the ECOG group and within the Cancer and Leukaemia Group B Clinical Trials Group (Cella and Cherin 1987), and is also recommended by the WHO (1979). Maguire and Selby (1989) state that it is less easy to use than the comparable WHO (1979) 5-point scale of physical performance, although the latter is very limited in scope. The Zubrod Scale, or ECOG, is probably the most widely used performance measure in oncology.

Pain scales

While single-item measures of pain frequency and intensity are popular, and frequently used, these are unidimensional and ignore the quality of the pain. The alternative is to use a multidimensional pain scale. The most frequently used measure of chronic pain is the McGill Pain Questionnaire. This is less often used for acute pain, as it is generally believed that most visual analogue scales (VASs) work adequately for acute pain (McQuay 1990).

THE MCGILL PAIN QUESTIONNAIRE (MPQ)

This was developed by Melzack and his colleagues at McGill University, Canada (Melzack and Torgerson 1971; Melzack 1975, 1980, 1987). It is the most frequently used measure of pain. It is used in particular in cancer studies (e.g. Morris and Sherwood 1987). Melzack and Torgerson (1971) selected 102 words from the literature describing the intensity and quality of pain (Melzack 1975). After a review by 20 judges, the final version to be tested contained 78 adjectives describing pain, arranged in 20 groups. A factor analysis during testing yielded four factors which led to the subsequent scale development based on these. These included sensory and evaluative sub-scales to designate perception of pain, and an affective sub-scale to denote emotional response.

A fuller pain assessment questionnaire was designed to elicit medical history, cause and location of pain, diagnosis, treatment, pain pattern and accompanying symptoms (e.g. nausea, headache). The measurement of these other domains is optional, and they are not included in the pain score. There have been several versions of the questionnaire, and a short version containing 15 groups of descriptions is available (Melzack 1987).

Content

The major part of the scale comprises 78 adjectives. The three major measures of the MPQ are the pain rating index, based on two types of numerical values that can be assigned to each word descriptor, the number of words chosen, and present pain intensity based on an intensity scale of 1–5. The advantage of the scale is that it quantifies pain, and it has been found to be sensitive to different treatment methods (Melzack 1975).

The short version contains 15 descriptors (11 sensory, 4 affective), which are rated on an intensity scale (0 = none, 1 = mild, 2 = moderate, 3 = severe). The 15 descriptors used are: throbbing, shooting, stabbing, sharp, cramping, gnawing, hot-burning, aching, heavy, tender, splitting, tiring–exhausting, sickening, fearful, punishing–cruel. Three pain scores are derived from the sum of the intensity rank values of the words chosen for sensory, affective and total descriptors. It also includes the Present Pain Intensity Index of the long version, and a VAS for assessing pain severity.

Administration and scoring

Although originally designed to be administered by an interviewer, the scale can be self-administered. The full-length scale takes 15–20 min to complete, but only 5–10 min on repeat testing (once respondents are familiar with its format), and the short version takes 2–5 min. The length of time required to complete the scale depends on the patient's familiarity with the words used as the descriptors.

Each description carries a weight corresponding to the severity of the pain, which was developed by panels of doctors, patients and students (Melzack and Torgerson 1971). Subjects then receive pain scores according to the number of descriptors selected to describe the pain and their assigned weights: 0 = no pain, 1 = mild pain, 2 = discomforting, 3 = distressing, 4 = horrible and 5 = excruciating.

There are four alternative scoring methods, ranging from number of words chosen to the sum of scale values (based on the scale weights) (for details, see Melzack 1975).

Examples from the MPQ

1 Flickering
   Quivering
   Pulsing
   Throbbing
   Beating
   Pounding
5 Pinching
   Pressing
   Gnawing
   Cramping
   Crushing
8 Tingling
   Itchy
   Smarting
   Stinging
16 Annoying
   Troublesome
   Miserable
   Intense
   Unbearable

Validity and factor structure

Several studies support the construct, concurrent and predictive validity of the MPQ. Melzack (1975) reported a study of 40 patients, which showed correlations between the pain question-naire score and a visual analogue rating of between 0.50 and 0.65. Reading (1983) has reviewed several studies and concludes that the MPQ is able to distinguish between patient groups. The specificity of the questionnaire was supported by a study of 536 cancer patients (Greenwald 1987). Dubuisson and Melzack (1976) reported that the questionnaire was able to correctly classify 77 per cent of their 95 patients with eight pain syndromes into diagnostic groups on the basis of the pain descriptors. How-ever, there is some evidence that the descriptors do

not include all those words used by patients with joint problems to describe their pain (Papageorgiou and Badley 1989).

Correlations between the long and short ver-sions were reported to be high and consistent in a study of 83 different types of patients tested before and 30 min after treatment for pain, the correlations ranging from 0.60 to 0.89 (Melzack 1987). Factor analyses of the questionnaire have yielded between four and five factors, with some overlap between the factors obtained (for a review, see Prieto and Geisinger 1983). There appears to be support for the distinction between affective and sensory di-mensions, but not for the distinctive evaluative component.

Cross-cultural applications of the questionnaire are reviewed by Naughton and Wiklund (1993).

Reliability

Data on the reliability of the long and short forms is limited. Although Melzack (1975) reported the results of test–retest exercises (three test com-pletions at intervals of 3–7 days between each), which showed a consistency of response of 70 per cent; the sample comprised 10 people only. No data have been published on the reliability of the short form.

Despite some questioning of its factor structure, and the limited data on the reliability of the scale, it is still the leading measure of pain.

Other symptom scales

SYMPTOM DISTRESS SCALE

The Symptom Distress Scale was designed for use with all types of cancer patients (McCorkle and Young 1978).

Content, administration and scoring

This scale is self-administered, usually in the pres-ence of an interviewer, and contains 13 items on symptoms of nausea, mood, loss of appetite, insomnia, pain, mobility, fatigue, bowel pattern, concentration and appearance. Responses are rated on a 5-point scale; scores are summed and high scores reflect more distress.

Examples from the Symptom Distress Scale

Nausea

| I feel as sick as I could possibly be | 5 | 4 | 3 | 2 | 1 | I do not feel sick at all |

Appetite

| Can't face food at all | 5 | 4 | 3 | 2 | 1 | Normal appetite |

Appearance

| The worst I've ever had | 5 | 4 | 3 | 2 | 1 | Appearance has not changed |

Validity and reliability

Construct validity was demonstrated in a study reporting a negative correlation between symptom distress and good quality of life (Young and Longman 1983). McCorkle and Young (1978) reported that it correlated well with global quality of life measures. McCorkle *et al.* (1986, 1989) reported that the instrument was sensitive to changes in treatment over time and between treatment groups. Sarna (1993) used a modified Symptom Distress Scale (McCorkle and Young 1978; McCorkle and Quint-Benoliel 1981) and the CARES-SF (Schag and Heinrich 1988; Ganz *et al.* 1990; Schag *et al.* 1991) among 69 women with lung cancer. The Symptom Distress Scale was strongly associated with the physical sub-scale of the CARES-SF ($r = 0.80$).

Reliability coefficients (coefficient alpha) of 0.78–0.89 have been reported (McCorkle and Young 1978; McCorkle and Quint-Benoliel 1983; McCorkle *et al.* 1986, 1989; McCorkle, 1987). McCorkle and Young (1978) tested the scale on 53 medical patients and reported a reliability coefficient alpha of 0.82.

The Symptom Distress Scale is one of the recommended instruments in the quality of life measurement package of the Southwest Oncology Group Cancer Control Research Committee (Moinpour *et al.* 1989).

LASRY SEXUAL FUNCTIONING SCALE FOR BREAST CANCER PATIENTS

This scale was developed after a review of the literature on the impact of breast cancer on body image. After tests for reliability, a scale of seven items was derived, with a Cronbach's alpha of 0.81 (Lasry *et al.* 1987; Lasry 1991). While further psychometric testing is required, the scale is reported here because of the lack of similar scales tapping the same dimensions.

Examples from the Lasry Scale

5 When you think of having sexual relations, how anxious do you feel?

   Not at all anxious / a little anxious / moderately anxious / very anxious

8 During lovemaking, do you keep some sort of clothing (nightgown, T-shirt, etc.) on you?

   No / sometimes / usually / nearly always

11 Since you had breast surgery, has there been any change in the following behaviours?

   In your mate's sexual drive

   Increase / same / decrease

Summary of other symptom scales

Other symptom scales are briefly described below, but they have either not been subjected to systematic psychometric testing or are relatively new scales at an early stage of development.

WORLD HEALTH ORGANIZATION (WHO) SYMPTOM CHECKLIST

The WHO checklist of treatment side-effects consists of 12 categories: nausea/vomiting, diarrhoea, constipation, haematuria, pulmonary function, fever, allergic reaction, skin reaction, hair loss, infection, neurological effects and pain. Each is coded on a 0–4 index, ranging from none, or no status change to severe (Miller *et al.* 1981).

MEDICAL RESEARCH COUNCIL (MRC) UK SCALE

The MRC in the UK has developed a 5-item scale that involves category rating techniques for vomiting, activity, mood anxiety and an overall score in a diary card (Fayers and Jones 1983). The scale has been criticized for lacking content validity (Selby and Robertson 1987), partly because it contains no questions about the toxic effects of treatment apart from vomiting, or disease complications. Reducing scales to such a small range of items inevitably leads to loss of information. It has been reported to be acceptable to cancer patients (Rieker *et al.* 1992).

THE QUALITATOR

This is an instrument developed for use with breast cancer patients by Fraser *et al.* (1990). Patients are able to decide themselves which symptom is most important to them. It is being tested for reliability and validity.

Disease-specific quality of life scales

EUROPEAN ORGANIZATION FOR RESEARCH ON TREATMENT OF CANCER (EORTC) MODULAR APPROACH

In 1980, a Study Group on Quality of Life was created within the European Organization for Research and Treatment of Cancer (EORTC). Its long-term goal was to develop a brief, standardized quality of life measure which could be used in international cancer trials. The EORTC quality of life scale was developed by this group. Most of the work of the group has related to cancer of the lung, oesophagus and breast, and development work is ongoing for other conditions (European Organization for Research on Treatment of Cancer 1983; van Dam *et al.* 1984; Aaronson 1986, 1987, 1993; Aaronson *et al.* 1988, 1991a, 1993).

The model of quality of life is multidimensional, and the questionnaire (based on self-report) covers cancer-specific symptoms of disease, the side-effects of treatment, psychological distress, physical functioning, social interaction, sexuality, body image, global health and quality of life, and satisfaction with medical care. The authors explicitly define quality of life in relation to the defined core elements of functional status, cancer and treatment-specific symptoms, psychological distress, social interaction, financial/economic impact, perceived health status and overall quality of life.

The original questionnaire tested contained 42 items, which were subsequently reduced to 36. The 36-item version was widely tested (Aaronson *et al.* 1991a). These 36 core items have recently been shortened to 30 (known as the QLQ-C30), and this is the current recommended version, although most published studies to date have used the 36-item version.

There are also 13 supplementary disease-specific items; for example, the first one developed was for lung cancer, and one has since been developed for breast cancer, and more recently for head and neck cancer (Aaronson *et al.* 1988; Bjordal and Kassa 1992). Thus the symptom checklist varies according to the type of cancer being studied. Most items are based on self-report methods, but there are also some observer rating items. The measure concentrates mainly on problem and symptom-specific items, with some global well-being and distress measures.

36-Item version

The earlier, longer versions of the scale have been subjected to fuller psychometric testing. The 36-item version is the best tested version of the EORTC, and was tested on 537 lung cancer patients drawn from 15 participating countries. The currently used EORTC-30 was derived from this and is very similar. In the core section of the EORTC-36, two Guttman scales measure functional status. The first is a 7-item scale of personal functioning, including self-care, mobility and physical activity. The items are similar to the Arthritis Impact Measurement Scales, a scale designed for use with patients with arthritis (Meenan *et al.* 1980). The second is composed of two items which reflect the extent to which patients can perform their usual work or housework activities. The response choices are dichotomous (yes/no).

In the core sections, physical symptoms frequently reported by cancer patients are assessed with a series of single items (for pain, breathlessness, constipation, diarrhoea, sleeplessness and cognitive disorder) and multiple item scales (for nausea and vomiting, fatigue and malaise). The symptom questions use a categorical format with response choices ranging from 'not at all' to 'quite a bit'. For the core psychological distress items, Aaronson *et al.* (1988) selected eight of the 14 items from the Hospital Anxiety and Depression (HAD) Scale (Zigmond and Snaith 1983), after inspecting the scale for its factor loadings and discussions with the scale's authors. This is regarded as the most appropriate of the depression scales for use with cancer patients (see pp. 76). The HAD response categories were adapted to the EORTC's uniform 4-point Likert scale. The core section contained two items on the perceived disruption of normal social activities, using the EORTC's uniform 4-point scale. The authors purposely avoided using the traditional social support items that focus on feelings of being loved/supported, as they felt that responses could be influenced by an under-reporting bias. A single question was included asking patients to report whether their condition had resulted in any financial difficulties, using the same 4-point scale. Finally, two global self-perceived quality of life items were also included in the core section. One question asks patients to rate, on a 7-point scale ranging from 'very poor' to 'excellent', their 'overall physical condition' during the past week. This is a similar item to those used in many other large studies (Ware et al. 1978). Using the same response categories, the second item asks patients to rate their 'overall quality of life during the past week'.

30-Item version

A shorter version than the 36-item version has been developed, known as the EORTC-30 (Tchek-medyian and Cella 1990; Aaronson 1993). It reflects the same basic structure as the 36-item version. The 30-item version covers five functional scales (physical functioning, role functioning, cognitive functioning, emotional functioning, social functioning), general quality of life, three symptom scales (fatigue, nausea and vomiting, pain) and six single items (Aaronson 1990, 1993).

The items on physical functioning have dichotomous yes/no responses. The sections on symptoms, anxiety and depression and limitations have 4-point response choices of 'not at all' (1), 'a little' (2), 'quite a bit' (3) and 'very much' (4). Categories 3 and 4 are regarded as indicators of clinically significant symptom levels. Finally, there are two items that ask respondents to rate their overall physical condition during the past week and overall quality of life during the past week (both using a 7-point VAS, where 1 = very poor and 7 =

excellent). The 30-item questionnaire has been published in full by Aaronson et al. (1993).

Modules

It was indicated earlier that the QLQ-C30 is now regarded as the version to be used, and it is seen as the core instrument, to be supplemented by more specific modules. Guidelines have been developed by the EORTC team for the development of the modules (Sprangers et al. 1993). The recommended domains include disease site, stage, symptoms, treatment (surgery, chemotherapy, radiotherapy, hormonal therapy), quality of life dimensions such as sexuality, body image and future perspective.

A tumour-specific supplement was designed regarding problems unique to lung cancer. Additional questions cover coughing, dyspnoea, the side-effects of chemotherapy, pain and use of medication for pain (total of 13 response items).

While it has been developed mainly with patients with cancer of the lung and breast, other investigators are beginning to use it to measure quality of life among patients with other types of cancer. For example, Sigurdardottir et al. (1993) used the Swedish translation (Bergman et al. 1991, 1992) to analyse the quality of life of 89 patients with generalized malignant melanoma, along with the Hospital Anxiety and Depression Scale (Zigmond and Snaith 1983), some of the items of which were already incorporated into the EORTC scale, and disease-specific items on melanoma. The measures differentiated between sub-groups of patients, and the authors reported that the EORTC questionnaire was feasible for use with melanoma patients. After piloting, the authors developed a core disease-specific supplement of 11 items, all of which experts felt were essential but missing from the core EORTC scale (e.g. temperature, sweating, stomach bloating, numbness in arms or legs, difficulties moving arms or legs, pain when moving around, pain when resting, use of painkillers, swellings, difficulties 'finding the right word', and hearing).

A breast cancer module to supplement the QLQ-C30 is also being tested. This covers dry mouth, changes in taste, hair loss, hot flushes and other cancer-specific symptoms, body image, worry about health, sexual functioning pain, problems of the breast, armpit, arm and shoulder, and skin problems (Sprangers *et al.* 1993).

A module on head and neck cancer, which includes symptoms, treatment-related side-effects, nutrition and social function, has been developed in Scandinavia (Bjordal and Kassa 1992), and is being pre-tested in other countries.

Administration and scoring

The scale is designed for self-administration, and is regarded as applicable across a range of cancer diagnoses. Although several investigators of quality of life have complained about poor compliance rates with questionnaires among cancer patients, Sadura *et al.* (1992) reported that over 95 per cent of their EORTC (36-item) questionnaires, and a breast cancer chemotherapy questionnaire, were returned and more than 99 per cent of the items were answered in three of the National Cancer Institute of Canada Clinical Trials. They attributed their success to having a comprehensive set of measures.

Scales are summed to produce sub-scale scores. The 30-item version takes about 10 min to administer. An English version is available, it is easy to complete, acceptable to patients and it has been translated into several languages.

Examples from the QLQ-C30

1 Do you have any trouble doing strenuous activities, like carrying a heavy shopping bag or a suitcase? No / yes
5 Do you need help with eating, dressing, washing yourself or using the toilet?   No / yes

During the past week:

8 Were you short of breath?
14 Have you felt nauseated?
15 Have you vomited?
19 Did pain interfere with your daily activities?
24 Did you feel depressed?
27 Has your physical condition or medical treatment interfered with your social activities?

   Not at all / a little / quite a bit / very much

30 How would you rate your overall quality of life during the past week?
   1   2   3   4   5   6   7
   very poor   excellent

Examples of items from the malignant melanoma module of the QLQ-C30

During the past week:

39 Has your stomach felt bloated?
45 Have you noticed swelling, e.g. on your neck, in your groin, on your skin?
47 Has your hearing been impaired?

Not at all / a little / quite a bit / very much

Validity and factor structure

The 36-item version was reported to be sensitive to differences in clinical status in a study of 62 adult patients with small cell lung cancer, and responded to clinical changes over time (Bergman *et al.* 1992). It has also been reported to be able to discriminate between different groups of patients receiving treatment for head and neck cancer, as each group reported different problem areas (Jones *et al.* 1992). The factor structure of the scale was confirmed by a series of factor analyses and multi-trait scaling analyses (Aaronson and Beckmann 1987).

Initial tests for validity with the current 30-item version were encouraging, and further testing and development is ongoing (particularly on lung cancer) with 305 patients with non-resectable lung cancer recruited from hospitals in 12 countries. The EORTC Study Group on Quality of Life is currently conducting a multi-centre study with participants from 15 member countries in order to test its psychometric properties and cross-cultural validity, and interim results are gradually being released (Aaronson 1987; Aaronson *et al.* 1988, 1991a). The 30-item version was also tested with 96 mixed cancer chemotherapy patients in Canada (Niezgoda and Pater 1993). Its sub-scales were reported to correlate moderately to strongly with comparable domains on the Sickness Impact Profile (SIP: Bergner *et al.* 1981): $r = 0.73$ (physical sub-scales), 0.48 (emotional), 0.48 (social), 0.58 (cognitive), 0.58 (fatigue) and 0.55 (role). The pain scale correlated moderately with the McGill Pain Scale (Melzack 1987): $r = 0.57$ (sensory/affective score) and 0.53 (present pain intensity score). Appropriate sub-scales correlated moderately to strongly with the Cancer Rehabilitation Evaluation System (CARES: Ganz *et al.* 1992) sub-scales: $r = 0.71$ (physical), 0.56 (emotional), 0.69 (pain), 0.61

(finance), 0.46 (social) and 0.55 (symptoms). These correlations were stronger than with the SIP, reflecting the fact that the EORTC and the CARES are both cancer-specific. Finally, the psychological functioning sub-scale correlated fairly strongly ($r = 0.61$) with the overall score of the General Health Questionnaire (GHQ: Goldberg 1972; Goldberg and Williams 1988). The authors commented that some sub-scales correlated with other scale sub-scales thought to be dissimilar (e.g. the social interaction sub-scale of the EORTC), and concluded that the question wording and specificity of these sub-scales required further investigation.

The 30-item version has been further tested on 177 heterogeneous cancer patients in Finland with good results which support the scalability of the instrument, although the cognitive and role functioning scales were below the acceptable level in terms of internal consistency. The depression sub-scale also correlated ($r = 0.71$) with the Hospital and Anxiety Depression Scale (HAD: Zigmond and Snaith 1983; Ringdal and Ringdal 1993).

Reliability

In relation to the 36-item version, Cronbach's alpha for internal consistency ranged from 0.69 for social interaction to 0.95 for symptoms of lung cancer. Scale intercorrelations ranged from 0.21 to 0.58 (Aaronson and Beckmann 1987). Sigurdardottir *et al.* (1993) reported that, with the exception of two items (role functioning, $r = 0.61$; nausea/vomiting, $r = 0.67$), all items satisfied criteria of internal consistency with reliability coefficients exceeding $r = 0.70$. A correlation matrix of the variables showed them to be high or moderate. The EORTC scale and sub-scales correlated moderately to strongly with the HAD sub-scores and total scores ($r = 0.40$–0.70); however, given that some of the items in the EORTC were from the HAD, this was only to be expected.

The practicality and reliability of the 30-item version was assessed in 305 resectable lung cancer patients from 12 countries. With the exception of role functioning, the data supported the scale structure of the questionnaire. Role functioning was the only multi-item scale that failed to meet the minimal standards for reliability (Cronbach's alpha coefficient ≥ 0.70). Internal consistency coefficients (Cronbach's alpha) reached criteria of acceptability at between $r = 0.52$–0.89. Most of the functional and symptom measures discriminated between patients differing in clinical status, and the questionnaire was responsive to changes in health status over time (Aaronson 1993). Inter-scale correlations between physical functioning, role functioning and fatigue scales ranged from 0.54 to 0.63; correlations of 0.43 and -0.42 were reported between the fatigue, emotional and social functioning scales. Weak correlations were reported between the emotional functioning scale and the physical and role functioning scales (0.25–0.27). The global quality of life scale correlated substantially with most other scales (0.41 to -0.62, but lower at -0.26 for nausea and vomiting). The authors noted that the moderate size of the inter-scale correlations indicated that they are assessing distinct components of quality of life. The reliability of the questionnaire was highly consistent across the three language/cultural group studies: Northern Europe, Southern Europe and patients from English-speaking countries. The 9-item tumour-specific questionnaire module supplemented the QLQ-C30, and addressed symptoms specific to lung cancer (Aaronson *et al.* 1991a).

Ringdal and Ringdal (1993) believe there is scope for improvement of the EORTC-30, to the extent that the instrument should be expanded in order that a minimum of 3–4 questions cover each dimension. The authors are also critical of the six single items which measure separate traits, such as sleeplessness and financial problems, arguing that it is difficult to use these sensibly and all dimensions should be multi-item or excluded.

In sum, it appears to reflect changes over time, and differences between treatment groups and type of cancer. Saunders and Baum (1992) describe it as a useful measure, but somewhat lengthy. Selby (1993) criticizes the use of analogue scales in the EORTC and the global ratings of overall physical condition and overall quality of life during the past week (7-point VAS, where 1 = very poor and 7 = excellent), and notes that in general in his experience, compliance is poor, as they are perceived as lengthy and onerous by doctors and patients, although researchers perceive them as brief. But it has been carefully developed to date and may be a useful instrument in the future. It has, however, been criticized as being too narrow in its focus with regard to ignoring much of the impact of cancer on social life (Siegrist and Junge 1990). While this is a valid criticism, the disadvantage of attempting to make disease-specific scales more comprehensive will be an inevitable lengthening of the scales. The argument can also be applied to a lack of focus on self-concept and self-esteem, coping and adjustment. The scales measuring these dimensions are long, and have to remain fairly lengthy in order to retain their psychometric properties. Disease-specific scales can aim to tap the major domains of quality of life, but where there is specific interest in a major or more peripheral domain, then a specialist scale will need to be used as a supplement.

The scale is not suitable for use with children and its sensitivity for use with elderly people with multiple pathology has yet to be assessed. In relation to all existing scales, more attention needs to be paid to the balance between the types of items contained in the scales, given that the balance of items can bias results and can increase or decrease the chances of obtaining a significant result in clinical trials (Hyland 1992a; 1992b).

ROTTERDAM SYMPTOM CHECKLIST

This is a 38-item scale which was developed by de Haes and his colleagues (de Haes et al. 1986, 1990) specifically to measure physical toxicity, social functioning, physical activity and psychological adjustment in cancer patients. It was constructed on the basis of analyses from three studies using different checklists of symptoms (Pruyn et al. 1980). The selection of items from the checklists was based on factor analyses, the distributions of answers and the judgements of oncologists (de Haes et al. 1990). The initial testing was carried out using eight items of daily living and 34 symptoms, and patients were asked to indicate the degree to which they had been bothered by the indicated symptoms during the past 3 days, on a 4-point Likert-type rating scale ('not at all', 'a little', 'quite a bit', 'very much') (de Haes et al. 1990). High scores indicate more discomfort.

It was originally validated in a Dutch study (de Haes et al. 1983), and has since been used in several Dutch and British investigations (Hopwood 1984; de Haes and Welvaart 1985; Fallowfield et al. 1986; Morris and Royle 1988). Principal components analysis was carried out by the authors based on

studies of 95 cancer out-patients receiving chemotherapy or being followed up, 56 patients participating in a trial comparing two chemotherapy regimens, and almost 400 cancer patients undergoing surgery or chemotherapy in the past 3 months, and 'normal' controls'. The analyses confirmed the instrument's stability and distinction between the psychological and physical dimensions (de Haes et al. 1990). An Italian study of 147 healthy women and 61 breast cancer out-patients by Paci (1992) reported a factor analysis of the Italian version of the scale with similar results to the English version. Paci also reported a correlation between the Rotterdam Symptom Checklist and the State–Trait Anxiety Inventory (Spielberger et al. 1983) of $r = 0.74$ (healthy sample).

Content

The items ask about appetite, worry, energy, nausea, headache, sexual interest, irritability, sore muscles, pain, despair, vomiting, tiredness, depression, nervousness, sleep, dizziness, tension, anxiety, dyspepsia, sore eyes, constipation, shivering, sore mouth, dyspnoea, diarrhoea, tingling, hair loss, dry mouth, stomach aches, concentration, self-care, walking, housekeeping, climbing stairs, odd jobs, shopping and work. Respondents are asked to indicate how much they have experienced particular symptoms over the last week.

The final version includes 30 symptoms in a category rating 4-point scale format (0 = not at all, 1 = a little, 2 = quite a bit, 3 = very much), and eight items which assess daily activities. One global quality of life item is included at the end.

Administration and scoring

It can be self-administered. It is easy to score and can be divided into different sub-sets for analysis. It is of value in the assessment of physical symptoms and treatment toxicity, and psychosocial morbidity. It takes 5–10 min to complete and appears to be acceptable. Scores are summed to provide two main sub-scales which measure physical and psychological dimensions.

Examples from the Rotterdam Symptom Checklist

Symptoms

In this questionnaire you will be asked about your symptoms. Read each item and place a firm tick in the box opposite the reply which comes closest to how you have been feeling during the past 3 days.

1 Lack of appetite

   Not at all / a little / quite a bit / very much

5 Worrying

   Not at all / a little / quite a bit / very much

9 Low back pain

   Not at all / a little / quite a bit / very much

15 Vomiting

   Not at all / a little / quite a bit / very much

21 Tension

   Not at all / a little / quite a bit / very much

All things considered, how would you describe your quality of life during the past week? Excellent / good / moderately good / neither good nor bad / rather poor / poor / extremely poor.

Others (e.g. Slevin *et al.* 1988) have adapted the questionnaire as follows:

Examples

In this questionnaire you will be asked about your symptoms. For each symptom mentioned below, we would like you to indicate to what extent you suffer from it, by encircling the answer most applicable to you. For each question please indicate how you have been feeling over the past 3 days.

● lack of appetite
● irritability
● tiredness
● worrying
● sore muscles

Not at all / a little / somewhat / very much

Validity

It was found to be sensitive to treatment in a study of 174 adult cancer patients (Greer *et al.* 1992),

although further testing for validity is required. It has been criticized for not covering adequately the sexual or social dimensions of quality of life, and it requires supplementation with additional physical symptom items (Slevin 1992). However, the question on sexual dysfunction has been used successfully within a battery of other measures by Fallowfield *et al.* (1990) in a study of the psychological outcomes of different treatment policies in women with early breast cancer. It was sensitive to improvements over time after treatment. It has been reported to be able to correctly identify 75 per cent of patients suffering from an affective disorder, as judged by a psychiatric clinical interview (Hopwood *et al.* 1991).

Slevin suggested that the scale should be used alongside the Hospital Anxiety and Depression Scale (Zigmond and Snaith 1983), and it has been used in conjunction with it by some investigators (Greer *et al.* 1992), although Maguire and Selby (1989) concluded that it had high specificity and sensitivity in measuring psychological dimensions, and that further testing of its physical and social dimensions is required. Saunders and Baum (1992) describe it as a useful scale, with good validity to date, and which is easy to administer. It is a clear questionnaire, and its advantage is its flexibility, which allows extra items to be included if additional illness or treatment variables require assessment.

Reliability

The internal reliability of the physical distress and the psychological components of the scales has been shown to be good (Cronbach's alpha = 0.71–0.88 and 0.88–0.94 respectively) (de Haes *et al.* 1990).

The MRC Working Party on quality of life assessments (Maguire and Selby 1989) recommended the use of the Rotterdam Symptom Checklist, supplemented by other items when needed, VAS items for symptoms and adverse effects, and the Hospital Anxiety and Depression Scale. However, since they made these recommendations much progress has been made with the increasingly popular EORTC questionnaire. A manual for the Rotterdam Symptom Checklist is available from de Haes.

FUNCTIONAL LIVING INDEX – CANCER (FLIC)

The FLIC is one of the most widely used self-completed cancer-specific quality of life indexes. The scale is sometimes called the Manitoba Cancer Treatment and Research Foundation Functional Living Index, reflecting its origins. It was developed by Schipper and his colleagues in Winnipeg (Schipper *et al.* 1984; Schipper and Levitt 1986) and is still in popular use (Cassileth *et al.* 1992; Lindley *et al.* 1992; Morrow *et al.* 1992). It is multidimensional in concept. It is a 22-item linear visual analogue scale, with a 7-point interval Likert scale format.

The scale was developed from a panel of 11 people (patients, spouses, doctors, nurses, psychologists and clergy). They produced 250 questions that they believed to be relevant to the assessment of quality of life in cancer patients. They were sorted into 92 items which did not overlap. After preliminary testing, a reduced pool of 42 items was tested on over 300 patients. The authors state this as evidence of the instrument's face validity.

It was further tested on over 800 patients in two cities. Three factor analyses generated relatively consistent findings with respect to physical status and psychological state. The factor analyses reduced the number of scale items to 20, and a final version was tested which contained 22 items.

Content

The domains of the final 22-item version include physical and occupational functioning, psychological state, sociability and somatic comfort (Schipper *et al.* 1984). It is apparently easy for patients to complete, and takes less than 15 min.

Administration and scoring

The scale is reported to be of value if administered in out-patient settings, as it has limited applicability for in-patients (e.g. some of the items relate to performance of household tasks, work satisfaction, etc.). Each VAS line covers either 'now' or 'the past 2 weeks'. The patient is instructed to answer all the questions by making a mark on the scoring line that best represents his or her response.

Responses are made on a 7-point VAS. For scoring, each interval is divided in half and responses are scored to the nearest even whole integer. The scores for each question are summed to give an overall score, the minimum being 22 (all 1 responses on each of the 22 scales) and the maximum being 154 (all 7 responses). A high score corresponds to a better quality of life.

Examples from the FLIC

Respondents are asked to indicate their rating with a cross on a 7-point VAS (e.g. none / a great deal or not at all / a great deal). The scale is reversed for some items.

1 Most people experience some feelings of depression at times. Rate how often you feel these feelings.

4 Rate your ability to maintain your usual recreation or leisure activities.

5 Has nausea affected your daily functioning?

6 How well do you feel today?

7 Do you feel well enough to make a meal or do minor household repairs today?

9 Rate how often you feel discouraged about your life?

11 How uncomfortable do you feel today?

21 Rate your confidence in your prescribed course of treatment.

Validity

More work has been published on the validity of the scale than on its reliability. The FLIC was tested for validity on 837 patients with different stages of cancer and on different treatments in two cities over 3 years (Schipper *et al.* 1984). Criteria for validity included stability of factor analysis, concurrent validation studies against the Karnofsky Performance Index (Karnofsky and Burchenal 1949), Beck Depression Inventory (Beck *et al.* 1961), Spielberger State–Trait Anxiety Inventory (Spielberger *et al.* 1983), Katz ADL Scale (Katz and Akpom 1976a, 1976b), the General Health Questionnaire (Goldberg and Hellier 1979) and the McGill Pain Questionnaire (Melzack 1975). The concurrent validity in these studies ranged from −0.30 with the Katz ADL Scale to −0.76 with the GHQ. It was reported to be free of social desirability bias when analysed with the Jackson Social Desirability Scale (see Schipper *et al.* 1984). Principal factor analysis with an orthogonal varimix rotation was used to reduce the items and define physical well-being, ability and emotional state factors.

Butow *et al.* (1991) used the scale with 103 cancer out-patients and compared the results with several other scales, including LASA items (Spitzer *et al.* 1981). They reported high correlations ($r = 0.63$–0.72) between the FLIC and selected LASA items on appetite loss, mood and physical well-being. The other dimensions on the scale have inconclusive validity. The scale was able to distinguish between different groups of cancer patients. However, as the validation samples were not severely disabled, tests of validity need to be repeated. It did not perform well against the Katz ADL Index. Major symptom-specific items are not included.

Ganz *et al.* (1988b) used the FLIC (cancer) and the Karnofsky performance status scale in a prospective, randomized Phase III clinical trial for the treatment of advanced metastatic non-small cell lung cancer. The response rate from patients was disappointing, as many were unwilling to complete the FLIC; some had problems reading it (due to poor vision or debilitation), and others refused to complete it unless it was read out to them. Among those who did respond, the correlation between the two scales was moderate but still significant at $r = 0.33$, although the correlation between the physical sub-scale of the FLIC and the Karnofsky Scale was higher at $r = 0.47$. The authors did not feel that the global assessment approach of the FLIC adequately detected the degree of difficulty experienced by their patients, and concluded that whereas the VAS has psychometric advantages, it may have inherent problems with administration. They recommended the use of scales that ask more specific questions about functional performance and psychosocial status, possibly the Cancer Inventory of Problem Situations (Schag *et al.* 1983). Finkelstein *et al.* (1988) also reported poor compliance with regard to the completion of the instrument among lung cancer patients.

The physical status section has been reported to correlate highly with the doctor-rated Karnofsky Performance Index, the McGill/Melzack Pain Index, and also with measures of psychiatric morbidity such as the General Health Questionnaire and the Beck Depression Inventory, and with the Spielberger State–Trait Anxiety Inventory (Schipper *et al.* 1984; Ganz *et al.* 1988b). More specifically, whereas the physical function and ability factor of the FLIC correlated well with the other instruments which measured physical attributes, it did not correlate as strongly with the psychosocial measures. Also, FLIC's emotional function factor correlated strongly with measures of depression and anxiety, but weakly with the physical ability measures. This provided evidence that the FLIC measures a composite of distinct factors contributing to overall 'functional living' and is presented as evidence of the measure's concurrent validity (Schipper *et al.* 1984). The measure did not correlate well with the Katz ADL Scale. The authors suggest that this was because the Katz Scale is appropriate for a more disabled population than that sampled (most of their study patients scored at the ceiling of the Katz Scale) and is restricted in its range of scores. There was a reasonable correlation of scores when only patients scoring at the lower levels on both scales were considered.

Reliability

Morrow *et al.* (1992) reported the results of psychometric analyses of the FLIC, based on 530 consecutive cancer patients, divided into two groups so as to cross-validate the results. Principal components analysis revealed a 5-factor solution, accounting for 70 per cent of the variance in a random half of the original sample, and 68 per cent in a cross-replication sample. Correlations testing for the stability of the factor structure (Carmine's theta, a special case of Cronbach's alpha) were $r = 0.90$ for the original sample and 0.94 for the validation sample. Cronbach's alpha correlations testing for the consistency of the individual items forming each factor ranged from $r = 0.65$ to $r = 0.87$. Convergent-discriminant validity was measured by testing for associations between the FLIC and the State–Trait Anxiety Inventory, and a symptom and nausea/emesis checklist designed by the authors for use with cancer patients (Morrow and Morrell 1982; Morrow 1984; Carnrike and Carey

1990). The Factor 4 loading (gastrointestinal symptoms and side-effects) correlated significantly with severity ratings of nausea ($r = 0.28$) and vomiting ($r = 0.27$). The Factor 2 loading (psychological factors) correlated more highly with state and trait anxiety measures ($r = -0.71$ and -0.63, respectively). The weakest section of the FLIC was the current 'well-being' sub-scale. It did not distinguish between patients with different diagnoses, and its internal consistency coefficient was slightly smaller than the others. On the whole, however, the authors concluded that the FLIC appears to be conceptually sound and internally consistent.

The FLIC has been criticized by Aaronson et al. (1988) for using an overall score to reflect the sum of the individual items, and the resulting score is probably too crude to be of clinical value. Saunders and Baum (1992) caution that it has not been fully assessed for reliability and validity, and other reviewers have pointed out that construct validation and other psychometric properties are yet to be carefully evaluated (van Knippenberg and de Haes 1988; Donovan et al. 1989; Cella and Tulsky 1990), although this has begun to be redressed (Morrow et al. 1992). Maguire and Selby (1989) and Selby (1993) have reported that the use of the word 'cancer' in the scale has distressed patients. A further criticism is that few physical symptom items are included. Its test for validity and sensitivity to change is not extensive enough. Maguire and Selby (1989) and Selby (1993) concluded that such considerations prevented the Medical Research Council's Cancer Therapy Committee Working Party on Quality of Life from recommending its use. The Cancer Control Research Committee of the Southwest Oncology Group in the USA also failed to recommend this measure, largely because of its reliance on VASs, which, it was felt, some patients have difficulty completing (Moinpour et al. 1989).

FUNCTIONAL LIVING INDEX – EMESIS (FLIE)

Most investigators ensure that an item or scale measuring nausea and vomiting has been included in their questionnaires. Several scales have been developed, although not widely used on an international basis, for example checklists of symptoms which include vomiting and nausea (Morrow 1984) and the Morrow Assessment of Nausea and Emesis (Morrow 1984; Carnrike and Carey 1990).

The FLIE scale was modelled after the FLIC by Lindley et al. (1992). The authors justified the need for a complete scale to measure emesis (vomiting) in view of the fact that nausea and vomiting following the administration of chemotherapy are common and often overlooked causes of impairment. An earlier study estimated that 30 per cent of cancer patients seen at Duke University refused chemotherapy and an additional 20 per cent delay treatment or miss clinic appointments because of nausea and vomiting (Laszlo 1983), although very few patients in Lindley and co-workers' study reported delayed treatments or missed appointments for these reasons.

The scale is illustrated below. It uses the same 7-point VAS response format as the original FLIC (e.g. none/a great deal or not at all/a great deal):

Examples from the FLIE

1 How much nausea have you had in the past 3 days?
4 How much has nausea affected your ability to enjoy a meal in the past 3 days?
10 How much vomiting have you had in the past 3 days?
11 Has vomiting affected your ability to maintain usual recreation or leisure activities during the past 3 days?
16 Has vomiting affected your daily functioning during the past 3 days?

The authors reported a study using the FLIC and their newly developed 18-item scale, FLIE, in which it was found that vomiting, and to a lesser extent nausea, substantially reduced patients' ability to carry out household tasks, enjoy meals, spend time with family and friends and carry out other daily functions and recreation. The scale was administered to 122 cancer patients. Correlations between the FLIE and patient-reported vomiting and severity of nausea (Pearson's coefficient) were $r = -0.65$ and -0.68, respectively (in the expected direction). Correlation of the FLIE nausea-related sub-scale with the FLIC nausea factor was $r = 0.83$. This provides evidence of the scale's construct validity. A factor analysis of FLIC by Lindley et al. reproduced the factors for the FLIC reported by Schipper et al. (1984). Reliability was assessed using Cronbach's alpha of inter-item correlation, and the item correlation within the FLIE was above 0.9.

CANCER INVENTORY OF PROBLEM SITUATIONS (CIPS) AND THE CANCER REHABILITATION EVALUATION SYSTEM (CARES)

Cancer Inventory of Problem Situations (CIPS)

This scale was developed by Schag and his colleagues (Schag *et al.* 1983; Heinrich *et al.* 1984). It was derived from a review of the literature and interviews with health professionals, patients and their families. Patients were a main source in generating the items.

Content

It covers the psychosocial and physical problems of cancer patients. It represents a move away from the concern with emotional distress, towards assessing the disease and treatment effects on behaviour. The scale consists of 131 problem statements grouped into more than 20 categories (reported variously in the authors' articles as between 20 and 27, depending on the stage of development) under four main headings: personal care, medical situations, interpersonal interactions, miscellaneous. In the 21-category version, the items fall into the following categories: activity, anxiety in medical situations, changes in physical appearance, cognitive difficulties, communication with medical staff, control in medical situations, dating relationships, domestic chores, eating, employment, finances, pain, physical abilities, prostheses, relationships with family and friends, self-care, side-effects of treatment, significant relationships, sleeping, transportation and worry.

Respondents read the problem statement and rate how much it applied to them during the previous month. The statements are quite specific. For example, for eating, three problems relate to the patient's perception of how appetizing the food is, how it tastes, and how well the respondent can swallow. Responses are made on a 5-point scale, ranging from 'not at all' to 'very much'.

Administration and scoring

The scale was designed for self-completion. It is reported to take 20 min to complete. The category score is an average intensity rating and is obtained for each category by summing the rankings of the statements endorsed in a given category and dividing it by the number of statements that received ratings greater than zero. The items are weighted. Three global scores can be obtained. These include the global severity rating, the total number of problems, and the global intensity rating.

Examples from the CIPS

Communication with medical staff

I have difficulty getting information from my doctor about my disease
I have difficulty understanding what the nurses tell me about my treatment or disease

Anxiety in medical/stressful situations

I get nervous when I am waiting to see the doctor
I get nervous when I get my blood drawn

Not at all / a little / a fair amount / much / very much

Validity and factor structure

The instrument was tested on over 2000 adults with cancer, including some with advanced lung cancer (Schag *et al.* 1983; Heinrich *et al.* 1984). These authors reported CIPS to have content and face validity, and presented normative data for the instrument. Factor analyses initially revealed 31 clinically useful sub-scales, and further analyses showed that it contains five higher-order factors representing the physical, psychosocial, medical interaction, marital and sexual problem areas characteristic of cancer and its treatment. The concurrent, discriminant and convergent validity of the scale were supported by its correlations with psychological distress, physical, marital and sexual functioning and quality of life (Schag *et al.* 1990). An early study carried out to test the validity and reliability of the CIPS was undertaken by Schag *et al.* (1983) among 306 heterogeneous cancer patients. Content validity was confirmed by this study. It correlated with a psychosocial index ($r = 0.69$). Factor analysis confirmed internal consistency. Most patients found the scale easy to complete and it took an average of 18 min.

Reliability

The CIPS achieved good test–retest reliability

coefficients of 0.89 (Schag *et al.* 1983), and the authors have reported that it is acceptable to patients. The CIPS was the developmental version of CARES (see below).

The Cancer Rehabilitation Evaluation System (CARES)

CARES is based on CIPS (see above) (Schag *et al.* 1983, 1990; Ganz *et al.* 1986, 1990, 1992; Schag and Heinrich 1988, 1990). CARES is a 139-item instrument used to assess the rehabilitation needs of cancer patients. It is also used as a measure of quality of life among all types of cancer patients (Ganz *et al.* 1990, 1992; Schag *et al.* 1993). It focuses on problems amenable to rehabilitative effort, and patients can identify areas where they would like more help. Its theoretical basis is a competency model of coping with cancer (Goldfried and D'Zurilla 1969). CARES provides a measurement of the problems with which cancer patients cope, and assesses behaviour as affected by cancer and its treatment, as opposed to emotional distress.

Content

The full version of the instrument contains 139 items. Some sub-sections apply only to patients who are at risk of specific problems (e.g. from chemotherapy). Patients complete the CARES by rating problem statements on a 5-point problem severity scale ranging from 0 (not at all) to 4 (applies very much). High scores indicate increased disruption. Patients rate a minimum of 93 and a maximum of 132 items. CARES is a relatively comprehensive instrument, and a shorter (59 items) and more popular version is available (Schag 1988; Schag and Heinrich 1988; Ganz *et al.* 1990). With the short version, patients complete between 38 and 57 items. The ratings are the same as for the full version. The short version produces the overall score and the five summary scale scores. Individual items can be analysed. The items overlap with CIPS (overleaf).

Administration and scoring

The scale was designed for self-completion. Scores are available for an overall assessment of disruptions in quality of life (global score), and the five summary scales: physical (disruptions in day-to-day activity and physical changes due to disease/treatment); psychosocial (emotional distress and anxiety, communication problems, body image); medical interaction (communication and interaction with health professionals); marital (communication with partner, expression of affection, concerns about neglect and over-protection); and sexual (disruptions in sexual interest and function for those who are sexually active).

Validity

Ganz *et al.* (1990) used the CARES with 109 newly diagnosed breast cancer patients. They reported that, in comparison with the Karnofsky Scale (Karnofsky *et al.* 1948) and the Global Adjustment to Illness Scale (Morrow *et al.* 1981), CARES was the best single predictor of patients' self-rated quality of life. Research in heterogeneous samples of out-patients and in over 200 breast cancer patients has demonstrated good reliability and validity (Schag *et al.* 1983). The CARES has been reported to correlate moderately with performance status and with quality of life as measured by a single global rating on a LASA scale (Gough *et al.* 1983; Schag *et al.* 1990).

Tests for validity among 109 newly diagnosed breast cancer patients using the Functional Living Index and the Karnofsky performance status scale yielded strong correlations with the CARES of -0.74 and -0.60, respectively (Ganz *et al.* 1990). A study by Ganz *et al.* (1992) of 277 colorectal cancer patients, 214 lung cancer patients and 288 prostate cancer patients reported that CARES was able to distinguish between patient type; for example, the prostate cancer patients had better overall CARES scores than the lung cancer patients in relation to localized disease, and the prostate cancer patients with extensive disease had significantly better CARES scores than the colorectal and lung cancer patients with extensive disease. The comparisons were similar for the five summary scales of the CARES. In relation to a second sample of 109 breast cancer patients, no overall score differences were found between women undergoing modified radical mastectomy and segmental mastectomy, although the clothing and body image sub-scale items of the CARES were able to distinguish between the two groups, with the former group having greater difficulties as would be predicted

(Ganz *et al.* 1992). The CARES was reported to be sensitive to changes over time with survivors of lung, colon and prostate cancer (Schag *et al.* 1994).

Sarna (1993) used the short version (CARES-SF) to measure quality of life among 69 women with lung cancer, and reported that the global CARES-SF score was moderately correlated with the Karnofsky Performance Index ($r = 0.69$) and with the modified Symptom Distress Scale (McCorkle and Young 1978; McCorkle and Quint-Benoliel 1981) ($r = 0.72$). The Symptom Distress Scale was strongly associated with the physical sub-scale of the CARES-SF ($r = 0.80$).

Little has been published on the reliability of the scale. In sum, CARES can provide detailed information about the type of problems associated with quality of life ratings. It is expensive to obtain, because it has been copyrighted on a commercial basis. A handbook is available for purchase (Schag and Heinrich 1988).

Visual analogue scales and other scales

Frequently used visual analogue scales (also known as linear analogue scales) in the assessment of quality of life are the Spitzer Quality of Life Scale and the Spitzer Uniscale (Spitzer *et al.* 1981), the Linear Analogue Self-Assessment Scale (LASA: Priestman and Baum 1976; Priestman 1984), the Quality of Life Tool (Padilla *et al.* 1983) and the LASA Quality of Life Assessment developed by Selby *et al.* (1984). These, and others, are reviewed briefly below.

SPITZER QUALITY OF LIFE (QL) INDEX

This scale was developed by Spitzer *et al.* (1981) specifically for doctors to measure the quality of life of their cancer patients. Ease of administration, simplicity and speed were paramount in their scale criteria. The instruments were designed for use by patients, health professionals and significant others. It was developed after questioning lay people and health professionals who formed three advisory panels for the questionnaire item construction. The factors that were rated as the most important by these groups formed the first draft of the QL Index, which was then tested on 339 out-patients.

Content

The resulting instrument covered the following five domains: activity, performance of activities of daily living, perception of health (e.g. energy level), support from family and friends, and outlook on life. It was designed for completion by health professionals (e.g. doctors) on behalf of patients. It apparently takes less than 1 min to complete. A global (Uniscale) VAS for rating overall quality of life the previous week is also included, which is often used separately (Spitzer *et al.* 1981).

Each question contains a number of items and thus confuses several domains within one, although respondents can only give one tick per question to imply that it applies to them (see examples below). There is also a 6-point scale for rating one's confidence in the ratings. It is apparently acceptable to professionals and patients. It has been modified for completion by patients.

Administration and scoring

It can be self-administered. Ratings for each are scored as 0, 1 or 2, resulting in a total QL score of 0–10 (higher scores = better QL).

Examples from the Spitzer Quality of Life Index

Patient-administered scale (scale item for professional in brackets)

Activity
(a) I do not work in any capacity nor do I study nor do I manage my own household

(Has not been working or studying in any capacity and not managing own household)

Daily living
(b) I am able to eat, wash, go to the toilet and dress without assistance. I drive a car or use public transport without assistance

(Has been self-reliant in eating, washing, toileting, and dressing; using public transport or driving own car)

Health
(c) I lack energy or only feel 'up to par' some of the time

(Has been lacking energy or not feeling entirely 'up to par' more than just occasionally)

Support

(p) I have good relationships with others and receive strong support from at least one family member and/or friend

(The patient has been having good relationships with others and receiving strong support from at least one family member and/or friend)

Outlook

(j) I am sometimes troubled and there are times when I do not feel fully in control of my personal life. I am anxious and depressed at times

(Has sometimes been troubled because not fully in control of personal circumstances or has been having periods of obvious anxiety or depression)

The Spitzer Quality of Life Uniscale

'Please mark with an X the appropriate place within the bar to indicate your rating of this person's quality of life during the past week. If more than a week please state the last time you saw this person.' Visual analogue scale (bar) is marked at the two extremes as 'lowest quality' and 'highest quality'. *Lowest quality* applies to someone completely dependent physically on others, seriously impaired mentally, unaware of surroundings and in a hopeless position. *Highest quality* applies to someone physically and mentally independent, communicating well with others, able to do most of the things enjoyed, pulling own weight, with a hopeful yet realistic attitude

Lowest quality —————————— Highest quality

Validity

Despite its crudity, this scale has been extremely popular, and has been used in numerous studies. In the initial full 5-item scale development, three panels of 43 people generated a large number of potential scale items which were reduced by examination and factor analysis into the five areas of activity: occupation, activities of daily living, perception of health, family support and outlook on life. However, only four members of each panel were cancer patients, and there is no record of independent interviews with patients at this stage.

The 5-item scale has been tested on healthy subjects, people with chronic diseases, cancer patients and other seriously ill patients. Content validity was reported on the basis of a literature review and on the basis of information provided by panels of patients, healthy people, health professionals, patients' relatives and clergy. It was reported to have convergent validity among patients with a diagnosed disease (Spitzer *et al.* 1981). The authors reported that just 59 per cent of doctors, in a study of the ratings of 150 doctors and 879 patients, said that they were 'very confident' in their ratings of patients' quality of life. Convergent validity was judged to be acceptable by a correlation of 0.61 between doctors' ratings and patients' self-ratings. The authors also demonstrated discriminant construct validity, as the scale discriminated between ill and healthy people, and between cancer and other chronically ill patients.

Levine *et al.* (1988) believe it is not sensitive enough to discriminate between treatment and completed treatment groups with breast cancer. It did reveal some lack of responsiveness, as relatively few of the cancer patients registered low scores. Spitzer *et al.* (1981) concluded that the scale could only discriminate between healthy and ill people, or between those with early- or middle-stage cancer and those who were seriously ill. The instrument was unable to detect differences within the seriously ill group, or within the group without physical symptoms. Coates *et al.* (1987), on the basis of a study of the outcome of breast cancer patients, reported that the scale could discriminate between patients on intermittent and continuous therapy.

Mor (1987) used the 5-item Spitzer Index with 397 newly diagnosed cancer patients and reported it to be a robust indicator. They had previously reported that the Spitzer Index was able to discriminate between the stages of decline as death approaches (Mor *et al.* 1984), but concluded in 1987 that the scale was probably not sufficiently sensitive for use as an outcome of care variable. On the basis of three samples of newly diagnosed cancer patients ($n = 2046$), they reported correlations of $r = 0.63$ between the Spitzer Index and the Karnofsky Performance Scale. Others have reported good correlations between the Spitzer Index and LASA Scale (Gough *et al.* 1983), and between the Spitzer Index and the Karnofsky Performance Scale (Morris and Sherwood 1987). The latter study included a very large sample of more than 2000 patients, and while it correlated with the Karnofsky Scale, the authors felt it was not sufficiently sensitive for use as an outcome measure of the impact of the disease on patients' lives, largely because of the insensitivity of the social-functioning index. Its sensitivity to changes over time has yet to be tested in full.

The scale is able to predict mortality among cancer patients (Mor *et al.* 1984; Morris *et al.* 1986; Mor 1987). Parker *et al.* (1989) conducted a study of 283 cancer patients, and their doctors, referred to a cancer rehabilitation service over a period of 1 year. They reported that the Spitzer Scale scores were lowest for patients with the worst prognosis. They reported score by type of cancer. Leukaemia patients had the highest total score (7.08), followed by breast cancer patients (6.39) and lymphoma patients (6.31). Lung cancer patients had the lowest total score (5.05). The difference between lung cancer and leukaemia and breast cancer patients was statistically significant. The clinical teams caring for the patients, however, did not feel that the index was sufficiently sensitive to detect differences in activity levels in individual patients. They also questioned the equal weighting of items, given that patients might weight activity levels and family support, for example, differently.

Wood-Dauphinee and Williams (1991) reviewed the literature on the Spitzer QL scale and the Uniscale and reported several studies supporting the validity of the scale as it correlates with other quality of life scales. It can distinguish between healthy and sick people, and is sensitive to the stage of the disease process. These authors presented a positive review, in contrast to the usual more cautious conclusions about the scale.

The single item overall quality of life rating ('uniscale') was reported to correlate over 0.60 with the Karnofsky Performance Index, and it is reported to be sufficiently reliable and valid (Gough *et al.* 1983). Coates *et al.* (1987) used the Spitzer Uniscale and LASA scales for the assessment of symptoms (physical well-being, mood, pain, nausea and vomiting and appetite: Priestman *et al.* 1977; Coates *et al.* 1983) in a trial of 308 breast cancer patients undergoing chemotherapy. They reported that scale scores were sensitive to intermittent versus continuous treatments, with the quality of life of patients receiving intermittent therapy being worse. The 'uniscale' is, however, not regarded as a serious quality of life measure on its own, because it does not provide information about the different dimensions (Maguire and Selby 1989).

Reliability

Large discrepancies in assessments between patients and doctors have also been reported by Slevin *et al.* (1988), who compared assessments using the Karnofsky Performance Index (Karnofsky and Burchenal 1949), the Spitzer Quality of Life Scale, LASA items (Aitken 1969; Spitzer *et al.* 1981) and the Hospital Anxiety and Depression Scale (Zigmond and Snaith 1983). Their study involved 108 patients with advanced malignant disease and their doctors. The patients completed the questionnaires on a single day, and then daily for five consecutive days. The Karnofsky Scale had the highest reproducibility (this correlated with the Spitzer Scale at $r = 0.49$). They also concluded that doctors' ratings on the scale were of questionable validity, and that the scale contained inappropriate questions for measuring the quality of life of cancer patients.

In their original testing of the scale, which involved 150 doctors' ratings of 879 patients, Spitzer *et al.* (1981) reported good internal consistency (Cronbach's alpha = 0.78). Inter-rater reliability between two doctors' independent ratings was statistically significant and high (Spearman's r = 0.81). Patients' and doctors' ratings were positively correlated, although more weakly (Spearman's $r = 0.61$), and social workers' and patients' ratings also correlated well (Kendall's tau = 0.72) (Spitzer *et al.* 1981; Gough *et al.* 1983). Inter-item correlations have been reported to be moderate (Mor *et al.* 1984; Morris *et al.* 1986; Mor 1987). Test–retest correlations were not reported.

Despite increasing criticism of the scale, it remains popular (Addington-Hall *et al.* 1990; Higginson 1992). It gives equal weighting to all scale items, which has been criticized as unrealistic by Clark and Fallowfield (1986), and its brevity has been criticized as not being able to do justice to the different aspects of quality of life (Maguire and Selby 1989). It has also been criticized as time-consuming (Fergusson and Cull 1991). Saunders and Baum (1992) argue that it may oversimplify the issue, it is not cancer-specific and does not reflect change over time. One of its weaknesses is that an observer usually rates the patient's quality of life.

Increasing recognition of its weaknesses has led most reviewers to no longer recommend its use. It is likely that the trend away from the use of this scale will continue given poor results for reliability, and the fact that each question asks about more than one aspect.

LINEAR ANALOGUE SELF-ASSESSMENT (LASA) SCALE

The Linear Analogue Self-Assessment (LASA) Scale was developed for use with cancer patients, and has been used successfully to evaluate quality of life of patients receiving cytotoxic therapy for advanced breast cancer (Priestman and Baum 1976). Although simple, it is apparently time-consuming in terms of its administration. It has been reported to be acceptable to cancer patients (Rieker et al. 1992). Despite the scepticism some-times voiced about the acceptability of visual analogue techniques to general population samples, it has been reported that cancer patients find them easy to use (Aitken 1969; Revill et al. 1976; Holmes and Dickerson 1987).

Content

The LASA questionnaire contains 25 items, 10 of which relate to the symptoms and effects of the disease and treatment (e.g. pain and nausea), 5 examine psychological consequences (e.g. anxiety and depression), 5 measure other physical indices (e.g. ability to perform household chores), and 5 items are concerned with personal relationships.

The LASA tests employ lines, the length of which are taken to indicate the continuum of emotional or physical experiences such as tiredness or anxiety (Priestman and Baum 1976). The lines are usually 10 cm long with stops at right angles to the line at its extremes, representing the limits of the experience being measured. The patient is instructed to mark along the line a point that corresponds to his or her perception of the experience. The original LASA Scale contains ten items covering pain, appetite, well-being, nausea, sleepi-ness, weakness, drowsiness, anxiety, mood and vomiting. Baum and his colleagues later increased the length of the scale to 25 items in a study of women receiving chemotherapy for advanced breast cancer (Baum et al. 1980). The number of

items in the sub-scales has varied over time, depending on the stage of the development of the scale. Generally, 10 items relate to symptoms and side effects (alopecia, anorexia, appetite, consti-pation, diarrhoea, dyspnoea, fatigue, nausea, pain, vomiting, and other), 5 relate to physical function-ing (daily activities, employment, level of activity, social activities), 5 (or more in some versions) relate to mood (apprehension, depression, insomnia, irritability, anxiety, mood and well-being), and 5 relate to social relationships (getting along with partners and others, sexual relationships, social relationships).

Administration and scoring

The scale can be self-administered. It differs from the FLIC in that there are no numbers placed along the analogue lines, so that while the FLIC scores range from 1 to 7, the LASA allows for continuous scores ranging from 0 to 100. The patient is instructed to mark along the line a point that corresponds to his or her perception of the experi-ence. The distance from the 'none at all' mark to the patient's mark provides a numeric score for the item. Priestman and Baum's (1976) scale scores to the nearest centimetre. The total score is then summed for all items, ranging from 0 to 100. Each item is given equal weighting in the scoring scheme, which the authors admit is probably unrealistic.

Examples from the LASA

Ability to perform shopping

None ├─────────────────┤ Better than ever

Nausea

Constant ├─────────────────┤ None

How would you rate your quality of life:

Very poor ├─────────────────┤ Very good

Have you had pain today?

Not at all ├─────────────────┤ Severe pain

Validity

There are many references in the literature about how valid the LASA is in the measurement of pain

(Melzack 1983). However, more recently, Slevin *et al.* (1988) reported that the LASA Scale correlated poorly with the Hospital Anxiety and Depression Scale. These authors suggested that this was due to the HAD items being less applicable to cancer patients. However, the scale has been shown to have discriminatory power between cancer patients receiving intermittent *vs* continuous therapy (Coates *et al.* 1987). Gough *et al.* (1983) reported that correlations testing for validity between a single QL LASA item, the LASA and the Spitzer QL Index ranged from moderate to good (0.38–0.86). It has also been reported that just two or three LASA scales can provide apparently reliable and valid measures of pain, nausea and mood (Scott and Huskisson 1976; Redd and Andrykowski 1982; Cella and Perry 1986). It was able to reflect clinical changes when used on a weekly basis among women with advanced breast cancer (Priestman and Baum 1976), and was reported to be sensitive to treatment of patients with malignant dysphagia (Barr and Krasner 1991) and to the treatment of patients with malignant melanoma, small cell bronchogenic carcinoma and ovarian cancer (Coates *et al.* 1983).

Butow *et al.* (1991) reported that the LASA items on physical well-being, mood, pain, nausea and vomiting and appetite (Priestman *et al.* 1977) were sensitive to patients undergoing either intermittent or continuous chemotherapy for advanced breast cancer in their trial of 308 patients. In another study of 103 cancer out-patients by Coates *et al.* (1990), correlations testing for validity between the FLIC and selected LASA items on appetite loss, mood and physical well-being were high ($r = 0.63$–0.72).

The scale is applicable to patients with breast cancer, although it has been used with patients with lung cancer and cancer of the ovary. The method was able to discriminate between different groups of patients with breast cancer, and between patients undergoing different doses of drug treatment. The issue of weighting has not been resolved (Selby and Robertson 1987).

Reliability

The test–retest correlation of the LASA was 0.73 (Priestman and Baum 1976). Slevin *et al.* (1988) tested LASA against the Hospital Anxiety and Depression Scale, the Karnofsky Index and the Spitzer Quality of Life Index among 108 cancer patients in London, and reported that the LASA Scale showed similar concordance coefficients when taken as a whole compared with being divided into four equal parts (i.e. the continuous scale is no more sensitive than the 4-point scale). Two different groups of 25 patients also filled in the same forms on a single day, and daily for five consecutive days, during a period when their clinical state was expected to remain stable. Professionals also completed the scales in relation to the same patients. The LASA was found to be easily reproducible, and had greater reproducibility than the other scales. Little other information about its reliability has been published.

Further testing for reliability in particular is required, as well as evidence on the case with which people across social groupings can conceptualize the items along such continuums. A major limitation with such scales is the ceiling effect. For example, as Clark and Fallowfield (1986) have pointed out, if at the outset of an outcome study the patient responds 'not at all' on the pain scale then he or she can only measurably achieve a different score at follow-up if they get worse. If a patient at the outset of the study places a mark at the extreme severe pain end of the continuum, then he or she cannot be measurably worse at follow-up, even though he or she may be. However, it appears to detect changes over time and to distinguish between different treatments, although its validity and reliability have not yet been satisfactorily established. It may be criticized on the grounds that it is a fairly superficial measure, but to be fair to its authors, they did state in their original article on LASA that they had not intended to create a scale capable of in-depth assessment, but that it was a convenient and reliable method of patient self-assessment of quality of life during and after treatment (Priestman and Baum 1976).

Other visual analogue scales

ONTARIO CANCER INSTITUTE/ROYAL MARSDEN LINEAR ANALOGUE SELF-ASSESSMENT SCALE

Selby and his colleagues at the Royal Marsden Hospital and the Ontario Cancer Institute (1984) developed a 32-item linear analogue scale in studies with over 230 women with breast cancer. This is also known as the Ontario Cancer Institute Quality of Life Scale. Eighteen of the items (those which relate to general aspects of health) were derived from the 12 categories of the Sickness Impact Profile (SIP: Bergner *et al.* 1981). The SIP items encompass work, housework, recreation, mobility, concentration, eating, sleep, social life, family relationships, self-care, physical activity, anxiety, depression, anger, speech and writing.

One of the items (a 'uniscale') gives an overall rating of quality of life. The other 13 items are disease-specific and were derived from clinical experience of patients with breast cancer: pain, breathing, sore mouth, nausea, vomiting, hair loss, attractiveness, breast appearance, burning on passing urine, diarrhoea, fatigue, satisfaction with information received. The uniscale and three of the specific items are illustrated below. While different versions have been published in the literature, this reflects the early stage of development of this scale and consequently it is being continually refined and improved. Test–retest reliability at 24 h and 7 days among breast cancer patients showed good agreement with correlations greater than 0.70. The scale was able to distinguish between clinically different groups of patients. A full report of the scale and its developmental testing awaits publication (Selby 1992).

Content

The five main domains of the questionnaire are emotional well-being, activities of daily living, appearance and attractiveness, symptoms, and nausea (the fifth factor, nausea, was not selected by the regression analysis). The details of the scale are given in Selby (1992). Selby (1992) also emphasizes the psychological and social problems of cancer patients – anxiety, depression at home and at work, job loss, marital break-up, financial loss, and career handicap due to loss of time for treatment.

Administration and scoring

The scale is self-administered and takes less than 5 min to complete. Each item is on a 10 cm line anchored at each end by descriptive phrases, with the right-hand end corresponding to absence of symptoms and the left-hand end to maximum symptoms.

Examples from the Ontario/Royal Marsden Scale

The overall score completed by patients and physicians

Please score how you feel your life has been affected by the state of your health (any disease or treatment) during today (24 h).

You may like to look back over the previous scales and consider the scores you have made and how much you feel they have affected your life.

My life is extremely unpleasant because of the state of my health ————————— My life is normal with no changes because of the state of my health

LASA scales are completed by patients and physicians

Nausea
To what extent have you experienced nausea or vomiting or both during the past 24 h?

Extremely severe nausea, vomiting or both ————————— No nausea or vomiting

How far do you feel that your appearance/attractiveness has been altered by your present illness or its treatment?

Extremely severe alteration ————————— No alteration at all

Other items

Physical activity
Completely unable to move my body ————————— Normal physical activity for me

Depression
Extremely depressed ————————— Not at all depressed

Validity and factor structure

It was initially tested with five distinct groups of breast cancer patients receiving different treatments. Correlations of patients' self-assessments and doctor assessments were high for functional status items ($r = 0.60$–0.88), but lower for psychological status ($r = 0.11$–0.58) and for symptoms ($r = -0.04$–0.62).

The uniscale overall quality of life rating scores correlated well with the SIP overall score ($r = 0.7$) and moderately with the Karnofsky indices ($r = 0.6$). The uniscale correlated significantly with medical global ratings ($r<0.70$). The scale was able to distinguish between patients with metastatic breast cancer receiving chemotherapy and those receiving adjuvant chemotherapy (Selby *et al.* 1984; Selby 1992).

A factor analysis yielded groups of items which were associated statistically; of particular importance was the result that clinically related items were associated with each other, which lends credibility to the validity of the instrument. The scale explained 58–70 per cent of the variation in overall quality of life ratings (Selby *et al.* 1984; Selby 1992). Another study by Bell *et al.* (1985) compared patients' and doctors' ratings in a study of 25 breast cancer patients, and reported item correlations between scores of just 0.50. Bell *et al.* (1985) also reported that the measure was able to discriminate between patients receiving high or low doses of chemotherapy.

Reliability

Selby *et al.* (1984) previously used the popular LASA format simultaneously with patients and raters and recommended its dual use given that only moderate coefficients of agreement were obtained (Selby *et al.* 1984; Bell *et al.* 1985).

The initial tests by the authors of the scale were with five distinct groups of breast cancer patients receiving different treatments. Test–retest and item consistency correlations gave coefficients of above 0.70 for most sub-scales. Test–retest reliability (at 7 days) for the uniscale was $r = 0.72$ (Selby *et al.* 1984; Selby 1992). The scales for nausea, vomiting and diarrhoea were less reliable, with coefficients of agreement of less than 0.40.

It requires much more testing before its use can be generally recommended. It has been criticized by Aaronson *et al.* (1988) because the scoring treats each item separately, and because the resulting absence of sub-scales to summarize the data may lead to 'information overload'. The Cancer Control Research Committee of the Southwest Oncology Group in the USA has included the Selby uniscale in its quality of life assessment package (Moinpour *et al.* 1989). However, they have

changed its response format from a visual analogue scale, which they felt was less acceptable to patients, to a categorical scale: it has five response categories ranging from extremely unpleasant to normal (no change). The scale is still regarded as underdeveloped (Selby 1993). While the committee recommends the use of this uniscale, its preferred instrument is the Short Form Rand Instrument (see pp. 281–5).

PADILLA QUALITY OF LIFE (QL) SCALE AND VARIANTS, INCLUDING THE MULTI-DIMENSIONAL QUALITY OF LIFE SCALE – CANCER (MQOLS-CA)

A 14-item visual analogue scale was developed by Padilla and his colleagues entitled the Padilla Quality of Life Scale or the Quality of Life Index (Padilla *et al.* 1981, 1983; Presant 1984; Padilla and Grant 1985; Ferrell *et al.* 1989; Ferrell 1990). Using different versions of the instrument, these investigators have described quality of life as a multidimensional construct characterized by psychological well-being, physical well-being, symptom control, nutritional concerns, social concerns, and affective states (Padilla *et al.* 1992a, 1992b). It has since been renamed the Multidimensional Quality of Life Scale – Cancer (MQOLS-CA: Padilla *et al.* 1992a) in order to distinguish it from the scales developed by Ferrans and Powers (1985) and Spitzer *et al.* (1981).

Site-specific extensions of it are called the Quality of Life Index – Cancer and, for patients with colostomies, the Quality of Life Index – Colostomy, and in cancer patients receiving radiation therapy, the Quality of Life Index – Radiation (Padilla *et al.* 1983; Padilla and Grant 1985; Padilla 1990). For example, the version for colostomy patients has 10 VAS items on eating, pain, sexual satisfaction, interpersonal and body image aspects of self-worth, in addition to the original 14 QL items. This was reproduced by Padilla and Grant (1985).

Content, administration and scoring

The current version of the scale (MQOLS-CA) contains 14 items which measure three areas:

side-effects (e.g. nausea, vomiting), daily activities (e.g. eating, working, sexual activity) and general quality of life (e.g. feelings of satisfaction, usefulness and fun). The MQOLS-CA uses 100 mm linear analogue scales as the response format. There are no numbered markings on the lines. The end-points of the lines carry words denoting the extremes of responses. Respondents place an X on the line to indicate how they feel.

Each item is scored by measuring the distance from the zero end (the poorest quality of life end) to the 'X', using a centimetre ruler. The measurement is carried out by two independent coders. The total score and sub-scale scores are obtained by adding together all the scores to the items in the MQOLS-CA or the relevant items for that sub-scale, and then dividing by the number of items in the total scale or sub-scale ($n = 14$). It is easy to score, and takes less than 5 min to administer.

Examples from the 23-item QLI for colostomy patients (items overlap with the MQOLS-CA)

1 How much strength do you have?

4 Do you feel your present weight is a problem?

9 How much fun do you have (hobbies, recreation, social activities)?

15 How satisfying is your life?

18 How good is the quality of your life?

19 How fearful are you of odour or leakage from your colostomy?

Not at all ——————————————— Extremely

Validity and factor structure

The scale was tested initially on a convenience sample of 130 cancer in-patients and out-patients, and with reported acceptable levels of reliability and validity. The current version has a factor structure relating to the properties of psychosocial well-being, physical well-being and disease and symptom distress. The correlation tests of validity with other scales were variable in strength. For example, the correlation between the MQOLS-CA and the POMS ranged from weak to moderate, despite them all being statistically significant (0.37–0.65). The correlations with a range of emotional well-being scales (measuring uncertainty in illness, appraisal, coping and mastery) ranged from $r = -0.16$ to 0.54. Discrepancies in assessments between professionals' and patients' ratings of quality of life were also reported by Padilla et al. (1983) and Presant (1984).

Reliability

The current version has good internal consistency coefficients (Cronbach's alpha), ranging from $r = 0.67$ to 0.96. Although it underwent some initial testing with satisfactory results, there has been insufficient testing of its psychometric properties despite the authors' reporting of acceptable basic levels of reliability and validity (Padilla et al. 1983; Presant 1984). The recommendation of this scale is not helped by its frequent modifications together with numerous changes of name, which creates confusion for new investigators searching for an appropriate scale.

HOLMES AND DICKERSON

Holmes and her colleague (Holmes and Dickerson 1987; Holmes 1989) have developed a simple, modified symptom distress scale using a LASA format. They experimented with an unnumbered visual analogue scale and with a visual analogue scale marked with either five or six numerical scale points. At each extreme were written statements representing the opposite extreme responses. They drew symptoms from the Symptom Distress Scale (McCorkle and Young 1978) and included a range of daily living items.

Items in the Holmes and Dickerson Scale

Symptoms

Pain
Nausea
Appetite
Sleep
Mobility

Bowel habits – diarrhoea
Bowel habits – constipation
Tiredness
Concentration
Mood
Appearance

ADL

Ability to eat
Flavour of food
Texture of food
Sleep
Respiration
Urination
Change in bowel pattern
Recreational activity
Changes in life as a whole
Worry about future
Concern over earning ability
Isolation
Communication with family
Communication with medical staff
Communication with nursing staff

Examples

Worst pain I
have ever had————————————— No pain

I cannot face   My appetite is
food at all   1 2 3 4 5   normal for me

I cannot sleep 1 2 3 4 5 6 I sleep as well
at all   as ever

Validity and reliability

There are few data on the validity of the scale. Some testing has been carried out, initially on a convenience sample of 72 oncology in-patients. The unnumbered VAS had the highest test–retest correlation coefficients ($r = 0.97$), the 6-point scale having the lowest ($r = 0.72$). The unnumbered scale was the most acceptable to patients, and, once explained, the simplest.

Reliability based on internal consistency was reported to be high (Cronbach's alpha=0.08, total instrument; 0.09 for symptoms and 0.07 for ADL). Patients commented that items relating to sex and work life should have been included, as these were two major areas of life affected by their illness.

GLOBAL QUALITY OF LIFE SCALE (COATES)

This LASA contains eight items: anxiety/depression, nausea/vomiting, numbness or pins and needles, loss of hair, tiredness, appetite or sense of taste, sexual interest or ability, thoughts on the idea of treatment. Responses to items are marked on a line between 'none' and 'worst as can imagine'.

Examples from the Global Quality of Life Scale

Pins and needles

None ——————————————— Worst as can imagine

Tiredness

None ——————————————— Worst as can imagine

Validity and reliability

In a study of 166 cancer patients, it correlated well with the older VAS scales (Coates *et al.* 1990); the test–retest correlations exceeded 0.80 for almost all items. One hour and 24 h test–retest correlations were higher than for the older LASA scales, but inter-item correlations were lower. There is little other information on its psychometric properties.

QUALITY OF LIFE INDEX

This scale was developed by Ferrans and Powers (1985) to measure morbidity in normal and ill populations. The scale was developed after an extensive literature review and factor analysis of items using patients on haemodialysis. It measures satisfaction with various domains of life and their importance to the respondent.

Content

The instrument has two parts, and both contain 32 items which assess domain satisfaction and importance for: health care, physical health and functioning, marriage, family, friends, stress, standard of living, occupation, education, leisure, future retirement, peace of mind, personal faith, life goals, personal appearance, self-acceptance, general happiness and general satisfaction. There are also some disease-specific items for use with dialysis patients. Subjects respond on a 6-point Likert-type scale from 'very satisfied' to 'very dissatisfied' and from 'very important' to 'very unimportant'. There are four underlying domains: health and functioning, socioeconomic, psychological/spiritual and family.

Administration and scoring

The scale can be self-administered. Scores are calculated by weighting each satisfaction item with its paired importance item. Thus high scores reflect high satisfaction/importance. The overall scoring is complicated: the scale is centred on zero for satisfaction items, and then one multiplies paired satisfaction and importance responses, sums the resulting weighted items, divides by the number of items answered, and adds 15 to every score to eliminate negative values. Although the authors offer a computer program for the scoring, the complexity of this task is inevitably going to put off potential users. The possible range for the overall and sub-scale scores is 0–30.

Modified version for cancer patients

The version modified by Ferrans and Ferrell (1990) for use with cancer patients consists of two parts: satisfaction with domains of life and the importance of the same domains to the respondent. Both parts contain 35 items that cover a broad range of life domains: physical health and functioning, stress, leisure activities, future retirement, friends and social support, socioeconomic aspects, peace of mind, personal faith, life goals, self-acceptance, general happiness, general satisfaction, control over life, marriage and family. It also includes an external item on satisfaction with the nation, which appears odd. Responses are on 6-point Likert scales ranging from very satisfied = 6 to very dissatisfied = 1 for Part 1 items, and from very important = 6 to very unimportant = 1 for Part 2 items.

Validity

The authors have reported its levels of reliability and validity to be appropriate, but it has not undergone extensive testing (Ferrans and Powers

Examples from the Quality of Life Index

Part 1

How satisfied are you with your health?

Very satisfied   6   5   4   3   2   1   Very dissatisfied

Part 2

How important is your health to you?

Very important   6   5   4   3   2   1   Very unimportant

1985; Ferrans and Ferrell 1990; Ferrell 1990). Ferrans and Ferrell (1990) reported the properties of the modified Ferrans and Powers Quality of Life Index, with a sample of 111 breast cancer patients. They reported concurrent validity was supported by a strong correlation of 0.88 between the QLI and life satisfaction. Construct validity was supported by an association in the expected direction between the index and pain, depression and coping with stress.

Reliability

The original index had a test–retest correlation coefficient at 2 weeks of 0.69 (students) and 0.81 (dialysis patients) (Ferrans and Powers 1985). Test–retest reliability and the internal consistency of the index was further supported with reported correlations of $r = 0.87$ and a Cronbach's alpha of $r = 0.93$ (Faris and Stotts 1990). It was reported to be sensitive to improvements in health following treatment (Faris and Stotts 1990). Ferrans and Ferrell's (1990) findings supported the internal consistency of the modified scale in relation to reliability (alpha = 0.95 for the total scale and 0.90, 0.84, 0.93 and 0.66 for the four sub-scales of health and functioning, socioeconomic, psychological/ spiritual, and family, respectively).

BREAST CANCER CHEMOTHERAPY QUESTIONNAIRE (BCCQ)

The BCCQ was developed by Levine *et al.* (1988) for use as an outcome measure of quality of life in relation to breast cancer and adjuvant chemotherapy. It is interviewer-administered and reported to be valid.

The items were generated from a literature review and discussions with health professionals and patients. The original 150 items were reduced to 99 and then to 30, according to their mean rating of importance allocated by 47 patients receiving adjuvant chemotherapy.

Content, administration and scoring

The scale was designed for administration by an interviewer. It contains 30 items, and these have been published in full by Levine *et al.* (1988). Seven dimensions have been identified including psychological distress and social interaction. Responses to questions are rated on a 7-point scale, and the scores are totalled; high scores reflect a better quality of life. The scores are transformed so that the final score ranges from 0 to 10. It takes 30 min to complete.

Examples from the BCCQ

1 How often during the past 2 weeks have you felt worried or upset as a result of thinning or loss of your hair? Please indicate how often you have felt worried or upset as a result of thinning or loss of your hair by choosing one of the following options from the card in front of you (blue card).

    All of the time / most of the time / a good bit of the time / some of the time / a little of the time / hardly any of the time / none of the time

8 How often during the last 2 weeks have you been troubled or upset as a result of feeling unattractive? Please indicate how often you have been troubled or upset as a result of feeling unattractive by choosing one of the following options from the card in front of you (blue card – options as Example 1 above).

16 How much help and support have you received from people outside your family during the last 2 weeks? Please indicate how much help and support you have received from people outside your family by choosing one of the following options from the card in front of you (yellow card).

    None of the time / a little of the time / some of the time / a good bit of the time / most of the time / almost all of the time / all of the time

17 How often during the last 2 weeks did you have the sensation that you smelled of chemicals? Please indicate how often you had the sensation you smelled of chemicals by choosing one of the following options from the card in front of you (blue card – options as Example 1 above).

29 How much trouble or distress have you had as a result of pain, soreness, or sores in your mouth, during the last 2 weeks? Please indicate how much trouble or distress you have had as a result of pain, soreness, or sores in your mouth during the last 2 weeks by choosing one of the following options from the card in front of you (green card).

    A great deal of trouble / a lot of trouble / a fair bit of trouble / some trouble / a little trouble / hardly any trouble / no trouble

Validity

It has been reported to correlate moderately well with the Rand emotional questionnaire (0.58), with the Rand physical questionnaire (0.60) and the Spitzer QL questionnaire (0.62) (Levine *et al.* 1988). In a comparative study among women with stage II breast cancer, the BCCQ, selected Rand instruments, and the Spitzer and Karnofsky instruments were used. Only the BCCQ and the Karnofsky Index were able to discriminate between the group who had completed treatment and the group still undergoing treatment (Levine *et al.* 1988). A study of treatment for breast cancer by Guyatt *et al.* (1989c), Levine *et al.* (1988) reported that the scale was valid as a measure of subjective health status, and was able to distinguish between long- and short-term treatments. Patient acceptability and completion rates are good (Sadura *et al.* 1992). Saunders and Baum (1992) report that it is useful in studies of breast cancer patients. There are few data on its reliability.

VISUAL ANALOGUE SCALE (VAS) FOR BONE MARROW TRANSPLANT PATIENTS

Grant *et al.* (1992) were concerned to measure the quality of life of their patients who had survived bone marrow transplantation. This is a procedure that, while potentially life-saving, is also known to produce physical and emotional stress due to the potential for toxicities, the conditioning regimen, the process itself and the long-term sequelae, and consequently has major implications for quality of life measurement (Brown and Kelly 1976; Wolcott *et al.* 1986, 1987; Folsom and Popkin 1987; Haberman 1988; Andrykowski *et al.* 1989, 1990; Mashberg *et al.* 1989; Wingard *et al.* 1991; Ferrell *et al.* 1992a, 1992b).

In an attempt to design a disease-specific scale, these investigators piloted five open-ended questions about what quality of life meant to these patients, how transplantation had affected their quality of life, what factors made quality of life better or worse and how health professionals could enhance it (Ferrell *et al.* 1992a, 1992b). This was taken a stage further by the same team (Grant *et al.* 1992) and a structured instrument, based on 100 mm visual analogue scales, was piloted on 205 allogenic bone marrow transplant survivors, aged 18 and over.

Content, administration and scoring

The instrument is based on a multidimensional definition of quality of life, and includes physical well-being (from functional ability to fertility, nutrition, etc.), psychological well-being (from depression to coping ability), social well-being (from relationships, activities and work to finances), and spiritual well-being (from hope to inner strength). Items for the VAS are shown below. It can be self-administered; the scale items are summed.

Examples from the VAS

How easy is it for you to adjust to your disease and treatment?

Very easy – not at all easy

How good is your quality of life?

Extremely poor – excellent

Do you have physical/emotional support if needed?

Not at all – a great deal

Factor structure and reliability

The authors tested the scale and reported a factor analysis which confirmed that the strongest three factors were consistent with the three central domains of the model and that it had good test–retest reliability and internal consistency. They report that further refinement of the scale is on-going.

EUROPEAN NEUROBLASTOMA STUDY GROUP QUALITY OF LIFE ASSESSMENT FORM – CHILDREN (QLAF-C)

Quality of life issues have not received the same attention in paediatric oncology as in adult oncology. The focus has in the main been on organ toxicity, pain, nausea, vomiting and the consequences of bone marrow suppression, although increasing attention is being given to psychological adjustment and consequences (Feeny *et al.* 1991).

Apart from the physical effects of cancer, the consequent medical interventions and associated treatment toxicities can have quite specific effects on the quality of life of children – for example, loss of desire and/or ability to play and to participate in games and sports, and loss of attendance at school for certain periods. This is in addition to the disruptions which they share with adults with cancer – effects on friendships and family relationships and effects on psychological well-being. All this can affect their physical, intellectual, social and emotional/affective development.

Current measurement of quality of life in children with cancer is heavily dependent upon assessments by proxies rather than assessments by the children themselves, with questionable reliability and validity. As the effects on everyday life are different for children, as compared with adults, it is important that questionnaires should be specifically designed for use with them, rather than the current reliance on adaptation of scales for adults and proxy assessments. Only in the area of psychological, educational and intellectual assessments have a large number of scales for use with children been carefully developed (see Chapter 3).

Content, administration and scoring

The European QLAF–C is also reliant on proxy assessment. It aims to assess the quality of life of children with cancer, and was reported by Fayers and Jones (1983). The form was designed for parents to complete. The form is structured, but also invites parents to make comments on the child's health, attitudes and treatment in order to assist with the refinement and development of the questionnaire. Clinicians also record their impressions of the child's quality of life. The closed questions are in categorical form, largely on a

4-point scale. Parents are asked to assess the degree to which the child's activity has been restricted by the illness, levels of pain, sickness, fever, appetite, hearing difficulty, sleeplessness, worry about hair loss and apprehension about the next hospital visit. Parents are also asked to make an assessment about the child's overall enjoyment of life, and about their own level of worry about the child's health, and their perception of the acceptability of the treatment Details of medication for pain, insomnia and vomiting are recorded. Items are summed.

Examples from the QLAF-C

During the week has your child been:

1 As active as normal in play / at school
Somewhat restricted in activity / not able to go to school
Very restricted in activity / confined to home
In bed at home / in hospital because of ill health
In hospital for treatment

3 Normal / no sickness
Feeling sick without being sick
Sick occasionally
Sick several times

10 Not worrying about the next hospital visit
Worrying about the next hospital visit
Not applicable / too young
In hospital

While the scale is crude, reliant on proxy assessment, and evidence of its psychometric ability is still lacking, it is reproduced here because there are so few scales applicable to children.

Brief details of other scales

Several other cancer-specific scales have been developed, but which require further development or use before an assessment can be made of their psychometric properties. The better known of these are described below. In addition to the scales below, there are several other cancer-specific quality of life scales that have been developed, or are in the process of being developed, that are still being tested. For example, Llewellyn-Thomas *et al.* (1984) have developed a scale to measure voice quality in laryngeal cancer patients receiving radiation therapy, based on 10 cm visual analogue scales on which patients are instructed to indicate the quality of their voices in relation to eight symptoms (e.g. voice fatigue) and eight functional areas (e.g. ability to use the telephone). Some basic tests for reliability were carried out and showed the scale to be adequate. Doctor and patient ratings were compared and found to be correlated but not identical (Sutherland *et al.* 1984). The Functional Assessment of Cancer Therapy (FACT) scale is under development and is fairly comprehensive in coverage, consisting of 38 core questions which are appropriate for all cancer patients and nine item modules for head and neck cancer, lung, breast and colon cancer (Cella *et al.* 1990).

CANCER LEUKAEMIA GROUP B STUDIES (CALGB)

In the USA, Holland *et al.* (1986) have been developing and evaluating a range of methods for more than a decade, which aim to assess psychiatric morbidity and disease-specific problems. The measurement of quality of life is not comprehensive, and their conclusions and the scales are really still at the developmental stage.

ABILITY INDEX

This is a series of simple rating scales which measure physical, social and psychological factors (Izsak and Medalie 1971). The index is cancer-specific, but cannot be used across a wide range of cancers. It has limited research applicability.

The scale evaluates quality of life longitudinally in relation to objective markers of the patient's condition (Izsak and Medalie 1971). It contains 15 items and is cancer-specific, with item ranges of 1–3; thus the highest possible score is 45. The items form three groups: subjective reactions and feelings of the patient (*n* = 7), working ability and earning capacity (*n* = 3), and social adjustment (*n* = 5). Seven of the 15 items assess the patient's subjective reactions, and these vary by disease site. For example, women with breast cancer rate their reaction to their breast prosthesis. For carcinoma of the rectum, this variable changes to 'control of bowel movements', and for carcinoma of the bladder or prostate it changes to 'disturbances of urination'. This facilitates comparisons across tumour sites. Its advantage is that it is brief and simple; it is also flexible. The Ability Index is an appealing measure, although there are no clear guidelines for its administration and there is no evidence of its reliability and validity (Cella and Cherin 1987).

BURGE QUALITY OF LIFE SEVERITY SCALE

Burge *et al.* (1975) used a scale which they designed to measure quality of life in patients with acute myeloid leukaemia, graded as follows.

Burge Quality of Life Severity Scale

- Hospital stay throughout illness
- Frequent admission to hospital, disabling symptoms
- Occasional admission to hospital, frequent or severe symptoms but not continuous
- Moderate symptoms, perhaps at work, living an independent life
- Mild symptoms at work (or equivalent way of life)
- No symptoms, normal life

This is simply an indicator of symptom severity and crude effects, rather than a quality of life scale.

AMNESTIC COMPARATIVE SELF-ASSESSMENT (ACSA)

This is a global measure of quality of life in which the patient is asked to rate overall quality of life on a scale of −5 to +5 (Bernheim and Buyse 1983). The end-points are determined by patients themselves on the basis of their life experiences, and these are then used for the evaluation of their current status. Patients use their own criteria for weighting. It has made provision for tapping the positive end of the quality of life spectrum. Using memories of the best and worst periods of their life, a personal scale of well-being is constructed for each patient.

WORLD HEALTH ORGANIZATION QUALITY OF LIFE ASSESSMENT INSTRUMENT (WHOQOL)

The World Health Organization's WHOQOL Group has an ongoing project to develop the WHOQOL for measuring quality of life, referred to in Chapter 1 of this volume. It is eventually intended to develop disease-specific modules to supplement it, particularly for use in oncology. The WHOQOL Group (1993a, 1994a) defined quality of life as 'an individual's perception of their position in life in the context of the culture and value systems in which they live and in relation to their goals, expectations, standards and concerns. It is a broad-ranging concept affected in a complex way by the person's physical health, psychological state, level of independence, social relationships, and their relationship to salient features of their environment'.

The instrument is currently under development using focus groups in several countries, with members reflecting users of health services and members of the general population. It is also planned to assemble an expert panel to generate questionnaire items, making use of the focus group transcripts. It will be tested for reliability and validity in different cultural settings around the world. It will encompass five broad domains: physical health, psychological health, level of independence, social relationships and environment. These core modules will remain the same across cultures, and additional culture-specific modules will be developed. It will measure respondents' perceived quality of life in relation to the effects of disease and health interventions. It is expected to be useful in clinical trials. Later, disease-specific and quality-of-life-specific modules will be developed and added (e.g. for cancer, diabetes, informal carers, the elderly, etc.).

Despite its apparent face validity, there are no comprehensive data on the reliability or validity of this scale. Some early testing was carried out on 65 patients with various malignancies (Bernheim and Buyse 1983). The authors proposed it should be used as one of the outcome measures in cancer clinical trials.

TWiST

Gelber and Goldhirsh (1986) introduced the concept of TWiST (Time Without Symptoms and Toxicity) into the amalgamation of quality and quantity of life; it was tested by Goldhirsh *et al.* (1989) and Gelber *et al.* (1989) on 463 early breast cancer patients undergoing adjuvant chemotherapy. The results are contentious.

TWiST is a quality-adjusted survival analysis,

and is a crude cost–benefit formula, rather than a quality of life measure. Overall survival time is divided into time with experience of toxicity, time without symptoms and toxicity (TWiST), and time after systemic relapse. Time with toxicity and time after systemic relapse are weighted by co-efficients of utility relative to TWiST, and the results are added to give a period of quality-adjusted survival.

The resulting TWiST times can be used to compare patients receiving different treatments. However, different weights are not given to differ-ent degrees of morbidity and patients' evaluations are not taken into account (Selby and Robertson 1987). Saunders and Baum (1992) also described it as complicated and lengthy, although it has proven useful in evaluations of cytotoxic drugs. While of considerable interest, the method must be viewed with caution, in the same way as QALYS. Such measures are crude rather than comprehensive indicators of quality of life, with insufficient testing for validity and reliability. They were developed for use in financial decision-making, rather than for clinical decision-making between treatments in relation to outcomes.

CONCLUSION

As with other conditions, the state of the art in relation to the assessment of quality of life in cancer patients is developmental. No measure satisfies a multidimensional model of quality of life. The disadvantage this poses for clinicians, other re-searchers and patients is that it implies that admin-istration of more than one scale is necessary in order to tap all the required dimensions. This means that several scores have to be interpreted indepen-dently. However, even with generic scales, sub-scale scores often need to be analysed separately in order to demonstrate sensitivity to change after interventions. Single number descriptions of qual-ity of life are even more conceptually and techni-cally elusive (Selby and Robertson 1987).

Most investigators have developed their own package of different scales and applied them to their studies of outcome of treatment for cancer. For example, Sugarbaker et al. (1982) used the Sickness Impact Profile (SIP: Bergner et al. 1981), the Katz ADL Scale (Katz and Akpom 1976a, 1976b), the Barthel Index (Mahoney and Barthel 1965), the Psychosocial Adjustment to Illness Scale (Dero-gatis et al. 1979) and their own derived items for the measurement of problems related to limb sarcomas (pain assessment, sexual relationships, mobility and treatment trauma). Such a huge battery would be impractical to administer to most healthy people, and cannot be recommended for frail people or people with a chronic or terminal con-dition. Not only are such combinations lengthy (the SIP alone has 136 items) they overlap, and can thus be tedious for the respondent. The use of a battery with a long instrument also limits the number of other instruments that can be used.

Saunders and Baum (1992) and Fallowfield (1990) recommend the EORTC or the Rotterdam Symptom Checklist as the instrument of choice, although both require supplementation with other instruments and items where appropriate; for ex-ample, the authors suggest the Hospital Anxiety and Depression Scale (Zigmond and Snaith 1983) is a good supplement. Maguire and Selby (1989) conclude their review of measures for the Medical Research Council by recommending the use of the Rotterdam Symptom Checklist in oncology trials (supplemented with additional disease-specific items where necessary), the Hospital Anxiety and Depression Scale, and the selective use of linear visual analogue scales where they are useful for eliciting adverse effects of treatments. But the promising development of the EORTC question-naire supersedes this recommendation.

The suggestion by some of using the SF-36 (Ware et al. 1993) as the core scale, to be sup-plemented with disease-specific items, also has potential, and mirrors developments in other specialities (Aaronson et al. 1993). For example, the Cancer Control Research Committee of the South-west Oncology Group in the USA has included the short form Rand instrument (the 20-item version, which has now been overtaken by the 36-item version), the Symptom Distress Scale (McCorkle and Young 1978) and the Selby LASA uniscale (Selby et al. 1984) in its list of preferred measure-ments (Moinpour et al. 1989). Most of the broader scales discussed here are reviewed in this volume, in their appropriate chapters, or in Bowling (1991). Finally, the earlier caution should be repeated – no one study can hope to measure adequately all the domains of health-related quality of life. The resulting battery of scales would be too lengthy and impossible to administer. The core instrument and/or the disease-specific measurement scale(s) should be chosen carefully, in relation to the aims of the study. If particular domains of relevance and of interest are judged to be missing, then supplementation with scales measuring these should be carried out – bearing in mind that the longer the battery, the higher the rate of item non-response (and the greater risk of tiring patients).

In sum, the best developed quality of life measure for use with cancer patients is currently the EORTC (Aaronson *et al.* 1993). This covers physical, social and psychological functioning as well as cancer-specific symptoms. It also has the advantage of site-specific modules, which are still being developed. It may require supplementation with domain-specific scales (e.g. adjustment and coping), depending on the aims of the study. The SF-36 (Ware *et al.* 1993) has also been recommended as a generic core for use with batteries of symptom- and domain-specific measures with cancer patients. Its appropriateness for use with these patients has still to be fully tested.

3

PSYCHIATRIC CONDITIONS AND PSYCHOLOGICAL MORBIDITY

QUALITY OF LIFE RESEARCH AND PSYCHIATRIC AND PSYCHOLOGICAL MORBIDITY

Quality of life research is firmly on the agenda in social psychiatry. There are promising and careful developments in measurement, and the World Health Organization Quality of Life Group is currently encouraging research into the quality of life of patients with psychiatric and other illnesses (WHOQOL Group 1991). More thought on conceptual and definitional issues has taken place in psychiatry than in any other clinical speciality.

Quality of life and human needs

Bigelow et al. (1991a) have developed a concept of quality of life relevant to mental health, basing it on the concepts of need and role:

Quality of life, as we view it, comes out of a social contract – fulfillment of needs in exchange for meeting of demands which society places upon its members. Needs are fulfilled through opportunities presented by the social environment. Demands are met through the exercise of basic psychological abilities – cognition, affect, perception, and motor. For example, a work role demands concentration and stress tolerance while it provides opportunities for meeting self-esteem, social affiliation, and basic needs.

Abilities compromised by mental illness deprive a person of the satisfaction of his or her needs due to impairment of the person's participation in the normal opportunity structure.

(Bigelow et al. 1991a: 44–5)

The needs of people with mental illnesses have been clearly described by Wing (1989). These authors also define quality of life in relation to measurable concepts such as physical necessities (heat, light, shelter, food, security, etc.), which need to be provided for those who cannot otherwise secure them, and they emphasize the importance of measuring the quality of these provisions, such as the quality of the environment and the choice available. They emphasize the quality of personal life (the extent of self-respect and autonomy, maintenance of interests, contribution to society and increase in self-knowledge). As the authors point out, in these respects 'quality of care and quality of life are two sides of the same coin'. However, assessments of need in relation to mental illness are complex due to their subjectivity (Bebbington 1992).

MEASURING QUALITY OF LIFE IN INSTITUTIONS

A key domain of quality of life is the quality of living arrangements in institutions or special housing. Its measurement is difficult, perhaps due to the inability or reluctance to communicate on the part of some patients (e.g. elderly people with dementia), although objective measures (e.g. the state of repair, facilities, decoration, etc.) can be made. Standards for assessing the quality of long-stay care have been drawn up (Sinclair 1988; Hibbs 1989).

Individual meaning is also important (Brown and Harris 1978). Questions on activities and environments should (but rarely do) relate to the respondents' value system. For example, question-naires should include open-ended items which ask respondents about where they want to go socially, and what they would like to do, rather than simply listing activities and asking respondents if, and how often, they have done them over a fixed period of time. Respondents could also be asked about what stops them pursuing things they want to do, and other appropriate probing questions. There have been some attempts to measure 'person–environ-ment fit' in this manner in social gerontology (see reviews by Kane and Kane 1988). Investigators at the MRC Social Psychiatry Unit, developed several questionnaires for assessing quality of life in relation to patients' everyday activities, such as the proportion of time (hours) spent having meals, etc., working/in occupational therapy, listening to the radio/watching TV, other leisure activities, in bed (day/night) and no leisure activities (Wykes 1982). Patients' attitudes to care were assessed by asking them if they had enough free time, privacy, freedom; whether they thought the place of resi-dence was pleasant, liked the food, the people they lived with, the bedroom/dormitory, the staff, how it was run; whether they wanted to stay there, go elsewhere; whether they had any definite plans; whether they liked living there and in their pre-vious residence (Wykes 1982). They also used a profile for measuring restrictive practices, which included assessing, for example, whether residents possessed adequate amounts of clothing, whether they could go out alone without telling staff where they were going, bed times, ability to lock toilet doors, facilities to make snacks, choice of main meals, facilities to do personal laundry and choice of clothing.

Innovative scales for use with elderly people who live in institutions are regularly being developed, given the additional problems of assessing people in wards or long-stay homes where there is little privacy. There is a constant striving for realistic and user-friendly assessment scales. An example of a new assessment scale is BASDEC, which is for the assessment of depression. It uses a deck of cards comprising statements relating to depression, to which the subject answers 'true' or 'false' (Adshead et al. 1992).

Where client groups or patients are not always able to communicate their needs (e.g. in the case of elderly people with dementia, very young children or patients in psychotic states), the only feasible method for assessing quality of life is by using observational methods. It is well known that institutions can have an effect on behaviour and well-being (Barton 1959; Goffman 1961; Towns-end 1962; Robb 1967; Wing and Brown 1970; Booth 1985; Clark and Bowling 1989, 1990; Sin-clair and Clarke 1991). Observational schedules can be drawn up to record both objective quantitative information (e.g. number of times patients' re-quests are acted upon by staff, time taken to attend to patients, liquid refreshment available, etc.) and qualitative data (e.g. recording events descrip-tively, recording conversations and voice tone, facial expressions, activity, detachment, etc.) (Clark and Bowling 1989, 1990). It is merely intended to point out this methodology, rather than detail it. Unfortunately, it is rare for a schedule to have universal applicability. Measures for use with people living in institutions may require the use of visual cues to stimulate response choices (e.g. pictures of different environments with the request that the patient chooses between them) rather than traditional questions (Peace et al. 1979).

COMMUNITY INDICATORS OF QUALITY OF LIFE

In research on mental health, some account needs to be taken of the community and the extent to which it might contribute to, or detract from, psychological well-being. Communities establish norms for human behaviour and define deviance, affect quality of life, and are in turn affected by the individuals who work, live and socialize in them and the organizations and institutions that they create (Klein 1970; Zautra and Goodhart 1979). Satisfaction with, and participation in, life is partly regulated by these organizations (Etzioni 1968). In addition, the community's ability to meet basic human needs (e.g. shelter, food, etc.) also determines quality of life. Therefore, for those interested in global quality of life, it is essential to assess these (Rossi 1972).

Routine data on quality of life in community settings tend to rely on social indicators of life, or statistics which 'facilitate concise, comprehensive and balanced judgements about the condition of a major aspect of society . . . a measure of welfare' (Bauer 1966a). There are numerous examples of such measures, although questions can usually be raised about their reliability and validity due to the way they have been collected (Kitsuse and Cicourel 1963), and because of the relativity of their meaning (Berger and Luckmann 1967). Commonly used indicators include unemployment figures, crime statistics, housing costs, average incomes, suicide figures, infant deaths, education levels, leisure facilities, transport costs and environmental indicators such as air pollution levels, etc. (see e.g. Flax 1972). Rates of change of such indicators are also relevant (Schneider 1976). Characteristics of communities that have long been reported to be associated with the use of psychiatric facilities include high proportions of divorced residents, residential mobility and rented accommodation (Bloom 1975). Similar findings have been reported by Stewart and Poaster (1975) and Zautra and Simons (1978). Areas with high levels of poverty also have high rates of use of psychiatric facilities, which affects the quality of life of the entire community (Zautra and Simons 1978). The ethnic mix of the area has also long been associated with psychiatric service needs (Rosen *et al.* 1975).

Such community indicators are of importance in so far as communities can target risk areas for improvement, as in the California (Quality of Life) Healthy Cities Project and the European Healthy Cities programmes (Stiff and Silver 1990; Ashton 1992). However, these indicators lack specificity in that they disregard the human meaning of events. Outcome measures of psychiatric care, while needing to take account of adverse social circumstances that might affect rehabilitation, need to concentrate on individual measurement scales. They should also be appropriate for use in the community, as most people with mental health problems live at home (Goldberg and Huxley, 1980).

MEASURING QUALITY OF LIFE IN INDIVIDUALS: THE DOMAINS OF MEASUREMENT

The quality of life instruments presented here, while adequately covering a number of relevant domains, may still require supplementation with instruments measuring symptoms, behaviour, functioning, coping and adjustment. Whether additional domains are selected for supplementary measurement depends on the aims of the study and the comprehensiveness of the quality of life instrument selected.

Symptoms

The symptoms of a psychiatric illness such as depression can include lack of motivation, concentration, decisiveness, sleep disturbances and other problems that may adversely affect relationships with others and role performance. Psychotic illnesses can have an even more severe impact on quality of life. A range of symptom scales are reviewed in the first part of this chapter (e.g. anxiety and depression). The quality of life scales will require supplementation with a symptom scale. Several of the anxiety and depression scales reviewed in this chapter are appropriate for use with elderly people, and some have been adapted for use with children. A review of psychiatric screening and psychological symptom scales was undertaken by Thompson (1989c).

Domain-specific measures of quality of life

Needs, functioning and coping

Functioning and abilities are impaired by psychiatric illness. Ultimately independent living and employment can be threatened. Lehman (1983, 1988) has described how people with chronic mental illnesses need help in several areas of life, such as housing, finances, family support, opportunities for social interaction and personal development, legal and safety problems, medical care and use of mental health services. These parameters require measurement in a study of quality of life of people with mental health problems. Adjustment and coping are important modifiers of outcome, and worthy of inclusion in scales or batteries. A range of single-domain instruments on need, functioning and behaviour, coping and adjustment are presented after the quality of life scales. They overlap with some of the quality of life instruments reviewed.

Self-esteem

The measurement of self-esteem is also important, although existing scales are less appropriate for use with people with severe mental illnesses than with other clinical populations. Some of the quality of life scales include self-esteem. Scales of self-esteem were reviewed by Bowling (1991) and are not presented here.

Stress

Stress is not an outcome variable, but the experience of stress has been implicated in disease onset. The experience of stress is also a response to the experience of illness. A few investigators have attempted to measure the degree of stress experienced as a result of physical disease, for example cancer (Vinokur et al. 1989, 1990). It has been argued that mental health and quality of life depend on the maintenance of internal homeostasis or equilibrium, which requires restoration if disrupted (Zautra and Goodhart 1979). Psychiatric disturbances have been reported to be associated with the experience of stressful life events, including unemployment (Holmes and Rahe 1967; Brenner 1973; Brown and Harris 1978). An epidemiological study would need to take account of such stressful agents by using domain-specific scales (e.g. of stress). Outcome studies are more focused, however, and stress scales are rarely used, while the individual's level of role functioning, adjustment and coping are.

Satisfaction

Life satisfaction, and satisfaction with services, are also important domains to include. Readers will note that most of the quality of life scales tap these domains - for example, Lehman et al.'s (1982) Quality of Life Interview - and borrow heavily from the scales of life satisfaction developed by Andrews and Withey (1976), Campbell et al. (1976) and Cantril (1965).

Social support

Social support may modify the impact of illness on the patient (Cohen and Wills 1985; Ganster and Victor 1988). There is some evidence, more generally, that a supportive family or social network is essential as a social buffer to the adverse health effects of social stress and for recovery (e.g. Holahan and Moos 1981), although the direction of relationships needs to be interpreted cautiously (Payne and Graham-Jones 1987; House et al. 1988). Social support may be instrumental in whether or not a person with a psychiatric problem is cared for in the community or in an institution, and is another important measure to include. It is also an outcome variable - psychological morbidity can impair a person's ability to initiate and maintain social relationships and activities.

The availability of social support is crucial for the success of community care, as opposed to hospitalization, of patients with mental health problems, and its accurate measurement is important. A selection of generic social support measures has been reviewed by Bowling (1991), and appropriate schedules for use with elderly people have been reviewed by Kane and Kane (1988). A measure developed for use with psychiatric patients is the TAPS Social Network Schedule (Leff 1988), although it is fairly unstructured and lengthy to administer. The Rand HIS Social Support Scale has been used as a predictor of use of mental health services (Sherbourne 1988; Sherbourne and Hays 1990), and has been used with people suffering from depression (Sherbourne et al. 1992). It is one of the most carefully developed scales of support, but it is probably too structured to be successful with people who are severely disturbed.

Probably the most robust of the in-depth schedules is the Self-Evaluation and Social Support Schedule (SESS) developed by O'Connor and Brown (1984) and Brown et al. (1986). The schedule prioritizes measuring the meaning of relationships to the individual, rather than simply network structure. This is important given that different network sizes and structures may meet the different needs of individuals (i.e. one person may be content with one close friend, others may need more than one for their emotional well-being). This instrument collects data on type of relationship, frequency of contact, quality and content of contact and respondents' view of cognitive/ affective quality of the relationship. It emphasizes very close relationships, and enquires about support in a crisis or life event. It also measures positive and negative self-esteem. As with Brown's measure of expressed emotion and life events (Brown and Harris 1978), the context and tone of spontaneous comments are noted. Ratings are made on a 4-point scale: marked, moderate, some, little/none. It is lengthy, taking 1–2 h to administer, but its authors claim a high degree of reliability. This makes it unsuitable for use with severely disturbed people. The interview is followed by 'panel' ratings based on audiotape recordings. It has a high degree of reliability between raters. Intensive interviewer training is required, which makes the use of the measure prohibitively expensive for most investigators.

On a different but related dimension is the measurement of negative social support, which receives little attention. There is a reported association between relapse rates in psychiatrically ill people and the emotional atmosphere in the home (Leff and Vaughan 1985). The Relatives Expressed Emotion Questionnaire was developed by Brown and Rutter (1966) for use with patients with schizophrenia and modified by Vaughan and Leff (1976). Associations were found with schizophrenia and the course of positive symptoms and expressed emotion (critical comments, hostility and over-involvement; Brown *et al.* 1972), although not all studies have been consistent (see review by Leff, 1991a). While the ratings of expressed emotion were initially based on the relatives' responses at interview, these were later based on observations of the relatives' interactions with the patients, and the questionnaire was validated. The studies showed a strong association between response to the questionnaire and observed interaction, except with over-involvement (Miklowitz *et al.* 1984; Strachan *et al.* 1986; Szmuckler *et al.* 1987).

There are also several scales for measuring the quality of marital/cohabiting relationships across all population groups (ill/normal) (Spanier 1976; Frank and Kupfer 1976, undated). Test corporations and distributors throughout the world also list several scales measuring the quality of relationships – versions exist for children, adults and married couples (see, for example, NFER-

Nelson's catalogue in England; and see the test critiques published by Keyser and Sweetland 1985b). These are usually too structured for use with psychotic patients. For the latter group scales need to be shorter (so that they can be completed before the patient becomes distracted or restless) and semi-structured in order that multiple probes can be used where necessary and information can be obtained from more than one (identified) source. The items contained in the more comprehensive quality of life scales for use with mentally ill people – for example, Lehman *et al.*'s (1982) Quality of Life Interview – are adequate for most purposes.

Loneliness

Loneliness is also an important variable to measure in relation to the quality of life of people with mental health problems. A widely used scale of loneliness is the UCLA (University of California at Los Angeles) Loneliness Scale (Russell *et al.* 1980). A wide range of loneliness measures have been reviewed by Shaver and Brennan (1991). Interested readers are referred to these sources. Such scales may be less suitable for people with psychotic conditions. The items included within the broader quality of life scales may suffice for most purposes.

Sleep

Many sleep items are contained in scales of psychological and health-related quality of life. However, in research aiming to investigate sleeping patterns as a particular outcome, a specific sleep scale may be required in order to ensure that the domain is reliably and validly measured. There are several sleep scales, although few have been fully tested. One such scale is the sleep dysfunction scale, which was adapted by Croog *et al.* (1986) from their previous work (Rose *et al.* 1978; Jenkins *et al.* 1983a, 1983b). It consists of four questions that measure the number of days in which there were problems in falling asleep, staying asleep, early awakening and awakening tired (Jenkins *et al.* 1983a, 1983b). Scores range from 4 (no sleep disturbance) to 20 (high sleep disturbance). Cronbach's alpha (reliability) is $r = 0.79$; otherwise, there has been little testing for reliability and validity.

SUBJECTIVE ACCOUNTS AND THE VALUE OF PATIENTS' RATINGS

In 1958, Jahoda identified six main themes which recurred in definitions of positive mental health, including positive attitudes towards the self, integration of personality, autonomy and environmental mastery. Jahoda noted their subjective element, and dependence on social and cultural values. Mechanic (1991) has pointed to the subjective elements of self-assessments of health, which are made in the context of self and other comparisons. He points out that, as people age, they may attribute some of their discomforts to the ageing process, and may normalize these. People who experience a feeling of well-being may perceive that they are doing better than others in their reference group and so on. However, while the subjectivity of assessments has been criticized as a methodological weakness of scales in the past, particularly in relation to reported life satisfaction and perceived social support, their subjectivity is regarded as their strength in the 1990s. What is important in predicting outcome is how the respondent actually feels and perceives life.

Direct assessment of people's perceptions of their psychological well-being and life circumstances are relevant when assessing outcome of psychiatric treatment. A major issue, which is rarely discussed, is the value that can be placed on patients' ratings. Many scales rely on interviewers' and third-party assessments of the patient's life circumstances and functioning. Patients are not always asked to give first-hand accounts due to the belief that their perception of 'reality' can be distorted. For example, those in low spirits may be inclined to underestimate the amount of social support available to them. Patients may sometimes feel inclined to give false responses, and research by Rosenhan (1973) demonstrated how successfully people can bluff psychiatric symptoms even before psychiatric staff. Scales do have to be administered carefully, often involving carers and staff in making dual assessments because of the potentially distorted perceptions of patients with certain conditions, which will in turn distort results. Many questions will need additional probing, which necessitates an open-ended format with interviewer-coding, but the patients' viewpoints should

never be dismissed – and only patients can judge whether they are satisfied with their care.

While there has been much scepticism about the value of patients' accounts, there is increasing evidence that patients with severe psychiatric conditions are able to give reliable and consistent accounts (MacCarthy *et al.* 1986; Brewin, 1992; Thornicroft *et al.* 1993). Lack of agreement between patients' and professionals' assessments should not be dismissed as being due to inadequacies on the part of patients (Babiker and Thorne 1993). There are also dangers in assuming that the values of raters are the same as the values of the respondents (Scheff 1961; Szasz 1971; Littlewood and Lipsedge 1982). While many clinicians accept the need to measure subjective health-related quality of life by also taking patients' assessments into account, long-held prejudices occasionally surface, echoing Bunge (1975) who argued that the use of subjective measures of quality of life may simply indicate the 'backward state' of research.

THE MEASUREMENT SCALES

PART I   SYMPTOM SCALES

BACKGROUND

The concept of mental illness itself is based on concepts of the symptoms and signs of 'dysfunction', resulting from perceptions of deviant behaviour (Wing *et al.* 1992). The application of the most rigorously tested and standardized assessment schedules generally results in fairly reliable diagnoses across the world. However, there is always capacity for cultural bias in psychiatric research. For example, Geil (1991) has pointed out that even some of the DSM-III-R categories may be interpretations of reality (i.e. culture-bound syndromes) rather than universal classes of disease (e.g. anorexia nervosa).

Classification systems

There is a need for instruments to have cross-cultural applicability and validity. Few achieve this status. Psychiatric epidemiology has striven for high standards in classification. Two systems, the American Diagnostic and Statistical Manual (American Psychiatric Association 1980, 1987)

(DSM-IV is the newest version (APA 1994)) and the International Classification of Diseases (ICD), 10th edition (WHO 1990, 1992), have gained increasing acceptance over the course of several editions. Diagnostic measurement scales should base their categories on one of the international diagnostic classifications.

The WHO (1978) issued a guide to the classification of mental disorders with previous editions of ICD, but the classification of mental disorders has been considerably improved with the 10th edition, facilitating its use in research. ICD-9 (WHO 1977) was extensively used in Europe, although it does not equate well with the DSM. However, ICD-10 was published in 1992 and the psychiatric section is more closely based on DSM-III, to facilitate international comparisons. These are regarded as the gold standards for psychiatric classification. Brugha and Bebbington (1992) reported that the DSM-III-R and the ICD-10-DCR depressive disorder research diagnostic criteria showed considerable similarities. However, their use of the Present State Examination, PSE-9, with 130 patients indicated considerable differences in actual subjects allocated to case categories, implying that research should utilize interval level scales (e.g. the PSE).

The introduction to ICD-10 includes a set of diagnostic guidelines and diagnostic criteria for research. The American Psychiatric Association's (APA) DSM-III and DSM-III-R (revised) diagnostic criteria for depressive disorders (APA 1980, 1987) were developed from the diagnostic rules published by Feighner et al. (1972) and the Research Diagnostic Criteria (Spitzer et al. 1975b, 1978). A structured clinical interview for the DSM-III-R has been developed (Spitzer and Williams 1988).

Psychiatric screening and diagnostic instruments

When carrying out a study of needs for psychiatric services, or quality of life among psychiatric patients as an outcome measure of care/treatment provided, a decision will be needed about whether to use a diagnostic screening tool or a self-report symptom questionnaire. In contrast to the psychiatric screening instruments that can yield a psychiatric diagnosis, the self-report questionnaires provide only descriptive data. Although the scoring cut-offs of some of these can point to likely psychiatric disorders, psychologists often view these cut-off points with some scepticism, preferring instead to analyse problems on a continuum.

When deciding whether to use a psychiatric screening (diagnostic) instrument or a self-report symptom questionnaire, investigators must ask what the former would achieve over the latter in relation to the study aims. While the psychiatric screening instrument can lead to the psychiatric classification of subjects, this may not be necessary in research on health outcomes. Such instruments are essential in epidemiological research, but for the assessment of health outcomes, self-reported feelings (e.g. of anxiety and depression) and self-reported and observed role functioning and behaviour may be sufficient as indexes of psychological morbidity and severity.

In relation to schizophrenia, psychotic symptoms such as dissociative thinking, hallucinations and delusions are dramatic and socially disruptive. They are responsive to treatment with antipsychotic drugs. It is therefore unsurprising that outcome measurement has focused mainly on psychotic symptomatology. Some of the diagnostic screening instruments popularly used are briefly described below. The next section concentrates on the self-report questionnaires and reviews them in more detail, given their greater relevance to the assessment of health-related quality of life.

Present State Examination (PSE)

One international standardized and well-tested screening tool is the Present State Examination (PSE: Wing 1992; Wing et al. in press). The PSE is a standardized clinical interview, and has a computer program called CATEGO (now CATEGO5) which provides a psychiatric classification based on ICD. A short and a computerized version have been developed (Wing and Sturt 1978; Wing 1991, 1992). The short 10-item version deals only with milder or 'neurotic' complaints (see Cooper and McKenzie 1981).

The 10th edition of the PSE has been published (Wing et al. 1990; Wing 1991), and is used within a package of instruments called SCAN (Schedules for Clinical Assessment in Neuropsychiatry) to assess psychotic and neurotic symptoms (Wing et al. 1991, in press). The disorders included in SCAN are defined in terms of the criteria contained in

DSM-III-R (Spitzer 1987) and ICD-10 (WHO 1992). Details are available from the WHO (1992) or from the Royal College of Psychiatrists' Research Unit.

The long version requires a week's training at a recognized centre, and it is open to non-psychiatrically trained interviewers (Brown *et al.* 1977). The PSE is usually used in epidemiological surveys (see Bebbington 1992). It has excellent properties of reliability and validity (with the exception of anxiety) (Wing *et al.* 1967, 1974, 1977a, 1977b; Kendell *et al.* 1968; Sartorius *et al.* 1970; Cooper *et al.* 1977; Luria and Berry 1979; Newson-Smith and Hirsch 1979; Rabins and Brooks 1981; Robinson and Price 1981; Banks 1983; Wilson *et al.* 1985; Hasin and Skodol 1989; Manchanda *et al.* 1989; Wing 1991).

Research Diagnostic criteria (RDC)

The RDC was developed under the auspices of the National Institute of Mental Health, in the USA, to enable researchers to apply a consistent set of criteria for the description or selection of samples of research subjects with functional psychiatric illnesses (Spitzer *et al.* 1978). This diagnostic schema is widely used internationally. There are several less frequently used diagnostic schema, and these have been reviewed by Dworkin (1992). Unlike the DSM, it was designed for use in research, not clinical practice. It is a semi-structured clinical interview.

There is less evidence of the validity of the scale, in comparison with its reliability. The results of tests for its reliability have been variable (Spitzer *et al.* 1975b, 1978; Dworkin 1992). Dworkin (1992) also points to the problems inherent in common clinical practice which, prior to the application of criteria to schemata, generally relies on unstructured, open-ended interviews to gather relevant data.

Schedule for Affective Disorders and Schizophrenia (SADS)

This instrument was developed by Endicott and Spitzer (1978) in the USA. The SADS is a semi-structured interview for clinical interviewer use (Endicott and Spitzer 1978). It was initially developed for use in studies of depression (Katz *et al.* 1979). SADS was designed as a companion to the RDC in order to evaluate the symptoms of disorders as defined by the RDC (Spitzer *et al.* 1978), which are the intermediate set of diagnostic criteria between the earlier Feighner Criteria (Feighner *et al.* 1972) and the DSM-III (APA 1980).

The SADS has been reported to have good validity and is sensitive to change (Woody *et al.* 1985), although more testing is required; it has a clear factor structure (see Hasin and Skodol 1989). It has excellent reliability (Spitzer *et al.* 1978; Shrout and Fleiss 1979), although it is lower among community populations and with long test-retest periods (see Bromet *et al.* 1986; Hasin and Skodol 1989).

Diagnostic Interview Schedule (DIS)

This schedule was developed by Robins *et al.* (1979, 1981), under the sponsorship of the National Institute of Mental Health, in the USA, for use in a set of large-scale epidemiological studies. It was developed in an attempt to produce a relatively inexpensive interview schedule (Regier *et al.* 1984). It is frequently used in American clinical and epidemiological research. Its development, reliability and validity, as well as translations into several languages (e.g. into Spanish), have been fully described (Robins *et al.* 1981, 1982; Burnham *et al.* 1983; Anthony *et al.* 1982; Helzer *et al.* 1985). The diagnoses by the three sets of criteria (Feighner, DSM-III and RDC) are generated by computer. It also provides a symptom count.

The DIS (Robins *et al.* 1981, 1985) is a rigid list of questions, administered by a trained interviewer, designed to reduce clinical judgement to a minimum. It is suitable for use by lay interviewers. The data obtained by the DIS (DIS-III) are used to establish diagnosis using the DSM-III (APA 1980), the Feighner Criteria (Feighner *et al.* 1972) and the RDC (Spitzer *et al.* 1978). It has been used in many large epidemiological surveys (see Bebbington 1992 for a brief review). It is an extension of the Renard Diagnostic Interview (Helzer *et al.* 1981). The validity of the scale has been reported to be variable, from moderate to good (Robins *et al.* 1981, 1982; see Hasin and Skodol 1989), and there is little evidence of its reliability.

Brief Psychiatric Rating Scale (BPRS)

This scale was developed in the USA by Overall and Gorham (1962) for use in recording clinical judgements based on information obtained in a brief semi-structured interview. The authors have made suggestions for lead questions (Rhoades and Overall 1988) and a semi-structured interview format (Overall and Hollister 1986). It has been widely used, and has been subjected to a substantial amount of methodological development and testing. It consists of 18 global, clinically familiar symptom and behaviour constructs and covers much of the range of manifest psychopathology (Rhoades and Overall 1988); two of the scales were incorporated later (Overall 1974). Definitions of severity have been discussed by Rhoades and Overall (1988). The original 14 scales were derived from factor analysis of psychiatric rating data. The scale has been reviewed by Hedlund and Vieweg (1980).

The use of the total score in measuring outcome can be misleading; for example, in studies of schizophrenics, as not all the items reflect psychotic phenomena, a change in overall scores leads to uncertainty as to what has changed (psychotic, neurotic or affective symptomatology) (Manchanda et al. 1989). A consistent factor structure has been replicated several times, although the scale has been criticized by Manchanda et al. (1989) for imprecisely defined items and for incompatible rating instructions from different investigators, which they feel account for differences in reported levels of reliability. They reported that ratings can be highly idiosyncratic and subjective. Although the scale has apparently been successfully used in research for recording the severity of manifest psychopathology, Manchanda et al. (1989) indicate that its weak construct validity does not justify its use.

Self-report symptom, functioning and behaviour scales

These are probably the most appropriate scales to use when assessing the broad outcome of illness and treatment. There are many self-report scales for the measurement of symptoms of depression. There are at least 30 in the English language (Snaith 1993). Many of the most popular scales are reviewed in this chapter. Notable omissions include the Montgomery–Asberg Depression Rating Scale (Montgomery and Asberg 1979), the Symptoms of Anxiety and Depression Scale (Bedford et al. 1976)

and other, older, instruments which were developed in the USA, including the Psychiatric Screening Inventory (22 items) developed for use in the Midtown Manhattan Study (Langner 1962), the Health Opinion Survey developed for use in the Stirling County Study (Leighton et al. 1963), the Gurin Scale (Schwartz et al. 1974) and the Cornell Medical Index (Gunderson and Ronson 1969). Interested readers are referred to the source material. Inevitably, in a book of this size some difficult decisions have to be made about exclusions. The scales presented have been selected on the grounds of their popularity and frequency of use in both clinical and psychiatric research. Critical reviews of a wide range of scales used in psychiatry can be found in Thompson (1989c).

Some symptom scales include blunted affect (Overall and Gorham 1962; Wing et al. 1974; Endicott and Spitzer 1978) and other scales focus on this dimension (Abrams and Taylor 1978; Andreasen, 1979). These often involve inferred judgements about the presence or absence of certain behaviours. Heinrichs et al. (1984) make this point and clarify it by the example of a student with a diagnosis of schizophrenia who deliberately reduces his or her number of social contacts because of the need to revise for exams, and hence would not be perceived to be exhibiting symptoms of social withdrawal in the same way as a patient with schizophrenia who begins to refuse to maintain social contacts and becomes increasingly isolated. Thus, scales which are limited to measuring such deficit symptoms are inadequate unless interpretation is allowed for in the coding.

SYMPTOM QUESTIONNAIRES

HOPKINS SYMPTOM CHECKLIST (SCL) AND THE SYMPTOM CHECKLIST-90

There are several scales of varying length entitled the Symptom Checklist which are widely used in the USA. These scales are derived from the earliest version, which was the Hopkins Symptom Checklist. The history and evolution of later versions has been described by Derogatis et al. (1974a, 1974b). The Hopkins Symptom Checklist was developed by Parloff et al. (1954) and revised by Frank et al. (1957). The version used most often is the 90-item version, known as the Symptom

Checklist-90 (SCL-90). The series also contains the Brief Symptom Inventory (BSI) checklist (Derogatis *et al.* 1976; Derogatis 1993a), which will be described later. Widely used sub-scales that have been developed by Derogatis include those which measure the distress of physical symptoms, based partly on symptom items used in the National Heart, Lung and Blood Institute Hypertension Detection and Follow-up Program (HDFP Co-operative Group 1982), and the distress related to impaired sexual functioning. These have been tested extensively and the latter, in particular, has good psychometric properties (Hogan *et al.* 1980). These scales are popular in the USA across a wide range of specialities.

Content

The SCL is comprised of items which, on the basis of clinical opinion, reflect the primary symptom dimensions underlying the majority of psychiatric disorders. Scales of varying length are available. Clinical researchers have often used the 90-item version, which comprises nine sub-scales – depression, anxiety, somatization, obsessive–compulsive, interpersonal sensitivity, hostility, phobic anxiety, paranoid ideation and psychoticism (Derogatis *et al.* 1974b, 1976; Wilson *et al.* 1985) – and the 58-item version, which has five sub-scales – depression, anxiety, somatization, obsessive–compulsive and irascibility (Derogatis *et al.* 1974a). A 35-item version is also available (Derogatis *et al.* 1971, 1974b). It is a self-report scale, and the 90-item version (the SCL-90) is one of the most popular.

The instrument is concerned with current state and each item is scored using a 5-point frequency distress scale, ranging from 'not at all' to 'extremely'. The response scores are coded as follows: 0 = no distress, 1 = a little distress, 2 = moderate distress, 3 = quite a bit of distress and 4 = moderate to extreme (high-intensity) distress. The scoring involves dividing the sum of the response scores by the number of questions answered, although not all researchers carry out the division and sum the scores.

Administration and scoring

The SCL-90 takes about 20 min to complete, and an interviewer is not necessary (it is a self-report scale). It was developed for use with out-patients, but can be used with in-patients (Derogatis *et al.* 1974b). The scoring details are available in the manual (Derogatis *et al.* 1977).

Examples from the SCL-90

Below is a list of problems and complaints that people sometimes have. Please read each carefully. After you have done so, please fill in one of the numbered spaces to the right that best describes HOW MUCH THAT PROBLEM HAS BOTHERED OR DISTRESSED YOU DURING THE PAST _____ INCLUDING TODAY . . .

How much were you bothered by:

1 Headaches
2 Nervousness or shakiness inside
9 Trouble remembering things
15 Thoughts of ending your life
26 Blaming yourself for things

Validity and factor structure

The sub-scales have undergone extensive testing on thousands of patients. The 35-item version correlates well with the GHQ and psychiatric assessment (0.70–0.78) (Goldberg *et al.* 1976). It is highly sensitive when compared with psychiatric interview (Feighner *et al.* 1972), and sub-scale scores correlate highly with the PSE (0.34–0.51) (Wilson *et al.* 1985). Derogatis *et al.* (1974a) reported the results of validity tests for the five sub-scales of the SCL-58 version. Testing was carried out on 1800 psychiatric out-patients and 700 'normals'. The instrument was reported to be sensitive to treatment effects, and also to withdrawal phenomena from minor tranquillizers. The authors also reference other studies which refer to the validity of the scale, and its associations with diagnostic groups. Derogatis *et al.* (1976) tested the validity of the SCL-90 with 209 'symptomatic volunteers'. Correlations of the SCL-90 and the Minnesota Multiphasic Personality Inventory scales (Hathaway and McKinley 1990) ranged from $r = 0.40$ to 0.75. These results support the scale's convergent validity. The scale has been reported to be sensitive to change (Edwards *et al.* 1978).

The main domains have been supported by factor analyses (Derogatis *et al.* 1974a, 1974b). The scales are sensitive to treatment type among outpatients (Derogatis *et al.* 1973, 1974b). Derogatis and Cleary (1977) reported that 5–6 items on each sub-scale were sufficiently loaded to sustain an effective operational definition of each syndrome construct.

Reliability

Derogatis *et al.* (1974a) reported the results of reliability tests for the five sub-scales of the SCL-58 version on the large samples reported above. The internal consistency coefficient alphas were uniformly high at 0.84–0.87. Item–total correlations were all above $r = 0.50$. Test–retest correlations 1 week apart were $r = 0.75–0.84$ for the five sub-scales, and inter-rater reliability (intra-class) coefficients ranged from $r = 0.64$ to 0.77. The SCL-90 has similar psychometric properties (Derogatis *et al.* 1976). A manual is available (Derogatis *et al.* 1977), as well as a bibliography (Derogatis 1993b). It has been used in over 700 research studies (Derogatis 1993b).

BRIEF SYMPTOM INVENTORY (BSI)

The Brief Symptom Inventory was designed to reflect the psychological symptom patterns of psychiatric and medical patients, as well as community (non-patient) samples (Derogatis 1993a). The BSI was developed by Derogatis and Spencer (1982), and an updated manual has been published by Derogatis (1993a).

It was developed from the Symptom Checklist-90 (see above) in an attempt to produce a more concise instrument for use in assessment settings with greater time constraints. The items that loaded highest on each dimension were selected to form the BSI (Derogatis and Cleary 1977; Derogatis 1993a).

Content, administration and scoring

The scale was designed for self-completion, after an introduction by an interviewer. It is a 53-item self-report symptom inventory. It is really a brief version of the SCL-90-R (revised). The time referent is 'the past 7 days, including today'. It contains nine primary symptom dimensions: somatization, obsessive–compulsive, interpersonal sensitivity, depression, anxiety, hostility, phobic anxiety, paranoid ideation and psychoticism. The BSI provides three global indexes: the Global Severity Index, the Positive Symptom Total and the Positive Symptom Distress Index. It takes 8–10 min to complete.

Each item is rated on a 5-point scale of distress, from 'not at all' (0) to 'extremely' (4). The items are summed and the sum for each symptom dimension is then divided by the number of endorsed items in that dimension. The raw scores are converted to standardized scores. The scoring details are included in the manual (Derogatis 1993a).

Examples from the BSI

16 Feeling lonely (depression)
21 Feeling that people are unfriendly or dislike you (interpersonal sensitivity)
36 Trouble concentrating (obsessive–compulsive)
37 Feeling weak in parts of your body (somatization)
41 Having urges to break or smash things (hostility)

Not at all (0) / a little bit (1) / moderately (2) / quite a bit (3) / extremely (4)

Validity and reliability

The BSI was reported by Derogatis *et al.* (1976) to correlate highly with the Minnesota Multiphasic Personality Inventory (MMPI) in a sample of 209 symptomatic volunteers (MMPI Dahlstrom and Welsh 1960; Hathaway and McKinley 1990). The correlations between the BSI, the MMPI and other similar scales range from 0.30 to 0.72 (Derogatis 1993a). Its predictive validity has been established in a wide range of studies, including studies of mental health, HIV, pain management and studies of cancer patients (for reviews, see Derogatis 1993a). Principal components analysis has confirmed the factor structure of the instrument (see Derogatis 1993a).

It has been widely used in studies of cancer patients and also in studies of cardiovascular disease. The Positive Symptom Distress Index was reported to be sensitive to differences in type of medication among 626 men with mild to moderate hypertension participating in a randomized controlled trial of hypertensive therapy, and the alpha coefficients for the Positive Symptoms Index ranged from 0.78 to 0.83. (Croog *et al.* 1986). Internal consistency coefficients ranged from 0.71 to 0.85 on the nine dimensions (Cronbach's alpha) in a study of 719 psychiatric patients (Derogatis 1993a). Test–retest reliability coefficents at 2 weeks retesting in 60 'non-patient' subjects ranged from $r = 0.78$ to 0.90. The scale is popular among clinicians across a range of specialities. A bibliography is available which lists more than 200 published reports relating to the scale (Derogatis 1993c).

SYMPTOM RATING TEST (SRT)

The Symptom Rating Test was developed to measure psychological state, including anxiety and depression (Kellner and Sheffield 1973), particularly as an outcome measure in drug trials. It was compiled on the basis of the complaints of 100 consecutive neurotic patients. The authors' aim was to produce a brief, comprehensive checklist of symptoms, easily understandable to most patients.

Content

The current version is a 37-item scale which provides sub-scores for depression, anxiety, somatic problems and inadequacy (later modified to replace the inadequacy score with questions on cognitive function and hostility). A short 30-item version is available, and is reproduced in Kellner and Sheffield (1973).

Administration and scoring

The 38-item scale is usually interviewer-administered. Items can be displayed on test cards shown during a semi-structured interview, or in a self-report questionnaire. Patients either select the test card that applies to them or tick the symptom on the questionnaire that applies to them, depending on the version used. Items are scored 0, 1, 2, 3 or 4

from left to right. The sub-scales are anxiety, depression, somatic problems and inadequacy or (later version) cognitive function and hostility. All sub-scale scores are summed to produce a scale score, and the cut-off for identifying cases is 7. Full scoring details are reported by Kellner and Sheffield (1973). Fava *et al.* (1982) reported that this cut-off point led to the misclassification of 9 of 40 depressed patients and 4 of 40 normal controls.

Examples: Short 30-item version (checklist)

Describe how you have felt during the past week . . .
If you have had the symptom describe how much it has bothered or troubled you . . .
Please answer all questions. Do not think long before answering.

1 Feeling dizzy or faint
2 Feeling tired or a lack of energy
6 Poor appetite
8 Feeling that there was no hope
10 Poor memory
13 Worrying
22 Irritable
26 Attacks of panic
30 Awakening too early and not being able to fall asleep again

Not at all / a little, slightly / a great deal, quite a bit / extremely / could not have been worse

---

Validity and reliability

The SRT (both versions) was validated by comparing the results with those from the Hamilton Depression Scale, and the authors reported acceptable levels of validity (Fava *et al.* 1982). They reported the correlation between the two instruments to be $r = 0.72$ among patients with depression and $r = 0.65$ among 'normal' sample members. There were similar misclassification rates for both scales. Its convergent validity was supported by a study of anxious patients, showing that respondents with lower levels of benzodiazepines in their blood had higher levels of distress with the SRT (Robin *et al.* 1974). In comparison with controls, the scale was reported to be sensitive to changes due to treatment at 1 month among 40 neurotic outpatients, but not after

2 months of treatment. It was able to discriminate between depressed and neurotic patients, as well as normal controls. It was able to discriminate between alcoholic patients and normal controls before treatment, but not after treatment. It also correlated in the expected direction with scales of neuroticism from a range of measures (Kellner and Sheffield 1973). The authors reported no differences in the results obtained with the two different versions of the scale, nor with observer ratings.

There is less evidence of its reliability. Kellner and Sheffield (1973) reported the test–retest reliability of the test card version of the scale at 24 h for 28 neurotic out-patients to be $r = 0.94$, and to be $r = 0.92$ for in-patients using the self-report version. Conventional split-half reliability tests were not possible due to the items not being psychometrically equivalent. The authors undertook a test of the split-half reliability of changes among 40 patients at 1 month, reporting a correlation of $r = 0.89$ (test card version).

CENTER FOR EPIDEMIOLOGICAL STUDIES DEPRESSION SCALE (CES-D)

This scale was developed by Radloff (1975, 1977) on the basis of the literature and factor analytic studies of existing measures. It was developed by the National Institute of Mental Health, Center for Epidemiological Studies to assess the frequency and severity with which symptoms of depression were experienced (over the past week) in the general population. It was not intended to be used as a diagnostic tool. During its development, it was tested on about 3000 randomly sampled people living in Kansas City and Washington County, and on over 100 psychiatric in- and out-patients. While it is widely used in the USA, its use in Europe is limited.

Content

It is a 20-item, self-report depression scale. The scale asks respondents about their feelings over the past week, and about the number of days so affected. The six major symptom areas covered are depressed mood, feelings of guilt/worthlessness, a sense of helplessness/hopelessness, psychomotor retardation, loss of appetite and sleep disturbance.

The 20 items can be reduced to 19 (the item omitted is 'I had crying spells').

Administration and scoring

The scale was designed for self-administration, although it is also often used in interview formats. Each item is rated on a scale of 0–3 in relation to frequency of occurrence during the past week (0 = rarely or none of the time, 3 = most or all of the time), with total scores ranging from 0 to 60; high scores indicate a higher frequency (symptomatology). A standard cut-off score of 16 has been defined to assess depressive symptomatology (Eaton and Kessler 1981; Radloff and Locke 1986).

Short version

A short version has been developed, which is composed of eight items, six of which were taken from the longer instrument to represent the six domains measured. The other two questions are summary questions about lifetime symptoms (Shumaker et al. 1990).

Children's version

A modified 19-item version (language and scoring) is available for use with children (a suggested cut-off point is 15), and a shortened scale for children with just four of the items from the full children's scale can be obtained.

Examples from the adults' and children's versions

Adults' scale

1 I was bothered by things that usually don't bother me
5 I had trouble keeping my mind on what I was doing
6 I felt depressed
12 I was happy
14 I felt lonely
19 I felt that people disliked me
20 I could not get 'going'

Rarely (<1 day) / some or a little of the time (1–2 days) / occasionally or a moderate amount of the time (3–4 days) / most or all of the time (5–7 days)

Children's scale

I did not feel like eating; I wasn't very hungry
I felt down and unhappy this week
I felt scared this week
I didn't sleep as well as I usually sleep this week
I had a good time this week
I felt people didn't like me this week

Not at all / a little / some / a lot

Validity and factor structure

Correlations with nurse-clinicians' ratings and clinicians' ratings based on other scales, including the Hamilton Depression Scale, indicated moderate convergent validity with correlations of 0.44–0.56 (see Shaver and Brennan 1991). However, Radloff (1977) notes that the correlations increased with treatment period to 0.69–0.75. It has been reported to correlate well with the Beck Depression Index ($r = 0.81$) and the Zung scales ($r = 0.90$) (Weissman *et al*. 1975). Radloff (1977) reported a low correlation with Crowne and Marlowe's (1960) Social Desirability Scale. The scale discriminated well between psychiatric in-patients and members of a general population, and discriminated moderately between levels of severity within patient groups (Radloff 1977). Clinical research has demonstrated its sensitivity to improvement after treatment (Weissman *et al*. 1975).

Principal components factor analysis of the 20-item scale was consistent across psychiatric patient and general population samples and, including items with loadings above 0.40, four factors were evident: depressed affect (blues, depressed, lonely, cry, sad); positive affect (good, hopeful, happy, enjoy); somatic and retarded activity (bothered, appetite, effort, sleep, get going); and interpersonal (unfriendly, dislike). The psychometric properties of the scale in relation to different cultures have been reviewed by Naughton and Wiklund (1993).

Reliability

In Radloff's (1977) developmental work, the inter-item, item–scale and inter-scale (personality and life satisfaction scales) correlations ranged widely (inter-item $r = 0.03–0.73$; item–scale $r = 0.29–0.79$; inter-scale $r = -0.3–0.74$). The inter-item and item–scale correlations were higher in the patient than in the general population samples, as would be expected given the heterogeneity of the latter. The coefficient alpha for internal consistency was 0.85 in the general population and even higher at 0.90 in the patient population. Radloff (1977) also reported test–retest reliabilities ranging from 0.32 at 12 months retesting and 0.67 at 4 weeks.

In sum, the scale has been validated as a screen for clinical depression in adults (Weissman *et al*. 1977; Myers and Weissman 1980). It has been used extensively (Zonderman *et al*. 1989). It is strongly correlated with other depression scales (Comstock and Helsing 1976) and discriminates well between clinically depressed and normal respondents (Weissman *et al*. 1977).

The children's version has obtained good psychometric properties (Fendrich *et al*. 1990). There is some evidence that it lacks specificity and performs better with older children, adolescents (12–18 years) and girls.

RAND DEPRESSION SCREENER

This short 8-item self-report measure was developed to screen for depression (major depression and dysthymia) in the Rand Medical Outcomes Study (MOS) in the USA. It was developed for use in a screening instrument of three chronic diseases, and it was intended that the whole battery should not take more than 10 min to complete (Burnam *et al*. 1988).

The scale was developed on more than 5000 people from a general population sample, mental health service and primary care users. The study measures included the 20-item Center for Epidemiological Studies Depression Scale (CES-D: Radloff 1977), which enquired about symptoms and frequency, and two items from the Diagnostic Interview Schedule (DIS) on duration of symptoms (Robins *et al*. 1981). The full DIS was also used to assess psychiatric disorders (as a gold standard). To select the best items for the screener, logistic regression analyses were employed. The final set of items selected for the screener included six CES-D items and the two DIS items. The latter two items were important predictors of depression and had the largest coefficients in the final regression model. A 6-item screener, with the latter two items removed, was also tested. However, the 8-item screener performed slightly better overall.

Content, administration and scoring

All the questions relate specifically to depressive symptoms. The response format ranges from 'yes/no' choices for the first three depression questions, to a 4-point response choice ranging from 0 = rarely or none of the time to 3 = most or all of the time (the scores are reversed for one positive item in the scale: 'I enjoyed life'). The individual items carry different weights, and two of the items relate to diagnostically relevant periods. These features distinguish it from other depression scales. There is, however, a complicated scoring equation because of the differential weights applied to the items (for details, see Burnam et al. 1988).

Examples

11 In the past year, have you had 2 weeks or more during which you felt sad, blue or depressed; or when you lost all interest or pleasure in things that you usually cared about or enjoyed?   Yes / no

12(a) Have you felt depressed or sad much of the time in the past year?   Yes / no

13 For each statement below, mark one circle that best describes how much of the time you felt or behaved this way during the past week. During the past week:

(b) I had crying spells
(d) I enjoyed life

Rarely or none of the time (< 1 day) / some or a little of the time (1–2 days) / occasionally or a moderate amount of the time (3–4 days) / most or all of the time (5–7 days)

Validity

The test results showed that the screener had high sensitivity and good positive predictive value for detecting recent depressive disorders and those that met full DSM-III criteria (APA 1987, 1993; Burnam et al. 1988). It was better at predicting depressive disorder in the past month than within the past 6–12 months. Varying the cut-off point for the screener improved the sensitivity for longer prevalence periods (6 months, 12 months and

lifetime). Detailed results for the specificity and sensitivity of the instrument by cut-off points have been published (Burnam et al. 1988).

Reliability

The test–retest reliability of the two DIS items from the screener were tested on 230 adults living in the community (baseline interview with the DIS and telephone follow-up of the depression subsection of the DIS). It was shown that the overall agreement between the two DIS items, asked on a lifetime basis, was 86 per cent for 2 weeks of feeling depressed and 91 per cent for 2 years of feeling depressed. The authors stated that the screener is suitable for population surveys and surveys of health service users. It is a promising development. However, some minor alterations to the wording (e.g. 'blue') will be required, and will need to be tested, before adoption elsewhere (Burnam et al. 1988).

Modifications and similar screeners from the Rand batteries

Three key items in the screener have been adapted for inclusion in one of the US versions of the SF-36 (the SF-36D). The items relate to: (1) depression in the past year for 2 weeks or more; (2) depression for most days over a 2-year period; and (3) depression for much of the time in the past year. The complex scoring of the screener has not been attempted, but instead the patterns of yes/no responses are used to identify patients *at risk* for major depression or dysthymia. A 'yes' reply to question 1 indicates a risk for major depression, and a 'yes' answer to questions 2 and 3 indicates a risk for dysthymia. Similar questions tested in large community studies identified 89 per cent of adults with a psychiatric diagnosis of major depresion or dysthymia (Health Outcomes Institute 1990).

Other attempts have been made to develop a short screening questionnaire based on the Rand Health Insurance Experiment Mental Health Inventory. Berwick et al. (1991) have developed a 5-item screening test which is able to detect the most significant DIS disorders, and it performed as well as the original 18-item version, and as well as Goldberg's (1972) General Health Questionnaire (30-item version).

HOSPITAL ANXIETY AND DEPRESSION (HAD) SCALE

The depression items in this scale were included if they made no reference to physical problems, ensuring that scores are independent of physical illness (Zigmond and Snaith 1983). Anxiety items were added from the Present State Examination, and analysis of the psychic manifestation of anxiety neurosis. The depression items were based on the anhedonic state, which the authors felt to be the likely central psychopathological feature of depression that responds to medication.

Content, administration and scoring

This scale consists of a brief scale of anxiety and one of depression. It can be self-administered, although Snaith (1987) recommends that an interviewer should administer it. Replies relate to feelings during the past week. The scale consists of 14 items on two sub-scales (7 = anxiety, 7 = depression). Ratings by subjects are made on 4-point scales, which represent the degree of distress: none = 0, a little = 1, a lot = 2, and unbearably = 3. Items are summed on each of the two sub-scales. High scores on each scale indicate the presence of problems (non-cases = 7 or less; doubtful cases = 8–10; definite cases = 11+).

Examples from the HAD

(D) I still enjoy the things I used to enjoy:

Definitely as much / not quite as much / only a little / hardly at all

(A) I get a sort of frightened feeling as if something awful is about to happen:

Very definitely and quite badly / yes, but not too badly / a little, but it doesn't worry me / not at all

(D) I can laugh and see the funny side of things:

As much as I always could / not quite so much now / definitely not so much now / not at all

(A) I feel restless as if I have to be on the move:

Very much indeed / quite a lot / not very much / not at all

Validity

Zigmond and Snaith (1983) reported good results for initial tests of reliability and validity, and scale scores were not affected by the presence of physical illness. This feature of the scale makes it extremely attractive in clinical research of physical conditions. The scale can be used to assess outcome during hospitalization. Tests on 50 patients found low misclassification rates (false-positive and false-negative rates ranged between 1 and 5 per cent); the severity ratings correlated highly with psychiatric assessments ($r = 0.70$ for depression and $r = 0.74$ for anxiety) (Zigmond and Snaith 1983; see also Snaith and Taylor 1985). There was evidence to suggest that the anxiety and depression items were tapping different dimensions. It was easily understood and acceptable to patients. Fallowfield et al. (1987) reported a good level of acceptability among general medical patients. Aylard et al. (1987) reported low misclassification rates for severe anxiety or depression. Correlations with other well-known depression and anxiety scales range from 0.67 to 0.77 (Aylard et al. 1987). It has been reported to perform better than the General Health Questionnaire (Goldberg 1972) in identifying cases against the criterion of a psychiatric assessment (Wilkinson and Barczak 1988).

Reliability

Zigmond and Snaith (1983) tested the internal consistency of the scale with a different group of 50 patients. The inter-item correlations on the anxiety scale ranged from $r = 0.41$ to 0.76; the inter-item correlations for the depression scale ranged from $r = 0.30$ to 0.60 (one item which fell below this during testing was removed from the scale, along with weak anxiety items). Test–retest reliability was not assessed.

This scale is increasing in popularity in clinical research, particularly in oncology, because of its brevity, simplicity and the lack of effect from physical conditions. It needs to be tested further for its psychometric properties, but appears to be one of the more promising of recent scale developments.

GOLDBERG'S GENERAL HEALTH QUESTIONNAIRE (GHQ)

The most commonly used international scale of general psychiatric morbidity, across a wide range of patients, is Goldberg's General Health Questionnaire (GHQ: Goldberg 1972, 1978; Goldberg and Williams 1988). It was developed in London during the 1960s and 1970s, and was intended for use in general practice settings as a screening questionnaire for detecting independently verifiable psychiatric morbidity (generally anxiety and depression). It does not make diagnoses. If these are necessary, a two-stage strategy must be employed. It is a measure of 'usual state', and not a measure of chronic (long-term) problems, although the authors argue that few of the latter are not detected (Goldberg and Williams 1988). It was not intended to detect functional psychoses, although it appears that these conditions may be detected (O'Riordan *et al.* 1990).

Content

An advantage of the GHQ is that scales of several lengths are available, ranging from 12 to 60 items (inevitably, the shorter versions are slightly less sensitive, although the 12-item version is as efficient as the 30-item version), and it has been translated into at least 38 languages. The 28-item version can also be analysed by sub-category (anxiety and insomnia, somatic symptoms, social dysfunction, and severe depression), which can be useful (Goldberg and Hillier 1979). Although the authors recommend the 60-item version, because of its superior validity, the most popular version appears to be the GHQ-30, probably because of its good psychometric properties and relative brevity.

Administration and scoring

The scale was designed for self-completion, and it has been administered by postal survey and by interview. There are several scoring systems (Goldberg and Williams 1988), which go in sequence from left to right across the response categories (for the latter, see the examples below). There is a Likert-type severity scoring system, a traditional method of counting problems (e.g. 0011) and also a newer version which allows for long-standing chronic problems (0111). The newer 0111 method has been said to give superior validity coefficients against caseness as measured by the Present State Examination (PSE), and more normal distributions as fewer respondents score 0 (Goodchild and Duncan-Jones 1985). However, its sensitivity is still unresolved and Goldberg and

Williams recommend that it be used in addition to the traditional scoring method, rather than as an alternative. The scale scores are summed to produce the total score.

Threshold scores on the GHQ are set to correspond to a case definition equivalent to the average patient referred to a psychiatrist. Scores above the threshold are probable cases. The authors' recommended threshold score is 4 or 5 (to be increased in cases where it is necessary to avoid a higher number of false-positives). Findlay-Jones and Murphy (1979) have shown that in order to identify 'cases' that correspond to standards derived from the PSE, it is necessary to increase the threshold score. A manual is available, which describes the scoring procedures.

Examples from the GHQ-28

Have you recently:

A2 Been feeling in need of a good tonic?

Not at all / no more than usual / rather more than usual / much more than usual

B1 Lost much sleep over worry?

Not at all / no more than usual / rather more than usual / much more than usual

C2 Been taking longer over things you do?

Quicker than usual / same as usual / longer than usual / much longer than usual

D2 Felt that life is entirely hopeless?

Not at all / no more than usual / rather more than usual / much more than usual

---

Validity and factor structure

The GHQ is probably the most extensively tested scale for reliability, validity and sensitivity to change across the world, and the results are good (Goldberg 1972, 1978; Goldberg and Huxley 1980; Goldberg and Williams 1988). Item analyses have confirmed the instrument's content validity and principle components analysis showed that there is a large general factor. Berwick *et al.* (1987) confirmed in a further factor analysis that the factors tended to cluster together.

Well over 50 studies have been carried out on the validity of the GHQ. Although it is not perfect, it correlates well with psychiatric diagnoses of morbidity and depression (Findlay-Jones and Murphy 1979; Williams 1987). Many studies have tested the GHQ against well-known psychiatric screening instruments and questionnaires with good results (e.g. Henderson *et al.* 1981; Cavanaugh 1983). The GHQ-60 has the highest correlations with the Present State Examination and the Clinical Interview Schedule, and the GHQ-30 the poorest (range = 0.45–0.83) (for a review, see Goldberg and Williams 1988).

The GHQ-30 is the most widely validated, with Goldberg and Williams (1988) citing 29 published validation studies. Using standardized psychiatric interviews as the gold standard, the reported sensitivities range between 0.55 and 0.92, and the specificities between 0.80 and 0.99, varying with the threshold score (Vieweg and Hedlund 1983).

There are some data to support its criterion validity. Those with the highest GHQ scores have been reported to use health services most (see Berwick *et al.* 1987; Goldberg and Williams 1988). Ford *et al.* (1989) also used the GHQ (20-item version) in a study of service use among 3389 respondents in the eastern Baltimore section of the Epidemiological Catchment Area study. The GHQ was able to discriminate well between service and non-service users, and was reported to be highly sensitive in this respect.

It has been used with people aged 65 and over and with very elderly people aged 85 and over, and reported to be acceptable to them, although some of the very elderly sample required assistance to complete it, due to stiff fingers or poor eyesight (Bowling 1990; Bowling and Browne 1991; Bowling *et al.* 1992; Bowling and Farquhar 1993). Self-completion questionnaires are always problematic in such cases, and will require the help of an interviewer (with an unknown degree of interviewer bias). High correlations ($r = 0.47$–0.67) have been reported with the GHQ and with scales of life satisfaction – the scales of Neugarten *et al.* (1961) and Andrews and Withey (1976) – in the authors' large population samples of people aged 85+ and, at follow-up, when they were aged 87+, supporting its construct validity among very elderly people.

There are concerns that, as the GHQ includes psychosomatic items, it may measure physical health status, not only psychiatric morbidity. Confidence in the use of the GHQ with frail or physically ill populations has been enhanced by the validation study recently conducted by Lewis and Wessely (1990), who used the GHQ and the Hospital Anxiety and Depression (HAD) Scale (Zigmond and Snaith 1983) with a sample of dermatology patients, and compared the results with a criterion – the Clinical Interview Schedule (Goldberg *et al.* 1970). The HAD, unlike the GHQ, does not include questions which overlap with physical illness. In this respect it is generally viewed as preferable to most other depression scales, although it has been less extensively tested than most. However, no difference was found between the GHQ and the HAD in their ability to detect cases of minor psychiatric disorder among a physically ill population. The psychometric properties of the cross-cultural versions have been reviewed by Naughton and Wiklund (1993).

Reliability

Test–retest reliability was assessed with respondents in whom independent assessors reported no change in condition, and the results were good (Goldberg 1978), although others have reported lower scores on the repeat testing suggesting a retest effect (Henderson *et al.* 1981; Ormel *et al.* 1989). Split-half reliability was tested with 853 respondents, and the correlations were high at $r = 0.95$. Internal consistency has been reported to range from 0.77 to −0.93 (Cronbach's alpha). Test–retest correlations range from $r = 0.51$ to 0.90 (Goldberg and Williams 1988).

BECK DEPRESSION INVENTORY (BDI)

The Beck Depression Inventory (BDI) was clinically derived, and covers sadness, pessimism/ discouragement, sense of failure, dissatisfaction, guilt, expectation of punishment, self-dislike, self-accusation, suicidal ideation, crying, irritability, social withdrawal, indecisiveness, body-image distortion, work retardation, insomnia, fatiguability, anorexia, weight loss, somatic preoccupation and loss of libido (Beck *et al.* 1961). The original BDI was revised, although little information is given on the background of item selection (Beck *et al.* 1961).

Content

The full BDI has 21 items which stress cognitive symptoms of depression, each with four Guttman-type response choices (the earlier version had between four and seven) in the form of statements, ranked in order of severity. The respondent selects the response that best fits the way he or she has been feeling during 'the past week, including today'.

Scale scores range from 0 to 3, reflecting severity. In the original version, in some categories, two alternative statements are assigned the same score. In the revised version, however, there is one alternative score for each level (so no statement is assigned the same weight), so that each of the 21 items has four alternatives ranging from 0 (low) to 3 (high). Total scores range from 0 to 63.

Administration and scoring

The scale can be self- or interviewer-administered. It takes 10–15 min to complete. The scale's authors did not provide cut-off points for the classification of depression. The ability to analyse scores as continuous data, rather than dichotomously with a rigid cut-off point to indicate a 'case', makes it preferable to a number of investigators who criticize cut-off points as artificial and unrealistic. Steer *et al.*(1986) argued that, although cut-off scores should be based on the purposes for which decisions about the intensity of depression are to be made – as the scale's authors intended – the following acts as an updated guide to cut-offs: no or minimal depression (<4), mild (5–13), moderate (14–20) and severe (21+). This is slightly different to the usual scoring guides based on normative data: 0–9 = normal; 10–15 = mild; 16–19 = mild/moderate; 20–29 = moderate/severe; >29 = severe. The BDI is available in a *computerized* scoring format from National Computer Systems, Minneapolis, MN.

Examples from the 21-item BDI

2 I am not particularly pessimistic or discouraged about the future
I feel I have nothing to look forward to

I feel that I won't ever get over my troubles
I feel that the future is hopeless and that things cannot improve

12 I have not lost interest in other people
I am less interested in other people now than I used to be
I have lost most of my interest in other people and have little feeling for them
I have lost all my interest in other people and don't care about them at all

Other versions

The BDI has been translated into several languages, and a version for children and adolescents is available (Kovacs and Beck 1977). Beck and co-workers (Beck and Beck 1972; Beck *et al.* 1974a) created a short form of the scale after re-examining earlier data based on 598 psychiatric patients. Thirteen items were selected based on their high correlations with the total BDI score and their correlation with clinical ratings. The short form correlated $r = 0.96$ with the total BDI score and $r = 0.61$ with clinical ratings. They suggested the following cut-off scores for the short form: none or minimal (0–4), mild (5–7), moderate (8–15), severe (16+). It has also undergone revisions (Beck *et al.* 1974a).

Examples from the short form of the BDI

1 I am so sad or unhappy that I can't stand it
I am blue or sad all the time and I can't snap out of it
I feel sad or blue
I do not feel sad

2 I get too tired to do anything
I get tired from doing anything
I get tired more easily than I used to
I don't get any more tired than usual

Validity and factor structure

There are numerous studies supporting the validity of the BDI. It correlates well with psychiatrists' assessments and with other depression scales. Beck *et al.* (1961) reported the agreement between the BDI and the ratings of psychiatrists on two groups of more than 300 patients to be 56 per cent, and agreement within one degree of specificity was 97 per cent. The agreement for severity ranged from 0.59 to 0.68. Correlations of between 0.66 and 0.75 were achieved against other depression and personality scales (Beck 1970), although correlations with the Hamilton Depression Scale (Hamilton 1976) were more moderate, probably reflecting the lack of congruence between the scales at the severe end (see Carroll *et al.* 1973).

A review of the literature from 1961 to 1986 by Beck *et al.* (1988) showed the concurrent validity of the BDI to be high. Mean correlations with the Hamilton Scale and clinical ratings for psychiatric patients were over 0.70, and for non-psychiatric patients they were over 0.74. It was sensitive to type of depression and able to distinguish depression from anxiety. It has been reported to be associated with suicidal behaviour and with alcoholism.

Other investigators have reported correlations between the BDI and global severity scores of 0.62–0.77 (Metcalfe and Goldman 1965; Crawford-Little and McPhail 1973; Bech *et al.* 1975). Against the Hamilton Scale, correlations of 0.58–0.82 have been reported (Schwab *et al.* 1967; Williams *et al.* 1972; Bech *et al.* 1975; Davies *et al.* 1975; Miller *et al.* 1985). Kearns *et al.* (1982) has reported the BDI to be weak in differentiating moderate from severe depression.

Factor analyses of the BDI generally reveal three intercorrelated factors: negative attitudes or suicide, physiological disturbance, and performance difficulty. When second-order factors are extracted, a single overall depression factor emerges (see Beck *et al.* 1988; Shaver and Brennan 1991). Another factor analysis has suggested that it measures depressive severity in almost a unidimensional manner, relying heavily on cognitive symptoms (Louks *et al.* 1989).

Reliability

Schwab *et al.* (1967) described a study of 153 medical in-patients, and reported a correlation of 0.75 between the BDI and Hamilton Scale; the intercorrelations on the BDI ranged from 0.32 to 0.62 and on the Hamilton Scale from 0.45 to 0.78. They concluded that the Hamilton Scale had greater internal consistency than the BDI and that the BDI was weighted towards pessimism, failure and self-punitive wishes, and thus that they measured different components of depression.

Among two groups of more than 300 patients, Beck *et al.* (1961) reported the scale to have high internal consistency. Split-half reliability using 97 of the cases was $r = 0.86$, although Weckowicz *et al.* (1967) achieved a lower reliability coefficient of 0.53. Beck *et al.* (1961) and Beck (1970) reported test–retest correlations at 2–5 week intervals, using 38 of the cases, of above 0.90. Gallagher *et al.* (1982) reported test–retest correlations (6 and 21 days apart) among 159 patients and volunteers from a 'senior centre' to range from 0.79 to 0.90, varying with diagnostic group. They reported coefficient alphas of internal consistency of 0.73–0.91. A meta-analysis of the reported internal consistency estimates yielded a mean coefficient alpha of 0.86 for psychiatric patients and 0.81 for non-psychiatric respondents (Beck *et al.* 1988).

There is some suggestion that the BDI suffers from a modest social desirability bias, and a small but modest correlation of 0.26 has been reported between the BDI and the Crowne and Marlowe Scale (1960) and the Social Desirability Scale (Reynolds and Gould 1981).

In sum, the BDI has good psychometric properties, although most of the tests have been conducted with psychiatric populations.

HAMILTON DEPRESSION SCALE (HDS)

The Hamilton Depression Scale (HDS) is an observer rating scale, which has an unstructured and a structured version. It cannot be used to establish a diagnosis, but it can assess severity once a diagnosis has been made (Hamilton 1960, 1967, 1969). The original unstructured version of the scale is the oldest and most frequently used.

Content

The scale items cover depressed mood, feelings of guilt, suicidal ideation, work and activities, insight, retardation, agitation, insomnia (early, middle and late), psychic anxiety, somatic anxiety, gastrointestinal symptoms, general somatic symptoms, genital symptoms (loss of libido or menstrual disturbances), hypochondriases and loss of weight. The rating is carried out by a trained interviewer and is based on the patient's condition in the last week or two.

It has 21 items on 3- to 5-point scales for the rater's use (0–2 or 0–4). The categories in the 5-point scale are 0 = absent, 1 = mild or trivial, 2–3 = moderate and 4 = severe; those in the 3-point scale are 0 = absent, 1 = slight or doubtful and 2 = clearly present (Hamilton 1967).

Administration and scoring

The scale is administered by trained interviewers. Total scores range from 0 to 100, representing the sum of two raters' scores, or double the score for the one rater. Some studies just report the single 0–50 rater score.

Examples from the original unstructured version of the HDS

Suicide (0–4)

Feels life is not worth living
Wishes he were dead
Suicidal ideas; attempts at suicide

Work and interests (0–4)

Feelings of incapacity
Listlessness, indecision and vacillation
Loss of interest in hobbies
Decreased social activities
Productivity decreased
Unable to work
Stopped work because of present illness only

Anxiety, somatic (0–4)

Gastrointestinal, wind, indigestion
Cardiovascular, palpitations, headaches
Respiratory, genito-urinary

Somatic symptoms, gastrointestinal (0–2)

Loss of appetite
Heavy feelings in abdomen
Constipation

Modifications

Although the scale is one of the most widely used in psychiatric research (Freemantle *et al.* 1993), many investigators have modified the scale (Paykel 1985). Potts *et al.* (1990) developed a fully structured interview version of the 17-item scale for use in the Rand MOS, the longitudinal study of the process and outcome of care for adults with a variety of conditions, including depression. Inter-rater reliability with two psychiatrists rating 20 subjects was good (Pearson's $r = 0.96$). The alpha correlations for internal consistency were 0.82–0.83. The test–retest correlations were high at 0.65 for the total score, although the item correlations varied between -0.04 and 0.77 (15-day retest). They omitted the items with low retest results and drew up a 14-item version to replace the 17-item one. They concluded that the 14-item scale produced good results, and had the advantage that it was structured and could be used by lay interviewers.

Examples from the 17-item structured version of the HDS

1 During the past month, have you been less able than usual to work or do your usual activities? If yes, probe with 1A–D

1A Do work or activities make you feel tired?
1B Have you lost interest in your work or activities?
1C Have you been getting less done at work, or have you been unable to complete as many activities?
1D Have you been spending less time at work or doing activities?

0 (No decrease in productivity or time spent at work and/or doing usual activities) to 4 (Yes, actual loss of interest and has stopped working)

11 List of physical problems:

11A Stomach or abdominal
11B Heart
11C Breathing
11D Urinary
11E Muscle aches, body aches
11F Unusual sensations
11G Flushing, pallor or sweating

1 (Moderate or trivial problems) to 4 (Severe or incapacitating problem)

13 During the past month, have you had thoughts that life is not worth living, or that you would rather be dead? Have you thought of hurting or killing yourself?

0 (No) to 4 (Suicide attempt)

15 During the past month, have you been feeling sad, depressed, helpless, hopeless, or worthless? If yes, probe with 15A:

15A How often do you feel this way?

0 (No, not at all) to 4 (Yes, almost all the time)

17 Rate speed of thoughts and speech, impairment in concentration, and motor activity at time of interview.

0 (Normal speech and thought) to 4 (Unresponsive, stuporous)

Validity and factor structure of original scale

The scale is reported to have good concurrent validity, and correlates well with the Beck Depression Inventory at $r = 0.70$ (Hamilton 1976). It is better able than the BDI to distinguish between groups of patients with varying degrees of severity of depression (Carroll et al. 1973). Schwab et al. (1967) compared the Hamilton Scale with the BDI on 153 medical in-patients. The correlation between these two scales was 0.75; the intercorrelations on the BDI ranged from 0.32 to 0.62 and on the Hamilton Scale from 0.45 to 0.78. They concluded that this suggested that the Hamilton Scale had greater internal consistency than the BDI, and that the Hamilton Scale is weighted towards somatic symptoms and the BDI towards pessimism, failure and self-punitive wishes, and thus that they measure different components of depression. Knesevich et al. (1977) reported that the Hamilton Scale correlated 0.68 with a change in global rating on a 10-point scale. Bech et al. (1975) reported a correlation of 0.73 using an 11-point global rating. Montgomery and Asberg (1979) reported the scale to be less sensitive than their own, especially at the severe end of the scale, a finding confirmed by Knesevich et al. (1977).

Factor analysis initially produced poor results, with a factor structure that bore little relationship to clinical practice (Hamilton 1960). Later factor analyses gave more satisfactory results (Hamilton 1967; Mowbray 1972). Bech (1981) reviewed the factor studies, and concluded that they shed little light on the dimensions of depression because of divergent results and different populations used for study. However, most of the factor analyses do isolate a dominant factor of general severity (see Hedlund and Vieweg 1979).

Reliability

The inter-rater reliability is consistently high at $r = 0.84–0.90$ (Hamilton 1960, 1976; see also Rehm 1981). Knesevich et al. (1977) reported a correlation of 0.94 and Bech et al. (1975) reported inter-rater correlations of 0.88–0.98. Results for the internal consistency of the scale are variable (Bech et al. 1975; Bech 1981). Hedlund and Vieweg (1979), in their review, criticized most of the reliability studies on methodological grounds. Moreover, it has been reported that just six of the scale items account for 31 per cent of the total scale score, which suggests more psychometric testing and refinement is needed (Williams 1984).

A brief review of the evidence on the psychometric properties of the scale was published by Potts et al. (1990). They reported research which showed that the Hamilton Scale has a high degree of scale reliability, concurrent, discriminant and construct validity, and is sensitive to treatment changes. However, they did point out that it has been criticized for its lower item reliability and its heavy reliance on the expertise of the interviewer, who is psychiatrically trained. This precludes its use in large-scale epidemiological surveys.

A review of outcome studies of depression by Freemantle et al. (1993) showed that the Hamilton Scale was the most consistently used measure by investigators. However, they did caution those designing outcome studies that a body of research evidence suggests that patients who receive support from their GPs, but no treatment, show a mean improvement in Hamilton Scale scores of 40–45 per cent at 4 weeks and of 60 per cent at 6 weeks.

ZUNG SELF-RATING DEPRESSION SCALE

This scale was constructed on the basis of clinical observations of the most common diagnostic criteria in relation to depressive disorders (Zung 1965). Factor analyses of initially developed items led to the retention of 20, which covered 'pervasive affect', 'physiological equivalents or concomitants' and 'psychological concomitants'.

Content

The scale contains 20 items, which include statements relating to affective, cognitive, behavioural and psychological symptoms of depression. Respondents are asked to rank each item as it applied to them during the previous week.

The response choices to the 20 items are 'None or a little of the time', 'some of the time', 'a good part of the time', 'most of the time' (scored 1–4, respectively). To counter agreement response set bias, half of the items are worded positively and half are worded negatively (with reverse scoring).

Administration and scoring

The instrument is self-administered, and takes about 5 min to complete. The scale items are summed. The sum of the raw scores is divided by the maximum possible score of 80, converted to a decimal and multiplied by 100 to obtain the final index (Zung *et al.* 1965). There has been some criticism of the scale's scoring and the dubious need to transform scores (Gurtman 1985).

The interpretation of scores is based on norms, which are given in the scale's manual. Below 50 = normal, 50–59 = minimal to mild depression, 60–69 = moderate to marked depression and 69+ = severe to extreme depression. The norms for these scores were based on adults aged 20–64 and may not be appropriate for younger or older people. The cut-off points are not agreed, and investigators have adopted a range of cut-offs from 50 to 60.

Examples from the Zung Scale

1 I feel down-hearted and blue
3 I have crying spells, or feel like it
5 I can eat as much as I used to
10 I get tired for no reason
15 I am more irritable than usual
17 I feel that I am useful and needed
20 I still enjoy the things I used to

Validity and factor structure

This scale is widely used (Zung 1986), and although there have been many studies of its validity, far fewer have studied its reliability. Zung *et al.* (1965) reported correlations of the scale with the three sub-scales of the Minnesota Multiphasic Personality Inventory (Hathaway and McKinley 1940a, 1940b, 1942a, 1942b; Dahlstrom and Welsh 1960; Dahlstrom *et al.* 1972), with new psychiatric out-patients, of $r = 0.13$, 0.68 and 0.70. Brown and Zung (1972) later reported a higher correlation of 0.79 against the Hamilton Depression Scale (Hamilton 1967). Zung *et al.* (1965) and Zung (1967b) reported that the scale was able to discriminate between different types of patients with depression and between those with confirmed and initial diagnoses of depression, although Carroll *et al.* (1973) reported that the Zung was unable to distinguish between patients with varying degrees of depression. Others have reported the Zung Scale to be unresponsive to changes in treatment (Hamilton 1976).

Davies *et al.* (1975) reported correlations between the Zung Scale and the Hamilton Scale, and a visual analogue scale of between 0.52 and 0.73. Biggs *et al.* (1978) reported a correlation between the Zung Scale and the Hamilton Scale of 0.80, although the correlation was lowest at the most severe levels. In comparison with clinical ratings of severity, Biggs *et al.* (1978) reported a correlation with the Zung Scale of 0.69, with differences at severity levels. Toner *et al.* (1988) reported a similar correlation against psychiatric judgements ($r = 0.65$).

Kutner *et al.* (1985) reported that the scale's large number of disease items led to an exaggerated score. Gurtman (1985) has criticized the scale for containing items that are inappropriate for use with elderly people as they are age-related (e.g. 'I find it easy to do the things I used to'). He pointed out that the scale items were not empirically evaluated or screened prior to their inclusion in the test, which leads to problems with content validity (inadequate item coverage) and poor discriminant validity.

The instrument was designed to be unidimensional, although a factor analysis by Morris *et al.* (1975) confirmed two dimensions: agitation and self-satisfaction. Blumenthal's (1975) factor analysis of the scale yielded four sub-scales: a well-being index, a depressed mood index, an optimism index and a somatic symptoms index.

The validity and sensitivity of the Zung Scale is in doubt. While the initial validation studies were reported to be satisfactory (Zung 1965), Downing and Rickels (1972) reported that the Scale failed to distinguish between depressed and non-depressed psychiatric patients. Cross-cultural applications have been reviewed by Naughton and Wiklund (1993).

Reliability

There is little information on the reliability of the scale. Zung (1986) reported split-half correlations of 0.92. Knight *et al.* (1983) reported a coefficient of 0.79. Kaszniak and Allender (1985) suggest that it is unsuitable for use with elderly people because of the large number of somatic items.

It is popular because it is short and easy to complete. Zung (1972) has developed an observer-rated scale to complement the Zung Scale, although Thompson (1989a) – in line with most reviewers of the scale – reports that it has no advantages.

STATE–TRAIT ANXIETY INVENTORY (STAI)

Anxiety has traditionally been viewed as taking two forms: the state form (transitory feelings of fear or worry) and the trait form (the stable tendency to respond anxiously to stressful situations, or proneness) (Chaplin 1984). The STAI was developed in the 1960s, and revised in 1983 (Spielberger *et al.* 1983). It measures in-built tendency to anxious response and current feelings of anxiety. It enables the investigator to distinguish between the transitory (state) and dispositional (trait) types of anxiety.

The pre-1983 versions of the STAI are known as Y1 and Y2 and the revised 1983 versions are known as X1 and X2. The STAI was developed from an item pool of 177 questions taken from existing anxiety scales. These were subjected to various tests to ensure acceptable levels of consistency and content. This was repeated in order to develop the items for 'state' and the items for 'trait'. Extensive testing of items was carried out, largely on college students (n = 5000+). The final version was subjected to item and factor analyses.

Content

The STAI consists of 20 items for measuring trait anxiety and 20 items for measuring state anxiety (Spielberger *et al.* 1983). The STAI is printed on a single sheet, with the state-anxiety scale on one side and the trait-anxiety scale on the other. Each state item is rated on a 4-point intensity scale, from 'not at all' to 'very much so'. Respondents are asked to blacken the circle of the appropriate response to indicate how they feel 'right now'. Each trait item is rated on a 4-point frequency scale, from 'almost never' to 'almost always'.

Administration and scoring

The instrument is self-administered, and takes less than 10 min. to complete. The state-anxiety scale should be administered first to avoid bias from the anxiety arising from test conditions. One score reflects the current level of state anxiety with scores between 20 and 80; high scores reflect greater levels of anxiety. The other score indicates the current level of trait anxiety, and also ranges from 20 to 80; high scores indicate more anxiety. The items are simply summed to obtain the scores, although the coding of some items requires prior reversal. A manual is available for purchase, and this includes a computer program for analysis written in Statistical Analysis Systems (SAS).

Children

There is a version of the STAI for children, which is regarded as one of the best available for research purposes (Walker and Kaufman 1984). It has the same 20:20 item format for trait and state as the adult version, and has good results for reliability and validity; it does depend on reading ability (Spielberger *et al.* 1973, 1983; Walker and Kaufman 1984).

An example of a state scale item is that children are asked about the presence of feeling upset ('I feel . . . very upset/upset/not upset'), and an example of a trait scale item is the indication of frequency of occurrence of behaviours such as sweaty hands ('My hands get sweaty') and worry ('I worry about school').

Examples from the STAI

Form Y1

1 I feel calm
3 I am tense
6 I feel upset
11 I feel self-confident
17 I am worried

Not at all (1) / somewhat (2) / moderately so (3) / very much so (4)

Form Y2

21 I feel pleasant
23 I feel satisfied with myself
29 I worry too much over something that really doesn't matter
30 I am happy
37 Some unimportant thought runs through my mind and bothers me

Almost never (1) / sometimes (2) / often (3) / almost always (4)

Validity

The testing of the original scale for construct validity against other anxiety scales produced correlations of between 0.52 and 0.80, with the lower correlation probably reflecting weaknesses in one of the other scales. It correlates well with other tests of personality. The scale is able to distinguish between normal adults and different groups of psychiatric patients (e.g. schizophrenia, anxiety reaction); and, in support of its construct validity, the STAI-state showed higher mean values in stressful situations than in neutral or relaxed situations (Spielberger *et al.* 1983; Chaplin 1984). In a study of 180 randomly sampled people living in Stockholm, Forsberg and Bjorvell (1993) reported that the STAI-state was significantly and negatively associated with reported health symptoms and the Rand Health Perceptions Battery (Ware 1976). It would be expected that the better the health and perception of health, the lower the rated anxiety. In a review of the scale evidence, Chaplin (1984) concludes that the measure of state anxiety is stronger (in terms of validity) than the measure of trait anxiety.

Reliability

The alpha coefficient has been reported to be high for both state ($r = 0.93$) and trait ($r = 0.90$) anxiety, indicating internal consistency. Test–retest correlations with college students at intervals from 1 h to 104 days showed stability for the trait scale (0.65–0.86), but less so for the state scale (0.16–0.62), although lower repeatability of the state scale would be expected as it measures responses to transient situations (Spielberger *et al.* 1983). Factor analyses with 2000+ students and Air Force recruits confirmed the scale's homogeneity.

There are several other measures of anxiety, although they are generally used less often in relation to clinical research (see review of anxiety scales by Thompson 1989b). The STAI is one of the most widely used measures of anxiety in psychological and clinical research.

PROFILE OF MOOD STATES (POMS)

The Profile of Mood States (POMS: McNair *et al.* 1971, 1992) measures mood by a list of adjectives not symptoms (which could reflect physical problems), and includes a measure of elevated well-being. It was developed from a literature review, and a series of factor analytic studies of mood state (McNair *et al.* 1971). Items were discarded after each factor analysis until the list of 65 items was finalized. It was originally developed to assess mood in psychiatric out-patient attenders.

Content

The POMS is a 65-item measure of present mood state (disturbance). It allows for a total score and sub-scale scores for six monopolar dimensions of affect or mood: tension–anxiety, depression–dejection, anger–hostility, vigour–activity, fatigue–inertia and confusion–bewilderment (McNair *et al.* 1971). It is self-administered, and is a popular scale among psychologists assessing mood change in experimental studies, in studies of the effects of drug treatments and among clinicians, including oncologists. It has been widely used in order to assess the psychological status of cancer patients before, during and after treatment and enables comparisons to be made across disease and treatment types.

Respondents rate 65 adjectives on a 5-point intensity scale, in terms of how they have been feeling during the past week (where 0 = not at all and 4 = extremely). Except for vigour/activity, the higher the score, the greater the mood disturbance/more distress (Derogatis 1986). The scale is contained on a single sheet. The time references for rating vary. For example, respondents are asked to rate their feelings 'during the past week including today' or 'rate your feelings during the last half hour'.

Administration and scoring

The scale is self-administered. Raw scores are converted to scaled scores for each of the six factors. These can be analysed by sub-scale or summed to give a total mood disturbance score. Because of the time reference variation in response choices, some researchers treat the scale cautiously and do not calculate sub-scale or total scores, but simply calculate average score per item (Peterson and Headen 1985). A manual is available (McNair et al. 1992).

Alternative version

Lorr et al. (1982) have developed a new 72-adjective POMS to assess bipolar mood states: composed–anxious, agreeable–hostile, elated–depressed, confident–unsure, energetic–tired, clear headed–confused. A 4-point scale is used: 0 = feeling 'much unlike this', 1 = 'slightly unlike this', 2 = 'slightly like this' and 3 = 'much like this'. A manual for the bipolar version of POMS is available commercially, which also lists population norms for the sub-scale scores, but not the total scores. This is an alternative to the 65-item POMS, not a replacement.

Short version

The POMS Short Form consists of 30 items and the same six scales as the long version (McNair et al. 1992). A briefer, but less often used, version of the scale has also been developed, which contains 11 items from the original instrument. Examples of items include: blue, discouraged, unhappy. The scoring is the same: 0 = not at all, 1 = a little, 2 = moderately, 3 = quite a bit, 4 = extremely. The 9

anxiety and 15 depression 5-point adjective ratings of the POMS are frequently used alone. Respondents are asked to mark the space (code) that best describes how they have been feeling 'during the past week including today'.

Examples from the 65-item POMS

Tension–anxiety

　2　Tense
　10　Shaky

Depression–dejection

　5　Unhappy
　35　Lonely

Vigour–activity

　7　Lively
　51　Alert

Fatigue–inertia

　4　Worn-out
　40　Exhausted

Not at all (1) / a little (1) / moderately (2) / quite a bit (3) / extremely (4)

Examples from the 72-item POMS

　1　Composed
　2　Angry
　3　Cheerful
　17　Nervous
　31　Energetic
　35　Powerful
　38　Bad tempered
　64　Inadequate

Much unlike this (0) to much like this (3)

Profile of Mood States (McNair et al. 1979). Reproduced with permission of EDITS, P.O. Box 7234, San Diego, CA, 92167, USA.

Validity and factor structure

Jenkins et al. (1983a, 1983b) used POMS, along with other scales, to evaluate the outcome of 318 patients undergoing coronary artery bypass surgery, and reported that the depression, fatigue and vigour sub-scale scores improved post-surgery.

Conn *et al.* (1991) used POMS, alongside other scales, in a study of 197 adults 1–2 years after their first myocardial infarction (MI), and reported that it was sensitive to age differences (older people had poorer scores). McNair *et al.* (1971) reported adequate test–retest reliability scores, and construct, concurrent and factorial validity for the POMS (McNair *et al.* 1971). However, use of its energy–fatigue sub-scales, while having good internal consistency, does not always demonstrate good discriminant validity (Reddon *et al.* 1985). Components analysis of the fatigue–inertia and vigour–activity (two of the six POMS scales) sub-scales has confirmed their factor structure (Norcross *et al.* 1984).

The authors report good validity for the six-factor structure of POMS, based on six independent factor analytic studies (McNair *et al.* 1992), although this still needs to be confirmed on other types of population (Peterson and Headen 1985). The manual provides these details, and also gives evidence of the scale's construct validity by providing evidence of its correlation with a number of other scales measuring emotional disturbance.

It has been widely used with cancer patients, and reliability, validity and sensitivity have been tested and norms provided for cancer patients (McNair *et al.* 1971; McCorkle and Quint-Benoliel 1983; Cassileth *et al.* 1985; Cella *et al.* 1987, 1989). Cella *et al.* (1989) tested it on 923 recently diagnosed cancer patients. The POMS scores were significantly different for the cancer patients in comparison with norms for other population groups, and Cella *et al.* advised investigators to use their norms for making comparisons with cancer patients. It correlates well with LASA mood and anxiety items (Rieker *et al.* 1992). It appears to have convergent validity. For example, Levy *et al.* (1989) reported that, using POMS, patients with breast cancer who chose lumpectomy as their treatment were more depressed, confused and angry at 3 months after the procedure than women who underwent mastectomy. They were also more distressed than women who had been randomly assigned to lumpectomy. This confirms other research on breast cancer – the psychological well-being of women who choose their treatment is affected in a complex way. A study of 159 patients with stage D cancer of the prostate, from 13 hospitals in the USA treated surgically or medically, showed POMS to be

sensitive to improvements in condition at 3 month follow-up. It showed an improvement in psychological status among those treated with goserelin acetate but no change in the group treated with orchiectomy (Cassileth *et al.* 1992). McNair *et al.* (1992) review several studies supporting the concurrent and construct validity of the POMS in a range of fields from studies of mood disturbance in cancer patients to studies of sports medicine.

Peterson and Headen (1985) have criticized the specificity of the scale in relation to the meaning of the different factor patterns – for example, the manual does not clarify how a subject profile should be interpreted if it has high scores on depression, anxiety and anger, and low scores on other domains (e.g. vigour and confusion).

Reliability

Data on test–retest reliability were initially obtained by the scale developers from a large psychiatric out-patient sample at 20 days retesting. The test–retest reliability coefficients were 0.70 for tension–anxiety, 0.74 for depression–dejection, 0.71 for anger–hostility, 0.65 for vigour–activity, 0.66 for fatigue–inertia and 0.68 for confusion–bewilderment. As it aims to measure present mood, it is sensitive to short-term changes in mood. This confounds the interpretation of test–retest data. Internal consistency coefficients of 0.90–0.92 for anxiety and 0.95 for depression have been reported (McNair *et al.* 1971). These results were confirmed by later studies of the reliability and validity of the scale (Reddon *et al.* 1985; McNair *et al.* 1992).

In sum, it appears to be a valid and solid measure of mood state and was recommended for use by Weckowicz (1978) and Peterson and Headen (1985), although the latter authors do caution about its use, in particular that it does not contain any items which check for social desirability bias or lying. This is thought to be problematic as the scale is easy to fake (or answered to avoid exposure).

SCALES FOR CHILDREN

Psychiatric screening and symptom scales

Some of the depression scales reviewed here have been adapted for use with children. The use of structured assessments of the psychiatric status of children and adolescents has developed rapidly over the last two and a half decades. These require a specialist knowledge of what is appropriate for each age group and reading ability group. A fairly wide range of depression scales for children exists (see Keyser and Sweetland 1984, 1985a, 1985b, 1988). One example has been reviewed above – the Center for Epidemiological Studies Depression Scale for Children (19-item and 4-item versions) (Radloff 1977; Fendrich et al. 1990). The scales available have been reviewed by Angold (1989) and Keyser and Sweetland (1984, 1985a, 1985b, 1988). Fuller reviews of depression and anxiety scales are given by Thompson (1989a, 1989b) and Shaver and Brennan (1991). A limited selection of different diagnostic tools for detecting depression in childhood has been reviewed and compared by Kronenberg et al. (1988). Scales for measuring psychopathology in children have been reviewed by Conners (1973), and other diagnostic and behavioural scales for use with children and adolescents have been reviewed by Angold (1989).

Adaptive behaviour, maladjustment and the quality of relationships

Several scales for children also assess adaptive behaviour, maladjustment and the quality of relationships. Lists of available scales, including educational ability scales and intelligence tests, can be obtained from the various test corporations and distributors (e.g. NFER-Nelson in the UK and the Test Corporation in the USA). Potentially useful scales which require further testing for their psychometric properties include the Paediatric Symptom Checklist, which is a one-page, 35-item parent-completed questionnaire that screens school-age children for psychosocial dysfunction (Jellinek and Murphy 1988), and the Newcastle Adolescent Behaviour Screening Questionnaire, which focuses on the mid-adolescent phase of development and is completed by teachers (Place et al. 1987).

Conclusion to Part I

Studies of the outcome of physical diseases and conditions, and studies of psychological morbidity, commonly use one of the several available self-report symptom scales. These are frequently used as quality of life indicators per se, although they only cover one domain of quality of life (e.g. anxiety and depression). Among the most popularly used self-report scales in the USA are the Center for Epidemiological Studies Depression Inventory (Radloff 1975, 1977), the Symptom Checklist-90 (Derogatis et al. 1974b) and the Symptom Rating Test (Kellner and Sheffield 1973). In the UK and Europe, popular scales include the General Health Questionnaire (Goldberg 1972), the Beck Depression Inventory (Beck et al. 1961), the Zung Self-Rating Scale (Zung 1965), the State–Trait Anxiety Inventory (Spielberger et al. 1983) and the Profile of Mood States (McNair et al. 1971). The latter two instruments are popular in studies of physical conditions (e.g. cancer and heart disease). The Hospital Anxiety and Depression Scale (Zigmond and Snaith 1983) is becoming increasingly popular for measuring the outcome of physical conditions, due to its omission of somatic items, although further testing is required of its reliability and validity.

PART II: QUALITY OF LIFE INSTRUMENTS

CONDITION-SPECIFIC QUALITY OF LIFE SCALES

For many patients with psychiatric diagnoses, psychological symptoms may fluctuate, while the social handicap remains fairly constant (Heinrichs et al. 1984). With improvements in medication and control of symptoms, and the emphasis on rehabilitation, prevention and community care there is an increasing interest in measuring impaired social, psychological and instrumental (activities of daily living) functioning. There is a large literature on scales of psychological and social functioning, covering not just symptomatology (Wing 1992), but social behaviour and role performance (Wykes and Hurry 1991), environmental restriction (Wykes et al. 1982), users' and carers' attitudes (Wykes 1982; Brewin et al. 1990) and community care needs (Brewin and Wing 1989; Team for Assessment of Psychiatric Services 1990). Some of these are called quality of life scales, and these are reviewed here, along with scales that assess need, due to the similarity of their domains, although they are based on different conceptual frameworks. Scales with other labels, but which overlap considerably with quality of life scales and tap some of the same domains (e.g. role functioning and behaviour), are reviewed in the next section.

QUALITY OF LIFE SCALE (QLS)

This scale, together with Lehman's (1983) Quality of Life Interview (see next section), is one of the most widely used scales with schizophrenic patients in the USA. It was developed by Heinrichs *et al.* (1984). The scale is applicable to patients in the community rather than in-patients. It has been used for people with schizophrenia, although its authors suggest that it can be used across a range of diagnostic groups (e.g. chronic affective illness or personality disorders). It is limited to the perceptions of the patient, justified by the authors' argument that while different perspectives may conflict, there is no evidence that the patient's perspective is not valid. However, it is also dependent on the interviewer's assessments.

Content

The scale provides information on symptoms and functioning over the previous month. It is a 21-item scale rated from a semi-structured interview designed to assess deficit symptoms. It incorporates multiple aspects of the deficit state into a single instrument by measuring the internal state and role performance (and thus allows for interpretation of performance). The scale items were derived from consideration of important manifestations of the deficit syndrome in schizophrenia, and can be categorized as intra-psychic foundations (items 13–17, 20, 21), interpersonal relations (1–8), instrumental role (9–12) and common objects and activities (18, 19). The 21 items are household, friends, acquaintances, social activity, social network, social initiative, withdrawal, sociosexual, occupational role, work functioning, work level, work satisfaction, sense of purpose, motivation, curiosity, anhedonia, aimless inactivity, commonplace objects, commonplace activities, empathy and emotional interaction.

Intra-psychic foundation items are based on

clinical judgements about the intra-psychic elements in cognition, conation and affect (the patient's sense of purpose, motivation, curiosity, empathy, ability to experience pleasure and emotional interaction are assessed). Interpersonal and instrumental role functioning are derived from these bases. Deficits in these areas are expected to be reflected in impairments measured by the other three categories. Interpersonal relations measures interpersonal and social experiences, and includes judgements about the capacity for intimacy, active *vs* passive participation, and avoidance and withdrawal tendencies. The instrumental role category measures the role of worker, student or housekeeper/parent. The extent of functioning is rated, and judgements are made about the level of accomplishment, amount of under-employment, and role satisfaction. The objects and activities section measures social activity, taking into account the context (e.g. physical illness leading to reduced social contacts cannot be perceived as reflecting increased deficit symptomatology).

Administration and scoring

It is intended to be administered by a trained clinician, and takes 45 min to complete. Each item has three parts: a brief descriptive statement to focus the interviewer on the judgement to be made, a set of suggested probes, and a 7-point interval scale with descriptive anchors for every other point to be used by the interviewer to judge the patient's functioning in each area. The interviewer is instructed to probe each item until he or she has an adequate basis for making assessments. The codes vary, but the high end of the scales (5 or 6) reflects normal/unimpaired functioning, and the low end (0 or 1) reflects severe impairment of the function being measured.

Examples from the QLS

2 Rate intimate relationships

This item is to rate close relationships with significant mutual caring and sharing, with people other than immediate family or household members. Exclude relationships with mental health workers. Suggested questions:

● Do you have friends with whom you are especially close other than your immediate family or the people you live with?

- Can you discuss personal matters with them?
- How many friends do you have?
- How often have you spoken with them recently, in person or by 'phone?
- What have these relationships been like?
- Can they discuss personal matters with you?

0 virtually absent
1
2 only sparse intermittent relations
3
4 some consistent intimate relations but reduced in number or intensity; or intimacy only present erratically
5
6 Adequate involvement; intimate relationships with more than one other person

6 *Rate social initiatives*

This item is to rate the degree to which the person is active in directing his or her social interactions – what, how much and with whom. Suggested questions:

- Have you often asked people to do something with you, or have you usually waited for others to ask you?
- When you have got together with friends, who decides what to do?
- When you have had an idea for a good time, have you sometimes missed out because it's hard to ask others to participate?
- Have you contacted people by 'phone?
- Have you tended to seek people out?

0 social activity almost completely dependent on initiatives by others
1
2 occasional social initiative, but social life significantly impoverished due to pattern of social passivity, or initiative limited to immediate family
3
4 evidence of some reduction by social initiative, but with only minimal adverse consequences on plans, both short- and long-range.

Validity and factor structure

The scale was tested on 111 recently discharged in-patients with a diagnosis of schizophrenia which satisfied the requirements of the Research Diagnostic Criteria (Spitzer *et al.* 1975b). A factor analysis of the items, carried out separately for men and women, yielded results compatible with the conceptual model on which the scale is based.

Reliability

Inter-rater reliability was tested using three raters with 24 of the 111 patients, and intra-class correlations ranged from 0.61 to 0.98, with percentage agreements ranging from 25 to 83 per cent. Further testing of five raters with 10 patients gave similar results ($r = 0.56$–0.94 for items; $r = 0.84$–0.94 for categories). Intra-class correlations between the categories and for the total were: intra-psychic foundations 0.91; interpersonal relations 0.94; instrumental role 0.97; common objects and activities 0.94; and the total score 0.94.

This is a popular and fairly comprehensive scale, tapping many of the relevant domains of quality of life. Further work is required to test the psychometric properties of the scale, but it is a promising development.

LEHMAN QUALITY OF LIFE INTERVIEW

This is an interview for the chronically mentally ill developed by Lehman *et al.* (1982) and Lehman (1988). It reflects a conceptual model based on personal characteristics, objective quality of life indicators and subjective quality of life indicators, all of which constitute global well-being. The schedule assesses the life circumstances of people with severe mental illnesses in terms of what they actually do and experience (objective quality of life) and their feelings about these experiences (subjective quality of life or life satisfaction).

The items were selected on the basis of literature reviews. Initially, eight life domains were selected: living situation, family relations, social relations, leisure, work, finances, safety and health. Subsequently, a ninth domain (religion) was added. A tenth domain, neighbourhood, was added to some versions on the basis of open-ended questioning of patients (Lehman *et al.* 1993).

Content

The scale, which has over 200 items, is oriented towards current feelings of satisfaction, functioning and access to resources in order to limit recall bias. It can produce relatively rich information about life domains. The objective quality of life scales include: living situation (security, privacy, autonomy, cohesion, independence, influence, comfort, current length of stay); frequency of family contacts; frequency of social contacts; number of leisure activities; work (current employment status); frequency of religious activity; finances (total monthly support, monthly spending money); safety (assaulted in past year, robbed in past year); health (perceived health status, amount of general/psychiatric care in past year). The subjective quality of life indicators include: general life satisfaction, and satisfaction with living situation, family relations, social relations, leisure, work, religious activity, finances, safety and health. The scale also uses Andrews and Withey's delighted–terrible scale to rate feelings about the domains of life included, and their ladder scale (with adapted questions).

Administration and scoring

The scale is interviewer-administered so as to avoid the difficulties experienced by some patients with self-completion scales. It takes about 45 min to administer. The interview is highly structured in order to minimize interviewer bias, and to enable its use by non-clinical interviewers. Some training in its use is required.

Different sections entail different scoring procedures. For example, the delighted–terrible scale uses a 7-point scale for responses (1 = terrible, 2 = unhappy, 3 = mostly dissatisfied, 4 = mixed, 5 = mostly satisfied, 6 = pleased and 7 = delighted). It is not possible here to detail the different coding and scoring procedures, but these are contained in the instruction pack available from the author.

Examples from the Lehman QLI

Overview

A The first question is a very general one.

1 How do you feel about your life as a whole? (Use the Delighted–Terrible (D–T) Scale)

1 = terrible, 2 = unhappy, 3 = mostly dissatisfied, 4 = mixed, 5 = mostly satisfied, 6 = pleased and 7 = delighted)

2 Here is a picture of a ladder. At the bottom of the ladder is the worst life you might expect to have. At the top is the best life you might expect to have (hand Ladder Scale to subject).

a) Where on the ladder would you put your life during the past month?

C1 Sheltered care environment scale (if the interview occurs in hospital, change 'residents' to 'patients')

3 Are the staff strict about rules and regulations?
10 Are residents taught how to deal with practical problems?
13 Are there a lot of social activities?
14 Are many new skills taught here?
20 Is it sometimes very noisy here?

YES/NO

3 Now look again at the D–T Scale and answer the following (hand subject the D–T Scale). How do you feel about:

1 The food here?
4 The rules here?
5 The amount of influence you have in what goes on here?
8 The privacy you have here?

1 = terrible, 2 = unhappy, 3 = mostly dissatisfied, 4 = mixed, 5 = mostly satisfied, 6 = pleased and 7 = delighted

Section F: Leisure activities

Now let's talk about some of the things you do with your time. Which of the things listed in this sheet have you done during the past week? Please say 'yes' or 'no'.

1 Went for a walk
2 Went to a movie or play
5 Went to a restaurant or coffee shop
6 Went to a bar
12 Worked on a hobby

Section K: Health

11 How do you feel about the following (use the D–T Scale):

1 Your health in general?
2 The medical care available to you if you need it?
4 The chance you have to talk with a therapist about your thoughts and feelings when you want to?

1 = terrible, 2 = unhappy, 3 = mostly dissatisfied, 4 = mixed, 5 = mostly satisfied, 6 = pleased and 7 = delighted

Section M: Closing questions

3 Can you think of one thing you'd like to change in your life . . . something that would make your life better?

Variations

Rand's modifications

The Delighted–Terrible Scale satisfaction items in relation to living situation, overall life satisfaction, satisfaction with finances, social life and health were used in a study of hospital recidivism carried out by Sullivan (1989) at the Rand Corporation in California, with minor wording modifications (see below). Respondents pick an answer to depict how they feel about certain things.

Examples from the Rand version of the QLI

How do you feel about your life as a whole?

How do you feel about:

- the living arrangements where you live?
- the privacy you have where you live?
- the amount of freedom you have where you live?

- how much money you get?
- how much money you have to spend for fun?

- your health in general?
- your physical condition?
- your mental or emotional well-being?

- the amount of fun in your life?
- the way you spend your free time?
- the amount of friendship in your life?

   1 = terrible, 2 = unhappy, 3 = mostly dissatisfied, 4 = mixed, 5 = mostly satisfied, 6 = pleased and 7 = delighted

---

Crosby's adaptation of the scale

Another adaptation of the scale was made by Crosby and Barry in an evaluation of resettlement into the community in North Wales. The Quality of Life Schedule used was adapted from Lehman *et al.* (1982). The initial studies indicated that sizeable amounts of non-response to the open-ended questions are experienced. Crosby (1990) first assessed quality of life among psychiatric in-patients who were subsequently discharged into the community and followed up at various intervals. This was within a larger evaluation study of resettlement. Subjective and objective quality of life were measured using patient reports, and checked for (objective measures) with staff and documentation. Sixty-two clients were studied in relation to quality

of life. In addition, Crosby used a global life satisfaction rating (satisfied/dissatisfied) and also asked clients to assess their satisfaction (satisfied/dissatisfied) in relation to their living situation, social relations, family relations, leisure, finance, work, religion, safety and health.

Interviewers sometimes reported that clients had resigned themselves to their present situations and had lowered their expectations accordingly. Crosby also used a number of open-ended questions to explore their perceptions of what was important in their lives, including sources of enjoyment, unhappiness, personal aspirations and hopes. The data in relation to in-patients are revealing. In relation to the question 'What is the most important thing to you in your life?', 27 per cent of the respondents did not reply, and a further 24 per cent said that they did not know or said 'nothing'. Among those who did respond, the domains most commonly mentioned included family, relationships and leisure activities. In reply to a question about what made them feel good, the most common responses related to smoking, eating and drinking (tea, coffee, etc.), followed by various leisure activities. Regarding the question about things that made them feel unhappy, 21 per cent failed to specify anything in particular. Most responses included reference to other residents and their habits/behaviour and to unpleasant aspects of hospital life. Few respondents replied or mentioned something in reply to the question about personal aspirations, but those who did respond most often mentioned leaving hospital.

The scale did have convergent validity. Crosby (1991) reported increases in expressed satisfaction post-discharge in relation to satisfaction with living conditions and medical treatment, a decrease in loneliness and an increase in reported social interactions. For further details of the battery of instruments used by Crosby and his colleagues in their further follow-up studies of the outcome of resettlement into the community, see Barry and Crosby (1993) and Crosby *et al.* (1993).

Another adaptation is the Lancashire Quality of Life Scale (Oliver 1991a, 1991b). This is a longer battery of scales and is reviewed separately.

Validity

Further testing of the Lehman QLI was carried out

against the Quality of Life Scale (Heinrichs *et al.* 1984), with 59 acute in- and out-patients with a diagnosis of schizophrenia. General Life Satisfaction from Lehman's QLI demonstrated low, but significant convergence with a related construct (Intra-psychic Foundations) from the Quality of Life Scale ($r = 0.26–0.38$). The scales relating to family and social relations on these two instruments showed generally moderate but significant correlations ($r = 0.23–0.75$). Test–retest correlations were moderate to high and ranged from 0.52 to 0.75.

Reliability

The Lehman QLI has been tested on three chronically ill 'board and care' populations in Los Angeles and New York (Lehman *et al.* 1982, 1986; Lehman 1983). Based on these studies of nearly 500 chronically ill psychiatric 'board and care' patients, in-patients and out-patients, the instrument was found to have satisfactory levels of reliability and validity. The internal consistency coefficients (Cronbach's alpha) ranged between 0.35 and 0.88 for each item, with most being above 0.70. One-week test–retest reliability coefficients were computed based on 45 of the patients ($r = 0.29–0.98$ for each item, with most being above 0.60). The correlations between the objective and subjective items ranged between -0.02 and 0.60, with most being weak or modest. These weaker correlations are consistent with the literature on associations between objective and subjective indicators (Andrews and Withey 1976).

Lehman (1988) recommended the use of psychiatric symptom measures, especially anxiety and depression, alongside the Quality of Life Interview. He concluded that chronically mentally ill patients can provide reasonably reliable information about their quality of life, although it is important to control for mental health effects on the quality of life data. This is probably the most widely used quality of life scale. A simplified version of the scale has been piloted by Peter Huxley and Joe Oliver in the Department of Psychiatry, University of Manchester (unpublished). Crosby (1990) criticized the scale for its inherent assumptions. The scale is based on a model of quality of life which integrates access to resources and opportunities, fulfilment of social

roles in multiple life domains, and expressed satisfaction with life in various domains, but access to resources is limited for hospitalized patients (Crosby 1990). Crosby and colleagues adapted the scale for use in a study of the outcome of patients resettled into the community, entitled the Quality of Life Schedule (Barry and Crosby 1993; Crosby *et al.* 1993). They reported that the Quality of Life items were able to distinguish between patients remaining in hospital and those who moved to the community (Crosby *et al.* 1993).

Lehman's scale is without doubt superior to other attempts to assess quality of life, although its length may lead to a large proportion of item non-response. It is one of the most popular scales of its type in the USA, and as pointed out above, has been adapted for use in other studies in the USA and UK.

LANCASHIRE QUALITY OF LIFE PROFILE

This instrument was developed by Oliver and co-workers (Oliver 1991a, 1991b; Huxley and Warner 1992; Oliver and Mohamad 1992) from existing British and American research instruments. It is based on Lehman's (1983) work and it retains eight of Lehman's life domains: health, social relations, law/safety, living situation, leisure, family, work and finances, and adds religion. It includes items on positive and negative affect and self-esteem. It was also derived from the measures used by Cantril (1965), Andrews and Withey (1976) and Campbell *et al* (1976) and is used to derive perceived quality of life. The Life Satisfaction Scale also includes a measure of global well-being (Andrews and Withey 1976).

Content

It includes objective and subjective indicators. Information is collected on personal details, work/education, leisure/participation, religion, finances, living situation, legal and safety, family relations, social relations, health, self-concept and global well-being.

Perceived quality of life was operationalized as a series of client judgements about objective life in each of the domains. The judgements were made using the Life Satisfaction Scale, which is a version of Andrews and Withey's (1976) Delighted–Terrible (D–T) Scale. This is a 7-point visual analogue scale, scored from low ('couldn't be worse') to high ('couldn't be better') with a variety of expressions in between ('displeased', 'mostly dissatisfied', 'mixed feelings', 'mostly satisfied' and 'pleased'). The interviewer also assesses the client's quality of life with a 10 cm visual analogue scale, the Uniscale (Spitzer *et al.* 1981).

Cantril's Ladder (Cantril 1965) is used to operationalize global well-being, together with items measuring happiness (Gurin *et al.* 1960). The client looks at the 10 cm ladder and marks an 'X' on it according to the degree to which their present life ranges from the 'worst' they could expect (point 1 on the scale) to the 'best' they could expect (point 9). It measures the degree to which life outcomes conform to the individual's expectations. The ladder has nine marked rungs for responses; Cantril's original scale had 11 (0 to 10).

Also included in the interview are two measures of psychological well-being: the 10-item Affect–Balance Scale (Bradburn 1969) and Rosenberg's 10-item Self-Esteem Scale. The Affect–Balance Scale contains two sections: negative affect (restlessness, boredom, depression, loneliness and upset) and positive affect (accomplishment, success, pride, interest and high spirits). The Self-Esteem Scale has two 5-item scales: positive self-esteem (high self-worth, good qualities, ability, positive attitude and self-satisfaction) and negative self-esteem (failure, lack of pride, lack of self-respect, uselessness and low self-worth).

Administration and scoring

The interviews take over 30 min. The quality of life domains are scored on a 7-point scale, with high scores indicating better quality of life. As can be seen from the description of the scale, several types of response forms and scoring systems for subscales are used. The package describing the content and scoring is available from the authors.

Examples from the Lancashire QLP

Section 4: Leisure participation

In the past fortnight, have you:

4.1 Been out to play or watch a sport?   Yes / no
4.4 Watched television or listened to radio?   Yes / no

How satisfied are you with (use life satisfaction scale):

4.6 The amount of pleasure you get from things you do at home?
4.7 The amount of pleasure you get from things you do outside your home?

Life Satisfaction Scale:
Can't be worse / displeased / mostly dissatisfied / mixed (about equally satisfied and dissatisfied) / mostly satisfied / pleased / can't be better

Section 12: Self-concept

How satisfied we are with ourselves is also a very important part of our lives. Do you agree that the following statements apply to you:

12.1   You feel that you're a person of worth.
12.3   All in all, you are inclined to feel that you are a failure.
12.6   You take a positive attitude toward yourself.
12.10   At times you think you are no good at all.

Yes / no / don't know

13.3 How happy has your life been overall?

(a) Very happy
(b) Pretty happy
(c) Not happy
(d) Don't know

Validity

The author felt that the instrument had face validity, and the significant and consistent correlations between the subjective general and psychological well-being items indicated that the instrument had construct validity (Cantril's Ladder, the Life Satisfaction Scale, the Happiness Scale, the Affect–Balance Scales and the Self-Esteem Scales had correlations in the various samples ranging from 0.24 to 0.63). Criterion validity was established by a three-stage hierarchical regression model using the Life Satisfaction and Delighted–Terrible Scale scores. The subjective well-being scores added significantly to their model, explaining half to two-thirds of the variance (Oliver 1991b).

In a study of 61 people who were residents of board-and-lodging schemes, group homes or residential hostels, all specifically catering for people with mental illnesses, the instrument was used along with the General Health Questionnaire.

Higher levels of psychiatric disorder were inversely correlated with global well-being (Spearman's $r = -0.50$) and with satisfaction in seven of the nine life domains (Oliver 1991b). In another study of 68 long-term psychiatric out-patients in Colorado, the scale was reported to be significantly, and inversely, related to total number of treatment contacts ($r = 0.47$). These results support the scale's convergent validity.

Reliability

Testing and scale development involved piloting with several samples totalling almost 1000 respondents in the UK and USA. Test–retest correlations ranged from 0.49 to 0.78 for life satisfaction. Inter–observer reliability correlations for the uniscale were modest at 0.44. In relation to perceived quality of life, mean inter-item correlations for life satisfaction were low (0.16–0.19), whereas Cronbach's alpha correlations were high (0.84–0.86) and split-half reliability coefficients were high (0.73–0.82). Mean inter-item correlations for the Affect–Balance Scale were relatively weak for the negative affect items ($r = 0.29$–0.32), with higher Cronbach's alpha ($r = 0.68$–0.70) and modest Guttman split-half coefficients ($r = 0.57$–0.64). Positive affect was stronger, with mean inter-item correlations of 0.33–0.37, alpha coeefficents of 0.71–0.75 and split-half coefficients of 0.61–0.70.

In relation to the Self-Esteem Scale, for negative self-esteem the mean inter-item correlations were 0.39–0.45, the alpha coefficients were 0.76–0.80 and the split-half coefficients were 0.73–0.76. Positive affect was more variable, with mean inter-item correlations of 0.38–0.53, alpha coefficients of 0.75–0.85, and split-half coefficients of 0.67–0.85. Further testing revealed more convincing evidence of reliability, with few correlations falling below 0.70 (Oliver 1991b).

It is a concise scale, although it ranks with Lehman's QLI and Becker and co-workers' QLI-MH in relation to its comprehensive coverage of quality of life domains. Results on the use of Oliver's scale to date indicate that the instrument can be successfully used in the USA and the UK (Huxley and Warner 1992). The authors have recently compiled a review of the instrument's psychometric properties (Oliver *et al*. in press).

SMITHKLINE BEECHAM QUALITY OF LIFE SCALE (SBQOL)

This is a scale developed in the UK based on a repertory-grid assessment (Dunbar *et al*. 1992; Stoker *et al*. 1992). It uses 23 predetermined constructs and three fixed elements: self now, ideal self and sick self. The authors argued that these distinctions recognize the subjectivity of quality of life assessment. Initially, on the basis of a literature review, 74 constructs covering ten domains of well-being were selected for study. Each construct was measured using a 10-point scale, the extremes of which were labelled with the positive and negative extremes of that construct. A street survey of 1000 volunteers in four areas in the UK was used for piloting. Principal components analysis and cluster analysis techniques were used to derive a subset of 28 constructs, which were combined to form the final instrument. The major domains defined by these constructs were psychic and physical well-being.

Content, administration and scoring

The scale has 23 VAS items covering sleeping, irritability, overwhelming problems, control over life, satisfaction with work, insecurity, physical mobility, hopefulness, desire to be alive, discomfort with self, pleasure from hobbies, worry, feelings of failure, coping at work, appetite, inferiority, energy, decision-making, helplessness, confidence, pain, worries about money and ability to maintain relationships. The scale was designed for self-completion. The respondent is presented with predefined elements and constructs: self now (i.e. experience at the present time), ideal self (i.e. experience in an imagined idealized state of well-being) and sick self (i.e. how one would feel as a person who is sick or unwell). Each construct is measured using a 10-point VAS scale, with the positive (0) and negative extremes (10) labelled at each end. Scores are summed. A computerized version can be obtained which contains all of the 28 original constructs, in contrast to the paper and pencil version which just contains 23 of the constructs.

Examples from the SBQOL

Physical well-being

I sleep well	☐☐☐☐☐☐☐☐☐	I sleep badly
I have reduced physical mobility	☐☐☐☐☐☐☐☐☐	I do not have reduced physical mobility
I am always full of energy	☐☐☐☐☐☐☐☐☐	I am lacking in energy
I experience physical pain	☐☐☐☐☐☐☐☐☐	I experience no physical pain
I have a good appetite	☐☐☐☐☐☐☐☐☐	I have a poor appetite

Locus of control

I feel in control of my life	☐☐☐☐☐☐☐☐☐	I do not feel in control of my life
I have no difficulty making decisions	☐☐☐☐☐☐☐☐☐	I have great difficulty making decisions
I feel helpless	☐☐☐☐☐☐☐☐☐	I do not feel helpless

Activities and interests

| I derive no pleasure from my hobbies | ☐☐☐☐☐☐☐☐☐ | I derive pleasure from my hobbies |

Validity

A study of the scale's reliability and validity was carried out by the authors with 129 patients presenting to their general practitioners with either major depression or generalized anxiety disorder, as defined by DSM-III-R. The investigators assessed patient outcome of treatment at 6 and 12 weeks. As well as the SBQOL, the investigators administered the Hamilton Depression Scale and the Hamilton Anxiety Scale, the Sickness Impact Questionnaire and the General Health Questionnaire. These scales provided evidence of construct and concurrent validity ($r = 0.33$–0.86). The scale's correlation with Eysenck's (1976) Personality Questionnaire was weak to modest ($r = 0.10$–0.47). The scale was sensitive to changes in patients' condition at 6 and 12 weeks.

Reliability

Reliability was assessed in the same study. Test–retest reliability coefficients were high ($r = 0.66$–0.83); internal consistency coefficients were also high ($r = 0.85$–0.95).

OREGON QUALITY OF LIFE SELF-REPORT QUESTIONNAIRE AND SEMI-STRUCTURED INTERVIEW RATING VERSION

These instruments were developed by Bigelow and colleagues (Bigelow *et al.* 1982, 1990, 1991a, 1991b, 1991c; Olson *et al.* 1991). The measures are based on a clearly stated theory of quality of life based on need and role. They were developed as outcome measures, specifically to assess the impact of psychiatric services on clients' quality of life.

A structured self-report questionnaire has been developed for use during interviews (Olson *et al.* 1991), as well as a semi-structured interview rating version, which includes ratings made by the interviewer from information obtained during the interview with the respondent (Bigelow *et al.* 1991b). The latter permits more interviewer discretion. Additional information can also be collected from significant others and professionals. The semi-structured instrument was developed with the awareness of the difficulties that can sometimes be experienced when asking chronically mentally ill people structured questions. The authors have reported that they found the semi-structured interview version easier to administer than the self-report structured questionnaire version (Bigelow *et al.* 1991a). A manual for this version has been produced by Bigelow *et al.* (1991b).

Content

The self-report questionnaire contains 263 items, and assesses satisfaction and performance in important domains represented by 14 scales:

- psychological distress scale (anxiety, depression, hostility and somatic disturbance);
- well-being scale (pleasure, optimism, calmness, and contentment);
- tolerance of stress;
- total basic need satisfaction (housing, food, income, transportation and medical care);
- independence;

- interpersonal interactions (including satisfaction);
- spouse role (the opportunity for affiliation, esteem, and other need satisfactions);
- social support (having people to share activities with and to rely on);
- work at home (domestic tasks);
- employability (skills required to obtain and keep a job);
- work on the job (attendance, cooperation);
- meaningful use of leisure time (creative or self-improving activities);
- negative consequences of alcohol use;
- negative consequences of drug use (problems with mood, health, control over behaviour and ability to perform social roles).

The semi-structured version contains 141 items in 15 quality of life domains, which cover housing, self- and home-maintenance, finances, employment, psychiatric medications, physical health, the meaningful use of time, psychological distress, psychological well-being and interpersonal functioning. Satisfaction of need and performance are included in assessments in the domains. Service items are also included in this version.

Administration and scoring

The self-report and the semi-structured scales are administered by a trained interviewer. The interview takes 30–40 min. Most items have 4-point response choices. With the interview version, items relating to services contain the codes: received service (1); received service, but inadequate (2); needed service, but didn't receive (3); and neither needed nor received service (4). The authors provide details of how these scores can be further combined to produce additional categories. In both versions, some item scores are reversed so that high scores reflect a better quality of life. Item scores are added within scales and transformed into a range from 0 to 100. Items can be analysed separately or sub-scales can be summed to produce sub-scale scores. The manual points out that as the scoring procedures have not been fully tested, there is flexibility for investigators to report the results in their own way.

Full details of the scale and scoring systems have been described by Olson *et al.* (1991) and Bigelow

et al. (1991b, 1991c) for the self-report and interview versions, respectively. Serious potential users can purchase the manuals from Bigelow.

Examples from the Oregon Scales: Interviewer rating version

Self- and home maintenance

Q.27 Do you cook your own meals?
Does anyone help?
How do you get your meals?

Subject's level of responsibility for cooking / providing meals for household or self:

Totally responsible / somewhat responsible / minimally responsible / not at all responsible / not applicable or unknown

Meaningful use of time

In the subject's daily life, how adequately are his or her following needs met?

What did you do: today? yesterday? this week?
Do you have places you go regularly?
Do you have any hobbies?
Do you do anything exciting?
Are you often bored?
What do you look forward to?

Q.108 Structuring of time:
Q.109 Productivity:

Very inadequately / inadequately / adequately / very adequately / not applicable or unknown

Psychiatric distress

Do you often feel tired? sad? excited? high?
Do you have trouble eating? sleeping?

Q.114 Rate subject's affective impairment:

Severely impaired / moderately impaired / slightly impaired / unimpaired / not applicable or unknown

Interpersonal domain

Who are the most important people in your life?
How often do you see them?
What do you do with them?
Do you have contact with your family?
How often?
Do you spend time feeling lonely?

When you are troubled is there anyone you can talk to?
Are there people who are supportive of you?
How adequately are the quality and quantity of the following types of support met?

Q.128 Information and advice:

Very adequately / adequately / inadequately / very inadequately / not applicable or unknown

---

Examples from the Oregon Scales: Self-report version

These questions ask about how you have been feeling in the past week. Pleasant and unpleasant feelings of several different kinds are covered.

PD-1 In the past week, how often have you felt very restless, unable to sit still, or fidgety?

All of the time / often / several times / none of the time

PQ-10 In the past week, how often have you found yourself really looking forward to things?

All of the time / often / several times / none of the time

These questions ask how you handle making decisions, dealing with conflict, asserting yourself, etc.

IN-2 In the past week, how did you find shopping, paying bills, preparing meals, and generally looking after your basic necessities?

Very easy / fairly easy / rather difficult / very difficult

IN-8 How often do you put off making important decisions until it is too late?

Always / often / occasionally / never

There are some things we share with family and friends; some things we can count on them for. These questions ask about your family and friends, as you see them now.

SS-3 How much would your family be of help and support if you were sick, or moving, or having any other kind of problem?

A great deal / a lot / a little / none

SR-3 In the last month, how much have you enjoyed your spouse's company?

A great deal / quite a bit / a little / not at all

Validity

The predictive validity of the structured questionnaire was demonstrated by its ability to discriminate between geographical areas (economically depressed *vs* other) and between clients undergoing different types of mental health programmes, and was sensitive to change in clients' condition (Bigelow *et al*. 1991a). The interviewer rating version was sensitive to outcome of care due to differences in service provision in a study of discharged patients, some of whom received intensive community services (Bigelow *et al*. 1991d).

Reliability

The structured questionnaire was tested in a 24-site study, which included 1154 pre-tests, 758 post-tests and 190 interviews with randomly sampled community residents. Internal consistency was good – Cronbach's alpha = 0.67–0.98, except with interpersonal interactions (0.05), independence (0.15) and meaningful use of time (0.17), where the correlations were weak (Bigelow *et al*. 1991a).

The semi-structured interview version was tested for reliability with six people with chronic mental disabilities, using six raters who participated in each interview. The raters agreed on between 58 and 100 per cent of their judgements. More than half of the items achieved more than 90 per cent agreement (Bigelow *et al*. 1990).

These are fairly comprehensive scales, tapping the main domains of quality of life. It is a promising development, although further testing of both the self-report questionnaire and the semi-structured interview is still required.

QUALITY OF LIFE INDEX FOR MENTAL HEALTH (QLI-MH)

This scale was recently developed by Becker *et al*. (1993). It is really a battery containing existing, and well-tested, scales which represent various domains of quality of life according to the literature. Additional items are also included. The index was initially designed for use in a drug trial of people with treatment-resistant schizophrenia. The item selection was theoretically driven, and based on existing well-tested health-related quality of life scales. The items were reviewed by a panel, which consisted of patients, their families, mental health professionals and university review groups.

Content

It assesses nine separate domains that together encompass quality of life. Each domain can be individually weighted depending on its relative importance to the respondents; thus the authors describe it as a 'patient-focused index'. Questions are addressed to the patient, the clinician and the family, when available. The patient-reported items form the core of the questionnaire. Items for the family (where available) and clinician to complete (using separate questionnaires) are used to supplement patient reports, and to examine discrepancies.

Some scale domains are entire scales developed by others. The nine domains of the index include: satisfaction levels for different objective quality of life indicators (10 questions); occupational activities (6); psychological well-being (12); physical health (12); social relations (5); economics (2); activities of daily living (24); symptoms (36); and goal attainment (6).

The life satisfaction items were derived from the items developed and validated by Andrews and Withey (1976). They cover the client's satisfaction with his or her living environment, housing, amount of fun, food, clothing and mental health services. Each satisfaction item is rated on an ordinal 7-point scale ranging from 'very dissatisfied' to 'very satisfied', and on a 5-point scale indicating importance ranging from 'not at all important' to 'extremely important'. A total score is summed, and sub-scale scores for each domain are summed.

The index also includes a global question for rating feelings about life as a whole. Responses are made on a 7-point scale ranging from 1 (very unhappy) to 7 (very happy). Six items relate to occupational activities: work, school or daytime activities (e.g. 'Do you feel you are working, or are in school . . . less than you would like; as much as you would like; more than you would like'). The emotional well-being items come from the Affect–Balance Scale (Bradburn 1969), which is a well-validated and frequently used scale of well-being. It includes separate assessments of positive and negative affect.

In addition to this scale, respondents are asked to rate their mental health on a scale ranging from excellent to poor, and how they feel about what they do for fun. Items on physical health include respondents' perception of their physical health over the past year, rated on a 5-point scale ranging from excellent to poor; another question asks about health over the past week. The activities of daily living items are the entire Life Skills Profile, which was developed and tested for its psychometric properties with good results by Rosen et al. (1989) for use with patients with schizophrenia. This was incorporated into the provider questionnaire. This section also includes Spitzer and co-workers' (1981) Quality of Life Index (see Chapter 2 for review). This was designed for use by clinicians, and was modified for patient completion. The Quality of Life Index consists of five questions with 3-point response choices, each scored as 0 ('activity essentially absent'), 1 ('activity partly present') and 2 ('activity fully present').

The family questionnaire also includes items on the amount of assistance required by the patients (respondents), and how family members feel about the amount of help they provide. Social relationships and social skills items include the entire International Pilot Study of Schizophrenia (IPSS) Scale (Strauss and Carpenter 1974) relating to type and frequency of social contact. Also included are two questions that ask respondents to rate the amount of support they have experienced from their relationships, and about perceived satisfaction with their social relationships. The economics items ask respondents about the adequacy of their financial support and about their satisfaction with, and the importance of, the amount of money they have.

The symptoms section includes the 24-item Brief Psychiatric Rating Scale, which was developed and tested by Overall and Gorham (1962; see also Overall 1974; Hedlund and Vieweg 1980). It is a brief, well-tested, and reasonably reliable and valid scale, although some psychometric properties are inevitably lost because of its brevity. It is one of the most widely used scales in research on schizophrenia. Also included are two additional global questions, one asking patients to rate the overall severity of their symptoms and another on the side-effects of anti-psychotic medication.

In relation to improvement, providers' assessments are based on open-ended questions for evaluating goals for improvement; these were also included in the family questionnaire. They were asked to specify the three most important goals for the patient's improvement. Two response scales are used: the first rates the relative importance of the goals from 1 ('not very') to 3 ('extremely important'); the second rates the extent to which it is felt that the goal has been achieved, from 1 ('not at all') to 3 ('completely achieved'). The family and provider questionnaires also contain comparable items on occupation, physical health, social relationships, activities of daily living, symptoms and goal attainment.

Administration and scoring

The scale was designed for self-completion, although the authors found that during testing some patients required assistance. The authors reported that clinicians took 10–20 min and the patients 20–30 min to complete the questionnaires. Becker *et al.* justify a structured, self-administered questionnaire with the argument that the bias due to patients' inability to complete questionnaires is untested and probably relates to a small proportion of people. The authors acknowledge that most investigators prefer third-party and/or semi-structure interviews with patients because they feel that people with severe mental illness cannot reliably complete questionnaires.

The sub-scale codes were described briefly above. Separate scores for each domain and a total score are calculated. Separate scores for the respondent (patient), clinician and family are calculated. For the existing scales that form part of the index, the original scoring methods of those scales are adhered to. For the total score, each item is rescaled on a common scale through a linear transformation, items within each domain are aggregated, and each of these domains is then aggregated to form the total score. The scale transformation is a common procedure among scale developers but it is based on the incorrect assumption that each scale is an interval scale.

Examples from the QLI-MH

Satisfaction

How satisfied are you with the way you spend your time?

Very dissatisfied / moderately dissatisfied / a little dissatis-fied / neither satisfied nor dissatisfied a little satisfied / moderately satisfied / very satisfied

Social relations

How do you feel about how you get along with other people?

Very dissatisfied / moderately dissatisfied / a little dissatis-fied / neither satisfied nor dissatisfied, a little satisfied / moderately satisfied / very satisfied

Activities of daily living

During the past week, have you:

● not been managing personal care and/or not leaving home or institution at all
● been requiring assistance for daily activities and transport, but performing very light tasks
● been self-reliant in daily tasks; using public transport or driving

Symptoms

Since you have been taking your medication, how have your symptoms been?

Substantially worse / much worse / somewhat worse / no change or same / somewhat better / much better / all better

Validity

The scale was initially tested as a whole on 40 patients and their clinicians at a local mental health centre, using patients with a diagnosis of schizophrenia who met the DSM-III-R criteria (Spitzer 1987). Some patients required assistance, the amount of which varied according to their degree of disorientation and their attention span. Three patients were unable to reliably or fully complete the questionnaire.

Becker *et al.* (1993) reported a correlation of 0.68 between the index and the global quality of life uniscale item, and a correlation of 0.98 between the index and the Spitzer Quality of Life (total) Scale (which contained the same items, and so this result should be viewed with caution). The correlations between the patient and clinician questionnaires were 0.57 and 0.50 for the total score and the global quality of life score respectively, and between the total clinical score and the Spitzer uniscale it was

0.79. In relation to construct validity, the investigators predicted on the basis of the literature that there would be little correlation between functional ability (activities of daily living) and psychiatric symptoms, and this was confirmed. No results for reliability and validity were reported for the family questionnaire.

The existing scales included in the index have already been tested for reliability and validity, with generally good results. The authors felt there were no known criteria variables against which they could test the entire index.

Reliability

Some testing for inter-scale and inter-item correlations were carried out by Becker *et al.* (1993). Inter-item correlations between each domain on the patient questionnaire ranged from 0.02 to 0.64, and between the clinicians' items they ranged from 0.16 to 0.73. Thus, while a number of items showed strong correlations, many were weak to moderate. Test–retest reliability was assessed by repeated administrations at 3–10 days with 10 out-patients with schizophrenia and their clinicians. The percentage matches between the scores ranged between 0.84 and 0.87 per cent.

This battery of items appears promising, but much more work needs to be carried out to test its psychometric properties and to further refine the scale where properties are weak. The advantage of the scale is the weighting of items according to their reported relative importance to the respondent, and the use of other well-tested batteries. After the Lehman QLI, this promises to be the next popular in relation to comprehensive coverage of quality of life domains.

INDEX OF HEALTH-RELATED QUALITY OF LIFE

This is a generic measurement scale, developed by Rosser *et al.* (1992, 1993). It is also known as the Health-Related Quality of Life Questionnaire. Although some of the questions have a psychiatric orientation, it was designed for use across all disease groupings (physical as well as psychiatric). The structure is hierarchical and multidimensional.

It was derived from a three-dimensional classification system from the original two-dimensional Rosser Index, which was based on disability and distress (Rosser and Watts 1972, 1978). Distress was divided into physical and emotional components to give the three dimensions of disability, physical discomfort and emotional distress. During development, 175 composite health states were valued; the dimensions of disability, discomfort and distress were subdivided into seven attributes – dependency, dysfunction, pain/discomfort, symptoms, dysphoria, disharmony and fulfilment. These in turn were subdivided into 44 scales. There are 107 descriptors with 225 descriptor levels between them. The descriptors were derived from the results of a questionnaire survey with a random sample of people in central London (sample size not given), interviews with professionals and others, and from literature reviews.

Content

The questionnaire begins with a broad question on whether health has caused any impairment to quality of life in the past week, categorized as none, mild, moderate, severe or extreme. The next section is on disability and asks respondents to select a description of their level of disability over the past week. More specific disability questions appear later in the questionnaire (the section topics are not grouped together) and relate to self-care (washing, dressing and feeding) and mobility (walking and travelling). The causes of disability are elicited, and use of services is asked about.

Discomfort and distress are separately rated on a 5-point scale, from none to extreme. Mental state, mood (e.g. single items on depression, anxiety and elation), sensory problems (e.g. sight, hearing) and body functions (e.g. incontinence) are elicited, as are various selective symptoms, ranging from disfigurement to eating disturbances (e.g. bingeing), communication impairments (e.g. speech) and items on social network and sexual functioning. There is a section on psychological feelings of fulfilment, with items ranging from feeling 'blamed' to 'loss of ambition', and one on attitudes to health, with items ranging from 'fighting' to 'disappointed'. A final item asks about perceived prognosis.

Values are attached to the health states which the instrument describes. Standard gamble techniques for states of 1 year's duration were used for this process, along with a six-stage category rating technique using a convenience sample of 40 people (Rosser *et al.* 1992). A single value for health-related quality of life was derived on a 0–1 scale, with 1 = no impairment and 0 = states equivalent to death.

Administration and scoring

Three versions of the scale are being developed: one for self-completion by the patient, one for completion by a trained observer and one for carers (relatives or friends). It has a five-level multidimensional classification system, and can also produce a unidimensional scale. Values are derived at each of the five levels through a multi-stage scaling process. Further details are given by Rosser *et al.* (1993).

Examples from the Index of Health-Related Quality of Life

Health-related quality of life

Has your state of health caused any impairment in your quality of life in the past week?

None / mild / moderate / severe / extreme

Distress

Which level of distress best describes the way things have been for you in the past week?

No distress
Slight distress
Moderate distress
Severe distress
Extremely distressed and/or actively suicidal

Occupational, social and family roles

In the past week, has your state of health impaired your ability to perform any of the following roles? If YES, please indicate . . .

- Main occupation, e.g. work, housework, study
- Other occupation(s), e.g. part-time job, housework
- Financial: providing income/financial resources
- Social: social activities, recreation, hobbies, holidays
- Family: family responsibilities and/or caring for dependents

No / mildly / moderately / severely / totally

Validity

Few data have been published on the instrument's reliability and validity as it is still being tested.

The authors have reported results from a study of 94 patients taking part in a psychotherapy trial after undergoing trauma (Rosser *et al.* 1993). A correlation of 0.65 was found between the instrument and the General Health Questionnaire (Goldberg and Hillies 1979). A correlation of 0.65 was found between the index and the symptom distress scale of the Symptom Checklist, the SCL-90 (Derogatis 1977).

Reliability

Rosser *et al.* (1993) reported good inter-rater reliability with Kendall's coefficient of concordance ($W = 0.89$) (details of study and sample size not given). Data are also needed on its applicability to samples of the general population.

PILOTING OF THE HEALTH OF THE NATION OUTCOME SCALES

The Department of Health in the UK has funded a major study to monitor the mental health of the nation, which is being carried out by Wing and colleagues at the Royal College of Psychiatrists' Research Unit in London. Health of the Nation (HoN) Outcome Scales have been developed on the basis of literature reviews and consultations with experts (Wing 1993). They have been designed for use as monitoring and outcome scales. They aim to be valid and reliable, brief and simple to use and score, usable in community, residential and institutional settings, sensitive to change and acceptable to users and carers. They will measure type and severity of health and social problems likely to be experienced by most people with mental disorders who are in contact with services.

Content

The scales currently being piloted include distressing or limiting subjective mental experiences (e.g. depression, anxiety, hallucinations and worry), with their immediate behavioural concomitants; deficits in basic functions (e.g. psychomotor slowness, cognitive and physical impairments), and their direct effects on personal functioning; behavioural problems that affect the individual and others (e.g. self-harm); environmental problems (e.g. housing, work, finance, social support and networks). Additional measures will include motivation and burden on carers (Wing 1993). Scales are being developed for use by professionals, with sections for completion by the user and carer. An overall scale for measuring incapacity is being used for piloting purposes, similar to the Global Assessment of Functioning of DSM-III-R (Spitzer 1987), although it relates only to ADL and has five anchor points. The scales are currently being tested and their likely final form has not yet been published.

TEAM FOR THE ASSESSMENT OF PSYCHIATRIC SERVICES (TAPS) MEASURES

The TAPS measures were developed for use by the research team assessing reprovision for psychiatric hospitals, specifically Friern Barnet and Claybury Hospitals, North East Thames Regional Health Authority (Leff 1991b, 1993). These measures are not labelled by their authors as quality of life measures, but as a battery of social, psychological and physical outcome measures. They do, however, tap most of the relevant dimensions of quality of life. The investigators developed the measures for the study, and used some existing scales, given the lack of a suitable and comprehensive battery (Anderson *et al.* 1993). The team of researchers aimed to measure the outcome of moving long-stay psychiatric patients into the community and their resulting quality of life. They therefore also included measurement of their opinions on their care and the degree of restrictiveness of their environment, as well as patients' social networks and the development of social links.

These scales, with some descriptive results, have been described by Leff (1991b, 1993). The TAPS study began in 1985 with about 900 patients, but study attrition brought the numbers participating down to 770 patients. The assessments on these patients took 2 years to complete. A lot of descriptive data have been reported, mostly at annual TAPS conferences organized by the investigators.

Content

The TAPS schedules contain over 500 questions. The measures included in the TAPS battery are:

1 *Present State Examination (PSE)* (Wing *et al.* 1974) (with the addition of two items on information from nursing staff about active psychotic symptoms to overcome the problem of patient denial of such symptoms). The PSE is a structured interview conducted with patients. It generates data relating to the previous month about a range of psychiatric symptoms, diagnostic information and the likelihood of being identified as a diagnostic 'case'. The scale produces a total score, a total negative features score, and sub-scores for delusions and hallucinations, behaviour and speech, specific neurotic features, non-specific neurotic features, and diagnostic group.

2 *Social Behaviour Schedule (SBS)* (Wykes and Sturt 1986) assesses social behaviour. The scale is answered by an informant and permits patients to be rated on a range of 20 problematic social behaviours covering two categories (communication problems and unsociable behaviours), and on 'other' items. Most items are rated on a 5-point scale, with the highest rating indicating a severe behavioural problem. A total social behaviour problem count is calculated (for each item score, 0 and 1 are recoded as 0, and 2, 3 and 4 are scored as 1 to give a total score of 0–20).

3 *BASIC Everyday Living Skills (BELS)*. This is a rating of the opportunity given to patients to undertake everyday tasks such as cooking, shopping and cleaning, and their performance of these. The scale produces a total score and items can be analysed separately (e.g. positive symptom items).

4 *Personal Data and Psychiatric History Schedule* (PDPH). This instrument collects sociodemographic data from medical notes and staff (e.g. ethnicity, primary diagnosis, length of stay, previous admissions).

5 *Physical Health Index (PHI)*. This extracts information from case-notes, as well as carer (e.g. staff) interviews, in relation to seven bodily systems – cardiovascular, respiratory, gastrointestinal, urogenital, locomotor, nervous and endocrine – and includes a rating of the level of disability and the level of medical and nursing care received. It also records problems with incontinence, immobility and dyskinesia (categorical data).

6 *Environmental Index (EI)*. This index was developed from existing scales for the study, and measures the degree of restrictiveness of the

patient's environment (it reflects institutional environment, but also asks about the community in relation to shops, launderettes, pubs, parks, day centres/hospitals). It is a measure of patients' opportunities for independent activity. A total score is calculated plus sub-scale scores for activity, possessions, meals, hygiene, rooms and services.

7 *Patient Attitude Questionnaire (PAQ)*. This questionnaire asks patients what they like/dislike about their caring environment; their desire to leave hospital or stay, and where they would prefer to live; helpfulness of medication; dislike of carers and present company; daytime occupation (categorical data). It was designed to assess attitudinal change during the transfer of patients from hospital.

8 *Social Network Schedule (SNS)*. The SNS is a measure of the quality and quantity of social contacts during the previous month and was designed for the study. Individuals are asked to name people they talk to regularly, who would be missed if not seen, who they would visit if they were separated, who is a friend and who can be confided in. The process can take up to an hour, as much in-depth probing is required to elicit the network structure. There is no equivalent scale for staff, as the researchers found that staff tended to over-report friendships between patients and under-reported out-of-ward contacts (Leff 1988). The scale produces scores for: total number of named social contacts in the last month number of social contacts named as friends; number of social contacts named as patients; number of social contacts named as professional staff; number of social contacts rated as active; number of social contacts rated as intermediate; number of social contacts rated as passive; intensity of network; social contacts with persons other than staff, patients, relatives, workmates or service contacts.

9 *Use of Community Facilities*. This lengthy schedule measures use of facilities such as day centres, community psychiatric nurses and general practitioners by discharged patients and permits a costing to be made by an economist.

Administration and scoring

Careful interviewer training is required at a recog-

nized centre. It is preferable that the interviewers are graduate psychologists or social scientists, as the interviews have to be administered, interpreted and coded with skill and care. Collecting all this information takes about half a day per patient.

The details of the scoring method of each scale are too lengthy to summarize here; full details can be purchased from the TAPS Team.

Examples from the TAPS Measures

Environmental Index

41 Are there shopping facilities available within . . .
42 Is there a pub within . . .
43 Is there a cafe within . . .
47 Is there a cinema within . . .

Response codes
(a) Walking distance without a main road to cross?
(b) Walking distance with one or more main roads to cross:
  (i)   with crossing or lights?
  (ii) without crossing or lights?
(c) One bus / tube / train journey without changing?
(d) Two or more buses / trains or changing on the underground?

Basic Everyday Living Skills

14 Shopping (clothes, shoes, personal, household items)

How independent is _____ in buying personal necessities other than food?

Opportunity rating
(i)   Open ward
(ii)   Locked ward but this particular patient is free to go out / or open ward but this particular patient has to inform staff if going out
(iii) Ward is locked to keep this particular patient in / or only allowed out with escort / or disabled and needs physical assistance

Performance rating
(a) Totally independent
(b) Partly independent. Has some assistance with more complex purchases (e.g. furnishing, furniture, etc.)
(c) Buys independently limited range of items (e.g. soap, cigarettes). Has help with other shopping (e.g. shoes). If no help given, evidence of neglecting needs or inappropriate purchase

(d) Shops with supervision only or relies on shop assistant for obtaining correct change even for simple purchases
(e) Does not purchase personal necessities at all

Social Network Schedule

E. *Confidant or not*
The respondent is asked whether the listed person is someone they confide in. Quite often this will need rephrasing as 'Are they someone you talk to about your personal worries/feelings?' If the respondent is only confiding the content of their delusions, this is also categorized as confiding, provided they are confiding to a selected few. If the respondent described the contact as a confidant and yet has already described him or her in terms of a passive or intermediate interaction, please go back to the section on level of interaction and reconsider with the respondent the amount of conversation that takes place.

Do you confide in . . .?
If you have a personal worry, do you share your feelings with . . . about it?

If they are a confidant: code 2
If they are not a confidant: code 1

Validity

Little information on the validity and reliability of the scales has been published (with the exception of existing scales, such as the PSE). Most of the published data are descriptive, although they can be used to support the battery's predictive validity.

One TAPS study analysed 278 patients who left hospital and matched them with an equal number of patients remaining in hospital. At follow-up, those who had left hospital had more diverse social networks and had more friends on the Social Network Schedule (although there was no change in the numbers of people in networks of either group, only in type of member), had more opportunities for autonomy (Environmental Index), were more likely to state during completion of the Patient Attitude Questionnaire that there was something they liked about their current placement and were more likely to find their medication helpful. The Social Behaviour Schedule also discriminated between the two groups of patients, indicating that subjects who were otherwise

clinically similar (this was confirmed by the PSE results) were more likely to leave hospital if they had fewer social behaviour problems. Both groups increased their scores over time, indicating an increase in social behaviour problems among both groups. The analyses of the Physical Health Index suggested that the more physically well subjects were more likely to be selected for discharge, although there was an increase in incontinence in both groups (Anderson *et al.* 1993).

Another TAPS study of 369 long-stay patients who were being resettled indicated that having a social network (as measured by the Social Network Schedule) – especially a large one – aided placement in the community (Dayson *et al.* 1992). A further study of the readmission rates of 357 previous long-stay patients showed that the PSE and the SBS were able to discriminate between those who were readmitted and those who remained in the community (the latter had higher levels of symptomatic and social behaviour disturbance) (Thornicroft *et al.* 1992).

Reliability

The TAPS measures have been used in a number of collaborative TAPS studies; for example, they were used in a study of patients (excluding those with senile dementia) occupying psychiatric beds for more than 6 months in City and Hackney Health District by O'Driscoll *et al.* (1990). Their work with long-stay patients also provided data on the validity and reliability of the Social Network Schedule (SNS). O'Driscoll *et al.* (1990) correlated scores on the SNS (patient-reported networks) with raters' observations of social behaviour and reported the inter-rater reliability coefficient to be $r = 0.95$. Correlations between the observed behaviour and the self-reports using the SNS items on network size and number of friends ranged from 0.54 to 0.74. Inter-rater reliability was also assessed. Independent exercises by these investigators using four raters with two patients, reported perfect agreement between all four raters in 94 and 99 per cent of cases; another patient was rated by five raters with 97 per cent perfect agreement (Dunn *et al.* 1990). Latent class analysis of the structure of the reported networks indicated the importance of non-verbal social contacts, and that patients may not have the same understanding as the investigators of the word 'confidant', which implies that data must be interpreted carefully (Leff *et al.* 1990).

An investigation of the reliability of the Social Behaviour Schedule (SBS) was carried out by members of the TAPS team across settings (community *vs* institution) and between informants (Dayson *et al.* (1990). These authors reported that hospital and community informants achieved a high level of agreement (the mean scores for hospital and community informants were 2.41 and 2.33, respectively; these were not statistically significant). There were also no significant differences between the informants' ratings of the individual items.

Thornicroft *et al.* (1993) assessed the reliability of the Patient Attitude Questionnaire with 43 long-stay patients (using the hospital version of the instrument) and four raters; one rater was used for test–retest reliability assessments at 6 months follow-up. The mean test–retest reliability value (kappa coefficient) was 0.51, and the average inter-rater value was 0.82. The authors concluded that the results demonstrated that long-term psychiatric patients are able to give clear and consistent views about their living arrangements.

An enormous amount of descriptive and outcome data have been reported from the TAPS studies (TAPS 1986 onwards; Leff 1988, 1993). In sum, population norms exist for the TAPS scales, and published data indicate that the TAPS instruments are able to discriminate between groups of patients on these dimensions. There is some limited published data on the scales' reliability and validity, but far more work is required and will no doubt emerge from the TAPS studies over the next few years.

GENERAL WELL-BEING SCHEDULE (GWBS)

This instrument, variously known as the General Well-being Schedule, the Psychological General Well-Being Index, or Schedule, is a measure of feelings of well-being or 'inner personal state' rather than of broader quality of life, but is often apparently used as a proxy measure of quality of life and outcome of medical care, and so is included here.

It is a concise, multidimensional measure of subjective feelings of well-being and distress. It was developed by Dupuy (1977; 1978) for use in the 1971 US Health and Nutrition Examination Survey (HANES I), and a modified version was incorporated into the Rand Health Insurance Experiment Mental Health Inventory (Brook *et al.* 1979a, 1979b). The Rand version is also increasingly popular. It was briefly reviewed by Bowling (1991) and will not be repeated here. Interested readers are referred to Brook *et al.* (1979a) and Stewart *et al.* (1992b).

Content

The initial instrument contained 68 items, although just 18 of these were used for the HANES (these were referred to as the General Well-Being Schedule). The most recent version has been reduced to 22 items. These items measure both positive and negative affect. It includes six domains of 3–5 items each: anxiety (e.g. bothered by nervousness; generally tense; anxious, worried, upset; relaxed, at ease *vs* highly strung; felt under strain, stress or pressure); depressed mood (e.g. felt depressed, felt downhearted and blue; sad, discouraged, hopeless); positive well-being (e.g. general spirits, happy, satisfied with personal life; interesting daily life; felt cheerful, light-hearted); self-control (e.g. in firm control; afraid of losing control; felt emotionally stable, sure of self); general health (e.g. bothered by illness, bodily disorders, or aches and pains; healthy enough to do things; concerned, worried about health); and vitality (e.g. energy, pep, waking feeling fresh, rested; felt active, vigorous *vs* dull, sluggish; felt tired, worn-out, used up). The time period of reference for questions is 'during the last month'.

Administration and scoring

This is a self-administered questionnaire, and takes about 12 min to complete. The first 14 questions have six different response choices, which are scored on a scale reflecting intensity or frequency from 0 (for the most negative response) to 5 (for the most positive response); four questions use a numbered visual analogue scale defined by adjectives at each end, ranging from 0 to 10. The range of scores is from 0 to 110 for the 14 questions, and for the sub-scales it varies from 0 to 15, 20 or 25. Overall or sub-scale scores can be used for analysis.

Scores of 0–60 reflect severe distress, 61–72 reflect moderate distress and 73–110 represent positive well-being.

Examples from the GWBS

5 Have you been under or felt you were under any strain, stress or presure? (DURING THE PAST MONTH)

Yes, almost more than I could bear or stand / yes, quite a bit of pressure / yes, some – more than usual / yes, some – but about the same as usual / yes, a little / not at all

6 How happy, satisfied or pleased have you been with your personal life? (DURING THE PAST MONTH)

Extremely happy, could not have been more satisfied or pleased / very happy / fairly happy / satisfied – pleased / somewhat dissatisfied / very dissatisfied

11 Has your daily life been full of things that were interesting to you? (DURING THE PAST MONTH)

All the time / most of the time / a good bit of the time / some of the time / a little of the time / none of the time

18 How DEPRESSED or CHEERFUL have you been? (DURING THE PAST MONTH)

Very   0 1 2 3 4 5 6 7 8 9 10   Very
depressed   cheerful

Variations

The GWBS has been adapted for use in the UK as a measure of outcome of depressive illness (the General Well-being Depression, GWB-D) by Hunt and colleagues (see Hunt and McKenna 1992, 1993; McKenna and Hunt 1992a). The English version of the questionnaire is almost identical, except for anglicization of the wording used for the 22 items that it contains on anxiety, self-control, positive well-being, depression, vitality and general health. The GWB-D asks respondents about their feelings over the past month. There are six response categories for each item, ranging from very positive to very negative.

Each sub-scale has been validated and the scale is associated with interviewers' ratings of depression, as well as with other instruments (see next section). The authors have also recently developed another indicator of quality of life in depression (see McKenna and Hunt 1992b). The Rand version was referred to earlier (Brook *et al*. 1979a).

Validity and factor structure

The GWBS has been reported to have good validity and reliability. It was reported to correlate moderately to very strongly ($r = 0.47$–0.90) with interviewers' ratings of depression and with various scales of anxiety and depression, such as the Zung (1965) Self-Rating Depression Scale (Fazio 1977; see review by Ware *et al*. 1979). National Center for Health Statistics 1978; the correlation between the GWB-D and the Center for Epidemiological Studies Depression Scale was 0.71 (Zonderman *et al*. 1989).

Edwards *et al*. (1978) reported that psychiatric patients achieved different scores on the scale in comparison with the national population norms from the HANES, and that it was sensitive to patients' progress. Kammann and Flett (1983) reported a correlation of $r = 0.74$ between the scale and their scale of general happiness and well-being.

Factor analyses of the HANES data have yielded three strong factors which explain 51 per cent of the variation: anxiety, tension and depression; health and energy; and positive well-being or life satisfaction (Wan and Livieratos 1977; Dupuy 1978). The six sub-scales of the schedule were also supported by multitrait and factor analysis (Ware *et al*. 1979). It is a psychometrically valid measure of depressive symptoms, and although it correlates with measures of clinical depression, it is not synonymous.

Reliability

Studies of students, the HANES and the HIS also afforded the opportunity to test the reliability of the GWBS. The test–retest reliability coefficients were reported to be 0.50–0.86, with variations according to the time period of retesting and the sample (Edwards *et al*. 1978; Monk 1981; see Brook *et al*. 1979a; 1979b). The internal consistency of the GWB-D was reported to be 0.78 among 2814 subjects in a large epidemiological survey in the USA (Zonderman *et al*. 1989). Monk (1981) also reported internal consistency coefficients of 0.93 on the basis of 6913 people from the HANES Survey.

A study of 195 college students by Fazio (1977) showed internal consistency coefficients of 0.91 for males and 0.95 for females, and inter-item correlations ranged from 0.16 to 0.72. Ware *et al.* (1979) reported three studies in which the internal consistency coefficients of the index were over 0.90, although Edwards *et al.* (1978) reported a lower coefficient ($r = 0.69$) for college graduates. In Fazio's study the coefficients were high (0.91 for males and 0.95 for females).

Although one sub-scale measures general health, the scale has the advantage of not including somatic items which may reflect psychometric morbidity. Population norms are widely available, and although the results of much of the early testing are unpublished, extensive reviews of the scale are available from the Rand Corporation (Brook *et al.* 1979a, 1979b). In sum, it appears to have excellent psychometric properties.

SCALES FOR ASSESSING NEEDS

Scales designed for assessing the need for psychiatric services overlap considerably with quality of life scales, although their aim is conceptually different. The measurement of human needs, and the extent to which these have been achieved, are the focus of both quality of life and assessment of need instruments. A number of the most well-known scales are presented below. Graham Thornicroft, at the Institute of Psychiatry in London, has recently developed the Camberwell Assessment of Need Questionnaires (clinical and research versions). These are likely to be extremely popular for the assessment of the needs of people with mental health problems. However, as the documentation is currently being compiled, it is not reviewed here. Interested readers can purchase the questionnaires, which are reasonably priced, from Dr Thornicroft. Outcome of health care is measured in relation to the quality of life of the individual, which includes the achievement of basic human needs (from housing to the maintenance of social relationships).

KEY INFORMANT SURVEY SCALES

This survey was designed to assess service need and delivery for people with chronic mental illness in several US cities, and was supplemented by using service utilization data, site visits, documentary evidence (e.g. annual reports, newspaper accounts) and analysis of organizational changes. The survey scales measure client needs and service adequacy and were designed for use with health professionals and clients (Goldman *et al.* 1992; Ridgely *et al.* 1992; Lehman *et al.* 1994; Morrissey *et al.* 1994). The instrument was developed on the basis of a literature review and an analysis of service goals, which were reviewed in order to identify the relevant domains of service interventions. The literature was also reviewed in order to inform the design and from which lists of survey items were developed.

It was designed to obtain performance ratings of local services from knowledgeable people in each study area. It therefore measures subjective perceptions of system capacity and performance. As the authors point out, there is no easy and reliable way of measuring service needs and adequacy of services (Ridgely *et al.* 1992).

Content, administration and scoring

The questionnaire was designed for use mainly with professionals. The first section identifies client needs and the experience of service delivery problems. Type of problem is probed for in relation to 11 areas: outreach services, emergency services, mental health treatment services, psychosocial rehabilitation services, case management, assistance with basic human needs, vocational and pre-vocational services, shelter/housing, medical/dental care, substance abuse services, and supportive services (peer and family support). Respondents are asked about the occurrence and severity of situations in their community.

In the next section, respondents are asked to rate the adequacy and quality of existing services within each of the 11 service categories. Adequacy is measured by asking how many of those who need each service receive it (all, most, some, few, none), and quality is measured by asking respondents to consider the technical and interpersonal aspects of care and the physical setting. The next section measures current service performance in terms of availability and accessibility, the level of coordination and information. The final section measures the administrative, planning and resource coordinating performance of the mental health authority.

This section collects qualitative data about the major accomplishments and shortcomings of the service programme.

This survey instrument is supplemented with client interviews asking them to report, in structured interviews, their needs (as identified by themselves and others), receipt of services to meet these needs, and feelings about the services received. The questionnaire yields both qualitative and quantitative data, the latter being derived from a series of Likert-type scale items. The scoring is too detailed to reproduce here, but it is available from the author.

Examples of the Key Informant Survey Scales

Examples of Knowledgeable Person Questionnaire

To what extent are the following problems occurring for chronically mentally ill (CMI) persons in City A:

(a) not having access to in-patient services because there are too few public in-patient beds
(b) not having access to adequate amounts of food and clean clothing
(c) lacking opportunities for vocational training or sheltered work

How well does the current service system for CMI persons in City A perform on these activities?

- avoiding excessive waiting lists or long delays in scheduling
- providing services at reasonable cost to CMI persons
- training staff to work caringly and comfortably with CMI persons
- developing agreements between agencies at the level of direct service delivery to avoid needless duplication of effort

Examples of Client Questions

The Delighted–Terrible Scale is used, where 1 = terrible, 2 = unhappy, 3 = mostly dissatisfied, 4 = mixed, 5 = mostly satisfied, 6 = pleased and 7 = delighted

F3 Now please look at the delighted / terrible scale again. How do you feel about . . .?

A The way you spend your spare time?
D The amount of fun you have?
E The amount of relaxation in your life?

G3 Please look at the delighted / terrible scale again. How do you feel about . . .?

B How often you have contact with your family?
D The way things are in general between you and your family?

H4 Look at the delighted / terrible scale again. How do you feel about . . .?

B The amount of time you spend with other people?
F The amount of friendship in your life?

L8 I'm going to read a list of places where people sometimes sleep when they have nowhere to stay. For each, please tell me if, in the past year, you have slept in . . . even for a night or two. PROBE FOR EXACT NUMBER OF NIGHTS IN EACH SETTING.

A Outside without shelter?
B Inside an empty building?
C In a public shelter?
D In a church?

No / Yes = How many times in the past year did you sleep in a place like this?

Validity and reliability

The instrument was pre-tested in Rochester, New York in a demonstration mental health project programme (Morrissey *et al.* 1990; Ridgely *et al.* 1992). This indicated that the instrument had face validity, and could be administered by post with an acceptable response rate after two follow-ups. Other analyses of reliability and validity are in progress.

THE MRC NEEDS FOR CARE ASSESSMENT

This schedule was derived from the work of John Wing on the planning and evaluation of psychiatric services (Mangen and Brewin 1991). There is also a community version for use with those with mild psychiatric conditions. Information is provided by subjects, if necessary backed up by general practitioners' notes, and staff are also interviewed. The assessment is made by a team of people involved with the care of the long-term mentally ill (particularly psychiatrists and psychologists), and requires a week's training. A manual is available (Brewin and Wing 1989). Social functioning is measured, in the community version, using the MRC Social Role Performance Schedule (Hurry and Sturt 1981; Hurry *et al.* 1983).

'Need' is treated by the authors of the instrument as 'normative' (expert-defined). They distinguish between needs for specific items of care (such as advice, treatment, shelter, etc.) and needs for services to supply these items of care. They distinguish between primary needs (the patient's functioning threatening to/falling below a minimum level which is due to a potentially remediable or preventable constraint) and secondary needs (the decision to take action will probably be more dependent on individual circumstances and on the policy of the unit or service, future needs, and possible needs in relation to social role performance) (Brewin and Wing 1989).

Content and scoring

The schedule divides needs into two broad sections: clinical state and social role performance. The clinical section covers nine areas of functioning: positive psychotic symptoms; slowness and under-activity; side-effects such as tardive dyskinesia; neurotic symptoms; dementia and organic psychosis; physical symptoms and disease; dangerous or destructive behaviour; socially embarrassing behaviour; and distress about long-term psychosocial problems. The section on social role performance covers basic skills and functional abilities regarded as necessary to live independently in society. There are five sub-sections, which are self-care skills, education, occupation, communication and money/household management. In the latest version of the schedule, the self-care sub-section is further subdivided into six areas: personal hygiene and appearance; shopping; cooking/getting meals; household tasks; use of public transport; and use of public amenities. The final sub-section is divided into the management of money and the management of household affairs (e.g. paying bills).

The process

The model involves a four-stage process. First the presence of clinical problems and level of social role performance are identified (lowered physical, psychological and social functioning below a minimum specified level). Social disablement is defined as a series of wants or problems presented by the patient (including relatives). The method of care thought to be acceptable and effective is next determined, and then therapeutic agents capable of undertaking these interventions are identified. Finally, the appropriate agencies for the coordinated delivery of care are considered. Need is defined in terms of social disablement together with an assessment that this is due to a (potentially) remediable cause.

Clinical

The ratings in the first part (clinical section) are made on 3-point scales: 0 = no/mild problem, 1 = no current problem but significant problem in recent past, usually within the past 2 years, and 2 = current significant problem. Codes 8 and 9 are included for 'insufficient information to make judgement' and 'not applicable', respectively. The handbook provides detailed instructions and guidance on how to make the assessments.

Social role performance

This assessment collects data on level of functioning and on appropriate actions required. In the original version (version 1), social functioning was assessed by using the Social Behaviour Schedule (Wykes and Sturt 1986; Wing 1989). The current MRC Needs for Care Assessment represents an attempt to standardize Wykes and colleagues' assessments, to increase the number of areas of functioning assessed and to analyse more specific types of care. Needs are then translated into needs for care (Brewin *et al.* 1987). It has been judged as unsuitable for the assessment of need in the homeless mentally ill (Hogg and Marshall 1992), due to its failure to take account of the views of hostel staff and residents.

The areas of role functioning assessed (version 2) are symptoms and behaviour problems (positive psychotic symptoms, retardation, side-effects of medication, neurotic symptoms, organic brain disorder, physical disease and disorders, violence or threats to self/others, socially embarrassing behaviour, distress about social circumstances) and personal and social skills (personal cleanliness, household shopping, cooking or buying meals, household chores, use of public transport, use of public amenities, basic literacy and arithmetic skills, occupational skills, social interaction skills, management of money and management of household affairs). The decisions about which skills to include in the assessments were validated by assessing the judgements of rehabilitation care staff and comparing the items (Brewin *et al.* 1987).

The scoring of symptoms and behaviour problems is as follows: 0 = no problem or mild problem; 1 = no current problem but significant problem in recent past and/or threat of a significant problem; 2 = current significant problem; 8 = insufficient information to make judgement; 9 = inadequate. Social skills and ability items are scored on 4-point scales (plus the 'does not apply' and 'inadequate reply' codes of 8 and 9), ranging from competence plus performance, skill demonstrated without prompting in the past month (0); currently shows competence plus performance but significant problem in recent past, usually within last 2 years, and/or threat of a significant problem (1); lack of competence, usually no evidence of a skill at any time in past year (2); lack of performance, skill performed competently during past year but not, or only with prompting, during past month (3).

Social disablement

The model defines social disablement as a series of wants or problems presented by the patient (including relatives); these wants/problems are then legitimized as 'needs' for care and services. This model assumes that the client cannot be the final arbiter of needs, as their definition depends on expert knowledge and the integration of information from patients, families and involved professionals and the reconciliation of conflicting assessments (Mangen and Brewin 1991). 'Need' is defined on the basis of the existence of effective treatments.

Items of care

In each area of social disablement, a list of 2–8 appropriate items of care (e.g. medication, behaviour programmes, etc.) is specified. The list is over- rather than under-inclusive, and was validated against the judgements of rehabilitation staff (Brewin *et al.* 1987). Each item of care is rated by the interviewer according to whether it has been tried, effectiveness, acceptability to the patient and current appropriateness. The rating is based on an interview with a key worker or other appropriate member of staff. Detailed interviewer training and instructions are required. Need status in each area of social disability is derived algorithmically from level of disability.

The assessment of items of care is made on an 8-point scale (plus the 'inadequate' and 'does not apply' categories), ranging from this item not appropriate and not provided, or provided because of some other problem (0); this item currently being provided and effective or potentially effective (1); this item currently being provided but has proved to be insufficient in itself after 3 months trial – it is still appropriate and worth continuing (2); this item offered during past year but refusal, premature termination, or non-attendance by patient (3); this item given adequate trial in past 2 years and proved ineffective – unlikely to be more effective if offered again (4); this item appropriate but not provided due to incapacitating symptoms or danger of overload – it will probably be required within the next 12 months (5); this item provided inappropriately and not worth continuing, overprovision (6); this item appropriate now but not given adequate or recent trial (7).

Primary and secondary need

Needs for short- and medium-term services are translated from needs for care. Five areas of intervention are assessed: symptomatology, behavioural problems and social skills deficits; occupational and industrial therapy requirements; leisure skills interventions; housing requirements; and deficits in material welfare. Where an unmet need is identified, agents are identified who can provide effective intervention.

Relatives' needs are also assessed in a similar way to patients' needs (MacCarthy *et al.* 1989). Seven problems related to living with a psychiatric patient are asked about, on the grounds that if present they may detract from the carer's quality of life: unwillingness to reside with the patient; financial hardship, failure to receive available social payments, or inadequate housing; unavailability of holiday relief; inadequate contact with care staff;

inadequate information and coping advice; excessive emotional burden; child–care difficulties due to the presence of the patients. Interventions are assessed as none employed, none even partly effective, some potentially fully effective, none fully effective/no alternatives, none fully effective/ alternatives available. The effectiveness of any interventions tried over the past year is assessed to permit judgements of 'met need', 'unmet need' and 'no need' to be made.

The assessment of primary and secondary need carries a 5-point scale (plus a 'not applicable' code), including no need (0), met need (1), unmet need – assessment (2), unmet need – treatment (3), no meetable need (4). Full coding details and essential instructions are provided by Brewin and Wing (1989).

Examples from the MRC Needs for Care Assessment

Section B: Skills and abilities

Rating instructions for Section B:
Rate level of functioning as follows:

0 = Competence plus performance (skill demonstrated without prompting in past month)
1 = Currently shows competence plus performance but significant problem in recent past (usually within past 2 years) AND/OR threat of a significant problem
2 = Lack of competence (usually no evidence of skill at any time in the past year)
3 = Lack of performance (skill performed competently during past year, but not, or only with prompting, during past month)
8 = Insufficient information to make judgement
9 = Not applicable

Rate ITEM OF CARE as in Section A whenever LEVEL OF FUNCTIONING is coded 1, 2, 3 or 8. (For example, assessment / medication / supervision, monitoring or medication / domiciliary visits / support, reassurance to subject / coping, advice to subject / coping, advice to relative / family intervention / sheltered environment / other. *Rate:* primary need status; over-provision; future need.)

Rate PRIMARY NEED STATUS as follows (summary codes without guidelines displayed here):

0 = No need
1 = Met need
2 = Unmet need (assessment)

3 = Unmet need (treatment)
4 = No meetable need
5 = Not applicable

B10 Self-care

(i) Personal hygiene

Rate LEVEL OF FUNCTIONING = 1, 2, 3, 8
Rate ITEM OF CARE *if* LEVEL OF FUNCTIONING = 1, 2, 3, 8

Assessment
Remedial training
Supervised baths or self-care
Sheltered residence
Other (specify)

Rate PRIMARY NEED STATUS
Rate POSSIBLE NEED (LACK OF PERFORMANCE)
Rate OVER-PROVISION (state item of care)
Rate FUTURE NEED (state item of care)

Validity

The results of studies of reliability and validity are presented by Brewin *et al.* (1987, 1988). However, testing for validity is limited because, as the authors point out, need involves making value judgements and no other comparable measures of need exist. They also point out that validity is limited by cultural factors which determine the appropriateness of domestic skills.

Reliability

Brewin *et al.* (1987, 1988) reported work on reliability in Italy in which 20 patients were independently rated by one London and two Italian assessors with a significant and high level of agreement (kappa = 0.92). Two other inner–city studies of 11 and 66 patients respectively reported similar results: the former identified a mean of 5.27 clinical and social problems per patient, of which 28 per cent were rated as unmet needs; the latter reported 6.4 clinical and social problems per patient, with 30 per cent rated as unmet needs (Brewin *et al.* 1988; Wainwright *et al.* 1988; Mangen and Brewin 1991).

One limitation of the assessment which the authors point out is that relatively little attention is paid to patients' assessments of their needs ('wants') (Mangen and Brewin 1991). The emphasis on professional assessments is due to the uncertainty expressed by the authors that all patients can equally articulate their needs. The manual, questionnaire, detailed instructions and training details are available from Brewin; recognized training is essential before the package can be used.

WYKE'S ASSESSMENT OF NEED QUESTIONNAIRE

This questionnaire was developed by Wykes et al. (1985) and was used in a large survey of psychiatric services. It was designed for completion by staff in respect of the sampled patient.

Content and scoring

The questionnaire contains 13 categories. The staff's assessment of need falls into one of four categories: 1 = no need, no service provided; 2 = over-provision, service provided but no need; 3 = need for and utilization of the service; and 4 = unmet need for service. Investigators analyse the results and then make a decision about the most appropriate service for the patient's needs. Other available information – on social performance, burden on relatives, etc. – is also taken into account before making a final decision.

Examples from Wyke's Assessment of Need Questionnaire

1 *Assessment:* Is there a need for some assessment either of the patient's medication or of his or her social behaviour in order to plan for changes in medication or in the provision of social support?

3 *Personal counselling:* Does the subject need advice on practical matters such as housing, welfare benefits, etc., or on any personal matters that are worrying him or her?

9 *Hotel services:* Does the subject need a supervised residential unit to provide meals and some laundry facilities?

10 *Behaviour modification:* Are there any behaviours which prevent or interfere with normal functioning which might be amenable to a behavioural programme?

Validity

There is little published information about the validity of the scale.

Reliability

Wykes et al. (1985) reported that there was good agreement between staff on patients' needs, the percentage agreement between staff ratings of the same patient ranging from 83 to 96 per cent, with a mean of 89 per cent. The values of weighted kappa ranged from 0.47 to 0.88, all indicating agreement that was significantly greater than chance (weighted kappa gives a value of zero to the level of agreement that would be expected by chance, and a value of 1 for 100 per cent agreement; Cohen, 1968). However, the research team judged more needs for assessment than did the staff. The investigators explain that this was because the team had access to more information about service availability than the staff. A difficulty arose because of staff assuming that where a service was needed but not received, the service had probably been tried and failed in the past (therefore, the staff recorded no need). Bowling and Parkman (1993) also found that staff reported this difficulty in decision-making about current need, and they were also uncertain about how to code services that were needed and offered but refused by clients. Wykes et al. state that the investigators should combine the questionnaire with an analysis of the case notes, and examine services received, before reaching a decision on need.

The scale has also been used in a large survey of psychiatric patients' needs by Bowling and Parkman (1993), with modifications in order to modernize it (e.g. the definition of occupational therapy was changed to reflect the current role of these professionals) and structure it (displaying it in a form).

A limitation of the scale is that it is administered to staff, and is thus dependent on staff's knowledge of service availability. However, its advantage is that it is easy to administer and, although it is not free from staff bias, it does give a crude but useful index of met and unmet need, and its reliability is enhanced if combined with investigators' assessments of case notes and actual service availability is taken into account.

SERVICES NEEDED, AVAILABLE, PLANNED, OFFERED, RENDERED INSTRUMENT

This was developed in New York by Levin *et al.* (1978) for a study of the met and unmet needs of 643 clients in six community mental health centres.

Content, administration and scoring

The instrument contains a list of 13 common services and modalities. The staff complete the first part of the instrument, immediately after being interviewed. The instrument asks them to identify which of 13 services clients need and to estimate the availability of the services. A later analysis of records at an appropriate time determines which were finally offered: the codes reflect which services were offered and which were actually rendered during the interval period (as clients do not always accept services). At follow-up analysis the response categories are: available, planned, offered, rendered (the investigators carried this out 8 weeks later). At baseline, the staff member indicates with a tick which of the 13 services the client should receive to meet fully his or her needs during the next 8 weeks if the programme has unlimited resources at its disposal. A service can be ticked even if the centre does not offer it. In the second column the staff member indicates which of the services would be readily available when needed. In the third column, the staff member indicates which services the programme actually plans to offer clients. It is a fairly general, and in effect, limited list of services. It would benefit from being more specific in places, in order to reflect the wide range of possible interventions. Items are analysed individually.

Examples of Levin and co-workers' instrument

The 13 services rated, with the codes, are:

Individual sessions
Group sessions
Family sessions
Home visits
Medication
ECT
Residential rehabilitation
Social rehabilitation
Vocational rehabilitation
Inter-agency collaboration
24 h hospitalization
Day hospitalization
Night hospitalization

No. of clients needing the service / Service: available / planned / offered / rendered / accepted

Validity and reliability

There is no published information about the scale's validity and reliability, but it is included here given the increasing interest in assessing need in a broad sense, incorporating quality of life issues, and the limited number of concise and inexpensive-to-administer instruments that are available.

Patient attitude scales

These are not well developed in relation to attitudes towards and satisfaction with care, partly because of the known difficulties in encouraging patients to be critical in structured surveys and partly because of the bias against patients' self-reports in psychiatric research. Some schedules are fairly basic, others are promising but there is limited published work on their psychometric properties. The Social Psychiatry Research Unit at the Institute of Psychiatry has a history of developing scales of patient functioning and patient attitudes (Wykes 1982). Further developmental work is urgently needed, especially given that satisfaction is likely to be sensitive to question wording (McPhee *et al.* 1975; Hargreaves *et al.* 1979). The best measures of patient attitude are those included within the quality of life measures reviewed earlier, in particular those that include the Delighted–Terrible Scale (Andrews and Withey 1976) items, such as Lehman's QLI. In social gerontology, several scales of 'person–environment fit' have been developed which measure elderly people's feelings about the institutions they reside in, the social climate within the homes and the extent of individual freedom of choice, for example Hulicka and co-workers' (1975) Perceived Latitude of Choice Questionnaire. Interested readers are referred to Kane and Kane (1988), who have reviewed these scales.

SOCIAL PROBLEM QUESTIONNAIRE

Corney (1988) developed a scale for use with patients in general practice to screen for psycho-social disorder (if used with the GHQ 12), the Social Problem Questionnaire. It contains items asking respondents to rate their satisfaction with various aspects of their lives.

Content

The questionnaire consists largely of 21 items on satisfaction with various dimensions of life.

Examples from the Social Problem Questionnaire

How satisfied are you with your present housing?

Satisfied / slightly dissatisfied / markedly dissatisfied / severely dissatisfied

Do you have any problems with your neighbours?

No problems / slight problems / marked problems / severe problems

How satisfied are you with your present job?

Satisfied / slightly dissatisfied / markedly dissatisfied / severely dissatisfied

How satisfied are you with not having a paid job?

Satisfied / slightly dissatisfied / markedly dissatisfied / severely dissatisfied

---

Validity and reliability

Some items are oddly worded (e.g. the last question above), and the scale has not been tested for reliability or validity. It is mentioned here because it is refreshing to see attempts to obtain people's feelings about aspects of their lives.

CLIENT SATISFACTION QUESTIONNAIRE (CSQ)

This questionnaire was developed by Larsen *et al.* (1979) in California due to the authors' belief that evaluation of mental health programmes was incomplete without an assessment of clients' perspectives, and the neglect of this area due to the common dismissal of clients' opinions because they tended to differ from those of therapists. They argue that clients may have different perspectives to therapists and that these are still valid. They point to the difficulties encountered in existing studies due to problems with the reporting of high rates of satisfaction, the difficulties of obtaining unbiased samples of patients, and the lack of a standardized satisfaction scale.

The scale was developed from a review of the literature, which identified nine possible determinants of satisfaction. For each category they created nine items. Each item has a 4-point anchored answer without a neutral point. A group of 32 health professionals ranked the nine items in each category according to how well they tapped the dimension in question, from 9 (best) to 1 (worst). Items receiving a mean rank of 5 or higher were retained. This left 45 items, with a minimum of four and a maximum of six per category. This reduced pool was then re-rated by members from various mental health boards. They were asked to select those about which they would most like to receive feedback. The three top ranked items in each category were selected, and four additional items to ensure some variation. This left 31 items, with a minimum of three items per category. This was then administered to 248 mental health clients in five out-patient service settings. As in previous research, responses were biased towards the 'satisfied' end of the scale. When the data were submitted to principal components factor analysis, one salient dimension was shown to account for 43 per cent of the total variance. Finally, item correlations and factor loadings were examined and eight items were selected for inclusion in the final questionnaire on the basis of those which loaded highly and which exhibited good item–total and inter-item correlations (Larsen *et al.* 1979).

Content

Several versions of the scale of varying length are in use. Investigators have tended to use either the 31-item version or the shorter 8-item version (see overleaf). An 18-item version is also still being used. The scale relates to satisfaction with services.

Administration and scoring

It takes 3–8 min to complete, and the authors suggest that it can be supplemented with other questions that are of interest to the investigator. It was designed for use with out-patients. A short 8-item version has been developed (CSQ-8). Item scores can be summed or analysed separately.

Examples from the CSQ-8

1 How would you rate the quality of service you have received?   (Circle your answers)

Excellent (4) / good (3) / fair (2) / poor (1)

3 To what extent has our programme met your needs?

Almost all of my needs have been met (4) / most of my needs have been met (3) / only a few of my needs have been met (2) / none of my needs have been met (1)

8 If you were to seek help again, would you come back to our programme?

No, definitely not (1) / No, I don't think so (2) / Yes, I think so (3) / Yes, definitely (4)

Client Satisfaction Questionnaire (Larsen *et al.* 1979). Copyright © 1989, 1990, Clifford Attkisson Ph.D. Reproduced with permission. Used with written permission.

Validity

Larsen *et al.* (1979) tested the 8-item scale with 49 out-patients, and found that it correlated moderately well with self-ratings of improvement after the onset of therapy ($r = 0.53$). The questionnaire also correlated moderately well ($r = 0.44$) with the Brief Psychiatric Rating Scale (Overall and Gorham 1962). Therapists' ratings of their satisfaction with their work with their clients correlated 0.42 with their clients' satisfaction ratings, and therapists' estimates of their clients' satisfaction correlated with the CSQ at 0.56, providing some evidence of the scale's concurrent validity. On the other hand, the scale has only low to moderate associations with measures of outcome after short-term follow-up periods, although it did correlate with early treatment drop-out (Larsen *et al.* 1979).

Reliability

Larsen *et al.* (1979) reported that the coefficient alpha for the final version was 0.93. The scale has also been used by Cox *et al.* (1978) on 213 clients after their first service contact; the authors reported a coefficient alpha of between 0.90 and 0.94 after a 90-day follow-up. The reliability of the 8-item version and an 18-item version of the scale was reported by Nguyen *et al.* (1983). The 18-item version was derived from the earlier 31-item version minus five items: it has 26 items on two parallel forms (18 each: CSQ-18, Forms A and B). The results again showed that the 8-item version had a high coefficient alpha (0.92) in the study of 49 out-patients prior to therapy. They also reported results from a study by Zwick (1982) on both the 8-item and the 18-item versions. The study was carried out with 62 clients in an urban community mental health centre. There was an association with treatment drop-out ($r = 0.61$). The CSQ had a high internal consistency (coefficient alpha = 0.91). The CSQ-8 performed as well as, and often better than, the CSQ-18. It was superior in terms of internal consistency, with a higher coefficient alpha value, inter-item correlations and item–total correlations.

The limitation of the scale is that its content was primarily determined by professionals rather than by clients, and was deliberately biased towards what service professionals wanted. The investigators have since developed several forms of a new Service Satisfaction Scale, designed to retain the 'generic' service capability of the CSQ but to assess multiple factors of service provision, the advantage being that distinguishable facets of a service are assessed. Factor analysis of 30 items used in primary care and mental health out-patient services yielded two well-replicated sub-scales: practitioner manner and skill, and perceived outcome (efficacy). Only pilot studies have been published to date (Greenfield and Attkisson 1989), and a version for use in residential settings has also been developed (Greenfield 1989).

Huxley (1988, 1990) and Huxley and Warner (1992) have developed a General Satisfaction Questionnaire based on the work of Larsen *et al.* (1979). The questionnaire contains 20 items, eight of which are rated on a 4-point scale and 12 on a 7-point scale. There are two sections for open-ended responses and a section for demographic data. Sub-scale items are summed. Responses yield four sub-scores related to general satisfaction, satisfaction with access to services, satisfaction with help given, and satisfaction with the acceptability of the service. The latter item relates to clients' perceptions of the quality of their reception and the competence of the case manager. There are few data on the psychometric properties of the scale. A study by Babiker and Thorne (1993) of 192 consecutively admitted psychiatric patients reported an inverse association between satisfaction and number of social problems. More work needs to be carried out on the reliability and validity of the scale.

SATISFACTION WITH LIFE DOMAINS SCALE

After a review of the literature on life satisfaction and well-being, Baker and Intagliata (1982) developed a model of quality of life domains based on the relationships between external environments (physical, social, economic, political, cultural), individual experience (*material*, e.g. housing, food, air, water, possessions, financial, transportation; *social*, e.g. family, friends, community; *activities*, e.g. work, leisure, creative, religious), individual physical and mental health status and quality of life responses (coping, adaptation, satisfaction, happiness, etc.). From this they constructed the Satisfaction with Life Domains Scale, for use with 118 clients in a community support programme for chronically mentally ill people in New York State.

Content, administration and scoring

The scale consists of an adapted Delighted–Terrible Faces Scale (Andrews and Withey 1976) to assess the client's satisfaction with 15 life domains. The scale is administered by an interviewer and the respondent is asked to indicate his or her feelings by choosing one of seven faces ranging from a delighted face with a large smile (scored 7) to a terrible face with a deep frown. Respondents pick the face that best represents their degree of satisfaction with various domains. The domains of satisfaction include:

- Their house/apartment/place of residence
- Their neighbourhood as a place to live
- The food they ate
- The clothing they wore
- Their health
- The people they lived with
- Their friends
- Their relationships with their family
- How they got on with other people
- Their job/work/day programme
- The way they spent their spare time

- What they did in the community for fun
- The services and facilities in their area
- Their economic situation
- The place they currently live in compared with the state hospital

Items can be analysed independently or as a total score. Item scores are summed.

Examples from the Satisfaction with Life Domains Scale

Life domain questions (some examples):

1 Which face comes closest to expressing how you feel about your house/apartment/place of residence?

6 Which face comes closest to expressing how you feel about the people you live wlth?

11 Which face comes closest to expressing how you feel about the way you spend your spare time?

15 Which face comes closest to expressing how you feel about the place you live now, compared with the state hospital?

Validity and reliability

The investigators also administered the Affect–Balance Scale (Bradburn 1969), and reported a significant correlation of 0.64. The scale showed the expected variation in responses on satisfaction, although the scale did display skewedness towards the higher end of positive feelings. The scale requires thorough psychometric testing.

Conclusion to Part II

More progress has been made in the field of mental health in developing broad indicators of quality of life than in any other area of medicine. In addition, several instruments for the assessment of need, role functioning, behaviour and adjustment have been developed which overlap with these instruments (also see next section).

The most popular quality of life scales in the USA are the Quality of Life Scale (Heinrichs *et al.* 1984), the Quality of Life Index for Mental Health (Becker *et al.* 1993), the Oregon Quality of Life Questionnaire (Bigelow *et al.* 1982, 1990, 1991a, 1991b, 1991c; Olson *et al.* 1991), and Lehman and co-workers' (1982) Quality of Life Interview. The latter is the most superior scale, although the others are all promising and admirable developments. In Britain, the best developed scales for measuring quality of life are based on Lehman and co-workers' (1982) Quality of Life Interview, and include Crosby's (1990) questionnaire and battery and Oliver's (1991a, 1991b) Lancashire Quality of Life Profile.

In addition, Leff's (1991b) TAPS assessment battery covers most of the domains of quality of life, although it was not described as a quality of life measure by its author. It was designed to measure the effects (on patients) of moving long-stay psychiatric patients into community settings. Scales of need also tap most of the relevant domains in quality of life assessment. The choice of scale will depend on the aims of the study and the resources available; the scales vary greatly in length and administration time.

There are several other brief quality of life scales that have been used with people with mental illnesses, but they are generally just checklists of problems, such as Malm *et al.* (1981), or modifications of life satisfaction scales, in particular the popular scales developed by Cantril (1965) (Cantril's ladder scale) and Andrews and Withey (1976) (Delighted–Terrible scale). Few of these other scales have been fully tested, and interested readers are referred to reviews by Boevink *et al.* (1994), Bullinger (1994) and Simmons (1994). Several investigators are currently assessing the applicability of the SF-36 (Ware *et al.* 1993) for use with mentally ill populations (Bullinger 1994; Crosby pers. comm.).

Although mental health investigators have devoted much thought and energy to the development of quality of life indicators, they face a fundamental methodological problem in that many of the scales are based on adaptations of life satisfaction scales. While these are useful instruments in cross-sectional population surveys, they are not generally sensitive to relatively short-term changes and can suffer from a certain degree of bias – people are notoriously reluctant to express dissatisfaction with their lives or with their health care in response to questionnaires, and therefore results are inevitably skewed towards the satisfaction end of scales. This makes improvements in life satisfaction, following interventions, even more difficult to detect. A more critical approach to their use is required.

PART III: ROLE FUNCTIONING AND RELATED INSTRUMENTS

ROLE FUNCTIONING, PERFORMANCE AND SOCIAL BEHAVIOUR SCALES

While social functioning may reflect many factors and not necessarily psychiatric disorder, the presence of symptoms tends to affect social functioning (see reviews by Tyrer 1990; Wykes and Hurry 1991). Scales of functioning, performance and behaviour are presented because of the large amount of overlap with quality of life scales. Although their focus is different, the content of several of these scales is remarkably similar.

Roles

Social role functioning or performance is assessed by asking patients and close others how they cope with major roles: work, relationships, home and self-care. However, cultural relativism will always present problems in such research, as with most activities of daily living scales. One recent scale – the Self-Care Measurement Schedule (Barnes and Benjamin 1987) – has been criticized by Wykes and Hurry (1991) for being particularly culture-specific, and assuming common norms for behaviour. The schedule includes items on eating a meal in bed, not getting up before 10.00 am, not going shopping, etc. Such instruments also rely on third-person accounts rather than self-report measures, despite evidence that patients can be good informants (MacCarthy *et al.* 1986). As Wing (1989) has also cautioned, a major problem with many structured formats is that expectations about an individual's level of functioning can vary, and there is no absolute standard against which to judge performance. It is important that measurement takes into account whether or not the individual wishes to perform up to a particular level, and if the opportunity exists for the performance in question. This is one reason why carefully trained raters' assessments are popular in psychiatry, so that all such factors can be taken into account when making an assessment.

Many of the instruments have not been thoroughly tested for reliability and validity

(Anthony and Farkas 1982), and have been developed for use in specific settings, such as institutional ones (Tyrer 1990; Wykes and Hurry 1991). Not all scales are reviewed here. Those that have been omitted include the ones developed by Cohler *et al.* (1974), Strauss and Carpenter (1974) and Willer and Biggin (1974). Several relevant scales have been reviewed by Weissman *et al.* (1981).

Social attainments, as opposed to performance, can generally be measured objectively in terms of major role areas of life, such as employment status. Key questions on job attainment, marital status and parental attainment are included in the Psychiatric Epidemiology Research Interview (PERI) developed by Dohrenwend *et al.* (1981). Such standardized assessments, however, are limited in that they assume individuals have the same major role values and are deficient without their attainment (e.g. child-rearing). Such roles, as the authors do point out, are also associated with social conditions, rather than psychiatric illness (e.g. employment).

Behaviour

Social behaviour measures are frequently used to assess need and also to assess quality of life among people with mental illnesses. These scales have been reviewed by Wykes and Hurry (1991). Some relevant scales are reviewed here.

SOCIAL FUNCTIONING SCHEDULE

This schedule was developed in the UK by Remington and Tyrer (1979). Its development was based on a literature review of existing scales, and from the authors' concerns about existing scales' assumptions of accepted norms of behaviour. It was designed for use with non-psychotic patients.

Content

The schedule is structured around 12 sections, which include functioning inside and outside the home: employment, household tasks, money, self-care, marital relationship, child-care, patient–child relationships, patient–parent relationships, household relationships, extra-marital relationships, social contacts, hobbies and leisure activities. For employment, household tasks, money and leisure

activities, the sections are divided into two: the patient's reports of behaviour are rated and then the patient is asked to describe feelings such as strain or worry within each area (stress sub-section).

Administration and scoring

The interview is semi-structured to permit the interviewer to adapt questions to elicit an adequate response. The sections and sub-sections make up 16 potential areas for questions and ratings. The interviewer summarizes the patients' reports on a 10 cm horizontal VAS for every item, ranging from no difficulties at one end to severe difficulties in functioning at the other. Sub-section scores are summed.

Examples from the Social Functioning Schedule

2 Household chores

Now I would like to discuss household chores – cooking, shopping, the washing, cleaning, gardening, decorating, household repairs and so on.
What household jobs do you usually do?
Give details:
Where necessary: does this mean you do something in the house every week?   (Yes / No)

2a Have you had any difficulties in managing the chores over this last month? Have you found that you cannot do as much as usual, or that others have had to take over/have you found it difficult to get things done? Have you been slow at doing things? Have you felt that you have done jobs well on the whole?

Rate problems with chores: Behaviour

None————————————————Severe difficulties

2b How do you feel about the chores? Have you found managing the chores a strain? Do chores get you down? Do the chores bore you, or irritate you?

Rate problems with chores: Stress

None————————————————Severe difficulties

Validity and factor structure

The scale was sensitive to type of diagnosis (personality disorders). The value of the scale is that it is brief, but it is difficult to corroborate the authors' claim that it is value-free. A factor analysis was carried out which produced four factors: domestic and leisure problems, reduced performance, domestic worries and occupational problems.

Reliability

The intra-class reliability correlation coefficients ranged from 0.45 to 0.81, with the exception of child-care which achieved near zero. Inter-rater correlations ranged between 0.48 and 0.88. The correlations between patient and informant assessments ranged between 0.45 and 0.80. It correlates well with observer ratings of functioning ($r = 0.68$ to 0.79) (Tyrer *et al*. 1990).

SOCIAL ROLE PERFORMANCE SCHEDULE (SRPS)

This is an early version of one of a series of scales developed at the MRC Social Psychiatry Unit in London. The early version of the scale was called the Social Performance Scale, which assessed leisure activities, domestic relationships, household tasks, child-care, dependence and overt behaviour disturbance. This early scale formed the basis for the Social Role Performance Schedule and the Social Behaviour Schedule (see Wing, 1989).

The early version was developed by John Wing and Til Wykes and their colleagues, and tested in several studies (e.g. Wing *et al*. 1972; see Wing 1989). A later version was subsequently tested (Creer and Wing 1974) and a third version emerged which has been used with patients both in hospital and in the community (Hurry and Sturt 1981; Hurry *et al*. 1983, 1987; Sturt and Wykes 1987; Hurry 1989; Wing 1989). The third version is based on the first version. An early version was used by Wykes (1982) in an evaluation of a 'hostel-ward' in Camberwell, and by Wykes *et al*. (1982) in a study of social behaviour in day and residential units. Wykes (1982) analysed the scale by collapsing each of the codes into problem *vs* no problem. Wing (1989) states that the SRPS should be used in conjunction with the Social Behaviour Schedule (Wykes and Sturt 1986), as the two instruments are complementary – one measures performance and the other measures behaviour. An account of the development of each of these scales can be found in Wing (1989).

Content

The first version of the schedule included one questionnaire for the subject and one for the relative. Eight types of role were covered, and a rating for satisfaction of each role was included. The second edition included some features of the Present State Examination (PSE). The third edition covers household management, employment, management of money, child-care, intimate relationships, other personal relationships, social presentation and coping with emergencies, plus overall ratings (Wing 1989). It is widely used. The WHO's (1988) Disability Assessment Schedule contains the Social Role Performance Section, which is derived from the third (latest) version of the SRPS.

The scale is administered by an interviewer and completed after discussion with a member of staff, and items are rated on 3-, 4- or 5-point scales, for example from 0 (no serious problem), 1 (occasional serious problem), 2 (serious problem most of the time) to 3 (virtually no contribution). Various scoring systems have been developed, but on the whole scores are summed and adjusted for the number of applicable sections and expressed as a percentage of the maximum score possible. If at least half of the items that make up each of the domains are defined as problems then the whole domain is regarded as a problem. The items can be grouped into 14 behavioural areas.

Examples of behavioural areas in the SRPS

Amount of interaction with staff
Type of interaction with staff
Amount of interaction with residents
Type of interaction with residents
Social contacts outside
Participation in unit affairs
Self-care
Manners and deportment
Abnormal behaviour
Violence or threats
Occupation during working hours
Self-confidence
Attitude to discharge
Specific behavioural problems (smoking, drinking, etc.)

Validity

Hurry and Sturt (1981) and Wing (1989) described the development and testing of the early version (Social Performance Scale) with psychotic patients. It correlated highly with the PSE ($r = 0.68$ in a population sample and $r = 0.57$ on an out-patient sample: Hurry and Sturt 1981). In a Medical Research Council (MRC) trial of drug treatments, data were collected on symptoms, adverse effects, relapses and return to hospital, and social functioning was measured using the Social Performance Scale (Stevens 1972). The scale proved to be sensitive to drug type (Shepherd and Watt 1975). This study clearly demonstrated the value of using social indicators of functioning as outcome measures.

Correlations between the PSE, which was designed to minimize the importance of any social component, and the latest version of the SRPS range between 0.57 and 0.68 (Hurry and Sturt 1981). The SRPS scores have been reported to be significantly associated with symptom type and severity, as measured by the PSE (Hurry *et al.* 1987; Wing 1989), suggesting that it has convergent validity.

Reliability

The reliability of the early Social Performance Scale was tested by the authors by comparing the information from two members of staff using one rater (number of patients not given). A total of 252 problems were assessed and there were 29 discrepancies when comparing dichotomized ratings (present/absent). The product–moment correlation coefficient for the two sets of scores was $r = 0.87$ (Wykes 1982). Further testing and development is required.

Tests for the reliability of the later SRPS were reported to be satisfactory (Wing 1989). Further evidence of the psychometric properties of the scale is required.

SOCIAL BEHAVIOUR SCHEDULE (SBS)

This scale is widely used and is one of a series that was developed at the MRC Social Psychiatry Unit in London, for use in a variety of day and residential settings. It was developed from the Social Performance Scale (Wing *et al.* 1972). Its development has been described by Wing (1989). It was designed initially for use with in-patients with a diagnosis of schizophrenia, although an expanded version was later developed to include non-psychotic items. The schedule underwent further modification as the trends towards community care increased, and was modified for use with patients in hostels and other community homes. The latest version is the fourth edition of the scale.

The items were derived from staff assessments of problems leading to dependency on care. It is biased towards patients with severe disabilities (Wykes and Hurry 1991). Two earlier sub-scales on social withdrawal and socially embarrassing behaviours have not been distinguished on statistical grounds in later versions of the scale (Wykes *et al.* 1982). The scale has provided the basis for a number of other schedules (e.g. REHAB: Hall and Baker 1983) and is recommended for use alongside needs assessment packages (e.g. the MRC Needs for Care Assessment: Brewin and Wing 1989; Wing 1989). The WHO's (1988) Disability Assessment Schedule includes the first version of the SBS.

Content, administration and scoring

The schedule is administered to a member of staff, who assesses the patient or resident. The schedule contains 30 questions and covers the following behaviours:

- *Communication:* initiative; coherence; oddity/inappropriateness of conversation; ability to make appropriate social contacts; hostility/friendliness; attention-seeking behaviour.
- *Other behaviours:* suicidal ideas and self-harm; panic attacks and phobias; overactivity and restlessness; laughing and talking to self; acting out bizarre ideas; posturing and mannerisms; socially unacceptable manners or habits; violent, threatening or destructive behaviour; depression; inappropriate sexual behaviour; personal appearance and hygiene; slowness; underactivity; concentration; and other behaviours ('that impede progress').
- *Occupation:* type of weekday occupation; leisure activities; restrictions on activity; unrealistic aims; reason for being in setting; the most difficult problem to deal with; physical and other extrinsic handicaps.

Sub–scale scores are summed. Further details of the scoring for severity are available from the author, and were briefly referred to by Wykes and Sturt (1986). A short version, and its scoring, has been used by Brewin and Wing (1989). Wing (1989) recommends that it should be used in conjunction with the Social Role Performance Schedule, as the two are complementary.

Examples from the SBS

11 Acting out of bizarre ideas

This rating is concerned with whether a subject decides on some action because of his or her delusions. For example: (a) going to the scene of some major catastrophe because subject feels his or her help is needed; (b) subject assumes that he or she has millions of pounds and so either spends it or tries to spend it on expensive items.

0 = No such behaviour
1 = Such behaviour has occurred once in past month
2 = Such behaviour has occurred more than once in past month

13 Socially unacceptable habits or manners

This rating concerns unacceptable habits, e.g. scratching genitals, passing loud flatus, picking nose, etc. Ask particularly about problems at meal times such as poor table manners.

0 = Has good manners and behaviour is socially acceptable
1 = Behaviour is not markedly unacceptable but subject has positive qualities in manner
2 = Occasional unacceptable behaviour (e.g. markedly unattractive habit, surliness, uncouthness). However much of the time subject is passively acceptable
3 = Frequent episodes of unacceptable behaviour as in (2) (e.g. once a week)
4 = Behaviour is markedly unacceptable most of the time

23 Leisure: Activities

Rate degree to which subject is able to occupy his leisure time, has active leisure interest, and goes out of the house (or hostel, etc.) to pursue these.

0 = Subject has an interest or interests which occupy his leisure time and which he pursues without encouragement from others

1 = Subject shows a bit of active interest in something, but it fluctuates considerably, or his interests are bizarre in nature
2 = Subject has some rather 'passive' leisure interest (e.g. watching TV) which occupies him to a limited extent
3 = Subject might respond fleetingly if somebody worked on engaging his interest in some leisure pursuits, but would not keep up interest if left to himself to pursue it on his own initiative
4 = Subject has no interest in anything. Even if a relative or professional carer tries to engage his interest in some leisure activity, he rejects this

Validity

The reliability and validity tests of the SBS were published by Wykes and Sturt (1986). The SBS has been able to discriminate between patients in short-stay psychiatric wards and patients in other residential settings, such as hostels, group homes, etc. (Wykes et al. 1982). It has been used in a wide range of research from pharmaceutical research to evaluations of patient provision (see review by Wykes and Hurry 1991). It is one of the instruments selected by the TAPS team (see pp. 103–6).

Reliability

The SBS was tested for reliability on an initial sample of 66 patients from a variety of settings. Inter-rater reliability, using two raters of 28 interviews, was significant using Kappa statistic (Cohen 1968), with 84 to 100 per cent agreement, and a mean of 94 per cent. Inter-informant reliability was also highly significant, with 70–90 per cent agreement, and a mean of 86 per cent. Test–retest reliability of the items at 9 months was good, with most items achieving significance, with 72 to 96 per cent agreement, and an average of 83 per cent.

Dayson et al. (1990) reported that hospital and community informants achieved a high level of agreement with individual items and total scores (the mean scores for hospital and community informants were 2.41 and 2.33, respectively; these were not statistically significant). It was used alongside the PSE-10 by Brewin et al. (1990) in a comparative study of staff members', relatives' and patients' assessments (sample of day hospital/

centre attenders). Their results showed that estimates of some symptoms and behavioural problems were highest when made by those who could observe the patient in a residential setting. This may have been due to the increased opportunities for observation or to differences in behaviours in different settings. Day-staff produced lower estimates of problem behaviours. The TAPS programme of research should provide further information on the psychometric properties of the scale when used in community settings. It is a popular and well-used scale.

REHABILITATION EVALUATION (REHAB)

This assesses instrumental behaviour. It is based on the scale developed by John Wing on rating ward behaviour and the later Social Behaviour Schedule (Wykes and Sturt 1986). It is used to assess rehabilitation status in psychiatric patients (Hall and Baker 1983).

Content

REHAB was designed to distinguish between socially embarrassing and socially withdrawn behaviour and also includes items on the management of money, care of possessions and use of community facilities (unlike the SBS). The scale provides five factor scores which are derived from the 16 items in the general behaviour scale. Part I measures difficult or embarrassing ('devient') behaviour, and Part II measures general social and everyday behaviours. Part I contains eight questions, seven of which have variously worded 3-point frequency scales. Seven of these questions ask about behaviour over the past week and cover: incontinence, violence, self-mutilation, sexually offensive behaviour, absence from the ward or hospital without arrangement, shouting or swearing at others, talking or laughing to self. The eighth question is a checklist of other deviant behaviours that occurred during the previous year. Part II contains 23 visual analogue scale ratings about general behaviour over the past week, anchored with extremes at each end, plus a middle statement, and one question on whether the behaviour was better, the same or worse than usual. The VAS covers: getting on with others on the ward or unit, mixing with others off the ward or unit, spare time activities, degree of activity, number of words in

speech, initiation of conversation, sensible content of speech, clarity of speech, table manners, self-care (washing), dressing, looking after own things, need for prompting or help, management of money, use of public facilities outside the hospital, and an overall rating.

Administration and scoring

The scale is completed by a member of staff. The scoring details and overlays (for the visual analogue scales) are included in the manual, and are too detailed to reproduce here.

Examples from the REHAB

7 Did the patient talk or laugh to himself/herself?

Episodes of talking to self, or outbursts of laughing/giggling more than once every day in the week ____
Talked or laughed to self on average once a day, or on only some days in the week ____
Did not talk to self ____

12 How many words did the patient use when he or she spoke?

| Mute, or occasional sounds | Spoke in short sentences only | Talked for a normal length of time |

Validity and factor structure

The reliability and validity of the scale are documented in the manual (Hall and Baker 1983), and in subsequent publications by the scale's authors. REHAB scores have been reported to be able to discriminate between day-hospital attenders and patients in long-stay wards (Baker and Hall 1988). Crosby et al. (1993) reported that the REHAB scores of patients resettled into the community had changed at 12 month follow-up, as would be expected, reflecting significant improvements for social activity, speech skills and community skills. Overall level of dependency had also improved, although level of deviant behaviour had not.

Factor analyses have been carried out and two main dimensions produced: general behaviour and deviant behaviour (infrequent behaviour such as violence). The latter did not achieve as strong reliability as the first part of the scale (Baker and Hall 1988).

Reliability

Baker and Hall (1983) reported good evidence of inter-rater reliability. They reported moderate to fairly strong reliability coefficients for comparisons of ratings of deviant behaviours and general behaviour. Comparable inter-rater coefficients were reported by Crosby et al. (1993) in their evaluation of resettlement into the community: 0.61–0.88 for ratings of deviant behaviours and 0.62–0.92 for general behaviour items.

It has been used in several organizational evaluations (Baker 1986; Baker and Hall 1988). REHAB was used by Hogg and Marshall (1992), in preference to the Social Behaviour Scale, in their study of homeless mentally ill people (hostel dwellers), as it offered several advantages: it was completed by hostel staff and therefore saved the investigators' time, it was designed for use with non-clinical raters, and it carries a structured training programme which facilitates the collection of high-quality data. REHAB was also used by Crosby (1990) in a study of the symptomatology, quality of environment and quality of life of discharged hospital patients (before and after discharge). He reported that the REHAB scale scores appeared to be outdated, given the trends towards community care which have left the most severely disabled patients in hospitals. Wykes and Hurry (1991) point out that there is little to choose between REHAB and the SBS, except that the SBS is cheaper to administer (Shepherd 1988) and more widely used.

SOCIAL BEHAVIOUR ASSESSMENT SCHEDULE (SBAS)

The Social Behaviour Assessment Schedule (SBAS) was designed on the basis of the literature and results from past research (Platt et al. 1980, 1983). It aims to assess psychiatric patients' disturbed behaviour, social functioning and the impact of their level of impairment on family and friends. It is a standardized, semi-structured instrument, designed to be conducted with the patient's closest relative or friend. It takes about 45 min to administer.

The SBAS consists of 239 defined and global items in six sections that assess the history and severity of the person's problems, current disturbed behaviour, social performance, adverse effects on others, other concurrent events and available social support for the informant. An earlier version of the scale was known as the Patient Behaviour Assessment Schedule (Hirsch et al. 1979).

Content

Section A (introduction) elicits sociodemographic characteristics of the informant; sections B–D (patient's behaviour, social performance and adverse effects on others) comprise the main part of the schedule. Twenty-two types of disturbed behaviour are assessed in section B, for example withdrawal, overdependence, obsessionality, overactivity and self-neglect. For each area of disturbance, three ratings are made: the presence or absence and severity of each disturbance on a 3-point scale; if present, the onset of each of the 22 areas of disturbed behaviour is made on a 6-point scale; finally, the amount of distress on the part of the informant in relation to each of the problem areas is recorded on a 5-point scale.

Section C evaluates 12 areas of social performance, or the impact of the patient's disturbance on his or her social functioning. The areas include household tasks, child-care, work or study, and the quality of the informant-patient relationship. Four ratings are made in each area using 3-point scales. Section D measures the adverse effects the patient's behaviour has had on others, including health, emotional well-being, social life, work or study. Section E assesses the presence of other important life-events in the lives of the patient, informant and close others, as a check that the distress rated in the schedule was not caused by other events (unconnected with the patient).

Administration and scoring

The scale is administered by the interviewer to a close informant of the patient without the patient being present and takes about 60–90 min to complete. The close informant is identified by the patient. Six summary scores are computed for the patient's disturbed behaviour, social performance, objective burden and distress arising from each of these. A manual comprising the scoring details has been published (Platt *et al.* 1983).

Examples from the SBAS

B2 Withdrawal

Q. In the last (time period) . . . did S keep him/herself to him/herself?
Was S untalkative?
Was S unsociable?
Did S reply when spoken to?
Did S refuse to meet people?
Was S like this all the time?

Rate patient's withdrawal

0 = normally sociable / 1 = socially withdrawn and solitary but will mix with others if encouraged to do so / 2 = never sociable even when encouraged to be so

Rate time of onset

1 (<1 week), 2 (>1 week and <3 months), 3 (>3 months and <1 year), 4 (>1 year), 5 (always), 9 (no withdrawal)

Rate informant's distress

0 = none / 1 = moderate / 2 = severe / 3 = resignation / 9 = no withdrawal

C1 Household tasks

Q. In the last (time period) . . . did S do any household tasks?
Did he/she do the shopping, cooking, cleaning?
Did he/she need to be reminded to do cooking, cleaning, etc?
Did he/she do the shopping, cooking, cleaning regularly?
Did he/she just do the (mention task, e.g. washing up) and nothing else?

Rate patient's performance of household tasks

0 = takes major part in performing household tasks; does cooking, shopping, cleaning, gardening, etc. regularly and without prompting / 1 = takes some part in household tasks; does tasks occasionally or does only minor tasks regularly or needs prompting to do household tasks / 2 = never does any household tasks

C6 Spare time activities

Q. In the last (time period) . . . did S do anything in his/her spare time?
Did he/she go out and visit friends? Or have friends in?
Did he/she go to any meetings or activities organized by church/local political party/local organizations/ sports club?
Did he/she have any hobbies?
Did he/she read, listen to music?
Did S regularly (mention the activities described by the informant) . . .?
Did S keep him/herself busy of his/her own accord or did he/she need encouragement to keep up activities and hobbies?

Rate patient's spare time activities

0 = regular spare time activities without prompting from others / 1 = some spare time activities; sometimes needs prompting from others / 2 = none – even if encouraged

Validity

Gibbons *et al.* (1984) reported a correlation of 0.43 between the schedule and the Present State Examination (Wing *et al.* 1974) in relation to 163 schizophrenic patients, providing support for the schedule's convergent validity.

Reliability

Platt and Hirsch (1981), together with other investigators (e.g. Gibbons *et al.* 1984), have reported population norms, although there are few published data on the psychometric properties of the scale. Platt *et al.* (1980) reported inter-rater reliability coefficients, using four raters and nine patients, of over 0.95 (weighted kappa was 0.7 or more for most items). Gibbons *et al.* (1984) assessed inter-rater reliability using two raters and 30 taped interviews and reported weighted kappas exceeding 0.97, 0.82 and 0.94 for disturbed behaviour, social performance and adverse effects, respectively.

The scale has been reviewed elsewhere, and has been described as impressive, but lacking in studies of reliability and validity (Weissman *et al.* 1981; Osberg 1985).

WHO PSYCHIATRIC DISABILITY ASSESSMENT SCHEDULE (WHODAS)

The WHO initiated a pilot study in seven countries in 1976 to develop these procedures for the evaluation of functional impairments and disabilities in patients with potentially severe psychiatric disorders (in their social and cultural context). The development was initiated because of the lack of easily applicable standardized assessment methods. Disability is defined as dysfunctional social behaviour and disturbance in the performance of social roles, resulting from mental disorder. The resulting schedule is reported to be applicable in a variety of cultural settings (WHO 1988). It comprises other well-known scales, including the PSE and the first version (ward behaviour scales) of the Social Behaviour Schedule (Wykes and Sturt 1986).

Content

The schedule consists of five parts: overall behaviour, social role performance, hospitalized patient section, modifying factors and global evaluation. There is also a summary of ratings and overall scoring.

The schedule is not a questionnaire. The rating of items assumes an ability to make a judgement on the basis of available information. The sources of information are: key informant, the patient, written records or data from other informants. Guidelines for the ratings are provided in relation to the choice of the appropriate point on a scale (e.g. 'no dysfunction' to 'maximum dysfunction'). The rater's criteria for selecting a rating includes severity of the behaviour and the proportion of time in the past month during which the behaviour was manifest. For most of the items, the patient's behaviour or functioning is evaluated against the assumed norms for the population.

Administration and scoring

The patient's behaviour and functioning is rated by a psychiatrist, psychologist, sociologist or social worker. Training and experience in making assessments is required. The aggregate scoring of the ratings is explained in the accompanying instructions. The scoring details vary for each sub-section, but basically involve adding the item ratings within each section, and in some cases dividing by the number of items in that section. The higher the score, the greater the severity of dysfunction.

Examples from the WHODAS

1 Patient's self-care during past month

Inquire about (i) personal hygiene (washing; shaving; keeping clothes, hair, fingernails, etc., clean and tidy; toilet habits); (ii) feeding habits; (iii) keeping living space (e.g. own room) tidy. (Rate 9 if no assessment possible)

0 = *No dysfunction:* level and pattern of self-care normal within patient's sociocultural context; patient takes a reasonable interest in his/her appearance

1 = *Minimum dysfunction:* patient maintains reasonable standards of (i), (ii) and (iii) with some (occasional) supervision; or standards are somewhat lowered when no supervision is available; some loss of interest in own appearance

2 = *Obvious dysfunction:* lack of self-care beyond minimum dysfunction is clearly established; patient likely to make an unfavourable impression; mild deterioration in appearance

3 = *Serious dysfunction:* marked decline in all aspects of self-care; evidence of neglect, e.g. vagrant or tramp-like appearance

4 = *Very serious dysfunction:* to the extent of exposing the patient to hazards such as malnutrition, dehydration or infection, and of a severity likely to necessitate social intervention

5 = *Maximum dysfunction:* patient totally uninterested in own appearance, unable to care for self; constant supervision is necessary for (i), (ii) and (iii); gross self-neglect when supervision is less intensive. (Use this code only in extreme cases, e.g. when patient wets or soils himself/herself if left unattended)

3 Patient in hospital

3.4 Contact with outside world

3.4.1 Being visited during past 3 months

0 = not visited during the past 3 months
1 = visited less often than once a week
2 = visited about once a week or more often
8 = patient in hospital for less than a week
9 = not applicable

4 Modifying factors

4.1 Specific assets

4.1.5 Does the patient have a stable confiding relationship with any person, other than parent or spouse (i.e. a person with whom the patient discusses personal problems, shares specific interests, asks advice, etc.)?

0 = no / 1 = yes (specify) / 8 = impossible to make a judgement / 9 = not known

Validity

While the handbook provides a description of the study and results for the collaborative study, and detailed rating instructions and guidelines, only limited information on validity and reliability is reported. The schedule was reported to be able to distinguish cases from controls.

Reliability

The results for inter-rater reliability were good. For social roles (self-care, interests and information, participation in household, underactivity, social withdrawal, work role and sexual relationship), the correlations for inter-rater reliability were 0.24 (sexual relationship) to 0.85 (social withdrawal), with all but sexual relationships being above 0.60.

The schedule is long at 31 pages and includes several scales and items. A glossary is included, and instructions for use. The instructions are also lengthy. It is available in a number of languages from the WHO.

GLOBAL ASSESSMENT SCALE (GAS)

The GAS is a single rating scale for evaluating the overall functioning of a subject over a specified time period or on a continuum (Endicott *et al.* 1976). The time period that is assessed is usually the last week prior to evaluation, although some studies employ 1 month, depending on the study aims and design.

Content

The GAS rating covers three major dimensions of psychopathology: impairment in daily functioning, reality testing, and potential for suicide or violence. The information for the rating can be derived from any source: direct patient interview, a reliable informant or medical notes. In making the

rating, the rater selects the lowest range describing the functioning during the 1 week time period.

The scale values range from 1, which represents the worst possible condition, to 100, which represents the healthiest condition. The scale is divided into ten equal interval ranges. The scale covers the entire range of severity and can be used where an overall assessment of severity of illness or degree of health is needed. The definitions for scoring functioning are given in the instruction sheets supplied by the authors on request.

Administration and scoring

The scale is administered by a trained interviewer, who extracts information from several sources. The two highest intervals (81–90 and 91–100) are for those people who are without significant psychopathology and who exhibit traits of 'positive mental health' (superior functioning, a wide range of interests, social effectiveness, warmth and integrity). The interval 71–80 is for individuals with no or only minimal psychopathology but who do not possess the features of positive mental health; the interval 61–70 is for those with some mild symptoms (e.g. depressed mood and mild insomnia); 51–60 is for those with moderate symptoms or who function generally with some difficulty; 41–50 is for those with any serious pathology or impairment in functioning that requires treatment or attention; 31–40 represents major impairment in several areas (e.g. work, family relations, judgement, thinking or mood); <30 represents those who are unable to function in almost all areas (e.g. stays in bed all day). Most out-patients will be rated between 31 and 70, and most in-patients between 1 and 40.

Children's GAS (CGAS)

A Children's Global Assessment Scale (CGAS) has also been developed (Shaffer *et al.* 1983). Each GAS scale was based on the model of the Health–Sickness Rating Scale (Luborsky 1962).

Examples from the GAS rating scale

100 = Superior functioning in a wide range of activities; life's problems never seem to get out of hand, is sought out by others because of his or her warmth and integrity. No symptoms

50 = Any serious symptomatology or impairment in functioning that most clinicians would think obviously requires treatment or attention (e.g. suicidal preoccupation or gesture; severe obsessional rituals; frequent anxiety attacks; serious antisocial behaviour; compulsive drinking; mild but definite manic syndrome)

10 = Needs constant supervision for several days to prevent hurting self or others (e.g. requires an intensive care unit with special observation by staff); makes no attempt to maintain minimal personal hygiene; or serious suicide act with clear intent and expectation of death

Validity

Validity for the GAS was assessed against three other structured psychiatric illness severity assessments and symptom dimension assessments. The scale correlations ranged from −0.25 to 0.67, and the symptom–item correlations ranged from −0.05 to −0.53. The GAS was reported to be sensitive to change in condition, and was able to predict readmissions (almost all the discrimination was in relation to scores below 40).

Reliability

Inter-rater reliability for the GAS was assessed in five studies described by Endicott et al. (1976). Three studies assessed inter-rater reliability with 41 in-patients, 120 in-patients' case notes and 38 out-patients, respectively. The reliability correlations ranged from 0.69 to 0.91. A fourth study of 18 parents of children at risk of schizophrenia involved clinicians making GAS ratings from transcripts of interviews, and the inter-rater correlation was 0.61. The fifth study involved the use of 34 brief case vignettes, involving 15 raters, with a rater correlation of 0.85.

GLOBAL ASSESSMENT OF FUNCTIONING SCALE (GAFS)

A revision of the GAS is the Global Assessment of Functioning Scale (GAFS) (see appendix of APA 1987). There have been some changes to the wording of scale definitions, although the meaning is essentially similar.

Examples from the GAFS rating scale

90 = Absent or minimal symptoms (e.g. mild anxiety before an exam); good functioning in all areas; interested and involved in a wide range of activities; socially effective; generally satisfied with life; no more than everyday problems or concerns (e.g. an occasional argument with family members).

50 = Serious symptoms (e.g. suicidal ideation, severe obsessional rituals, frequent shoplifting) OR any serious impairment in social, occupational, or school functioning (e.g. no friends, unable to keep a job)

10 = Persistent danger of severely hurting self or others (e.g. recurrent violence) OR persistent inability to maintain minimal personal hygiene OR serious suicidal act with clear expectation of death

ADJUSTMENT AND ADAPTATION SCALES FOR USE WITH PSYCHIATRICALLY AND/OR PHYSICALLY ILL PEOPLE

Social maladjustment is defined as ineffective performance in the roles and tasks for which an adult has been socialized (Parsons 1958), and dissatisfaction with that performance (Treanton 1962). It is therefore both an objective and subjective concept (Gurland et al. 1972a, 1972b). Several scales have been developed for use with psychiatric patients, but a number can also be used with people with physical conditions. An example of an adjustment scale in popular use in a wide range of specialities is the Vineland Adaptive Behaviour Scales (Sparrow et al. 1984a, 1984b, 1985). For fuller reviews of the many adjustment scales available, see Weissman et al. (1981). Scales developed specifically for psychiatric patients, or for use with other clinical populations as well, are reviewed here.

One approach to measuring a person's adjustment to his or her condition that has been advocated is the use of scales of social and occupational adjustment (Weissman et al. 1981). Schooler et al. (1979) designed a scale for use with schizophrenic populations. Scales that assess interpersonal contacts in relation not only to the patient's level of social withdrawal, but also by considering income, geographic area, physical health and mobility, community tolerance and the patient's appearance and social skills (manners), can be useful.

SOCIAL DYSFUNCTION RATING SCALE

The Social Dysfunction Rating Scale aims to measure maladaptation in relation to interpersonal dysfunction in elderly people and in psychiatric out-patients (Linn *et al.* 1969; Linn 1976, 1979). It concentrates on symptoms of low morale and reduced social participation. It focuses on negative aspects of social adjustment and on a model of social functioning based on equilibrium within the person and the social environment. Five factors define maladaptation: apathetic-detachment, dissatisfaction, hostility, health–finance concern and manipulative dependence.

Content

The scale contains 21 symptoms relating to social and emotional problems in three areas of concern: self, interpersonal relations and dissatisfaction in social situations.

Scoring

The 21 items have 6-point severity scales, which can be summed. High scores reflect more dysfunction, although it is unclear what the scores actually represent.

Examples from the Social Dysfunction Rating Scale

1 Low self-concept (feelings of inadequacy, not measuring up to self-ideal)
2 Goal-lessness (lack of inner motivation and sense of future orientation)
4 Self-health concern (preoccupation with physical health, somatic concerns)
8 Over-dependency (degree of parasitic attachment to others)
11 Lack of satisfying relationships with significant persons (spouse, children, kin, significant persons serving in a family role)
15 Lack of satisfaction from work
20 Financial insecurity

Validity

The correlation between the scale and independent social workers' judgements was 0.89 (Linn *et al.*

1969). Little information on the validity of the scale has been published.

Reliability

Inter-rater reliability was measured and intra-class correlations ranged from 0.54 to 0.86. Agreement between seven raters, rating ten patients with schizophrenia, was 0.91 (Kendall's index of concordance). A discriminant function analysis with schizophrenic out-patients and non-psychiatric subjects showed that 92 per cent were correctly classified (Linn *et al.* 1969). Although this is a well-known scale, relatively little is known about its psychometric properties.

STRUCTURED AND SCALED INTERVIEW TO ASSESS MALADJUSTMENT (SSIAM)

The SSIAM measures social maladjustment. Its authors accepted the definition of Parsons (1958) – 'ineffective performance in the roles and task for which an individual has been socialised' – and extended it to include Treanton's (1962) definition of 'failure in obtaining satisfaction from performance in these activities', in order to include both subjective and objective elements of the concept (Gurland *et al.* 1972a, 1972b).

It was designed to assess those aspects of maladjustment of clinical interest to psychiatrists. It includes three key dimensions of relevance to the aims of psychiatric treatment: distress, behaviour (normal–deviant) and interaction (friction) with others (the aims of psychiatric treatment being to reduce distress, to return behaviour to normal, and to smooth interaction with others). As items also include assets, its authors claim that it also contains measures of positive mental health. The authors justify their main focus on negative concepts on the grounds that 'since clinicians are more familiar with sickness than with health, their concern is with degrees of maladjustment rather than adjustment'. It was developed by a panel of senior psychotherapists and from the literature.

Content

The SSIAM contains 60 items. Each item includes a probing question which the interviewer puts to the patient. The patient's replies are rated by the interviewer on the scale. The 45 maladjustment items assess deviant behaviour, friction with others and subjective distress within five domains of maladjustment: work, social, family, marriage and sexual relationships. A further 15 items cover environmental stress, prognosis and positive mental health (Gurland *et al.* 1972a).

Administration and scoring

The questionnaire is administered by a trained interviewer. A training manual is available (Gurland and Yorkston 1971). The interview takes about 30–45 min to complete, and careful interviewer training is required.

Each of the 45 maladjustment items has a continuous response (VAS) scale with five anchoring definitions. The highest anchoring definition describes the maximum disturbance likely to be found in an out-patient psychoneurotic population; the lowest describes reasonable adjustment. The remaining three definitions represent successive levels of disturbance between the extremes. The interviewer acts as a rater and places a mark on the line to indicate the respondent's situation. The remaining 15 items on stress, prognosis and positive mental health require the rater to make more subjective judgements. For example, one item in each of the five areas of maladjustment asks the rater to make a judgement about the degree of stress in the respondent's environment. Other items ask the rater to judge aspects of the positive mental health of the respondent (e.g. talents and charm, resourcefulness, ability to apply energies constructively).

Each VAS scale has 11 points and ratings are scored at the numerical value of the nearest scale point. Each of the five sub-scales can be scored separately to give scores in each of the five areas of maladjustment; three separate sub-scale scores represent maladjustment in terms of deviant behaviour, friction and distress. The scale and instructions for administration can be obtained from its authors.

Examples from the SSIAM

Work

I'd like to talk now about your work and how you get along in your job. My first question is about the number of jobs you've had recently.

Unstable

Q. Do you have difficulty in holding down a job (or maintaining a course of study)? (For students, 'terminating a job' means failing or breaking off a course of study; housewives = not applicable)

10
9 Has terminated 6 jobs in last 4 months of working
8
7 Has terminated 4 jobs in last 4 months of working
6
5 Has terminated 2 jobs in last 4 months of working
4
3 Has terminated 1 job in last 4 months of working
2
1 Has not terminated any jobs in last 4 months of working
0

Friction

Q. Is there any tension, coolness or outright quarrelling in your (marital) family? (Disregard whether others are responsible. Include differences of opinion over sex, responsibilities and authority)

10
9 Marriage breaking up; gross incompatibility
8
7 Violence or marked estrangement or radical differences of opinion
6
5 Quite frequent quarrels or coolness or chronic differences of opinion
4
3 Some excessive tensions or misunderstandings or disagreements
2
1 Reasonably smooth and warm relationship
0

Lonely

Q. Do you feel the need for more companionship? ('Companionship' is a sense of shared social activity and warm mutual interest. This is independent of numbers of friends)

10
9 Feels companionship utterly lacking and desperately yearns for it
8
7 Feels a great need to fill a distinct gap in 'companionship'

6
5 Feels somewhat deprived of 'companionship'
4
3 Feels 'companionship' lacks a little fullness
2
1 Does not feel a lack of 'companionship'
0

Validity and factor structure

Evidence of the psychometric properties of the scale is limited. Correlations between the scale and structured psychiatric assessments for 100 schizophrenics have been reported to range between 0.21 and 0.41 (Serban 1979). It has been reported that the scale is able to discriminate between different types of schizophrenic patients (Serban and Gidynski 1979). Stern et al. (1977) reported that the SSIAM was strongly associated with depression, providing some evidence for its convergent validity.

Factor analysis has been carried out on the scale, based on 164 adults. Six factors emerged which do not fit with the three definitions of maladjustment: deviant behaviour, friction and subjective distress. The factors were social isolation, work inadequacy, friction with family, dependence on family, sexual dissatisfaction and friction outside the family (Gurland et al. 1972b).

Reliability

Intra-class correlations among raters ranged from 0.78 to 0.97 (Gurland et al. 1972b). The intra-class correlation coefficients of reliability of the six identified factors ranged from 0.78 to 0.97. Inter-rater agreement was reported to be adequate. There was significant agreement between ratings from patients and ratings from informants for all the factors except sexual dissatisfaction (Gurland et al. 1972b).

Despite the time-consuming nature of the scale, and the required training of interviewers, it has been used in several clinical studies and proved popular. It is one of the more promising adjustment scales, despite some psychometric problems.

VINELAND ADAPTIVE BEHAVIOUR SCALES

The Vineland Adaptive Behaviour Scales is a measure of adaptive behaviour from birth to adulthood (Sparrow et al. 1984a, 1984b, 1985). It was developed on the basis of a literature review, analysis of existing scale items, and development work involving field testing. The initial pool contained about 3000 items. It includes the assessment of social sufficiency, communication, daily living skills, socialization and motor skills (depending on age group), and provides a measure of maladaptive behaviour. It was developed for use with autistic children and adults, with good results for reliability and validity. It is suitable for use with handicapped and non-handicapped populations. It was designed for completion by a parent, teacher or care-giver during an interview. A shorter survey form and a longer expanded form for more detailed assessments are available.

Content

Three editions of the scale have been published: a survey form for a diagnostic and classification tool for normal to low functioning children or adults; an expanded form for use in the development of an individual's education or rehabilitation; and a classroom version for teachers (Sparrow et al. 1984a, 1984b, 1985). The survey form for diagnosis and classification is most often used in research in clinical outcomes. This is administered to the primary care-giver.

It has four domains, into which it is scored: communication, daily living skills, socialization and motor skills. The four domains (for those aged 5 and under) or the first three domains (for those aged 6 and above) are combined to form a composite adaptive behaviour score. The four domains can also be subdivided into receptive, expressive and written language (communication); personal, domestic and community (daily living skills); interpersonal relationships, play and leisure time and coping skills (socialization); and gross and fine motor skills (motor). An optional frequency and severity scale is available (maladaptive).

The communication domain assesses, for all ages, understanding of communication (receptive), expressive communication (expressive), reading and written communication (written). The daily living skills domain assesses, for all ages, eating, dressing, self-care skills (personal), household activities (domestic), use of time, money, telephone, job skills (community). The socialization domain assesses, for all ages, social interaction (interpersonal relationships), use of play and leisure time (play and leisure time), responsibility, sensitivity to others (coping skills). Motor skills for those aged under 6 assesses use of arms and legs for movement (gross), hand and finger movements (fine). The adaptive behaviour composite for all ages is the composite of the above, and the maladaptive behaviour composite for those aged under 5 assesses undesirable behaviours that interfere with adaptive functioning.

Administration and scoring

It is administered by a trained interviewer. The training of interviewers has to be particularly careful as some of the items are strangely worded and can be misinterpreted (e.g. item 5 of the communication domain is 'raises arms when caregiver says "come here" or "up"').

The instruction manual contains the scoring details for each section. Score *interpretations* are as follows: 2 = the activity is performed satisfactorily and habitually; 1 = there is emerging performance of an activity, or adequate but not habitual performance; 0 = the person is too young or immature to perform the activity, or can perform it but rarely does (plus N = no opportunity and DK = unknown). The standard scores from national samples are required in order to interpret scale scores (see the manual).

Validity and factor structure

Content validity was supported by the process of the scales' development, which was based on a literature review and analysis of other scale items, and developmental testing. The scales correlate with age, as would be expected, which supports the validity of the measure. It was tested against other behaviour scales with 39 non-handicapped children and 60 retarded adults living in institutions. Most correlations were moderate to strong ($r = 0.40$–0.70). It correlated weakly to moderately with intelligence test item scores ($r = 0.07$–0.52) in a study of 719 subjects aged 2–30 years (Sparrow *et al.* 1984a, 1984b, 1985). Principal components analysis and principal factor analyses confirmed the organization of the sub-domains into their respective categories.

Examples from the survey form of the Vineland Adaptive Behaviour Scales

Communication domain

18 Indicates preference when offered a choice
19 Says at least 50 recognizable words
25 Speaks in full sentences
31 Relates experiences in detail when asked

Living skills domain

41 Assists in food preparation requiring mixing and cooking
73 Straightens own room without being reminded
75 Looks after own health
91 Holds full-time job responsibly

Yes, usually (2) / sometimes or partly (1) / no, never (0) / no opportunity / don't know

In a study of 57 people aged 2–33 years attending a disabilities clinic in New Haven, Connecticut (Volkmar *et al.* 1987), it was reported that it was able to discriminate between autistic and non-autistic individuals.

Reliability

The authors demonstrated good levels of reliability for the scale (Sparrow *et al.* 1984a, 1984b, 1985). Split–half reliability coefficients range from 0.70 to 0.95 for the survey form for the sub-domains; test–retest correlations in the main range from 0.98 to 0.99, with a few in the 0.80s. Inter-rater reliability coefficients are also good, ranging from 0.62 to 0.78; these were based on the parents and carers of 160 subjects, who were interviewed twice by different interviewers (between 1 and 14 days apart; see manual for details). A manual, set of forms and scoring details are available for purchase.

SOCIAL ADJUSTMENT SCALE-II (SAS-II) AND SELF-REPORT VERSION

The SAS was initially developed by Paykel *et al.* (1971b, 1973), but revised for a study of depressed women and schizophrenic patients (see Weissman *et al.* 1971, 1974, 1978; Weissman and Paykel 1974; Weissman and Bothwell 1976; Schooler *et al.* 1979). Scale development has been described by Weissman and Paykel (1974). The scale is partly based on Gurland's SSIAM.

Content

The scale assesses interpersonal relationships in relation to feelings, satisfaction, friction and performance. Interviewer-administered and self-completion (SAS-SR) versions are both available from the author.

Both the original SAS and the SAS-SR versions contain 54 questions (42 answerable by any one respondent) covering six areas of functioning: work/school/housework (18 items), leisure activities (11 items), relationships with extended family (7 items), marital roles (9 items), parent role (4 items) and member of the family unit (4 items) (Weissman and Bothwell 1976; Weissman *et al.* 1978). The questions relate to the previous 2 weeks. In each area of functioning, the questions cover performance, amount of friction, other aspects of interpersonal relationships, inner feelings and satisfaction.

The SAS-II interview was developed from the original SAS by Schooler *et al.* (1979) and Glazer *et al.* (1980), for use with patients with schizophrenia, or a significant other. It contains two fewer questions (*n* = 52), which are administered in a semi-structured interview by a trained interviewer. Five global judgements are made by the interviewer on the basis of a 'community norm'. The areas assessed are work role, relationships, sexual adjustment, romantic involvement, social leisure activities and personal well-being. Both instrumental and affective areas are rated.

Administration and scoring

Both interviewer-administered and self-report versions have been developed. The interviewer-administered version takes an hour to complete, and the self-completion version about 10 min (in the presence of an interviewer). Interviewer training is required. Either 5- or 6-point response scales are used. An overall score is calculated by summing the item scores and dividing by the number of ticked items.

Examples from the SAS-SR

4 Have you had any arguments with people at work in the last two weeks?

I had no arguments and got along very well / I usually got along well but had minor arguments / I had more than one argument / I had many arguments / I was constantly in arguments

12 Have you found your housework interesting these last 2 weeks?

My work was almost always interesting / once or twice my work was not interesting / half the time my work was uninteresting / most of the time my work was uninteresting / my work was always uninteresting

15 During the last 2 weeks, have you been ashamed of how you do your schoolwork?

I never felt ashamed / once or twice I felt ashamed / about half the time I felt ashamed / I felt ashamed most of the time / I felt ashamed all of the time

Validity

The scale was weakly to strongly correlated with several depression scales; the correlations between these ranged from 0.18 to 0.84 for groups of community respondents, acute depressives, alcoholics and schizophrenics (Weissman *et al.* 1978). The agreement between the SAS and the self-report version in a study of 76 depressed outpatients was high, and the self-report version was reported to be sensitive to recovery.

Reliability

Agreement between 15 depressed patients' ratings and spouses' or others' ratings was reported to be $r = 0.74$, and between patients' and interviewers' assessments it was $r = 0.70$. Item–total score correlations ranged widely ($r = 0.09–0.83$) for the interview version. Inter-rater agreement for the interview version was 68 per cent.

Reliability was further tested on 56 schizophrenics and their informants (out-patients) and agreement between informants was high ($r = 0.98$). It has high internal consistency (mean alpha $= 0.74$) and test–retest reliability ($r = 0.80$) (Weissman and Bothwell 1976; Edwards *et al.* 1978;

Weissman *et al.* 1981). Agreement between 56 schizophrenic out-patients and their informants was reported to be high at 0.98 (Glazer *et al.* 1980). More evidence of its psychometric properties is still required. It has been extensively used in psychiatric research, and norms were developed with 200 hospitalized schizophrenics, and these have been published. A manual is available from the author.

KATZ ADJUSTMENT SCALES

These are among the most widely used self- and informant-report scales of adjustment for patients who are being reintegrated into normal living (Katz and Lyerly 1963). The authors defined adjustment in relation to the balance between the individual and the environment, freedom from psychopathology, absence of personal distress, suitable patterns of social interaction and adequate social role performance. Sub-scales cover symptoms, social roles and leisure activities. These were developed for use with patients with schizophrenia and have been successfully adapted for use with people with epilepsy (Vickrey *et al.* 1992a).

Content, administration and scoring

Social adjustment is evaluated by the subject (S scales) and by a close relative (R scales). Level of performance is measured and, on the R scale, performance with regard to expectations for performance. The scales are interviewer-administered.

The relative (R) has five forms to complete. Form R1 contains 127 items on the patient's psychiatric symptoms and social behaviour, which are scored on 4-point frequency scales (and which are summed). Form R2 contains 16 items on the performance of socially expected activities (social responsibilities, self-care, community activities), scored on 3-point frequency scales. Form R3 is identical to form R2 except that it covers expectations of performance. Satisfaction with performance is derived from computing the discrepancy between form R3 (expectations) and form R2 (actual). A pair of 23-item forms (R4 and R5) cover the relative's ratings of the patient's leisure activities (e.g. hobbies, social, community, self-improvement activities) and expectations for these.

The patient, or subject (S), completes five forms,

including S1, which contains 55 items derived from the Hopkins Symptom Checklist on somatic symptoms and mood (Derogatis *et al.* 1974a. Forms S2–5 correspond to the relative's forms (R2–5).

Examples of relative's forms from the Katz Adjustment Scales

R2 and R3

1 Helps with household chores
2 Visits his friends
3 Visits his relatives
4 Entertains friends at home
5 Dresses and takes care of himself

R2 response choices: is not doing / is doing some / is doing regularly

R3 response choices: did not expect him to be doing / expected him to be doing some / expected him to be doing regularly

Validity and factor structure

The symptom sub-scale is sensitive to treatment type, but the other sub-scales are less sensitive (Fiske 1974). The relative's forms are able to distinguish between patients judged by clinicians to be well or poorly adjusted. Psychometric analyses by Katz and Lyerly (1963) led to 13 factors. The scales were later reported to correlate well with clinical assessments of adjustment (Hogarty and Katz 1971).

Reliability

Internal consistency coefficients of 0.41–0.87 (median 0.72) were reported for the sub-scale scores; the coefficients were less than 0.70 for 6 of the 11 sub-scales which, according to Nunnally (1978), is not always regarded as acceptable.

There are relatively few other data on their validity or reliability. These are old scales, and in widespread and popular use.

PSYCHOSOCIAL ADJUSTMENT TO ILLNESS SCALE (PAIS)

This is a semi-structured interview designed to assess overall psychological and social adjustment to illness among medical patients, or their immediate relatives (Morrow *et al.* 1978; Derogatis *et al.* 1979; Derogatis and Lopez 1983; Derogatis 1977, 1986). It is a general measure and not disease-specific, although it is often used in oncology (Selby and Robertson 1987).

The instrument measures adjustments rather than overall quality of life, and is useful in longitudinal study design. There is no assessment of specific symptoms or side-effects. Investigators have found the measure of sexual functioning to be a useful outcome measure, and it has been reported that while overall quality of life measures may show improvement after certain cancer treatments, sexual functioning can simultaneously decrease (Chang *et al.* 1989).

Content

The PAIS interview version contains items grouped to measure specific domains of health-related quality of life. The authors have also developed a 46-item self-report analogue (PAIS-SR). The measures are almost identical and both measure seven areas of adjustment: health care orientation, vocational environment, domestic environment, sexual relationships, extended family relationships, social environment and psychological distress. Each is rated on a 4-point scale and then standardized, thus generating a total score.

Administration and scoring

A version for administration by an interviewer and a version for self-completion have been developed. Ratings for each question within each domain are made on a 4-point scale – for example, complete adequacy (0) to marked inadequacy (3) – which are summed and manipulated to generate standardized sub-scale scores and a total PAIS score. High scores reflect more distress. Both the interview and the self-report versions take about 30 min to complete.

Examples from the PAIS

Section I

1 Which of the following statements best describes your usual attitude about taking care of your health?

(a) I am very concerned and pay close attention to my personal health

(b) Most of the time I pay attention to my health care needs

(c) Usually, I try to take care of health matters but sometimes I just don't get round to it

(d) Health care is something that I just don't worry too much about

Section III

1 How would you describe your relationship with your husband or wife (partner, if not married) since your illness?

(a) Good
(b) Fair
(c) Poor
(d) Very poor

Section VI

1 Are you still as interested in your leisure time activities and hobbies as you were prior to your illness?

(a) Same level of interest as previously
(b) Slightly less interest than before
(c) Significantly less interest than before
(d) Little or no interest remaining

Validity and factor structure

Derogatis (1986) reported that the PAIS correlated highly ($r = 0.81$) with the Global Adjustment to Illness Scale (Morrow *et al.* 1981) and fairly highly ($r = 0.60$) with the Symptom Checklist-90 (Derogatis *et al.* 1976, 1977). It has also been reported to correlate well with physicians' assessments of renal dialysis patients (Kaplan–DeNour 1982). On the basis of a study of patients with Hodgkin's disease, Morrow *et al.* (1978) reported that the health care orientation sub-scale correlated with satisfaction with health care ($r = 0.27$), as would be expected; the psychological distress domain correlated with patients' self-assessments and observer ratings of anxiety and depression, and with other scales of anxiety and depression ($r = 0.47$–0.51). Derogatis (1986) reported that factor analyses generally supported the factor structure of the scale.

Reliability

Morrow *et al.* (1978) reported high inter-rater reliability coefficients ($r = 0.33$–0.83; all but one being over 0.60) in a study of 37 people with Hodgkin's disease. Good reliability coefficients were also reported by Derogatis (1986). The internal consistency coefficients (alpha) ranged from 0.63 to 0.87 with 269 renal dialysis patients, 0.47 to 0.85 with 61 cardiac patients and 0.68 to 0.93 with 89 lung cancer patients, except for the domain 'extended family', which only achieved 0.12. More examples of the scale items are given by Derogatis (1986).

The authors have provided norms for patients with lung cancer, patients undergoing renal dialysis, cardiac patients and heterogeneous groups of cancer patients (Derogatis and Lopez 1983). PAIS profiles are purchasable for patients with lung cancer, renal dialysis, burns, essential hypertension, mixed cancer patients, cardiac and diabetic patients. Sugarbaker *et al.* (1982) have reported norms for patients with soft tissue sarcoma undergoing different treatments.

GLOBAL ADJUSTMENT TO ILLNESS SCALE (GAIS)

The GAIS is a single global rating scale from 0 to 100, which was designed to record the judgement of a trained clinical observer in relation to the psychosocial adjustment of patients to a medical illness (Morrow *et al.* 1981). It is one of three scales developed from 25 videotaped interviews with cancer patients, undertaken by five site collaborators from the Psychosocial Collaborative Oncology Group and rated by 105 professionals (Morrow *et al.* 1981). The other two are the Rating of Psychosocial Function (RPF) and the Coping Adequacy Rating (CAR) scales.

Content, administration and scoring

The scale is an observer rating of psychosocial adjustment. On the rating scale (of 0 to 100), each decile describes a level of adjustment (e.g. 91–100 = excellent, 81–90 = very good, 51–60 = adequate with reservations, and so on).

Validity and reliability

The measure was reported to have adequate levels of validity. Pearson intercorrelations between the GAIS and the RPF and the CAR in four studies ranged from 0.55 to 0.80, suggesting a convergent validity of a 'psychosocial adjustment construct'. The GAIS was the scale of choice of the investigators because it coincided closely with their clinical impressions (Morrow *et al.* 1981). A study of 109 newly diagnosed breast cancer patients by Ganz *et al.* (1990) reported a moderate correlation between the GAIS and the Functional Living Index – Cancer ($r = 0.53$). There is little information about the scale's reliability.

ACCEPTANCE OF ILLNESS SCALE

Most scales of adjustment or acceptance measure broad outcomes such as mood or social functioning rather than illness-related adjustment (Wright *et al.* in press). The Acceptance of Illness Scale, in contrast, measures the extent to which people are able to accept their illness (Felton *et al.* 1984; Felton and Revenson 1984).

Content, administration and scoring

The Acceptance of Illness Scale is a brief self-report scale. It contains eight items, with a 5-point VAS response scale, anchored at one end with 'strongly agree' (1) and at the other with 'strongly disagree' (5). All items except one are negative. The coding for the one positive item is reversed. The scores are summed, with a total range of 8 (extremely low acceptance/adjustment) to 40 (extremely high acceptance/adjustment).

Examples from the Acceptance of Illness Scale

1 I have had a hard time adjusting to the limitations of my illness
3 My illness makes me feel useless at times
4 Health problems make me more dependent on others than I want to be
8 I think people are often uncomfortable being around me because of my illness

Strongly agree   1   2   3   4   5   Strongly disagree

Validity and reliability

There is little information available on the validity or factor structure of the scale. The authors used the scale on 151 patients with either hypertension, diabetes, arthritis or cancer. They reported the internal consistency of the scale to be high (Cronbach's alpha was 0.81–0.83). The test–retest reliability coefficent over 7 months was $r = 0.69$. Little other evidence of the psychometric properties of the scale has been published, but it appears to be a promising alternative to the lengthy generic adjustment scales. The scale was reviewed by Wright et al. (in press).

REINTEGRATION TO NORMAL LIVING (RNL) INDEX

Disease and treatment may result in disruption of activities and responsibilities. Wood-Dauphinee and Williams (1987) developed the RNL Index in order to measure reintegration, after forming three panels, each of which included professionals, patients and relatives and using interviewers to pilot questionnaires with them. The term 'quality of life' was not used by the interviewers. From this an 11-item index was developed.

Content

The RNL contains 11 VAS items. It measures nine domains of reintegration into normal living patterns: mobility, self-care abilities, daily activities, recreational activities, social activities, family roles, personal relationships, presentation of self, general coping skills.

Administration and scoring

The index was developed for patients to complete, and a similar index was designed for professionals and significant others to complete. The 11 items each have a 10-point VAS scale. The scores are proportionally converted to a 100-point system.

Examples from the RNL Index

2 I move around my community as I feel is necessary (wheelchairs, other equipment or resources may be used).

6 I am able to participate in recreational activities (hobbies, crafts, sports, reading, television, games, computers, etc.) as I want to (adaptive equipment, supervision and/or assistance may be used).

9 In general, I am comfortable with my personal relationships.

11 I feel that I can deal with life-events as they happen.

Validity and factor structure

Preliminary analyses demonstrated that the index had concurrent and discriminant validity, but further testing is required. The correlations between the Quality of Life Index (Spitzer et al. 1981) and the RNL sub-scales varied from 0.07 to 0.67. Principal components analysis demonstrated two theoretically meaningful factors: daily functioning and perception of self.

Reliability

The index was used with 109 patients with various diseases, and a Cronbach's alpha greater than 0.90 was recorded when the index was completed by patients, professionals and significant others (Wood-Dauphinee and Williams 1987). The correlations for significant others–patients was higher (0.62) than for professionals–patients (0.39).

The index has been criticized by Siegrist and Junge (1990) for failing to distinguish between the physical and social components of functioning – a person may be physically able but socially disinclined to perform certain activities. Many scales suffer from this weakness.

STRESS AND COPING SCALES FOR USE WITH PSYCHIATRICALLY AND/OR PHYSICALLY ILL PEOPLE

Social stress

It was pointed out earlier that few stress scales have been used in disease-specific studies. Stress is a response to an illness, or a predisposing variable, rather than a relevant factor in the assessment of outcome. However, some investigators have attempted to measure the stress experienced as the result of a disease, for example cancer (Vinokur et al. 1989, 1990).

Scales for the measurement of stress are only briefly referred to here. These scales are not disease-specific, and are of use mainly in epidemiological studies rather than in outcome studies. There are several frequently used life-events scales (e.g. Rahe et al. 1964; Paykel et al. 1971a; Horowitz et al. 1977; Dohrenwend et al. 1978; Sarason et al. 1978).

A brief review of the development of scales to measure stressful life-events is given by Leff (1991a). An initial approach was to develop checklists of events (e.g. divorce, marriage, bereavement), which respondents admit to having experienced or not.

The Schedule of Recent Experience, incorporating Holmes and Rahe's (1967) Social Readjustment Rating scale, is perhaps the best known, and also the most often criticized (Rahe 1969, 1974; Amundson et al. 1981; for reviews see Casey et al. 1967; McDonald et al. 1972; Tennen et al. 1985). This evolved from Meyer's (1919) Life Chart, and was initially developed by Hawkins et al. (1957). It includes a wide range of recent life changes in relation to personal, social, occupational and family events. It was further developed by Rahe et al. (1964) in their studies of life-events and coronary heart disease. A review of these studies has been published by Rahe (1988). Similar, but more suitable scales for children and also adolescents are available (e.g. Coddington 1972, 1981a, 1981b).

One problem with these scales relates to the lack of attention paid to the meaning of life-events to the individual (Brown 1974, 1991; Lazarus and Cohen 1977; Antonovsky 1979; O'Conner and Brown 1984). Another problem is the accuracy of recall of life-events (Paykel and Dowlatshahi 1988). Monroe (1982) found that 60 per cent of events 4 months previously are not recountable. Paykel (1983) reviewed the literature and reported that self-report schedules have low test–retest reliability, whereas interview questionnaires have moderately high test–retest reliability and high inter-rater reliability. Brown et al. (1973) and Brown and Harris (1982) reported about 80 per cent agreement for individual events using interview methods.

Trends in the measurement of stressful events

The widespread criticisms of measures of stress led to the movement towards semi-structured questionnaires (Brown and Birley 1968; Paykel et al. 1969; O'Conner and Brown 1984), and away from the early self-report questionnaires (Holmes and Rahe 1967). Several semi-structured interview schedules have been developed, the most detailed being the Life Events and Difficulties Schedule (Brown et al. 1973), which elicits life-events. These

investigators also developed a method for assessing the emotional impact of each event on an individual by taking the context into account (Brown and Harris 1978). This involves a tape-recording of the interview and a later rating (by coders in the office) of events (with inter-rater reliability checks). Brown and his colleagues also developed the Bedford College Self-Evaluation and Social Support Schedule, an intensive instrument which takes context into account in relation to social support (O'Conner and Brown 1984). While admirable for its methodological soundness, this method has been little used by other investigators because of its complexity and expense.

The Impact of Events Scale was developed by Horowitz et al. (1977, 1979, 1983) after a search of the literature revealed scales that consisted of checklists of events, without any attempt to take subjective experiences into consideration. This scale was developed with the aim of assessing current subjective stress for any life event. Thus the question wording is not anchored to a specific occurrence, but to qualities of the experience.

Paykel (1983) designed a shorter semi-structured interview, which covers 64 events and makes judgements of the degree of independence of the event, and its objective negative impact. This was based on earlier work (Paykel et al. 1969, 1971a; Paykel 1974). Interested readers are referred to Kasl and Cooper (1987) for further details of the measurement of social stress in relation to health.

Coping

While coping behaviour has been covered in part in the other measurement scales reviewed here (e.g. social behaviour and adjustment overlap with coping behaviour), coping behaviour scales tend to concentrate on the practical side of coping – what people do and think in order to cope with a stressful situation (e.g. illness).

Coping styles are important facets of health outcomes, given that they are thought to regulate emotions or distress, and manage the problem that caused the distress (Lazarus and Folkman 1984). The way in which people handle, or cope with, stressful events in life may be crucial in influencing and moderating the deleterious effects of these events on their health. An increasing literature exists on the individual's attempt to utilize personal and social resources to manage stress and to act on it (Lazarus 1966, 1980; Coelho *et al.* 1974; Pearlin and Schooler 1978; Billings and Moos 1981).

The hypothesized domains of coping have been reviewed by Billings and Moos (1981). The amount and quality of social support may also be associated with adequacy of functioning and coping, and act as a moderator of life stressors (Holahan and Moos 1981), although the literature is inconsistent on this point. Pearlin (1989) reviewed the theoretical literature on the mediating effects of coping behaviour on stress, and argued that research should move away from the study of single events and instead focus on stress and coping over time.

Coping scales

Coping scales tend to contain a large number of items, usually with the object of identifying the sub-dimensions of coping strategies used, given the psychological literature that individuals may have several coping styles which they employ in different situations. Recent interest in psychology has focused on cognitive and behavioural responses to external stressors, and the marked variations therein. Unless coping styles as modifying variables are of particular interest to the investigator, it is unlikely that coping scales will be routinely employed in outcomes research, although they have an impressive history of use in oncology (particularly the Ways of Coping Questionnaire or Scale: Folkman and Lazarus 1980).

Some investigators have developed disease-specific coping scales. One example is the Coping Questionnaire for Hypertensive Patients developed by Moum *et al.* (1990). They developed this on the basis of the psychological literature and discussions with hypertensive patients. It contains disease-specific items on coping strategies such as 'I talked to people whose blood pressure is too high', 'I tried to live a healthier life than I had done previously' and 'I tried to think about other things than sickness and health'. Unfortunately, the authors reported that the instrument lacked sensitivity and, if anything, active coping had a very slight counterproductive effect on emotional adjustment to a diagnosis of hypertension. Nicassio *et al.* (1985) have also developed a coping scale for use in rheumatology, with some testing of its psycho-

metric properties. It is more appropriate in outcome assessment than generic scales. It includes items such as 'I can reduce my pain by staying calm and relaxed' and 'I can do a lot of things myself to cope with my arthritis'. This is a promising scale, and it is to be hoped that the authors will test it further for reliability and validity.

Some of the most popular coping scales are presented here; however there are many others (see Cohen 1987). Several scales are also presented which measure single domains of coping, such as defensiveness (e.g. see Gleser and Ihilevich's, 1969, Defence Mechanism Inventory) and denial (e.g. Hacket and Cassem's, 1974, Denial Scale, which was developed to assess denial in myocardial infarction patients). Scales also exist which have been developed to measure the family's capacity to cope with stress (see Grotevant and Carlson 1989). For details of other scales, interested readers are referred to Aldwin and Revenson (1987), Cohen (1987), Endler and Parker (1990) and Parker and Endler (1992).

Hopelessness

At the opposite end of the spectrum to coping is hopelessness. While it is admittedly a slightly different concept, loss of control can lead to feelings of hopelessness and this can result in loss of self-concept and self-esteem (Charmaz 1983). Hopelessness is often included in mental health instruments (e.g. Lipman *et al.* 1969; Derogatis *et al.* 1971). The Hopelessness Scale, developed by Beck *et al.* (1974b), has been modified by some users (e.g. Jenkins *et al.* 1983a, 1983b), although it has not always been found to be sensitive to therapeutic intervention and improvements in the patient's condition (see Jenkins *et al.* 1983a, 1983b). This is an area in which more disease-specific measures are required.

WAYS OF COPING SCALE

The Ways of Coping Scale assesses how people cope with the stresses of everyday life, based on the cognitive–transactional theory of stress which was developed by the authors (Folkman and Lazarus 1980, 1988a, 1988b; Schaefer *et al.* 1982). This theory holds that, in the face of stress, individuals appraise the situation to assess its personal relevance, and then engage in secondary appraisal, which means they assess whether they can act to reduce the harmfulness of the stressor.

The original version (generally known as the Ways of Coping Checklist) contained 68 items, with 'yes/no' response choices. The scale was revised by Folkman and Lazarus (1985). The early revised version by Folkman and Lazarus (1985), referred to as the Ways of Coping Questionnaire, initially contained 66 items and a new response format (not a 'yes/no' response format but a 4-point Likert scale where 0 = does not apply/not used and 3 = used a great deal). The revisions were tested with 108 subjects. Factor analyses of the revised scale and analyses of skewness and variance led to the further deletion of items until 42 items were left to form the final, revised scale; however, the 66-item version is still in use.

Content

The scale covers three major coping domains: emotion-focused coping (aimed at reducing or managing the emotional distress associated with the situation), problem-focused coping (aimed at problem-solving) and seeks social support as a coping mechanism. These distinctions are important but have been criticized as too simple (Carver *et al.* 1989); research has found that responses to the scale form several factors (Folkman and Lazarus 1985; Folkman *et al.* 1986b).

Emotion-focused coping measures efforts to manage the emotions arising from a stressful situation (Lazarus and Folkman 1984). It is measured using responses to items on avoidance strategies to psychologically distance oneself from the situation (10 items), blamed self-strategies to hold oneself culpable for a situation (3 items), and wishful-thinking strategies to escape by using fantasy (8 items) (Lazarus *et al.* 1974).

Problem-focused coping aims to measure those strategies which are directed towards changing a stressful situation. It is measured by responses to items on the 'problem-focused sub-scale' (15 items). Social support seeking coping mechanisms are measured by the 'seeks social support sub-scale' (6 items), which describes both the problem-focused and emotion-focused coping strategies used (Lazarus and Folkman 1984). Subjects describe their coping responses in relation to the most

stressful episode they have experienced in the past week or month (Folkman and Lazarus 1988b).

Administration and scoring

The scale can be self-administered, although it is usually administered in the presence of an interviewer. Respondents indicate whether they use each of the given response choices in a given stressful situation, either by making a 'yes/no' response or by making a rating on a multi-point scale. There is no standard way to score the instrument, and different investigators have adopted their own techniques (Cohen 1987).

Modifications

There have been several modifications to the scale by a number of investigators (e.g. Vitaliano 1987; Larsson and Setterlind 1990). A modified Ways of Coping Scale was used by Redeker (1992) in a study of 129 patients recovering from coronary artery bypass surgery; it was reported that the most common method of coping was to seek social

---

Examples from the Ways of Coping Scale

Positive reappraisal

'Rediscover what is important in life'
'Pray'

Problem-solving plans

'Just concentrate on what I have to do next – the next step'
'Draw on past experiences; I was in a similar situation before'

Seeking social support

'Talk to someone to find out more about the situation'
'Talk to someone who can do something concrete about the problem'

Self-controlling

'I try to keep my feelings to myself'
'I go over in my mind what I will say or do'

---

support. Felton and Revenson (1984) and Felton *et al.* (1984) have adapted the Ways of Coping Scale for use with people with chronic illnesses (e.g. hypertension, diabetes, arthritis and cancer). Their two coping indexes were derived from the Ways of Coping Scale and, in order to elicit illness-specific responses rather than general dispositional answers, respondents were asked how frequently they had used each of the behaviours 'in reaction to being ill'. A 5-point response scale, ranging from 'never' (1) to 'most of the time' (5), was used because coping was assumed to be ongoing in chronic illnesses. They reported a satisfactory factor structure, and that the scale was associated with the independent adjustment items used. Several other scales have been designed which are similar to the Ways of Coping Scale, such as the Jalowiec Coping Scale (Jalowiec *et al.* 1984), but they have still not been fully tested for their psychometric properties (for a review, see Tennen and Herzberger 1985a).

Validity and factor structure

Vitaliano *et al.* (1985) reported that the scale had good construct and concurrent validity (and internal consistency); there is little evidence of its convergent validity. Principal components and factor analyses of the scale have variously reported it to produce 2–9 factors, or clusters of coping strategies (Aldwin *et al.* 1980; Folkman and Lazarus 1980, 1985, 1986; Revenson 1981; Collins *et al.* 1982; Felton *et al.* 1984; McCrae 1984; Parkes 1984; Vingerhoets and Flohr 1984; Vitaliano *et al.* 1985; Folkman *et al.* 1986a, 1986b; for a review, see Endler and Parker 1990). Clearly more testing is needed.

Reliability

Folkman and Lazarus (1980) used the original scale with 100 community residents aged 45–64 years in a study of how they coped with stressful events over a period of 1 year. They reported inter-rater reliability figures, using ten raters for classifying problem- or emotion-focused coping; there was 91 per cent agreement between raters. The internal consistency coefficients (Cronbach's alpha) were 0.80 and 0.81 for these two scales. Revisions were

undertaken with items showing weak (<0.25) item–total correlations.

The correlations for internal consistency were confirmed by Redeker (1992) in a study of 129 patients recovering from coronary artery bypass surgery (Cronbach's alpha 0.72–0.91). She reported that the most frequent coping strategy at 1 and 6 weeks after coronary artery bypass grafting was social support seeking, followed by problem-focused coping and the emotion-focused coping strategies of blamed self, wishful-thinking and avoidance.

The scale items have been criticized as ambiguous by Carver *et al.* (1989). For example, the item 'I did something which I didn't think would work, but at least I was doing something' is unclear in relation to which is more important – whether it was the fact that something was being done, or the fact that the respondent didn't think that the act would work.

Tennen and Herzberger (1985a) have reviewed the studies using the scale, and raised the question of whether respondents can really recall coping strategies. This criticism has been echoed by Stone *et al.* (1991). However, it has been the most popular coping scale among clinicians and social scientists. Endler and Parker (1990) concluded that the scale has been used more often by researchers than its psychometric properties warrant.

HEALTH AND DAILY LIVING FORM

This form was designed and widely used, by Moos and colleagues (Billings and Moos 1981, 1984; Moos *et al.* 1982, 1986, 1990). It is similar to the Ways of Coping Scale (see above) and was developed from the literature and existing scales. It includes questions on personal, social and health characteristics, and a series of questions on coping, adapted from the existing literature. It was developed for an investigation of coping behaviours of adults who were entering treatment for depression.

The original coping questions consisted of 19 'yes/no' items probing how people coped with identified life-events. The authors later expanded the number of items to 28, and then to 32 using a 4-point Likert scale instead of a 'yes/no' format (Billings and Moos 1984). The items were grouped into three methods of coping categories: active–cognitive (6 items), active–behavioural (6) and avoidance (5) (approach coping can also be calculated from items in the active–cognitive coping index, active–behavioural coping index and two additional items). They could also be grouped into two foci of coping categories: problem-focused (7 items) and emotion-focused (11). The new classification was grouped into three categories: appraisal-focused coping, problem-focused coping and emotion-focused coping, although little empirical evidence was presented to support this (Billings and Moos 1985; Moos *et al.* 1986)

Content, administration and scoring

The scale is usually completed in the presence of an interviewer. With the current version of the coping scale, respondents indicate whether they have experienced any stressful events (from a list), and then they are asked to rate their use of coping strategies in relation to 32 different coping re-

---

Examples from the Health and Daily Living – Adult Form B

Events in the past year

1 Here is a list of events that may happen to anyone. Have you experienced any of them personally DURING THE LAST 12 MONTHS?

If YES, please indicate:

(a) how many months ago the event occurred
(b) whether you had any control over it

List of events (examples)
Moved to a new residence
Marriage
Separation
Went deeply into debt
Assaulted or robbed

2 Sometimes when people have problems they turn to certain persons for help. HAVE YOU EVER GONE to any of the people on this list for advice or help with marriage or family problems, or other personal problems. If you have, was it in the last 12 months?

(a) Minister, priest, rabbi or other spiritual counsellor?
(b) Medical doctor?
(c) Self-help or sensitivity help?
(d) Lawyer?

---

sponses (33 questions), using a 4-point scale. The scoring details are lengthy, but a manual with full details of the scoring is available (Moos *et al.* 1986).

Validity

In a study of 294 randomly selected individuals, the authors reported only a modest association between types of event and coping behaviours (Billings and Moos 1981).

Reliability

The internal consistencies (Cronbach's alpha) of the coping categories were reported to be 0.72 for active–cognitive coping, 0.80 for active–behavioural coping and 0.44 for avoidance coping. This suggests moderate internal homogeneity. Inter-correlations between the items were low (the average was $r = 0.21$), suggesting that the categories were relatively independent.

Billings and Moos (1984) carried out an item analysis from which five scales emerged: appraisal-focused coping; problem-focused coping – information-seeking; problem-focused coping – problem-solving; emotion-focused coping – affective regulation; and emotion-focused coping – emotional discharge. The alphas were reported to be 0.53, 0.63, 0.66, 0.63 and 0.41, respectively. These moderate alphas reflect relatively poor internal consistency, and make the scale less attractive than other frequently used scales (see Tennen and Herzberger 1985a).

STRESS IN LIFE COPING SCALE

This scale was developed by Pearlin and Schooler (1978) to measure the diverse coping strategies used in response to conflicts and frustrations in four role areas. During its development, over 100 subjects were asked to identify the daily problems they faced and how they dealt with them.

Thematic examination of the results yielded several coping patterns which were tested for use in the scale. Factor analyses yielded 19 factors in three main categories: those which change the situation from that in which the stress occurred; those which control the meaning of the stressful experience after it occurs but before the stress emerges; and those which control the stress after it has been experienced. Subsequently, it was used on a larger sample of 2300 residents in Chicago (Pearlin and Lieberman 1978).

The four role areas covered by the scale are: marital coping responses (21 items), parental coping responses (21 items), household economics coping responses (15 items) and occupational coping responses (16 items). Factor analyses were carried out by the authors in each of the four areas. The marital coping responses cover six factors: self-reliance *vs* advice seeking; controlled reflectiveness *vs* emotional discharge; positive comparisons; negotiations; self-assertion *vs* passive forbearance; and selective ignoring. The parental coping responses cover five factors: selective ignoring; non-punitiveness *vs* reliance on discipline; self-reliance *vs* advice-seeking; positive comparisons; and exercise of potency *vs* helpless resignation. The household economic coping responses cover four factors: devaluation of money; selective ignoring; positive comparisons; and optimistic faith. Finally, the occupational coping responses cover four factors: substitution of rewards; positive comparisons; optimistic action; and selective ignoring (these factors make up the 19 contained in the scale).

Content

This is a 73-item scale, covering the four role areas of marriage, parenthood, household economics and occupation. The scale is contained within a larger interview schedule on the impact of psychological resources, strain and coping response on stress. This is known as a trait measure of coping, since it asks how people usually, rather than actually, coped in specific situations.

Administration and scoring

The scale is interviewer-administered. The 19 coping response factors in the instrument are scored by weighting the standardized item score by its factor loading and then summing. Scores within the four role areas (marriage, parenthood, household economics and occupation) can then be computed by summing the factor scores for each role.

The response choices vary from whether a particular coping response has been adopted (over the past year) to the frequency of coping responses.

Examples from the Stress in Life Coping Scale

Parental coping responses with children

Non-punitiveness vs reliance on discipline: When your children's behaviour is troublesome, how often do you:

2 Scold them?
3 Threaten some kind of punishment?

Positive comparisons

1 As time goes by, has being a parent generally become easier or more difficult?
3 How would you compare your experiences as a parent with other parents?

Household economic coping responses

Devaluation of money

1 When you are short of money, how often do you borrow?
2 During a typical week, about how much are money problems on your mind?

Selective ignoring: When you are short of money, how often do you:

1 Concentrate on more important things in life?
2 Notice people around who are worse off than you?
3 Tell yourself that money isn't worth getting upset about?

Occupational coping responses

Positive comparisons

1 How does your work life compare with what it was about a year ago?
2 When you think of the future, what would you say your work life will be like a year or so from now?

Selective ignoring: How often do you:

1 Just wait for difficulties to sort themselves out?
3 Try to pay attention only to your duties in order to overlook difficulties in your work situation?

Validity and reliability

There are few data on the validity and reliability of the scale, although the strong factor loadings suggest internal consistency (Pearlin and Schooler 1978). This scale has been influential in the coping field, although it is limited to chronic, rather than acute, strains on life.

COPE

COPE was designed by Carver *et al.* (1989) after a review of existing scales and a critical analysis of the most popular scales – for example, the Ways of Coping Scale (Folkman and Lazarus 1980) as well as other popular scales developed by Billings and Moos (1981, 1984) and Stone and Neale (1984). It has two formats: dispositional and situational.

Content, administration and scoring

The final version of COPE contains 13 conceptually distinct sub-scales, based on the theoretical literature about functional coping strategies. The instrument can be self-administered. Five sub-scales (four items per sub-scale) measure conceptually distinct aspects of problem-focused coping: active coping, planning, suppression of competing activities, restraint coping, seeking of instrumental social support. Five sub-scales (four items per sub-scale) measure emotion-focused coping: seeking emotional support, positive reinterpretation, acceptance, denial, turning to religion. And three sub-scales (three items per sub-scale) measure other, less useful, coping responses: focus on and venting of emotions, behavioural disengagement, mental disengagement. The responses to items are scored 1 to 4 and the sub-scale items are summed.

Examples from COPE

We are interested in how people respond when they confront difficult or stressful events in their lives. There are lots of ways to try to deal with stress. This questionnaire asks you to indicate what *you* generally do and feel, when *you* experience stressful events. Obviously, different events bring out somewhat different responses, but think about what you *usually* do when you are under a lot of stress.

Planning

I try to come up with a strategy about what to do
I make a plan of action
I think hard about what steps to take
I think about how I might best handle the problem

Seeking social support for instrumental reasons

I ask people who have had similar experiences what they did

I try to get advice from someone about what to do
I talk to someone to find out more about the situation
I talk to someone who could do something concrete about the problem

Denial

I refuse to believe that it has happened
I pretend that it hasn't really happened
I act as though it hasn't even happened
I say to myself 'this isn't real'

Validity and factor structure

Three phases of testing were carried out during the development and refinement of the scale, and the developmental versions of the scale were administered to several hundred college students. The final item set was first completed by 978 undergraduates in group sessions. In further studies of validity, between 162–476 students completed the COPE and a range of other personality scales. As would be expected, there were significant, although modest, correlations between the COPE active coping and planning sub-scale and scales of optimism, control, self-esteem, hardiness and Type A personality ($r = 0.20$–0.32). Active coping was inversely associated with trait anxiety ($r = -0.25$).

Principal factor analysis yielded 12 factors, all of which were in accord with the a priori assignment of items to scales, except the active coping and the planning items, which all loaded together on one factor; and all the social support items loaded on one factor, independent of the basis for seeking support. Weak loadings were reported for the mental disengagement factor and the positive reinterpretation factor. A second factor analysis based on 156 subjects mostly confirmed this structure, with some higher scale alphas than those achieved in study 1.

Reliability

The internal consistency coefficients (Cronbach's alpha) were high (0.62–0.92), but one fell below this at 0.45. Test–retest reliability was tested with a further 89 students (8-week retest) and 166 students (6-week retest) with correlations of between 0.42 and 0.77. The correlation between scale items was not strong, (0.02–0.69), with most falling below 0.30. The authors interpret this as supporting the empirically distinct domains of the scales.

Endler and Parker (1990) have criticized the scale for emphasizing gender differences and have pointed to the psychometric problems of scales consisting of four items. Endler and Parker (1990) have developed their own scale, the Multidimensional Coping Inventory, later revised and renamed the Coping Inventory for Stressful Situations (Endler and Parker 1992). Intitial testing indicated good psychometric properties, but it has yet to be widely used.

CONTROL OVER LIFE

A different, but overlapping dimension to coping and adjustment, is feelings of control over one's life. This is relevant to the outcome of illness and treatment because feelings of control may affect adherence to therapy and preventive health behaviour. Feelings of helplessness and fatalism may also be accompaniments of illness (e.g. Cousins 1979). There is increasing interest in the sense of personal control and its effect on health (e.g. Brenner 1977).

The most well-known and used scale is Rotter's (1966) Internal–External Locus of Control Scale. It is frequently employed in research on health behaviour (e.g. smoking habits, alcohol intake, diet and exercise; use of preventive services). Health behaviour is sometimes measured in outcome studies (e.g. after intervention in cardiovascular disease, where lifestyle factors are particularly important in recovery as well as in causation). A popular development is the Multidimensional Health Locus of Control Scales by Wallston *et al.* (1976, 1978). The locus of control model has apparently been responsible for some of the more successful reformulations of the 'health belief model' which attempts to describe the determinants of health behaviour (Becker 1974). Generic locus of control scales, including scales for children, have been reviewed by Lefcourt (1991). Few disease-specific locus of control scales have been developed, an exception being scales measuring personal control for use with patients with diabetes (see Bradley *et al.* 1990).

ROTTER'S INTERNAL–EXTERNAL LOCUS OF CONTROL SCALE

The most well-known scale is Rotter's Locus of Control Scale (Rotter 1966), including the many adaptations of it. Rotter's theory of internal *vs* external control holds that an individual's belief system is 'in internal control' when the person perceives that events depend on his or her own behaviour. The belief system is 'in external control' when a person believes that he or she is not the master of his or her own destiny.

Content

Rotter's scale is based on a series of paired items about control over life and health. It is a 23-item forced-choice internal–external statement instrument, with six additional filler items. Respondents choose one of a pair of statements as indicative of his or her beliefs. Some adaptations of the scale include five categorical response choices from 'strongly disagree' to 'strongly agree'. The items address the respondent's beliefs about the nature of the world. Modified versions have been developed for use with different age and social groups (Lefcourt 1991).

Administration and scoring

Rotter stipulates that the scale has to be administered by an interviewer who is trained to give and interpret personality measures or is supervised by someone with such training. It takes about 15 min to complete. The scale is scored by giving 1 point for each external statement selected from the paired items (internal–external). Scores range from 0 (most internal) to 23 (most external).

Examples from Rotter's Scale

1a Children get into trouble because their parents punish them too much
 b The trouble with most children nowadays is that their parents are too easy with them

11a Becoming a success is a matter of hard work; luck has little or nothing to do with it
 b Getting a good job depends mainly on being in the right place at the right time

25a Many times I feel that I have little influence over the things that happen to me

  b It is impossible for me to believe that chance or luck plays an important role in my life

28a What happens to me is my own doing

  b Sometimes I feel that I don't have enough control over the direction my life is taking

Validity and factor structure

The scale has an impressive history of use, although it has not been subjected to rigorous testing, despite its popularity. Items from it have frequently been used in clinical research, for example with cancer patients (Vinokur et al. 1989, 1990).

Rotter (1966) developed the scale with 575 male and 605 female students at Ohio State University. Despite earlier attempts to improve upon the scale, Rotter (1966) reported that the scale correlated with social desirability ($r = -0.21$ to -0.41; Crowne and Marlowe 1960). More recent studies have reported even higher associations (see Lefcourt 1991). Positive correlations between the scale and intellectual performance and anxiety have also been reported (see Rotter 1966).

Two factor analyses were reported by Rotter that yielded a general factor which accounted for much of the scale variance, and several additional factors. A factor analysis based on 159 male and 157 female psychology undergraduates resulted in two dimensions: control over one's destiny and impact of socio-political affairs. Several more recent factor analyses have also confirmed a two-factor solution (for a review, see Lefcourt 1991).

Reliability

Internal consistency estimates range from $r = 0.65$ to 0.79, depending on gender and estimation procedure. Item–total correlations ranged from 0.004 to 0.521, depending on item and gender. Test–retest reliabilities range from 0.49 (for males with a 2 month interval) to 0.83 (for females with a 1 month interval) (Rotter 1966).

Over half of all investigations of locus of control have used the Rotter scale (Lefcourt 1991). The scale is sensitive to individual differences in perception of control over destiny.

MULTIDIMENSIONAL HEALTH LOCUS OF CONTROL SCALES

This instrument was originally developed by Wallston et al. (1976, 1978) as a unidimensional measure of the extent of belief that health is determined by behaviour. It was based on Rotter's (1966) more general scale. Wallston and co-workers' original scale contained 11 items, which yielded a single score, with high scores reflecting 'health-external' beliefs (the belief that health is caused by luck, fate, chance, 'powerful others' and factors over which a person has little control), and low scores reflecting 'health–internal' beliefs (the belief that health is determined by one's own behaviour). The unidimensionality of the scale was questioned, and it was argued that internal beliefs are orthogonal to external beliefs (Levinson 1974, 1975).

A later development of the scale (Wallston et al. 1978) included new items to reflect, on an a priori basis, three dimensions of health locus of control beliefs: internal, powerful others and chance externality. This later version consisted of 25 internal items, 30 powerful other items and 26 chance external locus of control items. All items used a 6-point Likert scale for responses, ranging from 'strongly disagree' (1) to 'strongly agree' (6). These were tested on 125 people waiting at an airport, and items were retained according to the following criteria: those with an item mean close to 3.5 (the midpoint), a wide distribution of response alternatives on the item, scale desirability and item wording. This led to six pairs of items selected for each of the three new sub-scales. Equivalence forms for each scale were constructed (Form A and Form B), and the items assigned to each form were as identical as possible.

Content, administration and scoring

It was reported in the previous section that the current version of the scale contains three sub-scales, with six pairs of items within each. Six-point Likert-type response scales are used to measure agreement. The items are summed. Scores on each dimension of belief range from 6 to 36. It can be self-administered.

Examples from the Locus of Control Scales

Internal health locus of control

Form A

If I get sick, it is my own behaviour which determines how soon I get well again

I am in control of my health

Form B

I am directly responsible for my health

When I feel ill, I know it is because I have not been taking care of myself properly

Powerful others health locus of control

Form A

Whenever I don't feel well, I should consult a medically trained professional

Regarding my health, I can only do what my doctor tells me to do

Form B

Other people play a big part in whether I stay sick or healthy

Following the doctor's orders to the letter is the best way for me to stay healthy

Chance health locus of control

Form A

No matter what I do, if I am going to get sick, I will get sick

Luck plays a big part in determining how soon I will recover from an illness

Form B

Often I feel that no matter what I do, if I am going to get sick, I will get sick

When I am sick, I just have to let nature run its course

Strongly disagree – strongly agree

Validity and factor structure

Winefield (1982) tested the scale with 53 males under 65 years of age who had recently been discharged from hospital after surviving their first myocardial infarction, and compared their responses with 52 men in community and sports organizations. They reported that the heart attack patients were more likely than the 'normal' controls to report feeling dependent on health professionals, supporting the construct validity (convergent validity) of the scale. Associations between the scale and with recovery and health habits were weak or non-existent. Early factor analyses yielded two scales: internal and external (MacDonald 1973). Winefield *et al.* (1982) also reported that factor analysis supported the concept of internal and powerful others as separate sub-scales, but there was less coherence for the external (chance) sub-scale.

Reliability

More data exist on its reliability. Wallston *et al.* (1978) reported variable internal consistency alphas (0.40–0.72) for the original 11-item scale depending on the sample type. In Winefield's (1982) study, the scale was readministered to surviving patients at 30.6 weeks on average, with test–retest correlations of 0.58 for internal locus of control, 0.10 for external (chance) locus of control, and 0.76 for powerful others locus of control scales. Thus the external locus of control sub-scale once again appeared weak.

The later, longer scale (Wallston *et al.* 1978) was tested on a convenience sample of 125 people waiting at an airport, along with Levinson's (1974, 1975) similar scale items and the short version of the Marlowe–Crowne Social Desirability Scale (Strahan and Gerbasi 1972). The alpha reliabilities for this 81-item version of the scale ranged from 0.67 to 0.77, an improvement on the shorter, earlier version. Sub-scale correlations ranged from −0.07 to 0.64. Inter-item correlations ranged from 0.12 to 0.95 (the highest correlations were obtained between items within the same sub-scale, and the lowest were obtained across sub-scales, suggesting that the sub-scales had some independence). Each sub-scale correlated highly with the comparable sub-scales of Levinson's (1974, 1975) scale. Correlations in the expected direction with health status supported the construct validity of the scale. There was little correlation with social desirability – only the total scale score (negatively) correlated, and the total amount of shared variance between the two scales was less than 6 per cent.

Winefield (1982) further tested the longer version of the scale with 152 medical and dental students. Cronbach's alpha for internal consistency was 0.49 for the external (chance) control sub-scale, 0.58 for the powerful others sub-scale, and 0.70 for internal control.

The earlier and later versions of the scales have been widely used (e.g. Seeman and Seeman 1983; Pill and Stott 1985; Calnan 1988), and there are several adaptations and reformulations of the scale in existence (e.g. Cox *et al*. 1987). Despite widespread use, there are less data about the psychometric properties of the scales. Wallston *et al*. (1978) cautioned that the scale alone will not explain much of the variance in health behaviours, but will do so in interaction with other relevant variables (e.g. social support, perceived costs and benefits of alternative actions, the value of health as a reinforcement, etc.). Some studies have reported modest associations between beliefs and behaviour (Calnan 1988).

Conclusion to Part III

The scales of performance, role functioning, behaviour, adjustment and coping that were reviewed in this section overlap with quality of life scales. The choice of scale depends on the aims of the study. Some investigators may wish to supplement the quality of life scales with scales that emphasize a particular domain in more detail (e.g. adjustment and coping). Many of the adjustment scales reviewed here are popular in studies of physical conditions (e.g. cancer and heart disease). In relation to mental health, the Structured and Scaled Interview to Assess Maladjustment (Gurland 1972a, 1972b) is popular in the USA. Most of these scales cover a broad range of domains, from role functioning to personal relationships. The Vineland Adaptive Behaviour Scales (Sparrow *et al*. 1984a, 1984b) are popular among investigators assessing the outcome of physical conditions (e.g. in neurology). Of the coping scales, the Ways of Coping Scale (Folkman and Lazarus 1980) is the most popular in medical studies, and there are several disease-specific adaptations of it. It is unsuitable for use with severely psychiatrically disturbed people. Finally, the locus of control has been more commonly used in health promotion research than in clinical studies, but it may be influential in determining outcome (e.g. in influencing adherence to medical therapy and advice).

4

RESPIRATORY
CONDITIONS

QUALITY OF LIFE IN RESPIRATORY DISEASE SUFFERERS

Chronic obstructive airways disease (COAD), chronic obstructive pulmonary disease (COPD) and chronic airflow limitation (CAL) are all terms which describe chronic obstructive bronchitis, emphysema and some cases of chronic asthma, although there is disagreement about the inclusion of the latter (Williams 1989). The distinction between these conditions was clarified by the Medical Research Council (1965), and it was suggested that COAD refers to all those respiratory conditions characterized by abnormally high resistance to airflow in intrapulmonary airways.

The physical effects of COPD include chronic shortness of breath, or dyspnoea, which reduces energy and vitality, and which can lead to anxiety, dependency, loss of self-esteem, and other psychosocial and psychiatric problems (Rutter 1977; Dudley et al. 1980; McSweeny et al. 1982; Rosser et al. 1983; McSweeny 1984). It is potentially life-threatening, although most deaths occur after the age of 65, and after years of worsening disability. Fear of attacks may lead sufferers to limit their activities and consequently increase their dependency on others, with adverse effects on their quality of life (Ries 1990; Eakin et al. 1993).

Bronchitis, chronic bronchitis and emphysema are major reasons for days off work (Office of Health Economics 1977; Royal College of Physicians 1981; Williams 1989). Asthma sufferers also experience difficulties controlling their symptoms (Charlton et al. 1991), and have reported a wide range of restrictions due to their condition. These include holiday arrangements, housework (exhaustion and needing to do it slowly), work (time off), avoidance of certain foods, getting rid of pets, and extra expenditure (e.g. allergenic bedding) (Nocon and Booth 1991). School-age children have reported difficulties with sporting activities and walking (Nocon and Booth 1991).

Despite its handicapping and eventually potentially life-threatening nature, there is relatively little research on the overall quality of life of people with respiratory disease. Treatment is often palliative rather than curative, with the aim of enhancing quality of life, although most outcome measurement has focused on survival and/or pathophysiological measures which often correlate poorly with general quality of life indicators (Jones 1991a).

THE DOMAINS OF MEASUREMENT

Symptoms

The most frequently used measures of outcome have been the dyspnoea scales, together with various clinical tests and indicators of pulmonary function. These are reviewed in this chapter.

Generic measures

Generic health-related quality of life instruments usually measure physical, social and emotional well-being. They include sub-scales on physical functioning, the scores of which should be analysed independently for people with respiratory conditions. As respiratory disease may lead to inability to undertake everyday and social activities requiring exertion, generic scales can generate useful data.

Frequently used scales with COPD patients are the Sickness Impact Profile (SIP: Bergner *et al.* 1981), known as the Functional Limitations Profile in the UK, the Quality of Well-being Schedule (Kaplan *et al.* 1984), the Nottingham Health Profile (Hunt *et al.* 1986) and the SF-36 (Ware *et al.* 1993). There is concern that generic measures may not be sufficiently sensitive for use in research on outcomes. This is illustrated by Schrier and co-workers' (1990) study in which they found no correlation between lung function tests and SIP scores, although there were correlations between symptoms of wheezing and dyspnoea and SIP scores. In studies of treatment outcomes, general measures must always be supplemented with disease-specific and other relevant items that are judged to be missing. These generic scales are described more fully by Bowling (1991).

Nottingham Health Profile (NHP)

The Nottingham Health Profile (Hunt *et al.* 1986) has been used with respiratory disease patients with mixed results. Alonso *et al.* (1992) assessed 76 males who were attending an out-patient clinic. The patients with COPD had worse scores for energy, physical mobility and sleep disturbance in comparison with the general population. Dyspnoea was the variable that correlated highest with several of the NHP sub-scale scores, including energy and physical mobility. Patients with very low levels of dyspnoea, however, reported high levels of sleep disturbance. Traditional measures of respiratory function were not significantly correlated with the NHP sub-scale scores. The scale may not be sufficiently sensitive with respiratory conditions. The severe nature of the NHP was pointed out by Kind and Carr-Hill (1987).

The Short Form 36-Item Questionnaire (SF-36)

The SF-36 (Ware *et al.* 1993) is short, multidimensional, reliable, valid and more sensitive to low morbidity levels than scales of similar length (Brazier *et al.* 1992). The full Rand batteries, from which the SF-36 is derived, were able to distinguish between patients with chronic respiratory problems and members of the general (normal) population (Stewart *et al.* 1989). Brazier *et al.* (1993a) reported that, in a follow-up study of 200 COPD out-patients, the SF-36 had good validity and correlated highly with clinical tests of respiratory function. It performed better than the St George's Respiratory Questionnaire (Jones 1991a).

Quality of Well-Being Scale (QWBS)

The Quality of Well-Being Scale is a general outcome scale that is used to produce an overall health status score that can be transformed into a quality adjusted life year (QALY) (Kaplan and Bush 1982; Kaplan *et al.* 1984). It has been shown to correlate moderately with lung function, but more strongly with shortness of breath (Kaplan *et al.* 1984). It has high repeatability and discriminates between different levels of ill-health. Changes in scores have been reported to be associated with exercise tests and arterial oxygen consumption changes in intervention trials with patients with COPD. However, it was not associated with standard measures of respiratory function (Kaplan *et al.* 1984).

Sickness Impact Profile (SIP)/Functional Limitations Profile (FLP)

There are more data on the use of the Sickness Impact Profile with patients with respiratory disease, and its extensive use merits further discussion. The SIP assesses sickness-related dysfunction (Bergner *et al.* 1981). It is a comprehensive instrument, although lengthy (136 items). The UK version is known as the Functional Limitations Profile (Patrick 1982a, 1982b; Charlton *et al.* 1983).

Prigatano *et al.* (1983) used the SIP with 985 patients with mild hypoxaemia and COPD. Mildly impaired patients were significantly impaired on most SIP sub-scales, except body movement and eating. SIP/FLP scores correlate well with several indexes of disease activity, disability and distress, although not with spirometric measures (Jones *et al.* 1989; Williams and Bury 1989; Schrier *et al.* 1990). In contrast, the 6 min walking distance test has been shown to account for 40 per cent of the variance in the SIP (Jones *et al.* 1989). It correlates well with the MRC Dyspnoea Scale and the oxygen cost diagram (Jones *et al.* 1989; Williams and Bury 1989). McSweeny (1984) and McSweeny and Labuhn (1990) compared 203 patients with COPD with 73 healthy controls, and reported that SIP scores were significantly associated with a disease severity index that incorporated forced expiratory volume, maximum exercise intolerance, resting heart rate, oxygen saturation before exercise and pulmonary artery pressure (Pearson correlations between the SIP and these and other physiological and neurophysiological measures ranged between −0.12 and 0.45). The SIP is not always sensitive with respiratory disease (Jones *et al.* 1991b). Some SIP scales are more sensitive than others, which indicates the importance of the separate analysis of sub-scales scores (McSweeny *et al.* 1982).

The FLP was used by Williams and Bury (1989) in a study of 92 out-patients with COAD. They reported that only 14 per cent of the variance in FLP function sub-scale scores could be explained by lung function. Their results were broadly similar to those of McSweeny *et al.* (1982) in the USA. The main problem areas for sufferers (note that they were out-patients) were with household management, ambulation, sleep and rest, recreation and pastimes, and work. Williams and Bury (1989) reported that the various measures of dyspnoea they used correlated significantly with each other and with global FLP physical disability scores (e.g. the correlation between the oxygen cost diagram and global FLP of physical disability was −0.90, indicating a close relationship between breathlessness and degree of physical disability). They also reported significant differences in mean global FLP disability scores with the different Fletcher breathlessness gradings they used. The FLP global physical disability measure did not correlate so well with spirometric measures of lung function ($r = -0.38$).

The SIP/FLP is not a disease-specific measure and requires supplementation with disease-specific items which, in view of the length of the scale, lessens its attractiveness. There is some question regarding the sensitivity of the SIP/FLP in COAD patients with mild to moderate as opposed to severe disease (Nocturnal Oxygen Therapy Trial Group 1980; Jones 1991b, 1993). Jones (1993) also reported high item non-response to the SIP among COAD patients. McColl *et al.* (1993; in press), in a large study of the outcomes of asthma and diabetes and primary care, discontinued their use of the SIP in favour of the SF-36, as it had a high item non-response (95 of the 136 items were completed by less than 10 per cent of respondents) and showed ceiling effects.

Rather than using a generic tool, some investigators have compiled a battery of single domain measures, supplemented with disease and severity items (e.g. McSweeny 1984; Moody *et al.* 1990). While batteries are useful when the scale of choice omits areas of research interest and relevance, they can be lengthy and include overlapping items which may lead to patient fatigue and irritation.

Functional status

Functional status is an essential variable to include in disease-specific scales, given the reported associations between dyspnoea and the 12 min walking test (McGavin *et al.* 1978; Williams and McGavin 1980; Mahler *et al.* 1984; Guyatt *et al.* 1985a), although the nature of functional limitations other than walking still requires further exploration (Eakin *et al.* 1993). Williams (1989) has argued that most disability and health status scales tend to be more oriented to musculoskeletal based problems and to be more extreme, missing the less severe and more subtle impairments and disabilities of respiratory disease sufferers. He supports his point by reference to surveys which vary in the proportion of difficulties detected (i.e. 33–87 per cent), according to the scales they use (Sommerville 1982). This indicates a need for the development of disease-specific scales of functioning to supplement the scales and tests of dyspnoea.

Domain-specific measures

Anxiety and depression, mood and personality disturbances

It was pointed out earlier that poor physical functioning, and an inability to work among younger patients, can have adverse psychological consequences (Rubeck 1971). Common features are the anxiety and depression, isolation and loneliness stemming from withdrawal into the home, and avoidance of normal roles and social interactions (Lustig *et al.* 1972; Lester 1973; Agle and

Baum 1977; Dudley *et al.* 1980; McSweeny *et al.* 1982; Rosser *et al.* 1983; Grant and Heaton 1985; Gift *et al.* 1986; Renfroe 1988). Some popular scales are described here.

State–Trait Anxiety Inventory (STAI)
Spielberger and co-workers' (1983) State–Trait Anxiety Inventory is a popular measure in research on respiratory problems and has detected moderate levels of anxiety among sufferers (Swinburn *et al.* 1988). Renfroe (1988) reported a correlation of $r = 0.60$ between Spielberger's State Anxiety Scale scores and visual analogue scale ratings of dyspnoea. Others have also reported associations between dyspnoea and anxiety and depression (Gift *et al.* 1986). In a study which controlled for confounding variables, Moody *et al.* (1990) reported that dyspnoea was more strongly associated with patient psychology (e.g. mastery) than with disease severity. The results suggest that associations with psychological status are complex, and no study to date has demonstrated sufficiently the nature of the relationships (Eakin *et al.* 1993). The experience of these problems has been reported to be associated with those of a younger age and those from lower socio-economic groups (Fletcher *et al.* 1976; Guyatt *et al.* 1987c).

General Health Questionnaire (GHQ)
The General Health Questionnaire is a widely used scale of psychological morbidity (i.e. anxiety and depression) (Goldberg 1972). Several versions of varying length are available. Rosser *et al.* (1983) used the 30-item GHQ in a study evaluating the outcome of psychotherapy with 65 COAD patients and reported that 60 per cent were classified as 'cases' (i.e. disturbed). The GHQ was sensitive to different types of therapy, with lower scores being achieved by those receiving supportive but not analytical psychotherapy. The GHQ-12 was also used by Williams and Bury (1989) in a study of 92 out-patients with COAD, along with the Functional Limitations Profile (Charlton *et al.* 1983). It correlated well with disability scores, and with measures of dyspnoea (e.g. oxygen cost diagram $r = -0.68$), implying that the lesser the magnitude of the tasks provoking breathlessness on the oxygen cost diagram, the higher the patient's score on the GHQ-12, indicating anxiety/depression.

Hospital Anxiety and Depression Scale
The Hospital Anxiety and Depression Scale is a measure of anxiety and depression, but is becoming increasingly popular due to its lack of somatic items which could indicate physical rather than psychological morbidity (Zigmond and Snaith 1983). Jones *et al.* (1989) used it with patients with respiratory disease, and reported that almost half of the patients had an anxiety score at or above the borderline of clinical significance and almost a third had depression scores in this range.

Profile of Mood States
The Profile of Mood States is another popularly used scale with people with respiratory diseases (McNair *et al.* 1971). It contains a list of 65 adjectives, rated on a 5-point scale to indicate recent mood. This is but one dimension of the psychological domain of quality of life, but is usually regarded as important. It can produce fairly skewed results, although it is relatively easy to administer to COPD patients (McSweeny 1984).

Minnesota Multiphasic Personality Inventory (MMPI)
Personality is not an outcome variable, but a modifier of response to illness and treatment. The Minnesota Multiphasic Personality Inventory (Dahlstrom *et al.* 1972; Hathaway and McKinley 1990) has a long history of use in clinical research on COPD in the USA (Fishman and Petty 1971; McSweeny 1984). Personality assessment in studies of the outcome of these patients is less common in the UK. In the UK, the personality measure of choice among psychologists is the Eysenck Personality Questionnaire (Eysenck and Eysenck 1985), although it is not necessarily appropriate to include it in assessments of outcome (as opposed to studies of predisposing factors to the onset of disease).

Investigators should be cautious about using personality assessments in their outcome batteries. The MMPI in particular is lengthy and contains many irrelevant items and domains. The full inventory of the MMPI contains 556 items that measure ten major dimensions of emotional distress and personality disturbance. McSweeny *et al.* (1982) assessed the personalities of 150 COAD patients using the MMPI and reported that 42 per cent exhibited significant depression in comparison with 9 per cent of matched controls. However, there are much shorter and more appropriate scales of psychological morbidity that could have detected these differences. McSweeny did criticize the MMPI on the grounds of its heterogeneity, and the fact that its depression scale includes a variety of physical symptoms with the result that the meaning of scores is confounded with the effects of physical rather than mental disturbances.

Adjustment and coping

Adjustment and coping are worthy of consideration for use in broader outcome studies, given their modifying influences on outcome. A number of scales measuring adjustment and coping were reviewed in Chapter 3. A popular scale used with respiratory patients is the Katz Adjustment Scale (Katz and Lyerly 1963).

Katz Adjustment Scale

The Katz Adjustment Scale contains five major sub-scales that measure social adjustment, recreational activities and general psychological disturbances (Katz and Lyerly 1963; Hogarty and Katz 1971). It necessitates the involvement of a third party, such as a relative or friend in order to give another perspective. Problems have been reported in its administration with COPD patients, given that many are older and have lost their friends and relatives through bereavement, and thus there is no third party to administer it to (McSweeny 1984).

Self-esteem and self-concept

Another important dimension of psychological well-being to measure is self-esteem or self-concept. Rosenberg's (1965) Self-Esteem Scale is popular among clinicians in other specialities, although these scales are seldom used with respiratory patients.

Life satisfaction

Life satisfaction and well-being are also essential components of outcome. Use of life satisfaction scales is not common in respiratory medicine. The main scales used in measuring life satisfaction are the Neugarten Life Satisfaction Scales (Neugarten et al. 1961), the Delighted–Terrible Faces Scale (Andrews and Withey 1976), the Philadelphia Geriatric Morale Scale (Lawton 1972, 1975), the Affect–Balance Scale (Bradburn 1969) and the General Well-Being Schedule (Dupuy 1978). Most of these scales were developed for use with elderly people. Anderson (1992) used the Delighted–Terrible Faces Scale with stroke patients with good results. The most popular scale among gerontologists is the Philadelphia Geriatric Morale Scale, on the grounds of its superior results for reliability and validity.

Social support

Other important indicators include social support as well as effects on social activities and life. The use of these indicators is less common in respiratory medicine. Social support is a modifying and an outcome variable, as it may help to protect the individual from the stressful effects of illness, and illness may also impair the ability to maintain social relationships and activities. A range of social support scales is reviewed by Bowling (1991); also see Sherbourne and Stewart (1991) for details of the Rand Medical Outcomes Study Social Support Scale.

Other domains

It is important to measure the effects on social roles and activities. Generic and broad disease-specific scales will include sub-scales or items of relevance to these areas. Items on patient satisfaction should also be included (see Chapter 1).

MEASUREMENT SCALES

SYMPTOM-SPECIFIC SCALES: DYSPNOEA

Dyspnoea is the clinical term for shortness of breath (the subjective sensation of difficult or laboured breathing). It is probably the most disabling and distressing symptom of COPD/COAD, leading to much anxiety (Dudley et al. 1980; Kinsman et al. 1983; Rosser et al. 1983), and yet scales to measure breathlessness are often inadequate (Mahler et al. 1984).

The measurement of dyspnoea is not straight-forward, hence the proliferation of methods. Numerous studies have shown that dyspnoea is not strongly correlated with objective measures of pulmonary function (Stark *et al.* 1982; Shandu 1986; Schrier *et al.* 1990; Alonso *et al.* 1992). A review by Eakin *et al.* (1993) confirmed that dyspnoea measures across studies are at best moderately correlated with pulmonary function (e.g. forced expiratory volume in one second (FEV_1), forced vital capacity (FVC)), psychological function and 6 min walking tests. With the latter, people are asked to cover as much ground as they can in 6 min; they are then usually asked to indicate their level of dyspnoea using a 10 cm visual analogue scale anchored by the descriptions 'extremely short of breath' (0) and 'no shortness of breath' (10). There is a strong argument in favour of their standardization (Eakin *et al.* 1993). The implication of these at best moderate correlations, is that patients with mildly impaired lung function may report extreme breathlessness and vice versa (Eakin *et al.* 1993). This is discussed later.

Subjective reports of dyspnoea

Subjective reports are measured using symptom checklists and visual analogue scales. There are wide variations between individuals in the perceived intensity of dyspnoea in relation to ventilation (Stark *et al.* 1981; Adams *et al.* 1986; Wilson and Jones 1989). The level of distress from breathlessness that has been reported among normal subjects is unrelated to their perception of its intensity (Wilson and Jones 1991). Which aspects of breathlessness limit activities of daily living is largely unknown (Jones 1991a).

Symptom checklists have been developed. For example, Kinsman *et al.* (1983) constructed a checklist, based on patient interviews, of 89 symptoms commonly experienced by COAD patients. It was tested on 149 consecutively admitted hospital patients. Dyspnoea, fatigue and difficulties with sleeping were most often reported. The correlation between pulmonary dysfunction and quality of life impairment was relatively weak. As this was a sample of in-patients, any interpretation must be viewed with caution, as hospitalization may have influenced the responses (e.g. difficulties sleeping) (Williams 1989).

The clinical measurement of dyspnoea

Mahler and Harver (1990) reviewed the clinical measurement of dyspnoea, and reproduced the most widely used scales (including subjective patient report scales). Because dyspnoea is a subjective symptom, it is difficult to measure. There is no gold standard against which the validity of its measurement can be assessed. However, numerous scales have been developed. It has been assessed by clinical structured interviews, self-report questionnaires and visual analogue scales; with the latter, the subject rates the perceived magnitude of dyspnoea on a vertical or horizontal line, usually 10 cm in length, with the extremes labelled 'not at all breathless' and 'very breathless'. People may be asked about their experience of dyspnoea over a period of time, or asked to report on its severity while undertaking everyday activities. Exercise tests of various types are often used.

Typically, the measurement of functional status in respiratory disease patients is measured by exercise tests such as stair climbing and 6 and 12 min walking tests that simulate everyday activities (McGavin *et al.* 1976; Johnson *et al.* 1977; Guyatt *et al.* 1984). These types of scales are limited to the symptom, rather than its associated limitations on functioning. Clinical measures thus focus on the magnitude of the exertive task that evokes breathlessness, rather than the amount of effort involved (Mahler *et al.* 1984; Williams 1989).

Jones (1991a) has pointed to the limitations of routine clinical tests. In patients with obstructive airways disease, the association between the results of spirometry tests and walking distance are poor (McGavin *et al.* 1976; Swinburn *et al.* 1985). With symptom-limited ergometer stress tests, the maximum achievable exercise ventilation cannot be predicted reliably from FEV_1 (Carter *et al.* 1987; Matthews *et al.* 1989). It was pointed out earlier that the various subjective (patient's perceptions) dyspnoea scales correlate poorly with spirometry tests, although they correlate better, although still modestly, with measures of walking distances (McGavin *et al.* 1978; O'Reilly *et al.* 1982; Mahler *et al.* 1984; Guyatt *et al.* 1985a, 1985b; Mahler and Wells 1988; Wolkove *et al.* 1989).

Mahler and Harver (1990) recommended the use of visual analogue scales for assessing the impact of dyspnoea on the patient's daily activities, a quality of life measure (e.g. Guyatt *et al.* 1987a), and did not recommend exercise testing given its questionable reliability and sensitivity, nor psychophysics (perceptual sensation of breathlessness in relation to standard physical stimuli) outside the laboratory. Eakin *et al.* (1993) recommended the use of a visual analogue scale, or the Borg scale for assessing dyspnoea during exercise testing; they also recommended Mahler's Baseline Dyspnoea Index and the Medical Research Council/American Thoracic Society Scale (see below) for measuring overall impairment due to dyspnoea. They called for further research into the relationship between dyspnoea and everyday activities.

THE FLETCHER SCALE AND THE MRC DYSPNOEA GRADE AND RESPIRATORY SYMPTOMS QUESTIONNAIRE

Fletcher Scale

Fletcher *et al.* (1959) developed a dyspnoea questionnaire which has been adapted by Rose and Blackburn (1968) and Rose *et al.* (1982) for use by WHO, and has been further revised by the British Medical Research Council (MRC 1986). These scales are used extensively in research on respiratory disease, and also in cardiovascular disease. The variations on the Fletcher Scale, particularly Rose's version, are presented in more detail in Chapter 7 on cardiovascular diseases. In respiratory disease, the most commonly used versions appear to be that of the MRC and the American Thoracic Society (Brooks 1982). These are presented here.

The original Fletcher Scale has an ordinal 5-point scale for grading breathlessness (Fletcher 1952, Fletcher *et al.* 1959). This version has also been called the Medical Research Council Scale, because the Council funded its development, although the MRC scale is really the later version (see next section). The Fletcher Scale is based on patients' history of developing dyspnoea while walking on the flat or while climbing. It relates primarily to the magnitude of the task that provokes dyspnoea. There is little provision for measuring the effort involved. The Fletcher Scale is commonly used. Williams and Bury (1989) reported that the Fletcher Scale's gradings of breathlessness were significantly correlated with disability scores.

Medical Research Council Scale: Dyspnoea

The Fletcher scale was further developed by the MRC in Britain (MRC 1960, 1966, 1986), who proposed a 5-item questionnaire with 'yes/no' answers, which can be transformed into a 5-point scale. Like the Fletcher Scale, on which it is based, it relates primarily to the magnitude of the task that provokes dyspnoea. A very similar scale, also based on Fletcher's questions, was designed by Rose and Blackburn (1968; see also Rose *et al.* 1982) for the WHO. Rose and Blackburn's (1968) version of the MRC Scale was further modified for use in the USA by the Rand Corporation for their Health Insurance Study and Medical Outcomes Study (Rosenthal *et al.* 1981).

Based on the respondent's replies to the questions, dyspnoea is rated on a scale of 1–5.

MRC Scale: Grades of dyspnoea

Grade 1: Not troubled by breathlessness, except on strenuous exertion

Grade 2: Short of breath when hurrying on the level or walking up slight hill

Grade 3: Patient walks slower than most people on the level

Grade 4: Patient has to stop for breath after walking about 100 yards on the level

Grade 5: Too breathless to leave home, or breathless after undressing

Content and administration

The 1966 MRC Respiratory Symptoms Questionnaire was revised in 1986 (MRC 1986). The questionnaire contains a set of standard questions, based on the Fletcher Scale, for eliciting the presence or absence of common respiratory symptoms (e.g. chronic bronchitis). The revised instrument emphasizes the need for the careful wording of questions in order to avoid bias due to different techniques of questioning. Although it has been used as part of a self-completion questionnaire with satisfactory results (MRC 1965), most applications have used interviewer administration. Interviewer training is recommended and the MRC supplies training tapes for this. The instruction leaflet for interviewers provides guidance on the interpretation of symptoms such as cough, phlegm, breathlessness and wheezing. Instructions on measuring ventilatory capacity are also provided.

The questionnaire starts by collecting basic sociodemographic information, and then continues with three items on coughing, three items on phlegm, two items on periods of cough and phlegm, three items on breathlessness, three items on wheezing, three items on chest illness, nine items on past chest illnesses, and then a standard battery on smoking. Each question simply carries a 'yes' or 'no' answer. Finally, the interviewer measures and records ventilatory capacity.

Examples of items from the MRC Scale

Cough

1 Do you usually cough first thing in the morning in winter?   Yes / no
2 Do you usually cough during the day – or at night – in the winter?   Yes / no

IF YES TO 1 OR 2

3 Do you cough like this on most days for as much as 3 months each year?

Breathlessness

8a Are you troubled by shortness of breath when hurrying on level ground or walking up a slight hill?   Yes / no
8b IF YES, Do you get short of breath walking with other people of your own age on level ground?   Yes / no
8c IF YES, Do you have to stop for breath when walking at your own pace on level ground?   Yes / no

Validity and reliability

The MRC Scale was recommended for use by Eakin *et al.* (1993). It has been used extensively in epidemiological and clinical research (e.g. Brundin 1974; Murphy *et al.* 1976), although it has been tested less frequently for reliability and validity. It correlates well with the Sickness Impact Profile (Jones *et al.* 1989; Williams and Bury 1989). It has been reported to correlate strongly with other measures of dyspnoea impairment ($r = -0.53$ to 0.83) and modestly with lung function measures ($r = -0.41$ to -0.42) (Mahler and Wells 1988). Mahler *et al.* (1987) compared the MRC Scale with

the Oxygen-Cost Diagram (McGavin *et al.* 1978) and the Baseline Dyspnoea Index (Mahler *et al.* 1984) for subjective ratings of breathlessness among 24 patients with obstructive airways disease. They reported that the three clinical methods were interrelated and correlated moderately well with lung function, forced vital capacity (FVC) and forced expiratory volume in 1 sec (FEV_1) ($r = 0.43$–0.49) – but not with patients' estimates of difficulty breathing during psychophysical testing, using the Borg (1982a, 1982b) category scale of intensity (nothing at all = 0 to maximal = 10).

Lebowitz and Burrows (1976) compared the MRC Scale and the National Heart and Lung Institute (1971) version of the respiratory questionnaire in a study of 2350 adults. Some respondents completed the questionnaire at home, others completed it with a nurse interviewer in a clinic. Despite slight differences in wording and question order, the two scales produced very similar results in relation to overall prevalence of elicited symptoms. However, despite this, there was a 10 per cent level of disagreement between questionnaire responses to individual symptom questions, regardless of the time between tests or mode of administration. The authors reported very low rates of non-completion. Comstock *et al.* (1979) also reported no differences in results between the MRC Scale and the American Thoracic Society (1978) version in a study of 946 male smokers and non-smokers. Mahler and Harver (1990), on the basis of a literature review, criticized these scales for being too coarse to be able to demonstrate reliable changes in breathlessness following an intervention.

Other variations

AMERICAN THORACIC SOCIETY (ATS) RESPIRATORY QUESTIONNAIRE AND GRADE OF BREATHLESSNESS SCALE

The American Thoracic Society (Brooks 1982) developed a respiratory questionnaire, which is regarded as an improvement on an earlier version developed by the National Heart and Lung and Blood Institute. They both based the recommended respiratory questionnaire on the British MRC dyspnoea questionnaire (National Heart and Lung Institute 1971; National Heart, Lung and

Blood Institute 1978; American Thoracic Society 1978; Brooks 1982; Brown 1985). There are slight changes to wording and question order, and the MRC questions are briefer.

It is a self-report questionnaire which contains five 'yes/no' questions eliciting information about dyspnoea. It has been reported to be easy to administer and acceptable to interviewers and respondents. Dyspnoea is graded from 0 (none, not troubled with breathlessness except with strenuous exercise) to 4 (very severe, too breathless to leave the house or breathless when dressing or undressing) (Brooks 1982; for reproduction of the grades and categories, see Mahler and Harver 1990).

Examples from the ATS Questionnaire

Cough

9A Do you usually have a cough?   Yes / no
9D Do you usually cough at all during the rest of the day or night?   Yes or no

Breathlessness

15A Are you troubled by shortness of breath when hurrying on the level or walking up a slight hill?   Yes / no
15B Do you have to walk slower than people of your age on the level because of breathlessness? Yes / no
15D Do you ever have to stop for breath after walking about 100 yards (or after a few minutes) on the level?   Yes / no

Validity and reliability

Both the MRC and ATS scales have been widely used, sometimes in adapted form where the number of points on the rating scales, or the wording, has been changed. Concurrent validity has been reported (with correlations of 0.50 and above) between the MRC/ATS and other measures of dyspnoea, together with moderate correlations with lung function (Mahler *et al.* 1987; Mahler and Wells 1988). There are few published data on its reliability.

The MRC and ATS scales have been criticized because they measure dyspnoea only in relation to the magnitude of the task, but they ignore the magnitude of effort and functional impairment

resulting from the performance of everyday activities (Mahler *et al.* 1987; Harver and Mahler 1990), although they do address walking. It was reported earlier that the prevalence of symptoms is essentially the same when measured with the MRC or the ATS scales (Lebowitz and Burrows 1976). Comstock *et al.* (1979) also reported no differences in results between the two respiratory questionnaires in a study of 946 male smokers and non-smokers.

HORSLEY RESPIRATORY SYMPTOMS QUESTIONNAIRE

This respiratory symptoms questionnaire was designed by Horsley and his colleagues (Horsley 1985; Horsley *et al.* 1991, 1993) for use with elderly people. Like the MRC questionnaire, it is also based on the original Fletcher Scale/Rose Dyspnoea Questionnaire (Rose and Blackburn 1968), but with additional disease-specific questions.

Examples from the Horsley Questionnaire

4 When you have shortness of breath or chest tightness at rest, do you get at the same time:

(d) Dizziness or lightheadedness?
(e) Pins and needles in the hands?

5 Does anyone in your family have, or have they had, (bronchial) asthma?   Yes / no

7 Do any of the following affect your chest? If yes, what are the effects?
(a) Going from a warm room to a cold one
(b) Going into a room where people are/were smoking
(c) Traffic fumes
(d) Chemical such as hair spray, bleach, perfumes, etc.

Short of breath / wheezing / cough

(e) None of the above affect my chest

Validity and reliability

The scale was tested on a random sample of almost 2000 people aged 65+ (96 per cent response rate). Over half had a respiratory problem according to the questionnaire. A random sample were invited to attend for a medical examination and further testing in order to test the validity of the questionnaire. The authors reported no significant discrepancies between the symptoms reported by the respondents on the screening questionnaire and those reported at clinical interview. They also reported that no cluster of symptoms, nor number of symptoms, could reliably identify elderly subjects with highly reactive airways. However, the questionnaire was not designed to assess severity. They concluded that the questionnaire was not sufficiently sensitive to be used as an alternative to clinical interview and pulmonary function testing. It was judged to be useful, however, in separating respondents with a low risk of bronchial reactivity and those who had good lung function (the first two groups) from those in whom abnormal lung function and bronchial hyper-reactivity were more common. Little was published on its reliability.

Summary of other indexes of dyspnoea

AMERICAN LUNG ASSOCIATION SEVERITY OF DISABILITY (COAD)

This is an index which assesses disability as a result of dyspnoea, and not a dyspnoea scale in itself. The American Lung Association (1975) has suggested the disability due to COAD can be classified on five levels. While well known, this scale does not appear to be widely used, and there is little data about its psychometric properties.

Disability Index of the American Lung Association

1 Patient has recognized disease but has no restriction; is able to do what peers can do and continues usual lifestyle
2 Patient has minimally restricted activity, is able to do productive work; has some difficulty keeping up with peers and has begun to modify lifestyle
3 Patient has moderately restricted activity; is not housebound but may not be able to do productive work, but is still able to care for self
4 Patient has markedly / severely restricted activity; limited outdoor mobility, unable to do productive work but is still able to care for self but with difficulty
5 Patient has very severely restricted activity; is essentially / totally housebound, needs help with personal care / is unable to care for self

---

FEINSTEIN'S INDEX OF DYSPNOEA

Feinstein et al. (1989) developed a clinical index of dyspnoea and fatigue specifically for people with congestive heart failure, although it has also been used among patients with respiratory disease. It was developed from a scale previously developed by Mahler et al. (1984). The authors described it as an *index of quality of life* for people with heart failure, although it is really just an index of dyspnoea.

Content, administration and scoring

The index has three components: magnitude of the task that causes the shortness of breath, magnitude of the pace or effort that evokes the problem, and functional impairment. Each dimension is rated on a 5-point scale, from 0 (very severe impairment) to 4 (no impairment). The scores are summed to form a composite score. It is simple and easy to administer, and takes a few minutes to complete. It is completed by the health professional.

Example from Feinstein's Index of Dyspnoea

Magnitude of task (at normal pace) rating

4 *Extraordinary:* Becomes short of breath or fatigued (hereafter called 'symptomatic') only with extraordinary activity, such as carrying very heavy loads on level ground, lighter loads uphill or running. No symptoms with ordinary tasks
3 *Major:* Becomes symptomatic only with such major activities as walking up a steep hill, climbing more than three flights of stairs or carrying a light load on level ground
2 *Moderate:* Becomes symptomatic with moderate or average tasks such as walking up a gradual hill, climbing less than three flights of stairs or carrying a light load on level ground
1 *Light:* Becomes symptomatic with light activities, such as walking on the level, washing or standing
0 *None:* Symptomatic at rest, while sitting or lying down

Validity and reliability

The scale was initially tested on 362 patients with congestive heart failure before and after treatment. It was shown to be sensitive to improvement with medical treatment (Feinstein *et al.* 1989). It is probably also appropriate for use with people with respiratory diseases. There are few published data on its psychometric properties.

SEVERITY OF SYMPTOMS VISUAL ANALOGUE SCALE (VAS)

This consists of a measured line (visual analogue scale) with descriptive phrases at various points along the line (usually 10 cm in length). The respondent is instructed to make a mark on the line corresponding to the severity of the symptoms. The location of the mark provides quantification of the patient's dyspnoea ('extremely short of breath' = 0, 'no shortness of breath' = 10). The scale has been criticized for its lack of standardized criteria (there are no standards for anchoring the end-points), which inhibits consistent use between raters (Mahler *et al.* 1984; Eakin *et al.* 1993), although it is used widely (e.g. Guyatt *et al.* 1991).

Example of VAS

---

0   10
extremely short of breath   no shortness of breath

Validity and reliability

VAS dyspnoea ratings have been reported to increase as the resistive load of breathing is experimentally increased (Aitken 1969). It has also been shown to be associated with treadmill ratings, heart rate, oxygen uptake and respiratory rate (Stark *et al.* 1981, 1982). Concurrent validity has been demonstrated among asthma patients with correlations between the scale and peak expiratory flow rate of −0.85 (Gift 1989). Dyspnoea ratings have been found to vary in the expected direction at times of severe and little airways obstruction among patients, indicating it has discriminant validity (Gift 1989). Its reliability was assessed by Wilson and Jones (1989) in exercise tests 2 weeks apart, and was found to be weak.

The review by Eakin *et al.* (1993) concluded that half of all studies exploring the correlates of visual analogue scale ratings of dyspnoea have been carried out with asthma patients. Given that they have acute episodic attacks of dyspnoea, it may not

be appropriate to generalize the findings to patients with COPD, who have chronic unremitting dyspnoea at rest or at moderate levels of exercise (Schrier *et al.* 1990; Eakin *et al.* 1993).

OXYGEN COST DIAGRAM

The VAS has been used for an 'oxygen cost diagram' where daily activities are ranked along the 10 cm line in proportion to their associated oxygen cost (Durnin and Passmore 1967; McGavin *et al.* 1976, 1978). The patient marks the line at the point above which a task would have to be stopped because of breathlessness.

Examples of activities on the diagram are 'brisk walking uphill', 'medium walking on the level', 'bedmaking', 'standing' and 'sleeping'. Values for oxygen uptake for the various activities have been developed by Durnin and Passmore (1967).

Oxygen Cost Diagram

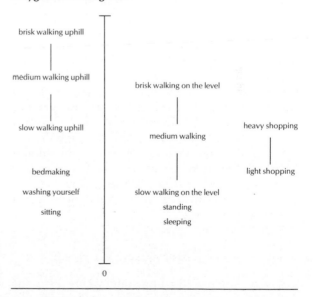

Validity and reliability

McGavin *et al.* (1978) reported that patients' ratings of breathlessness on this scale were significantly correlated with the 12 min walking test ($r = 0.68$), but not with FEV_1. It does correlate well with other measures of dyspnoea ($r = -0.53$ to -0.79) (Mahler *et al.* 1984, 1987).

It was used by Williams and Bury (1989) in a study of 92 out-patients with COAD. They reported that anxiety and depression and physical disability scores correlated well with the oxygen cost diagram: $r = -0.68$ and -0.90, respectively. Spirometric measures of lung function correlated poorly with dyspnoea using the oxygen cost diagram ($r = 0.38$), in line with other studies (McGavin *et al.* 1978). There is little information about its reliability.

Eakin *et al.* (1993) reported that in their experience many patients do not understand how to rate the scale according to its printed instructions, necessitating further explanations and consequent lack of standardization.

THE 6 AND 12 MINUTE WALKING TESTS AND STAIR CLIMBING

With the 6 min walking test, people are asked to cover as much ground as they can in 6 min; they are then usually asked to indicate their level of dyspnoea immediately following the test using a 10 cm visual analogue scale anchored by the descriptors 'extremely short of breath' (0) and 'no shortness of breath' (10) (Guyatt *et al.* 1985b). Other tests include stair climbing and a 12 min walking test. Using these tests is common practice (McGavin *et al.* 1976; Johnson *et al.* 1977; Guyatt *et al.* 1984, 1991; Eakin *et al.* 1993), although there is little information on their reliability and validity apart from the associations with the Oxygen Cost Diagram (McGavin *et al.* 1978; see p. 159), and the moderate correlations with lung function reported earlier (see Eakin *et al.* 1993).

BORG RATIO OF PERCEIVED EXERTION

This is a simple 0–10 rating scale (where 0 = none and 10 = maximum) on which respondents rate their degree of breathlessness (Borg 1982a, 1982b). The original scale ranged from 6 to 20 (as opposed to 0 to 10 on the revised scale) and was revised to give the categorical scale the properties of a ratio scale (Borg 1970). The 20-point scale is still in use (WHO 1993). It is also known as the Borg Property Scale.

The modified version is used to obtain dyspnoea ratings during a task that produces breathlessness, such as an exercise test, or over a given period of time (Borg 1982a, 1982b). Written descriptors are placed so that a doubling of the numerical rating corresponds to a two-fold increase in sensation intensity.

Versions of the Borg Scale

Original 20-item scale

Perceived exertion	Rating
Very, very light	6
Very light	9
Light	11
Somewhat hard	13
Hard	5
Very hard	17
Very, very hard	19
	20

Current 10-item scale

Perceived exertion	Rating
Nothing at all	0
Very, very slight (just noticeable)	0.5
Very slight	1
Slight	2
Moderate	3
Somewhat severe	4
Severe	5
	6
Very severe	7
	8
Very, very severe (almost maximal)	9
Maximal	10

Validity and reliability

Correlations between the Borg Scale and heart rate across various studies range from $r = 0.80–0.85$ (Borg 1982a). Burdon *et al.* (1982) reported a correlation between breathlessness ratings and FEV_1 of 0.88, although they reported substantial variations in the ratings of breathlessness at any given level of FEV_1. A modified Borg Scale was compared with a visual analogue rating by Wilson and Jones (1989), who found wide variations between patients. They reported that test–retest reliability correlations were good for repeat testing on the same day, but poor at retest at 2 weeks. Reliability has not been demonstrated.

MAHLER BASELINE AND TRANSITION DYSPNOEA INDEX

Mahler *et al.* (1984) designed an index to rate the severity of dyspnoea at a single point in time, and a transition dyspnoea index to denote changes from the baseline condition. The baseline and transition indexes consist of three categories: functional impairment, magnitude of task and magnitude of effort. The functional impairment section assesses whether the respondent has reduced or given up activities or work due to shortness of breath. The magnitude of task section rates the type of task that causes the breathlessness (e.g. light *vs* moderate *vs* strenuous tasks). The magnitude of effort section assesses how much effort the respondent exerts before becoming breathless (e.g. breathless only after extraordinary exertion *vs* so breathless that he or she has to pause frequently during most tasks). The baseline measure is used to rate the severity of dyspnoea at a single point in time, whereas the transitional index is used to assess changes from that baseline.

At baseline, dyspnoea in each of the three categories is rated on a 5-point scale from 0 (severe) to 4 (unimpaired). The ratings for each of the three categories can be summed to form a total score (0–12). The transition index is used to rate changes in each of the three categories using a 7-point scale from −3 (major deterioration) to +3 (major improvement). The ratings from the transition index can be summed to form a dyspnoea transition total score (−9 to +9). A modified version has also been produced (Stoller *et al.* 1986; for a reproduction of the index, see Mahler and Harver 1990).

Examples from Mahler's Indexes

Transition Dyspnoea Index

Change in functional impairment

−3 *Major deterioration:* Formerly working and has had to stop working and has completely abandoned some of usual activities due to shortness of breath.

−2 *Moderate deterioration:* Formerly working and has had to stop working or has completely abandoned some of usual activities due to shortness of breath

−1 *Minor deterioration:* Has changed to a lighter job and/or has reduced activities in number or duration due to shortness of breath. Any deterioration less than preceding categories

0 *No change:* No change in functional status due to shortness of breath

+1 *Minor improvement:* Able to return to work at reduced pace or has resumed some customary activities with more vigour than previously due to improvement in shortness of breath

+2 *Moderate improvement:* Able to return to work at nearly usual pace and/or able to return to most activities with modest restriction only

+3 *Major improvement:* Able to return to work at former pace and able to return to full activities with only mild restriction due to improvement in shortness of breath

Validity and reliability

The authors reported a correlation of $r = 0.60$ between the baseline total score and a 12 min walk test, and the transitional total score was significantly correlated with the change in the 12 min walk test ($r = 0.33$: Mahler *et al.* 1987). This was consistent with previous research (Fletcher *et al.* 1959; Leiner *et al.* 1965; McGavin *et al.* 1978). At baseline, the scale correlated moderately well with the MRC scale and the Oxygen Cost Diagram ($r = 0.53$–0.83), and with lung function measures such as FEV_1 and FVC ($r = 0.43$ and 0.41, respectively) (Mahler *et al.* 1987; Mahler and Wells 1988). Dyspnoea ratings did not, however, correlate well with all results of pulmonary function tests, but this was not unexpected given that dyspnoea is a subjective symptom and has not correlated with spirometric measures in other studies (Mahler *et al.* 1984).

The authors evaluated reliability by assessing agreement between multiple observers who graded dyspnoea in 38 male patients aged 42–82 years with various respiratory diseases (COPD, asthma and interstitial fibrosis). The percentage observer agreements using the indexes ranged from 84 to 94 per cent (Mahler *et al.* 1984). Test–retest reliability has not been reported.

The Mahler baseline and transitional dyspnoea

indexes were modified by Stoller *et al*. (1986). They clarified the rating scale points, and supplied more examples. The functional impairment sub-scale was split into impairment at work and impairment at home. The rating scale for each sub-scale was changed from a 5-point to a 4-point scale. It correlated significantly with FEV_1 and FVC ($r = 0.71$ and 0.69, respectively), but not with the 12 min walking test. Reliability was not reported. The raw scores are summed to form a total score, which gives equal weighting to items. The equal weighting has been criticized by Eakin *et al*. (1993). This modified scale has rarely been used.

The main advantage of Mahler and co-workers' (1984) scale is that it provides for the measurement of change. The instrument is easy to administer by physicians and non-physicians, but further testing is required.

DISEASE-SPECIFIC QUALITY OF LIFE MEASURES

There is no agreement over the relevant quality of life domains that should be measured in respiratory disease, and the criteria for assessment vary between studies (Najman and Levine 1981). The wider social problems of COAD sufferers have largely been ignored in outcome studies, but an understanding of the broader quality of life outcomes in relation to COAD is important in relation to the delivery of optimum care (Williams and Bury 1989). The lack of consensus is partly due to the lack of qualitative descriptive data of the lives of these patients. Without such data the relevance of existing scales remains problematic and unassessed (Williams 1989).

The social sciences have much to offer in relation to descriptive studies of disease processes and effects. A good example is physical disability. One such study is Blaxter's (1976) work on the meaning of disability, which provides many insights on the dimensions to be measured in relation to the practical, vocational, financial and social aspects of life and its associated problems. Similar studies are needed with respiratory disease in order to inform the further development of disease-specific scales. Without these, the content validity of existing scales is questionable.

Quality of life assessment in COPD/COAD patients: Disease-specific scales

GUYATT'S McMASTER CHRONIC RESPIRATORY QUESTIONNAIRE (CRQ)

The CRQ is a 20-item questionnaire compiled from an initial pool of 108 items. It was designed as an outcome measure for use with people with respiratory disease (Guyatt *et al*. 1987a). The scale's authors have given considerable thought to the measurement of health-related quality of life (Guyatt *et al*. 1987b, 1989b, 1989c).

The scale was developed to measure the frequency and importance of all areas of COAD-related dysfunction: fatigue, mastery (in control of disease), sleep disturbance, social disruption, cognition, anger, depression, anxiety, frustration and irritability. The items were drawn from unstructured interviews with patients with chronic airflow limitation, discussions with specialist nurses, literature reviews, other quality of life questionnaires and clinical experience. During testing, 100 patients were also asked how their quality of life was affected as a result of their chest disease by listing all the physical, emotional and social problems they experienced. Subjects were finally asked to rate items in order of importance on a 5-point Likert scale, from 'not very important' to 'extremely important' (Guyatt *et al*. 1987c). Dyspnoea in everyday activities, fatigue, embarrassment, frustration, anxiety and depression were most frequently reported and rated important by patients. Older patients had slightly fewer problems in relation to emotional disturbance and social limitations. Patients with lower spirometry experienced greater dyspnoea and were more depressed, angry and anxious, and experienced more cognitive problems.

During the scale's development, a sub-sample of patients' relatives also completed the questionnaire. The mean importance assigned to problems by relatives was greater than that assigned by patients. Pearson's correlations between the relatives' and the patients' total scores for the major dimensions were: dyspnoea 0.50; mastery 0.45; fatigue 0.42; sleep disturbance 0.60; emotional problems 0.44; social problems 0.40; cognitive function 0.47 (in each case the significance value was less than 0.01) (Guyatt *et al*. 1987c).

The 19-question/20-item version was developed from the study of 100 patients. The items were serially pre-tested in order to clarify wording and eliminate ambiguities.

Content

The final version contains 19 questions (20 items). It measures dyspnoea, fatigue and emotional function. Dyspnoea is measured by asking subjects to specify five important and frequent daily activities during which they experience shortness of breath. The intensity of dyspnoea they experience doing these five activities is measured serially using a 7-point Likert scale. The same five activities, identified on first administration of the questionnaire, are used for all subsequent (outcome) administrations.

As the questionnaire was designed for use as an outcome instrument, the scale also asks respondents to make a global rating of change in their dyspnoea – they are asked if their overall dyspnoea during day-to-day activities was the same, better or worse after each study period in comparison to the previous one. Those who say that their dyspnoea is worse or better are asked to quantify the change using a 7-point Likert scale varying from 'hardly any better (worse)' to 'a great deal better (worse)'.

Following the dyspnoea questions, the rest of the questionnaire comprises 15 standardized questions which are identical for each subject. These cover fatigue and emotional function, and all have the same 7-point response choice from 'all of the time' (1) to 'none of the time' (7).

Administration and scoring

Administration by an interviewer takes 15–25 min. This questionnaire is not completely standardized as it allows patients to tailor the questionnaire to suit their state. This method does not permit a standard score to be calculated. The questionnaire, scoring details, a training manual and training tape for the administration of the questionnaire are available from the authors.

Examples from the CRQ

The questionnaire begins by eliciting the five activities in which the patient experienced dyspnoea during day-to-day activities:

1 I would like you to think of the activities that you have done during the last 2 weeks that have made you feel short of breath. These should be activities which you do frequently and which are important in your day-to-day life. Please list as many activities as you can that you have done during the last 2 weeks that have made you feel short of breath.

3 (a) Of the items which you have listed, which is the most important to you in your day-to-day life?

I will read through the items, and when I am finished I would like you to tell me which is the most important.

(Read through all items spontaneously volunteered and those from the list (Q. 2) which patient mentioned)

(b) Which of these items is most important to you in your day-to-day life? (List items on response sheet)

(This process is continued until the five most important activities are determined . . .)

4 I would now like you to describe how much shortness of breath you have experienced during the last 2 weeks while doing the five most important activities you have selected.

(a) Please indicate how much shortness of breath you have had during the last 2 weeks while (Interviewer insert activity list in 3a) by choosing one of the following options from the card in front of you (green card):

Extremely short of breath / very short of breath / quite a bit short of breath / moderate shortness of breath / some shortness of breath / a little shortness of breath / not at all short of breath

This process continues until the subject's degree of dyspnoea on all five of his or her most important activities has been determined . . .

Validity

The questionnaire's construction ensures that the items are relevant to patients, and that it is a measure of the dysfunction most important to patients with chronic airflow limitation. The authors compared the performance of the instrument with the Rand Dyspnoea Scale, the Oxygen Cost Diagram, a transition dyspnoea index and Rand measures of physical and emotional functioning which were designed as part of the health-related quality of life assessments for their Health Insurance Study/Medical Outcomes Study (Stewart and Ware 1992). The respondents were 24 patients with primarily fixed chronic airflow limitation. The responsiveness of the instrument was confirmed (Guyatt *et al.* 1987a, 1989a, 1989b, 1991). Its validity was tested with these 24 patients by comparing all the test results before and after rehabilitation programmes and then serially over 6 months. There were moderate and significant correlations between changes in the questionnaire responses and changes in the other instruments ($r = 0.35$ and 0.62, respectively), except with less closely related dimensions, i.e. the correlation between emotional functioning and the walk test was 0.19 and with the global rating of fatigue 0.27 (Guyatt *et al.* 1987a, 1989a, 1989b, 1991). It was shown to be sensitive to treatment (with bronchodilators) (Guyatt *et al.* 1987b).

Reliability

Test–retest coefficients of variation at 6 weeks with 25 patients with stable chronic airflow limitation ranged between 6 and 12 per cent for each dimension, which the authors regarded as good. It was able to detect slight improvements in condition among a further 13 patients with chronic lung disease followed up between 2 and 6 weeks, who were participating in a drug treatment protocol. Similar results were reported with a comparable study of 28 patients participating in a respiratory rehabilitation programme (Guyatt *et al.* 1987a).

The scale has been criticized by Jones (1993) on the grounds that different cut-off scores appear to apply to different patient groups, limiting comparisons between patient groups (Guyatt *et al.* 1989a, 1989b; Morgan 1991). Its advantage over most scales is that it does not simply focus on shortness of breath, but includes other areas of dysfunction as well. The scale is regarded as the most comprehensive disease-specific measure for respiratory conditions (Jones *et al.* 1992).

It is almost identical to the Chronic Heart Failure Questionnaire (Guyatt *et al.* 1988, 1989a); the dyspnoea questions are identical, and the remaining questions overlap except for mastery, which is not asked of heart failure patients.

ST. GEORGE'S RESPIRATORY QUESTIONNAIRE (SGRQ)

This is a self-administered measure of impaired health in people with diseases that cause airways obstruction, i.e. asthma and COAD (Quirk and Jones 1990; Jones 1991a, 1991b, 1993; Jones *et al.* 1992; Jones 1994).

Content

It is divided into three parts:

1 *Symptoms:* frequency of cough, sputum production, wheeze, breathlessness, and duration and frequency of attacks of breathlessness or wheeze.
2 *Activity:* physical activities that either cause or are limited by breathlessness.
3 *Impact:* employment, being in control of health, panic, stigma, the need for medication and side-effects, health expectations, disturbances in daily life.

This division was supported by principal components analysis (Jones *et al.* 1992).

It contains 76 items and was recommended for use to complement, not replace, physiological measurement (Jones 1991a). While the impact section covers social and emotional disturbances due to the disease, it does not include anxiety and depression. The scale requires supplementation with an anxiety/depression scale for the assessment of these domains. Response categories vary from frequency codes, 'yes/no', 'true/false' to multiple-choice items (to be ticked).

Administration and scoring

The scale can be self-administered and takes about 10 min to complete. Each item is given a weight for the amount of distress associated with the symptom or state. The weights were derived empirically and based on studies of 141 patients, aged 31–75 years in six countries. The weights were found to be similar for patients with asthma and COAD; age, sex, duration of disease and various clinical measures accounted for a very small part of the variation between patients in the weights (Quirk and Jones 1990; Quirk *et al.* 1991; Jones *et al.* 1992).

Each of the three sections is scored separately (0–100 per cent), with a zero score indicating no impairment to life quality. A total score can be calculated for all item responses. The SGRQ scores are calculated using weights attached to each questionnaire item. These provide an estimate of the degree of distress associated with the symptom/state. The details of the weights and scoring are available from the authors.

Examples from the SGRQ

This questionnaire is designed to help us learn much more about how your breathing is troubling you and how it affects your life. We are using it to find out which aspects of your illness cause you most problems, rather than what the doctors and nurses think your problems are.

Part 1

Symptoms

7 Over the last year, in an average week, how many good days (with little chest trouble) have you had?

None __ One or two __ Three or four __ Nearly every day __ Every day __

8 If you have a wheeze, is it worse in the morning? Yes/no

Part 2
Section 5

Medication

My medication does not help me very much
I get embarrassed using my medication in public
I have unpleasant side-effects from my medication
My medication interferes with my life a lot

True/false

Section 6

Activity

I take a long time to get washed or dressed
I cannot take a bath or shower, or I take a long time

I walk slower than other people, or I stop for rests
Jobs such as housework take a long time, or I have to stop for rests
If I walk up one flight of stairs, I have to go slowly or stop
If I hurry or walk fast, I have to stop or slow down

True/false

Validity

The questionnaire was compared with spirometric measurements, bronchodilator responses, the results of oximetry during exercise, 6 min walking distance tests, the MRC respiratory questionnaire, the Hospital Anxiety and Depression Scale (Zigmond and Snaith 1983) and the Sickness Impact Profile (SIP: Bergner *et al.* 1981) among 141 patients with a wide spectrum of airflow obstruction. The component parts of the questionnaire correlated with appropriate reference measures, and followed the pattern of the SIP, except that it was over twice as sensitive to differences in disease severity as the SIP. Its skewness was less than 0.7 in all cases and the scores were all normally distributed (Jones *et al.* 1992). It was sensitive to changes in the reference measures over a period of 12 months. However, changes in quality of life as measured by the questionnaire correlated poorly with change in FEV_1, but better with walking distances and the MRC dyspnoea grade. The activity score correlated well with the MRC questionnaire items on cough and wheeze. The MRC dyspnoea grade and 6 min walking test were closely associated with the activity score but not to the symptoms score. The Hospital Anxiety and Depression (HAD) Scale scores correlated best with the impact section but there was little association with the symptom section (Jones *et al.* 1992). Thus, the SGRQ was more sensitive than the SIP, while covering similar domains (Jones 1993).

Brazier *et al.* (1993a) used the SGRQ with a sample of patients with chronic obstructive pulmonary disease, along with Guyatt's McMaster Chronic Disease Questionnaire (CRQ), the Rand SF-36, the Euroqol and clinical tests such as spirometry, the 6 min walk test, pulse oximetry and the Fletcher Scale/MRC Symptoms Questionnaire. They reported good results for the SF-36, which correlated well with the 6 min walk test, but poor results for the Euroqol, which was not significantly associated with the SF-36 or the SGRQ. The SF-36 and the CRQ both had greater internal consistency than the SGRQ.

Reliability

Jones *et al.* (1992) reported good reliability in relation to 2-week retest repeatability among 40 stable asthmatic patients and 20 patients with stable COPD, the coefficient of variation being 19 per cent. The intra-class correlation for the total score on the two occasions was 0.91 for the asthmatic patients and 0.92 for the COPD patients. The repeatability of the component sections was similar for both groups of patients, and for the patients combined ($r = 0.91$ for symptoms, 0.87 for activity, and 0.88 for impact).

CHRONIC DISEASE ASSESSMENT TOOL (CDAT)

This is a battery of largely existing measures developed by Moody and colleagues (Moody 1988; Moody *et al.* 1990, 1991). It was initially piloted with 21 people with chronic bronchitis and emphysema (CBE), and assessed by a panel of health professionals for content validity and then retested on 45 people with CBE. Inter-scale reliability coefficients ranged from 0.31 to 0.72. Not all results were as expected. While the anxiety trait correlated significantly with depression state, severity of dyspnoea, fatigue, mastery (control over everyday affairs) and quality of life, it was not associated with functional status. No direct link was found between severity of disease and severity of dyspnoea. The results indicated that while severity of dyspnoea had a clear effect on functional status, severity of disease affected quality of life through indirect links.

Content, administration and scoring

Part I contains 106 self-report items in five sections and takes 25–30 min to complete. The sections in Part I include:

● *General health and medical history:* perceived severity of dyspnoea measured with a visual analogue scale (Guyatt *et al.* 1986) and the American Thoracic Society Grade of Breathlessness Scale (GBS: Brown 1985).

● *Environmental risk:* air quality and active/passive tobacco exposure measured by the Task Force on Health Risk Assessment (1986); the Quality of Life Index (Spitzer *et al.* 1981), which is usually used in oncology research (a five-item index); and demographic data.

● *Impact on health:* measured with a modified version of the Arthritis Impact Measurement Scales (AIMS) and health service use (Liang *et al.* 1985).

● *A standard measure* of neuroticism (Costa and McCrae 1985) and the Chronic Disease Respiratory Questionnaire (CDRQ: Guyatt *et al.* 1986, 1987a, 1987c) which together measure functional status (mobility, physical activity, dexterity, household activity and ADL), cognitive ability, anxiety, depression, social support, fatigue, dyspnoea, mastery, health status and other health problems.

Part II is a clinical section for the recording of the results of physical assessment and pulmonary function tests and severity of disease, graded as mild, moderate or severe: type of pulmonary disease, history, chronicity, treatment, spirometry tests and maximum inspiratory pressure test results according to the American Thoracic Society (1987), clinical examination results and information given. Most of these scales are partly displayed elsewhere in this book.

Validity

In tests for convergent validity, the authors reported moderate to strong correlations between severity of disease and functional status, and between severity of dyspnoea and fatigue, depression and quality of life. The correlations were in the expected direction − as severity of disease increased, functional status declined ($r = -0.28$); as severity of dyspnoea increased, fatigue increased ($r = -0.47$), depression increased ($r = 0.67$) and quality of life decreased ($r = -0.75$).

Reliability

On the basis of a study of 45 patients, Moody *et al.* (1990) reported the reliability coefficients of the scales for functional status, depression, anxiety, mastery and fatigue (coefficient alpha) to be 0.65–0.96; for environmental risk it was 0.76; for health service use 0.93; for Spitzer quality of life 0.89; and the correlation between the American Thoracic Society Grade of Breathlessness Scale and the dyspnoea severity visual analogue scale self-rating was 0.40 (see also Walz *et al.* 1984). The authors suggested that further research using this battery with larger samples is needed (Moody 1990; Moody *et al.* 1990, 1991).

This measure is a simple battery of existing measures, although the justification for this particular selection is unclear and requires further testing and exploratory development.

HEALTH OUTCOMES INSTITUTE TyPE SCALES (HOI-TyPE) – COPD

The Health Outcomes Institute, previously known as Interstudy (2001 Killebrew Drive, Suite 122, Bloomington, MN 55425, USA) has also produced condition-specific specifications (TyPE) for COPD. The forms are designed for repeated application (at follow-up assessments) unless otherwise stated.

COPD Form

The patient's form comprises 22 questions, some of which are multi-item. The questions include items on smoking (2 items), service use (3), phlegm (4), medication (3), use of oxygen at home (3), use of machine for breathing (2), the SF-36 physical functioning subscale (10) (Ware *et al.* 1993), other disabilities (1), symptoms (13), employment status (1), days off work (2), side effects (8), height and weight (2) and peak flow rate (1).

The clinician has two forms to complete (total three sides) on diagnosis, results of tests and medical history.

Examples from the HOI COPD Form

Patient's form

6 Do you cough up phlegm?   Yes/no
10 Do attacks of shortness of breath, cough, or wheezing awaken you at night?   Yes/no
     (a) How often do such attacks awaken you?

Less than once a night/about once a night/more than once a night

11 Do you have to prop yourself up to breathe more easily?   Yes/no
14(a) (if employed). Has your COPD caused you to miss work in the past 4 weeks?   Yes (frequency) / no
16(b) How many hours a day do you use oxygen on average?

Only at night / 0–12 hours / 13–18 hours / 19–24 hours

18 Do you require a machine to breathe for you all the time?   Yes / no
19 Do you take a steroid . . . by pill for your COPD?   Yes / no

IF YES, have you developed any of the following side-effects?

(a) Round face, 'buffalo hump'
(e) High blood pressure
(g) Diabetes

Clinician's form

First request results for FEV_1 and FVC, peak flow, arterial blood gases, etc.

4 Does the patient meet the diagnostic criteria for chronic bronchitis (daily cough and sputum production for more than 3 months a year for at least 2 successive years)?   Yes / no / uncertain
10 Does the patient have:

(a) Other lung diseases (what?)
(d) Left ventricular failure
(j) Dementia, confusion, memory changes

Quality of life assessment in asthma patients: Disease-specific scales

Most studies of outcome of asthma care have used symptoms (wheezing, cough, sputum production, nocturnal waking, early morning chest tightness, etc.), frequency, consultations for acute wheezing, hospitalization, spirometry, peak flow rate, medication use and/or relapse as typical indicators of outcome (e.g. Strunk *et al.* 1989; Charlton *et al.* 1990; Fitzgerald and Hargreave 1990; Butz *et al.* 1991). Outcome batteries for use with adult asthma patients, which have built on existing scales (the Living with Asthma Questionnaire and the Self-

Efficacy Scale), have been developed for the Outcome Measures in Ambulatory Programme at the University of Newcastle upon Tyne (see below) and the Grampian Asthma Study of Integrated Care (Drummond *et al.* 1994). Asthma quality of life scales are presented below after the severity scale.

ASTHMA SEVERITY SCALE

A severity scale for adults and a scale for children was designed and reported by Nocon and Booth (1989, 1991). Its function was to assist with data analysis.

Content, administration and scoring

The scale for adults contains seven points, from 'effective control of symptoms' to 'severe chronic asthma, with further admissions to hospital in past 12 months, and getting worse'. The scale for children contains six points, from 'improved control of mild symptoms' to 'severe symptoms and getting worse'. Replies can be graded as mild, moderate or severe. It is usually interviewer-administered. It is short, simple and easily analysed.

Examples from the Asthma Severity Scale

Children

2 Improved control of moderately severe symptoms
4 Severe symptoms still occur, though infrequently
6 Severe symptoms, and getting worse

Adults

1 Effective control of symptoms
4 Severe chronic asthma, but no further admissions in past 12 months, but getting worse
7 Severe chronic asthma, with further admissions to hospital in past 12 months, and getting worse

---

Validity and reliability

The authors used it in a study of 32 children and 18 adults, but did not report on the psychometric properties of the scale. The authors did not develop this scale with the intention that other investigators use it and, therefore, it is largely untested. It is included here as it has potential.

LIVING WITH ASTHMA QUESTIONNAIRE

This instrument was designed by Hyland and colleagues (Hyland 1991; Hyland *et al.* 1991) as a quality of life scale which could be used when evaluating the outcome of treatment management programmes for adult asthma sufferers. It was therefore designed to contain asthma-specific items and to be sensitive to changes expected during clinical trials with asthma patients.

The first version of the questionnaire, generated from six patient focus groups, contained 101 items in 11 domains. The groups had omitted sexual behaviour, which was later added by the researchers who felt that the patients may have been inhibited from mentioning this in the group discussions. This increased the number of domains to 12.

The questionnaire was given to 18 general practitioners to test on their adult patients with asthma. Psychometric testing of the results of 101 asthma sufferers showed the test to be unidimensional, despite having several domains, a finding that was replicated during three further stages of the instrument's testing with 783 patients. Following this, poor discriminators were deleted or modified and a further 150 patients recruited by 23 general practitioners completed a new version of the questionnaire. The version contained 43 negative items and 29 positive items. A further version was developed and tested on 405 patients recruited by 78 general practitioners and via an advert in a newsletter for asthma sufferers. As a result some items were dropped and the testing of a final version involved 228 asthma sufferers who had participated earlier. The design stages and testing of the questionnaire have been described in detail by Hyland *et al.* (1991).

Content

The final version of the questionnaire is a 68-item quality of life scale, covering 12 domains: social/leisure, sport, holidays, sleep, work and other activities, colds, mobility, effects on others, medication use, sex, and dysphoric states and attitudes.

Administration and scoring

The scale can be self- or interviewer-administered (the latter method reportedly takes 15–20 min). The response to each of the items is made on a 4-point category scale from 'untrue of me' to 'very true of me'. For each domain, the scale scores are calculated by adding the values of each negative item (1–3) to the values of each positive item reversed in polarity (3–1), and dividing by the number of positive and negative items.

Examples from the Living with Asthma Questionnaire

I can take part in any sports I want

I tend to be more conscious than other people of the early symptoms of a cold

I feel that I miss out because there are some sporting activities I cannot join in with

Because of my asthma I feel drained after a cold

Untrue of me / slightly true of me / very true of me (does not apply = 8)

Validity and factor structure

Tests of the questionnaire's validity were conducted during its development. The questionnaire was administered to 76 patients along with the Sickness Impact Profile, and the correlation between the two scales was high ($r = 0.66$), indicating convergent validity. Predictive validity was supported by moderate correlations of the questionnaire with steroid prescribing ($r = 0.35$) and with peak flow ($r = 0.44$) in a study of 40 out-patients with asthma. More evidence of its validity is required.

Initial psychometric testing with the 228 asthma sufferers confirmed the unifactorial solution. The factor loadings were slightly lower for females than males. Later analyses of the scale's factor loadings identified a problem construct and an evaluation construct, with the former having greater sensitivity to longitudinal change (Hyland et al. 1994). Further testing is being carried out by McColl et al. (in press), who have identified several factors.

Reliability

Reliability was assessed with patients recruited by GPs who had participated earlier (final usable number of returned questionnaires = 95). Test–retest at 2 months using a postal method showed a correlation of $r = 0.95$.

The scale is shorter than Guyatt's CRQ, but it is also fairly broad. As the authors point out, however, it does not have as many items on emotional experience as the CRQ, nor does it cover cognitive impairment (Hyland et al. 1991). It requires further testing.

OUTCOME MEASURES IN AMBULATORY CARE (ASTHMA AND DIABETES) (OMAC)

Some of the items of Hyland's Living with Asthma Questionnaire have been incorporated into a battery of questionnaires for use in outcome studies of care of asthma patients in general practice by Allen Hutchinson and his colleagues at the universities of Newcastle upon Tyne and Hull. The researchers are developing outcome tools for use in general practice for patients with diabetes as well as asthma. The research team aim to develop 'practical, condition-specific outcome measurement methodologies for routine application in judging the effectiveness of care in ambulatory settings (general practice and hospital outpatients)' (McColl et al. 1993). They reviewed over 500 measures of general health status and quality of life, and asthma and diabetes condition-specific measures.

The selected instruments are being tested on 700 asthma and 700 diabetes patients. Apart from disease-specific items, the investigators are assessing the appropriateness of the Rand SF-36 (Ware et al. 1993a), the Functional Limitations Profile (FLP: Charlton et al. 1983), the Duke 17-Item Health Profile (Parkerson et al. 1990), the Hospital Anxiety and Depression Scale (HAD: Zigmond and Snaith 1983), the Euroqol (Euroqol Group 1990), and the Dartmouth COOP Charts (Nelson et al. 1990). The disease-specific items also include questions on co-morbidity and complications.

Content of battery

The domains considered for inclusion in their test battery of measures were: clinical (clinical control of symptoms, complications, iatrogenic problems, severity and co-morbidity); functional (ambulation/mobility, body care/activities of daily living, pain, sleep/energy); psychosocial ('quality of life', social function, role function, mental health, health and sickness perceptions). The scales which were initially selected for inclusion were listed earlier. The condition-specific measures they selected for use with asthma patients were the Living with Asthma Questionnaire and, following consensus reviews with specialists, a 38-item symptom questionnaire for asthma (see Chapter 8 for their diabetes battery).

Analyses of the initial results from preliminary investigations showed that the FLP had a high rate of item non-response and also had ceiling effects, and so this was excluded from further study; the Duke 17-Item Health Profile was found to have poor internal consistency and convergent validity and was excluded. All other measures were judged to be psychometrically sound and included in the next stage of analysis.

Administration and scoring

The remaining questionnaire battery is estimated to take 15 min to complete. Given the need for brevity in clinical practice, the investigators are conducting further analysis aimed at item reduction. The scales all have their separate scoring formats (see source references).

Examples from the OMAC

Asthma symptoms

2 In the last month, on how many days have you been short of breath during the day at times when you were not exercising?

Never – Every day

3 In the last month, on how many days have you wheezed during the day?

Never – Every day

8 In the last month, on how many nights have you had problems sleeping because of your asthma (for example, bother getting to sleep or being woken in the night)?

Never – Every day

9 In the last month, on how many days have you felt frightened because of your asthma?

Never – Every day

These questions are about the things that happen to people with asthma in their day-to-day life . . .

3 I feel that I miss out because there are some sporting activities I cannot join in with.

Untrue of me / slightly true of me / very true of me

Asthma care

45 Thinking about the doctor/practice nurse who looks after your asthma, could you tell me whether you agree or disagree with the following statements:

My doctor has helped me to make my asthma better
I wish that my doctor talked to me more about my asthma

Strongly disagree – strongly agree

Validity and reliability

The SF-36 (physical function and energy sub-scales), the HAD and condition-specific items were reported to explain 68 per cent of the variation in health perceptions among asthma patients. The factor structure of the SF-36 was confirmed (McColl *et al.* 1995). As the research is currently ongoing and many of the data are in preparation for publication, further details can be obtained from the authors. The battery is also being tested by Dr G. Feder and colleagues at St. Bartholomew's Hospital Medical College in the Department of General Practice (pers. comm.).

HEALTH OUTCOMES INSTITUTE TyPE SCALES (HOI-TyPE) – ASTHMA FORM

This is one of the many disease-specific outcome questionnaires developed for the Health Outcomes Institute (HOI). The scale items await the results of psychometric testing, which is not conducted by the HOI. Like most of the disease-specific batteries, the asthma outcomes measure requires the administration of the Rand SF-36 (Ware *et al.* 1993) as its core. The Health Outcomes Institute, previously known as Interstudy (2001 Killebrew Drive, Suite 122, Bloomington, MN 55425, USA), has published the forms.

Content

The patient's form contains 13 questions, some of which are multi-item in nature (e.g. the SF-36 physical functioning sub-scale at question 5 has 10 items). The form comprises two double-sided pages and covers health service use (2 items), night disturbance (1 item), the SF-36 physical functioning sub-scale (10 items), emotional problems due to asthma (1 item), difficulties in daily activities due to asthma (1 item) and cause (1 item), interference with social activities due to asthma (1 item), medication (4 items), and symptoms (8 items).

The clinician's questionnaire is a four-sided form requiring the doctor to record FEV_1 and FVC, peak flow, medication use, consultation rate, complications of corticosteroids, characterization of asthma (e.g. specific triggers of asthma attacks – animal danders, mites, seasonal inhaled antigens – allergic rhinitis, family history, etc.) and co-morbidity, including smoking.

Administration and scoring

The batteries are self-administered. The forms are designed for repeated application (at follow-ups), unless otherwise stated and another follow-up form provided. Each item is scored differently and analysed separately.

Validity and reliability

There are no published data on the psychometric properties of the questions included, apart from the core SF-36, which has good psychometric properties (Ware *et al.* 1993), although it needs further testing for sensitivity and predictive validity with this patient group.

ASTHMA QUALITY OF LIFE QUESTIONNAIRE

This is a new questionnaire being developed by Juniper *et al.* (1992, 1993a, 1993b, 1994) for use with asthma patients and which is capable of measuring change over time within individuals. In total, 152 items were generated from a literature search on asthma and on health-related quality of life measures, patients' experiences, discussions with chest physicians and unstructured interviews with six asthma patients. A study of 150 adult male and female asthma patients was conducted in order to identify which of the 152 items were most important. The items chosen most often and labelled as most important were selected for

Examples from the HOI Asthma Form

Patient's form

(This includes the physical functioning sub-scale of the SF-36).

2 How many times have you been hospitalized in the past six months for asthma?   0–4+

7 During the past 4 weeks, to what extent did your asthma cause difficulty to you in doing your daily work, both inside and outside the house?

Not at all / a little bit / some / quite a bit / could not do daily work

8 During the past 4 weeks, to what extent did your asthma interfere with your normal social activities with family, friends, neighbours, or groups?

Not at all / slightly / moderately / quite a bit / extremely

13 Over the past 4 weeks, how frequently have you had the following symptoms?

   (a) How often do you cough?
   (d) Did you have wheezing?
   (f) Did you have heartburn?
   (h) Did you have heart palpitations?

Never / occasionally / once or twice a day / many times a day / all the time

inclusion in the final questionnaire. Other criteria for inclusion were adequate representation of both physical and emotional function and a minimum of four items per domain. Responses are recorded on a 7-point scale. This questionnaire was pre-tested on 30 patients.

Content

The version currently being tested contains 32 questions, each of which has one of four sets of seven response options, displayed on cards (organized by colour coding). The domains covered are activity limitations (11 items), symptoms (12 items), emotional function (5 items) and exposure to environmental stimuli (4 items).

First, respondents are asked to identify activities in which they are limited by their asthma. If more than five activities are mentioned, they are asked to choose the five most important. Prompts are given from a list of 26 activities, ranging from housework to talking. When five activities have been identified, the subjects are asked about the extent to which they have been limited in each of the activities: 'Please indicate how much you have been limited by your asthma in [insert activity] during the last 2 weeks by choosing one of the following options. Green card: Totally limited, couldn't do activity at all/extremely limited/very limited/ moderate limitation/some limitation/a little limitation/not at all limited'. After this has been asked for each of the five items, the remaining 27 questions are asked of all respondents.

Administration and scoring

The questionnaire can be self- or interviewer-administered and takes about 5 to 10 min to complete. No weighting of scores is carried out. The authors calculated the scores on the domains as averages of all items on that domain.

Examples from the Asthma Quality of Life Questionnaire

6 How much discomfort or distress have you felt over the last two weeks as a result of chest tightness? (Red card)

A very great deal of discomfort or distress / a great deal / a moderate amount / some / very little / no discomfort or distress

7 In general, how often during the last 2 weeks have you felt concerned about having asthma? (Blue card)

All of the time / most of the time / a good bit of the time / some of the time / a little of the time / hardly any of the time / none of the time

9 How often during the past 2 weeks did you experience asthma symptoms as a result of being exposed to cigarette smoke? (Blue card)

19 How often during the past 2 weeks did you feel you had to avoid a situation or environment because of dust? (Blue card)

24 How often during the past two weeks have you been woken at night by your asthma? (Blue card)

31 Think of the overall range of activities that you would have liked to have done during the past 2 weeks. How much has your range of activities been limited by your asthma? (Yellow card)

Severely limited – most activities not done / very limited / moderately limited – several activities not done / slightly limited / very slightly limited – very few activities not done / hardly limited at all / not limited at all – have done all activities that I wanted to do.

Validity and reliability

The advantage of this scale is that, not only is it disease-specific, but the first five items are also patient-specific, and generate data meaningful at the individual level. It is presented here as an exciting development, although the authors have yet to publish full results on its psychometric properties. The scale has been reported to correlate significantly with conventional measures of asthma severity and generic quality of life measures (Rowe 1991; Juniper et al. 1993a). Data on change at 0, 4 and 8 weeks have been reported for 39 adults with asthma, not for the purposes of making test–retest assessments, but for determining minimally important levels of change in questionnaire scores for use as an outcome measure (Juniper et al. 1994). The questionnaire has been reported to be responsive to change in before/after studies and in clinical trials (Rowe 1991; Juniper et al. 1993a, 1993b).

ASTHMA SYMPTOM CHECKLIST

This is a symptom checklist, rather than a quality of life scale, although effects on some aspects of life are included (Kinsman et al. 1973, 1977; Avner and Kinsman 1987).

Content

The current version consists of ten symptom categories (sub-scales), containing 50 items about symptoms which can occur during asthma attacks (e.g. mood – worried, frightened; somatic: hard to breathe, coughing) (Kinsman et al. 1973, 1977). These were selected from items listed during patient interviews. The pool of 36 items was reduced from a larger pool. The symptom categories are dyspnoea, fatigue, sleep difficulties, congestion, irritability, anxiety, decathexis, helplessness/hopelessness, poor memory, peripheral/ sensory complaints and alienation. Responses are made on a 5-point scale: never (1), almost never (2), sometimes (3), almost always (4), and always (5). Positive items are summed, and divided by the total number of symptoms within the category.

Examples from the Asthma Symptom Checklist

Short of breath
Irritable
Dizzy
Tired
Panting
Angry
Afraid of dying
Scared
Lonely

Validity and reliability

Psychometric analysis showed the scale to be multidimensional (Kinsman *et al.* 1973). The factors were panic–fear, irritability, hyperventilation–hypnocapnia, bronchoconstriction and fatigue. The scale has stable psychometric properties, and the factor structure was confirmed in a further study (Brooks *et al.* 1989). In a study of 146 patients with lung disease, it was sensitive to type of lung disease and self-reported functional incapacity (Kinsman *et al.* 1983). The correlations of items within the sub-scales ranged from 0.81 to 0.94 (Kinsman *et al.* 1983). Despite the scale being limited to symptoms, Hyland *et al.* (1991) state that it is a valid scale for use with a restricted range of problems. It is a promising symptom scale, although more testing is required.

Summary of other scales which await full psychometric testing

ASTHMA SELF-EFFICACY SCALE

The literature on asthma indicates that the personality of asthma sufferers can influence the outcome of their care. For example, their confidence in relation to the self-management of asthma can affect their efficiency (Creer 1987). Various scales have been designed for assessing attitudes to performance (Creer *et al.* 1986a, 1986b; Creer 1987). Self-efficacy refers to a person's conviction that he

or she can successfully execute behaviours required to control an outcome, such as an asthma attack (Bandura 1986; Creer 1987). It is an essential variable to assess in outcome studies of asthma where much depends on the patient's management of the condition.

The Self-Efficacy Scale was developed by Tobin *et al.* (1987). It was developed in two experiments. In the first, 40 adults with asthma were asked to describe at least ten situations in which they might experience asthma. From this a questionnaire containing 80 items was developed. The second experiment involved tests for reliability. During its development and testing, the test was administered to 65 adults with asthma, and repeated at 2 months. The product–moment correlation between administrations was $r = 0.77$; the internal consistency of the scale for both administrations was $r = 0.97$.

ATTITUDES TO ASTHMA SCALE

The Attitudes to Asthma Scale consists of 31 statements relating to those attitudes and beliefs relevant to illness behaviour in people with asthma (Sibbald *et al.* 1986, 1988; Sibbald 1989). The items were determined by the investigators and other doctors on the basis of the literature and their knowledge. The scale initially contained 40 statements about attitudes and beliefs thought to be important in governing illness behaviour in chronic disease; the latest version contains 31 statements within seven sub-scales of 3–5 items each. The scales cover emotional impact of asthma (5 items), the effect of asthma on relationships with others (3 items), severity (5 items), the effect of asthma on activities (4 items), coping with an attack (5 items), feelings about medication (4 items) and satisfaction with medical care (5 items). Examples of items include: 'I feel different from other people because I am an asthmatic', 'I avoid letting people know I am an asthmatic', 'I worry that I might die from asthma', 'I can't enjoy a full life because of my asthma', 'I can prevent asthma attacks', 'My doctor has helped to make my asthma better' (Sibbald *et al.* 1986). Respondents were initially asked to mark their response on a 100 mm visual analogue scale. However, 22 per cent incorrectly completed the visual analogue scale, so this was subsequently changed to a 4-point Likert response scale from 'strongly disagree' to 'strongly agree'.

Factor analysis revealed a three-factor solution of the scale: stigma, confidence in the doctor and self-confidence in self-care. Hyland *et al.* (1991) reported data which failed to replicate this three-factor solution. Sibbald *et al.* (1986) reported that the scale had good repeatability at 4 weeks with 31 adult asthma patients, and self-completion responses were similar to those obtained at interview. The scale requires further evaluation of its psychometric properties.

CONCLUSION

While generic measures have been popular in outcomes studies of patients with respiratory disease, progress has been made over the past decade in developing disease-specific measures of quality of life. Probably the best disease-specific quality of life measure in relation to lung disease is Guyatt and co-workers' (1987a, 1987b) McMaster Chronic Respiratory Questionnaire. This has the advantage of taking into account individuals' assessments of the relevant quality of life domains that should be analysed in relation to outcome. It also contains an assessment of change. In relation to asthma, the OMAC batteries being tested by McColl *et al.* (in press) appear to be the most promising, which also includes Hyland's (1991) Living with Asthma Questionnaire. The specific asthma quality of life scales are fairly limited in scope, and need to be used as part of a battery of measures. Hyland (1992a, 1993) has cautioned potential investigators against selecting a scale on the basis of its content validity, in the absence of a theoretical description of the construct of quality of life. The quality of life questionnaires that have been developed for use with patients with respiratory problems are so diverse in their content, style and inclusion criteria for items, that their claims for content validity are suspect (Hyland 1992a).

5
NEUROLOGICAL CONDITIONS

MEASURING HEALTH-RELATED QUALITY OF LIFE IN NEUROLOGY

There are numerous areas within neurology where the application of broader outcome measures would be appropriate. For example, there is a rapidly increasing psychological literature on the measurement of outcome of head injury (Brooks 1984). This is an area which has moved towards more comprehensive assessments of outcome and away from fairly crude, albeit useful, indicators of outcome such as the Glasgow Outcome Scale. The latter has often been used to classify outcome into vegetative state, severe disability, moderate disability and good recovery (Jennett and Bond 1975; Jennett 1984). There are also numerous psychological texts reviewing various assessment tools of intellectual functioning and personality in children and in adults (see Mangen and Peterson 1982; Brooks 1984; Lezak 1989). A selection of cognitive scales is reviewed in the last section of this chapter; they are frequently used across all medical specialities. Subjective well-being is less commonly assessed in neurological patients, although this domain should not be overlooked.

Clearly, criteria for assessing outcome of care will differ for different disease syndromes within neurology. For example, a cerebrovascular accident (CVA) will affect different dimensions of functioning, than head injury or epilepsy. The specific effects of care and treatment will also require consideration. Beyond the identification of the specific types of patient outcomes which will require measurement for the particular disease syndrome, a general measure of health status should be included in order to assess patients' perceptions and facilitate comparisons with other population groups. Such a tool should be selected carefully, as a wide variety of tools exist which tap different dimensions (see review by Bowling 1991). Dye (1982) has reviewed tests of intellectual functioning, including tests used with brain-damaged older patients. Wade (1992) has reviewed measures of outcome commonly used by researchers among people with multiple sclerosis, Parkinson's disease, head injury, diseases of motor units and spinal injuries. However, these are mainly concerned with physical and mental functioning, aphasia and speech, rather than the effects of the condition on broader aspects of life and social functioning.

For the purposes of this text, two main disease syndromes, cerebrovascular accident and epilepsy, will be highlighted. In each of these areas, progress is being made by psychologists, neurologists and neurosurgeons on developing appropriate indicators of broader health status. This chapter is based on a briefer review by Bowling and Normand (in press). The final section briefly reviews well-known scales of neurophysiological functioning.

CEREBROVASCULAR ACCIDENT (CVA/STROKE)

The incidence of cerebrovascular accident (CVA), or stroke as it is commonly known, increases with age, and is an important cause of mortality and morbidity in the Western world. In the UK, about 75 per cent of stroke patients are admitted to hospital, and about 12 per cent who survive are admitted to institutional care 1 year after their stroke (see review by Freemantle *et al.* 1992). Over half of all stroke patients have continuing problems with mobility (Collin and Wade 1990).

The organization of services for stroke is diverse, and can include gereral medical wards in hospital, special stroke units, special rehabilitation units and community services. Many different professionals may be involved – doctors, nurses, physiotherapists, occupational therapists, speech therapists, social workers, counsellors, psychologists, chiropodists, etc. A review of the known effectiveness of these services in the care of stroke patients has been published by Freemantle *et al.* (1992). There is a continuing need to evaluate the effectiveness of services for stroke patients, hence the importance of careful selection of outcome indicators. Freemantle *et al.* (1992) concluded that more research, and of better quality, is required to establish which aspects of rehabilitation are most effective and what form of organization it should take.

THE DOMAINS OF MEASUREMENT

Apart from pathological measurements and neurological tests, there are several pertinent outcome indicators for stroke, including degree and type of motor and speech impairment, social, physical and mental handicap, and social and psychological well-being. Spontaneous recovery should also be included, which may occur with or without formal care. Those who recover from stroke do so in the first 3 months (this should be noted as a time reference for a follow-up assessment), regardless of rehabilitation, although it is unusual for improvement to continue beyond 1 year (another time reference for follow-up) (Freemantle *et al.* 1992).

Disease-specific measurements of functioning

Functional ability is one specific domain of health status, or health-related quality of life. When assessing the outcome of a disabling condition such as stroke, the areas that will need to be catered for by measurement tools include pathology, impairment (e.g. central nervous system, skeletal, muscular, etc.), the resulting disability (e.g. speaking, walking, etc.) and the handicap (e.g. communication, mobility, etc.) (WHO 1980). In any health-related quality of life outcome study, clinical markers for prognosis will also need to be included (e.g. urinary incontinence, loss of consciousness, severity of paralysis, etc.).

The problems which stroke sufferers may experience include difficulties performing activities of daily living (e.g. washing and dressing oneself), mobility (e.g. walking) and aphasia. These are obvious dimensions to include on an outcome instrument. The impact of the condition and its treatment on the performance of social roles (e.g. work, parent, care-giver), as well as activities, also requires measurement.

Studies of stroke patients and their prognosis and outcome have used a wide range of measurement scales for physical and mental functioning, including prognostic scores, assessments of motor deficits (e.g. in arm) and power, proprioception, ability to locate thumb, balance while walking, standing and sitting and cognition (see Kalra and Crome 1993) and aphasia batteries (Kertesz and Poole 1974).

Gait speed

Gait speed was chosen as the primary outcome measure by Wade *et al.* (1992) in their evaluation of physiotherapy with stroke patients. They asked the patients to cover a fixed distance of 20 m and recorded distance covered at 2, 6 and 12 min (Butland *et al.* 1982). The various time referents produce similar results; Wade (1992) recommends the 6 min test. This is a simple and reliable test, with obvious face validity, and is sensitive to change in patients with stroke, motor neuron disease and Parkinson's disease (see Wade, 1992). A further advantage of including gait speed in a battery of measures of outcome is that it achieves the criteria of a ratio scale, as well as being simple. Wade and his colleagues reported that gait speed was, in fact, the only outcome measure which showed improvement (an 8 per cent improvement in gait speed associated with treatment), confirming other research that gait speed is a more sensitive measure than scales of functional ability (Stewart et al. 1990; Wade et al. 1992). Wade et al. (1992) also recommend including a measure of starting and stopping to 'walk outside' in future studies, although large numbers of study patients would be needed in order to detect any changes in behaviour. A comprehensive range of indices is presented by Wade (1992).

Other clinical tests

Wade and his colleagues used a group of functional indicators, due to their concern that the measures should detect the useful benefits of therapy that might be achieved, particularly in quality of walking and gait speed (Butland et al. 1982; for descriptions of these scales see Wade 1992). These indicators included a nine-hole peg test of manual dexterity (the patient sits at a table and places pegs in holes and performance is timed: Mathiowetz et al. 1985); the motricity index (e.g. pinch grip, elbow flexion, shoulder abduction, ankle dorsiflexion, knee extension, hip flexion; rolling, sitting and balance: Demeurisse et al. 1980) and functional ambulation categories (Holden et al. 1984; Heller et al. 1987; Collin and Wade 1990; Collen et al. 1990; for a review, see Wade 1992).

Stroke scales

A number of fairly concise scales have been developed, which provide a simple and quick assessment of the level of stroke disability, handicap and/or severity (i.e. the severity of neurological deficits), sometimes encompassing a prognostic score. These vary in their prognostic accuracy and, while useful, provide only rudimentary information. Examples include the Rankin Disability Scale (Rankin 1957), the Scandinavian Stroke Scale (Scandinavian Stroke Study Group 1985, 1987; Lindenstrom et al. 1991; Boysen 1992), the Hemispheric Stroke Scale (Adams et al. 1987), the Canadian Neurological Scale (Côté et al. 1986, 1988, 1989; Côté and Hachinski 1992), the Oxford

Handicap Scale, which is a modified Rankin scale (Bamford et al. 1988, 1989) and the National Institute of Health (NIH) Stroke Scale (Brott et al. 1989; Brott 1992). A few of these are reviewed briefly later. Wade (1992) reviewed the most commonly used stroke scales, and stated a preference for the NIH Stroke Scale, the Canadian Neurological Scale and the Hemispheric Stroke Scale. He is, however, fairly critical of them, and argues that such scales are probably not needed, as a CT scan will diagnose stroke type more accurately.

Scales of functional ability and recommended clinical batteries

In 1987, the British Stroke Research Group (see Wade 1992) recommended a series of functional ability scales for assessing functioning in stroke, including the Barthel Index (Mahoney and Barthel 1965), the Nottingham Extended Activities of Daily Living Questionnaire (Nouri and Lincoln 1987), the Frenchay Activities Index (Holbrook and Skilbeck 1983) and the Rivermead Mobility Index (Collen et al. 1991). They also recommended scales encompassing death, level of consciousness, motor loss, visual field loss, difficulty with swallowing, neglect, memory, sensation and perception, walking tests and arm dexterity.

Generic measures

The most popular scales of quality of life in neurology are functional ability scales and measures of neurological functioning. However, these require supplementation with scales measuring other domains. Disease-specific quality of life scales (in the broader sense) have been slow to develop. Some investigators have consequently used broader measures of health-related quality of life, for example the Quality of Well-Being Scale (Kaplan et al. 1976). However, this is of limited value in research on outcomes, as it produces a single score by design and is therefore not informative in relation to the different domains of improvement or deterioration. More promising is the Short Form-36, which was developed from the Rand Health Insurance Study (HIS) and Medical Outcomes Study (MOS) batteries (Ware et al. 1993). It has not been tested for its appropriateness with stroke patients (its physical functioning sub-scale is unlikely to be sufficiently sensitive as it concentrates on mobility), although it is recommended for use with people with epilepsy (see pp. 195–6).

Domain-specific measures

Anxiety and depression

Psychological morbidity is a component of health status and health-related quality of life. Moreover, if the researcher wishes to tap this dimension of health directly, it is wise to select a specific scale, rather than rely solely on the mental health items in a health status scale. In relation to psychological morbidity (e.g. anxiety, depression) there are several popular scales in use. The type of scale selected partly depends on the severity of the patient's condition, and his or her ability to communicate. For patients with severe physical handicaps, assistance will be needed with questionnaires designed for self-completion, and simpler scales may be preferred for ease of administration.

Scales of psychological morbidity and functioning that have been used with stroke patients include Goldberg's (1972) General Health Questionnaire (GHQ), the Beck Depression Inventory (BDI: Beck *et al.* 1961) and the Hospital Anxiety and Depression Scale (HAD: Zigmond and Snaith 1983). The latter is preferable as it does not contain any somatic items that could reflect physical, rather than psychological morbidity. The HAD has been used with stroke patients by Wade *et al.* (1992). Another promising depression scale, which is very short and easy to complete, is the Rand depression screener (Burnham *et al.* 1988). The British Stroke Research Group (see Wade 1992) recommended using the HAD or the GHQ.

Cognitive impairment

A measure of cognitive impairment is likely to be required. Such measures are used routinely in research among people aged 65+, in order to assess for any effects on outcome and the validity of replies to questionnaires. Among the concise indicators of cognitive impairment, the most widely

used include the Mental Status Questionnaire (MSQ: Kahn *et al.* 1960a, 1960b), the Abbreviated Mental Test Score (AMTS: Hodkinson 1972), and the Mini-Mental State Examination (Folstein *et al.* 1975). The AMTS has been described by Wade (1992) as the most well-established test to be validated against neuro-pathological evidence, and describes the MSQ as the second most widely used test. As he pointed out, there is little to choose between them, although he prefers the variants of the MSQ. More comprehensive and much more lengthy instruments include CAMDEX for use with elderly patients (Roth *et al.* 1986). For those concerned to assess cognitive impairment fully among older people, the most extensively tested scale is the Geriatric Mental State, with its associated AGECAT computer package (Copeland *et al.* 1976; Dewey and Copeland 1986). Its disadvantage is its length.

In relation to mental functioning (e.g. intelligence and memory) in adults and children, the best tested and most frequently used scales are the Wechsler scales – the Wechsler Adult Intelligence Scale (WAIS: Wechsler 1981a, 1981b) and the Wechsler Memory Scale (WMS: Wechsler 1945). However, Wade (1992) points out that the WAIS is difficult to administer in cases of major motor impairments and the WMS is very lengthy, and has the disadvantage of requiring a psychologist for its administration. A more practical test in terms of ease of administration is the Rivermead Behaviour Memory Test, which is shorter, more specific and can be administered by a trained lay interviewer. The Rivermead is more specific than the WMS in distinguishing between patients who live independently. It takes 20–25 min to complete, is valid and does not need a trained interviewer to administer it. A children's version is being developed. It consists of 11 items (or 12 if the two prose items are counted separately) covering remembering names, objects, appointments, object recognition, immediate and delayed prose recall, face recognition, immediate and delayed route remembrance, remembering a question, orientation and date. Various scoring methods have been devised (Wilson *et al.* 1985, 1989). In 1987, the British Stroke Research Group (see Wade 1992) recommended using scales relating to aphasia, confusion (e.g. the AMTS) and memory (e.g. the Rivermead Behaviour Memory Test).

Self-esteem and self-concept

Other important dimensions of psychological well-being include self-esteem and self-concept (see Chapter 2 for distinction). There are numerous, but fairly long scales of self-esteem, some of which were reviewed by Bowling (1991). Self-image or self-esteem has been investigated successfully in neurology patients by Collings (1990a, 1990b) using more concise 7-point semantic differential rating scales (Osgood et al. 1957).

Life satisfaction

An important dimension to include is life satisfaction. Life satisfaction refers to an assessment of one's life, or a comparison, reflecting some perceived discrepancy between one's aspirations and achievement. Instruments that assess life satisfaction are increasing in popularity among researchers, thus shifting the balance of health status measures from a focus on negative aspects to the more positive ones. Life satisfaction measures include a balance of negative and positive items. Scales of morale and well-being tap overlapping dimensions. The most commonly used scales are the Neugarten Life Satisfaction Scales (Neugarten et al. 1961), the Delighted–Terrible Faces Scale (Andrews and Withey 1976), the Philadelphia Geriatric Morale Scale (Lawton 1972, 1975), the Affect–Balance Scale (Bradburn 1969) and the General Well-Being Schedule (Dupuy 1978). Most of these scales were developed for use with elderly people. Anderson (1992) used the Delighted-Terrible Faces Scale with stroke patients with good results and found it to be acceptable. The most popular scale among gerontologists is the Philadelphia Geriatric Morale Scale, on the grounds of its superior results for reliability and validity. There is insufficent space here to describe these scales and they have been reviewed more fully elsewhere (Bowling 1991).

Social support

A dimension of social health that should be included in outcome scales is social support, including social activity. Social support and activity are both modifying and outcome variables. If these are missing in the disease-specific indicator selected, the investigator may wish to use a separate scale. A review of the most commonly used scales can be found again in Bowling (1991) (see also the Rand MOS Social Support Scale in Sherbourne and Stewart 1991).

Other domains

Other relevant domains include coping and adjustment as modifying variables (see Chapter 3), and patient satisfaction (see Anderson 1992; Pound et al. 1994), although these have rarely been employed in neurology.

Self-report instruments

The selection of patient self-report scales depends on the ability of the patient to complete them or to indicate his or her responses to an interviewer. In some cases, questionnaires will need to be adapted for proxy interviews with 'significant others'. The effects of looking after the patient on the carer may be an important outcome measure in some cases. Carer satisfaction with services in cases where they suffer the burden of caring will require measurement in service evaluation. Few disease-specific satisfaction questionnaires have been designed. Pound et al. (1993) have developed a questionnaire to measure carer satisfaction in relation to stroke patients, with good results for reliability and validity.

MEASUREMENT SCALES

STROKE SCALES

RANKIN HANDICAP SCALE

Rankin (1957) developed this scale on the basis of research on the prognosis of patients with a cerebrovascular accident (CVA). No results of psychometric testing were given in the orginal paper on the scale, only frequency distributions. The Rankin Scale is the stroke equivalent of the Glasgow Outcome Scale, which is the most widely used outcome measure of head injury (Jennett and Bond 1975), but like that scale it is crude and has low sensitivity (Wade 1992), which is the price one has to pay for its brevity and simplicity.

Several versions and scoring methods exist. The scale comprises five grades, although it has been modified (see below), and requires further modification to improve its reliability.

The Rankin Handicap Scale Grades

Grade 1   No significant disability: able to carry out all usual duties

Grade II   Slight disability: unable to carry out some of previous activities but able to look after own affairs without assistance

Grade III Moderate disability: requiring some help but able to walk without assistance

Grade IV   Moderately severe disability: unable to walk without assistance and unable to attend to own bodily needs without assistance

Grade V   Severe disability: bedridden, incontinent, and requiring constant nursing care and attention

Modified Rankin Handicap Scale

Van Swieten et al. (1988) used a modified Rankin Handicap Scale (Rankin 1957; UK–TIA Study Group 1988) for the grading of stroke patients. In addition to the Glasgow Outcome Scale (Jennett and Bond 1975), they chose the Rankin Scale because it measures independence rather than being task-oriented, gives a better impression of self-care than disability indexes such as the Barthel Index, and represents handicap rather than disability. They reported that 100 pairs of observers agreed about the degree of handicap in 65 of 100 patients (κ = 0.56; weighted κ = 0.91). They suggested that a reduction in the number of grades would improve its reliability, as would removing the assessment of walking and converting the scale to simple pro-forma questions on restriction; however, reduction is always at the expense of sensitivity. It is completed by health professionals.

The Modified Rankin Handicap Scale Grades

0 = No symptoms at all

1 = No significant disability despite symptoms: able to carry out all usual duties and activities

2 = Slight disability: unable to carry out all previous activities but able to look after own affairs without assistance

3 = Moderate disability: requiring some help, but able to walk without assistance

4 = Moderately severe disability: unable to walk without assistance, and unable to attend to own bodily needs without assistance

5 = Severe disability: bedridden, incontinent, and requiring constant nursing care and attention

(N.B. the Original Rankin scale did not contain grade 0, defined grade 1 as 'No significant disability: able to carry out all usual duties', and defined grade 2 as 'Slight disability: unable to carry out some of previous activities . . .'

Oxford Handicap Scale

Bamford et al. (1988, 1989) also modified the Rankin Handicap Scale and called their version the Oxford Handicap Scale. They attempted to remove ambiguities in wording from the original scale and focused on handicap rather than disability. Inter-observer agreement for the modified version was moderate to strong (κ = 0.42; weighted κ = 0.72)

Oxford Handicap Scale Grades

0 = No symptoms

1 = Minor symptoms that do not interfere with lifestyle

2 = Minor handicap: symptoms that lead to some restriction in lifestyle but do not interfere with the patient's capacity to look after him or herself

3 = Moderate handicap: symptoms that significantly restrict lifestyle and prevent totally independent existence

4 = Moderately severe handicap: symptoms that clearly prevent independent existence though not needing constant attention

5 = Severe handicap: totally dependent patient requiring constant attention night and day

There are numerous examples of the use of the scale and its modified version (e.g. Gijn *et al.* 1991). While it may be of use as a crude index in busy clinical settings, it is no substitute for a full scale of functional ability for use in research studies.

NATIONAL INSTITUTE OF HEALTH STROKE SCALE

This is broader than the disability and handicap scales outlined above (Brott *et al.* 1989; Brott 1992). It is a 15-item scale that covers level of consciousness, pupillary response, gaze, visual loss, facial palsy, motor-arm, motor-leg, plantar reflex, limb ataxia, sensory loss, neglect, dysarthria, language and changes. It is observer-rated and takes 5–8 min to complete. Items have 3- or 4-point response scales, scored from 0 to 3 (0=normal). Change is measured as same, better or worse.

It was initially tested on 65 acute stroke patients over a period of 3 months with variable results for validity (Brott *et al.* 1989). Brott *et al.* reported a correlation of 0.74 between the total stroke scale at 7 days and the CT scan lesion volume. The stroke scale scores at 7 days corresponded to eventual patient clinical outcome ($r = 0.71$). They reported that the mean inter-rater agreement among four assessors was $\kappa = 0.69$. The test–retest reliability for the neurologist was 0.77, and slightly lower than this for the other assessors. Wade (1992) criticizes the scale for trying to summarize all impairments, making it too simplistic, despite some claims of reliability and validity.

Examples of the NIH Stroke Scale

Level of consciousness – questions

Ask the patient the month and his or her age. Score first answer.

0 = answers both correctly / 1 = answers one correctly / 2 = incorrect

Facial palsy

0 = normal / 1 = minor / 2 = partial / 3 = complete

Dysarthria

0 = normal articulation / 1 = mild to moderate dysarthria, slurring some words / 2 = near unintelligible or worse

CANADIAN NEUROLOGICAL SCALE (CNS)

This scale measures cognition and motor response in stroke patients, and takes 5 min to complete (Côté *et al.* 1986, 1988, 1989; Côté and Hachinski 1992). The content and weighting of the scale was agreed by a panel of 'experts'. It relies on judgements of functioning. Items are weighted and summed.

Côté *et al.* (1989) initially assessed validity and reliability with 157 patients with an acute CVA. They reported that the scale was sensitive to change and was able to predict satisfactorily death within 6 months, any cardiovascular or cerebrovascular events within 6 months and independence at 6 months. The internal consistency of the scale was reported to be $\alpha = 0.79$. The kappa statistics for agreement between two nurse raters ranged from 0.54 for level of consciousness to 0.84 for orientation. The agreement in total scores was $r = 0.92$. While adequate levels of reliability and validity are claimed for the scale, it is still crude.

Examples from the CNS

Mentation

Level of consciousness

3.0 Alert
1.5 Drowsy

Speech

1.0 Normal
0.5 Expressive deficit
0.0 Repetitive deficit

Motor function (no comprehension deficit)

Face

0.5 None
0.0 Present

Arm, proximal

1.5 None
1.0 Mild
0.5 Significant
0.0 Total

HEMISPHERIC STROKE SCALE

This is a mixed-concept scale for use with acute stroke patients (Adams *et al.* 1987). The items are variously scored on 2- through to 8-point scales. The items are summed, with 0 = good and increasing scores equalling worse conditions (100 = bad).

It was assessed among 16 acute stroke patients, with ratings provided by two clinicians. It correlated ($r = 0.89$) with the neurologist's or neurosurgeon's assessments, and inter-observer reliability was reported to be $r = 0.95$. Again, while adequate levels of reliability and validity are claimed for the scale, it is still crude and partly reliant on subjective observers' judgements.

Examples from the Hemispheric Stroke Scale

Repetition

Ask the patient to repeat the following: a single word, such as 'dog' or 'cat'; 'the president lives in Washington', 'no ifs, ands or buts'.

Score on number repeated:

0 = 5 / 1 = 4 / 2 = 2 / 3 = 0

Gaze

Score eye movements:

2 = gaze palsy, or persistent deviation / 1 = gaze preference, or difficulty with far lateral gaze / 0 = normal

Dysphagia

Score swallow of glass of water:

2 = severe dysphagia / 1 = moderate dysphagia / 0 = normal

Muscle tone

2 = increased or decreased / 0 = normal

Disease-specific measures of quality of life: Functional ability

In relation to health-related quality of life outcomes, the UK Clearing House for Information on the Assessment of Health Outcomes database cites the following as frequently used outcome measures for stroke: the Katz ADL scale (Katz and Akpom 1976a, 1976b), the Barthel Index (Mahoney and Barthel 1965; revised by Granger *et al*. 1979b), the Quality of Well-Being Scale (Bush 1984; Bush *et al*. 1973), and the Karnofsky Performance Status Scale

or Index (Karnofsky and Burchenal 1949). The most popular functional ability scale in this area is the Barthel Index. Others include the Frenchay Activities Index (see Wade *et al*. 1992), the Rivermead Mobility Index (Collen *et al*. 1991), and the Nottingham Extended Activities of Daily Living Index (Nouri and Lincoln 1987).

BARTHEL INDEX

The Barthel Index was developed by Mahoney and Barthel (1965). It is based on observed functions. The index was developed to measure functional ability before and after treatment, and to indicate the amount of nursing care required. It was designed for use with long-term hospital patients with neuromuscular or musculoskeletal disorders. It has since been used more generally to evaluate treatment outcomes. The Barthel Index is extremely popular among neurologists.

Content

The scale covers the following dimensions: feeding, mobility from bed to chair, personal toilet (washing etc.), getting on/off the toilet, bathing, walking on level surface, going up/down stairs, dressing and incontinence (bladder and bowel). It omits tasks of daily living such as cooking and shopping, and other 'elective' activities, as well as other everyday tasks essential for life in the community. It thus appears suitable only for institutionalized populations (for whom it was designed). It requires supplementation with items reflecting domestic (or 'elective') activities if used in community settings.

Administration and scoring

The Barthel Index is based on a rating scale completed by a therapist or other observer. The scale takes approximately 30 sec to score. Different values are assigned to different abilities. Individuals are scored on ten activities which are summed to give a score of 0 (totally dependent) to 100 (fully independent). The authors of the scale provide detailed instructions for assessing and scoring patients. For example:

Doing personal toilet: 5 = patient can wash hands and face, comb hair, clean teeth, and shave. He may use any kind of razor but must put in blade or plug in razor without help as well as get it from drawer or cabinet. Female patients must put on own make up, if used, but need not braid or style hair.

The modified scoring gives a maximum score of 20 to patients who are continent, able to wash, feed and dress themselves and are independently mobile (Collin *et al.* 1988). The scores are intended to reflect the amount of time and assistance a patient requires. However, the scoring method is inconsistent in that changes in a given number of points do not reflect equivalent changes in disability across different activities. Moreover, changes can occur beyond the scale end-points ('floor' and 'ceiling' effects).

Granger's modified Barthel Index

Granger and McNamara (1984), Granger (1982) and Fortinsky *et al.* (1981) have developed extensions of the Barthel Index, covering 15 topics. Good results for inter-rater agreement have been reported (Granger 1979a), although insufficient evidence of the reliability and validity of these extensions exists. Granger and his colleagues now regard their early adaptation of the Barthel as obsolete and have replaced it with the Functional Independence Measure (Stineman *et al.* 1994). It is

Examples from Granger's modified Barthel Index

Self-care

1 Drinking from a cup
2 Eating
5 Putting on brace or artificial limb
7 Washing or bathing
9 Controlling bowel movements

Mobility

10 Getting in and out of chair
11 Getting on and off toilet
13 Walking 50 yards on the level
15 If not walking, propelling or pushing wheelchair

Can do by myself / can do with help of someone else / cannot do at all

similar in scope to the original version, concentrating on personal care, mobility and walking, communication and cognition to the neglect of domestic functioning.

Gompertz's modified Barthel Index

Gompertz *et al.* (1993a, 1993b) adapted the Barthel Index for self-completion (where appropriate) or administration by a lay interviewer. It is a great improvement, particularly as the detailed instructions which accompany the original scale are not needed. It still requires a little refinement. While the original Barthel Index assessed need for help, this revised version asks whether the person does a task 'without any help'. However, interpretation is unclear as to whether people falling into this group undertake activities 'without any help' because they do not need it, or because they do need help but do not receive it. This problem is easily rectifiable with the provision of an additional category.

Examples from Gompertz's modified Barthel Index

Dressing

Do you get dressed:

Without any help
Just with help with buttons
With someone helping you most of the time

Mobility

Do you walk indoors:

Without any help (e.g. apart from a frame)
With one person watching over you
With one person helping you
With more than one person helping
Not at all

The comparable items from the original Barthel Index (Mahoney and Barthel 1965), which need to be accompanied by scoring guidelines and definitions, are:

Examples from the original Barthel Index

Dressing

0 = dependent
1 = needs help but can do about half unaided
2 = independent (including buttons, zips, laces, etc)

Mobility

0 = immobile
1 = wheelchair independent, including corners
2 = walks with help of one person (verbal or physical)
3 = independent (but may use any aid, e.g. stick)

Validity and factor structure

The original Barthel Index has been tested for validity by Wade *et al.* (1985, 1992) and Collen *et al.* (1990) in their evaluations of therapies for stroke patients. The results have been more fully described by Wade (1992). Wade and Collin (1988) stated that the Barthel Index has face validity – it appears to assess ADL. It correlates with other measures as expected (e.g. motor loss) and therefore has concurrent and predictive validity (Wade and Langton-Hewer 1987). Factor analysis has confirmed that it measures a single domain, and it has been reported to be sensitive to recovery (Wade and Langton-Hewer 1987).

There have been a number of studies reporting predictive validity for the Barthel Index. It is able to distinguish between patients with stroke who are discharged home and those who require extended care facilities. The Barthel Index has been reported to correlate well with various prognostic scores of stroke patients (Kalra and Crome 1993). It can predict mortality among stroke patients, length of stay and progress as independently rated by a physician (Wylie and White 1964). Evidence of its correlational validity with other scales comes mainly from studies comparing it with the PULSES profile, which give correlations of −0.74 to −0.90 (Granger *et al.* 1979a).

Rodgers *et al.* (1993) pointed out that the scale, and its scoring, while suitable for hospital patients, is less appropriate for disabled people who live at home. For example, in a home setting the patient and/or the carer may consider incontinence and regular night-time disturbance to be greater problems than lack of mobility. In addition, other disabilities (e.g. communication) are not included. Also, as the Barthel Index is a measure of what the patient actually does, rather than ability, scoring may be location-dependent.

In a controlled trial of exercise among 49 residents of four old people's homes, McMurdo and

Rennie (1993) reported that the interpretation of the Barthel Index was affected by the setting. For example, in such institutions elderly people are not usually permitted to bathe unassisted, thus reducing scale scores. In addition, respondents who walk independently with a frame, a stick or without any walking aid score the same in the appropriate section of the index, although the aids used reflect different levels of walking ability.

Mattison *et al.* (1991) used the Barthel Index with 364 patients attending day centres for the physically disabled. They compared it with the PULSES Scale and the Edinburgh Rehabilitation Status Scale (ERSS: Affleck *et al.* 1988) and reported correlations of −0.65 and −0.69, respectively. Mattison *et al.* (1991) reported that these scales had similar levels of validity, and that the Barthel Index requires supplementation with broader measures (e.g. those contained in the ERSS). Granger *et al.* (1979b) had earlier supported the supplementation of the Barthel Index with PULSES. Intending users need to be aware that this scale measures just one dimension of quality of life – physical functioning – and this is covered very narrowly.

Reliability

Shah *et al.* (1989) suggested that the sensitivity of the original Barthel Index can be improved by expanding the number of categories used to record improvement in each ADL function. Their modification, used with 258 stroke patients, led to improved reliability: the internal consistency reliability coefficient was 0.90, compared with 0.87 for the original scoring.

Sherwood *et al.* (1977) reported alpha reliability coefficients of 0.95–0.97 for three samples of hospital patients, suggesting that the scale is internally consistent. Collin *et al.* (1988) tested it for reliability on 25 stroke patients, and analysed observer agreement, using 2–4 observers. While overall their results suggested that the index was reliable, and observer agreement was generally high, observer agreement was lower for transfers, feeding, dressing, grooming and toileting. The difficulties in agreement arose in relation to the middle category. As a result of studying possible ambiguities in scale wording, they refined the instructions for observers. Granger *et al.* (1979b) reported a test–retest reliability of 0.89 with severely disabled adults, and an inter-rater agreement exceeding 0.95.

Ranhoff and Laake (1993) compared the scores of 59 elderly nursing home patients as rated by physicians based on clinical interviews and by nurses based on observation of the patients over time. The doctors' scores were higher than the nurses' scores, particularly for patients with some degree of cognitive impairment, and in general agreement was poor. Although it is a popular scale among clinicians worldwide, further evidence of its reliability is required.

Wade and Collin (1988) acknowledged that the scale is crude, but point out that it is sensitive enough to detect need for help, and they caution against the increasing number of modifications to the scale. In sum, while simplicity is an attraction of the scale, it also poses a major limitation on its use. The problem with such observed assessments is that they do not necessarily reflect what the person usually does in everyday life. It is limited in scope and may not be sensitive to improvements or deteriorations beyond the end-points of the scale ('floor' and 'ceiling' effects; McDowell and Newell 1987), or within dimensions not represented by the scale, e.g. domestic tasks, role functioning (work, parent, etc.) and socio-psychological functioning, mental status and well-being (Granger *et al.* 1979a).

NOTTINGHAM EXTENDED ACTIVITIES OF DAILY LIVING QUESTIONNAIRE

The Nottingham Extended Activities of Daily Living Questionnaire (Nouri and Lincoln 1987) includes many items related to mobility and also many 'elective mobility' items. Collen *et al.* (1991) suggest it could be used instead of the elective section of the Rivermead Scale. In the developmental work for the original version, Guttman scaling techniques were used, and 52 per cent of questionnaires were returned from a postal survey. The questionnaire was subsequently reordered according to the rankings and retested.

Content, administration and scoring

This 22-item, interviewer-administered questionnaire comprises four sections, with five or six items per section, and 4-point response choices scored 0

or 1, where 0 represents major difficulties. The section scales cover mobility, kitchen tasks, other domestic tasks and leisure activities. Respondents are asked whether they do the activity, rather than if they *can* do it, in order to assess level of activity rather than capability.

Examples from the original Nottingham Questionnaire

In the kitchen

Do you:

Manage to feed yourself?
Manage to make yourself a hot drink?
Take hot drinks from one room to another?
Do the washing up?
Make yourself a hot snack?

Leisure activities

Do you:

Read newspapers or books?
Use the telephone?
Write letters?
Go out socially?
Manage your own garden?
Drive a car?

Each question carries the same response choices:

0 = not at all / with help
1 = alone with difficulty / alone easily

Gompertz's modified Nottingham Questionnaire

An extended version of this scale was included in Gompertz and co-workers' (1993b) pack for use with stroke patients, with a self-administration format. It is intended to supplement the Barthel Index. However, several of the items on mobility and self-care are similar. It might be preferable to omit those items and adapt the instrument as a sub-scale of items on domestic chores (e.g. make a hot drink, take hot drinks from one room to another, washing up, make a hot snack, manage money, wash small items of clothing, housework, shopping, full clothes wash) and social/leisure activities (reading, telephone, writing, go out socially, gardening, driving). This suggestion requires testing.

A common problem with such concise ADL scales is that the response categories are ambiguous. For example, a 'no' response in Gompertz and co-workers' modification can mean that respondents do not do an activity because they cannot do it *or* because they do not want to do it. This problem is easily solved with the provision of an additional category.

Examples from Gompertz's modified Nottingham Questionnaire

Do you make yourself a hot snack?

On my own / on my own with difficulty / with help / no

Do you do your own shopping?

On my own / on my own with difficulty / with help / no

Do you go out socially?

On my own / on my own with difficulty / with help / no

Do you drive a car?

On my own / on my own with difficulty / with help / no, or don't have one

Reliability

Nouri and Lincoln's (1987) final version of the questionnaire was sent by post to 20 stroke patients discharged from the investigators' stroke unit, with a retest form at 2 weeks (12 patients returned both). The kappa coefficients of agreement ranged from poor (0.29) to excellent (1.0). Nineteen of the 22 items had an excellent kappa coefficient of 0.76 or above. The agreement was worse on the housework question, although the authors were not sure why. There are few studies of the scale's validity.

FRENCHAY ACTIVITIES INDEX

The aim of this scale is to measure activities which require the use of initiative. It measures frequency of activity over the recent past. It was initially developed by a social worker for practical use, and has since been revised (Holbrook and Skilbeck 1983; Wade *et al.* 1985). It requires further testing (Wade 1992).

Content, administration and scoring

This is a 15-item questionnaire which covers mainly domestic, leisure and social activities, and also work. It is interviewer-administered, has 4-point frequency scales, and carries fairly detailed guidelines for its completion (coding and scoring). Time periods asked about are either 3 or 6 months.

Examples from the Frenchay Activities Index

Frequency

In the last 3 months

- preparing main meals
- washing up

0 = never/1 = under once weekly/2 = 1–2 times per week/3 = most days

- washing clothes
- light housework
- heavy housework
- local shopping
- social occasions
- walking outside > 15 min
- actively pursuing hobby
- driving care/going on bus

0 = never / 1 = 1–2 times in 3 months / 2 = 3–12 times in three months / 3 = at least weekly

Validity, factor structure and reliability

Data from 976 patients with acute stroke were used to test the validity and reliability of the index (Wade *et al.* 1985). The construct validity (the degree to which the items could be shown to relate to a single 'idea') was tested with a factor analysis which showed a high degree of communality attributable to each item. Inter-rater reliability coefficients of 0.80 were obtained (tested using just 14 of the patients and two raters). Validation studies, particularly with elderly people, are still required.

RIVERMEAD MOBILITY INDEX (RMI)

This index concentrates on fundamental activities (which people will undertake if they can), such as walking or going up stairs. It focuses intentionally on disability, not impairment. The index is suitable for use in hospital or at home. The scale is reproduced in Collen *et al.* (1991).

Content, administration and scoring

The RMI is interviewer-administered, and contains 15 items with 'yes/no' answers, which are summed. A reply of 'yes' carries a score of 1. The items cover movement in bed, balance, transfers, walking, picking items up off the floor, bathing, going up and down steps, and running. It is simple to use and reliable (Collen *et al.* 1991; Wade 1992). Item 5 (see below) is observed by the interviewer. It is difficult to see how patients can reliably answer some of the items without necessarily having a good knowledge of distance and speed (e.g. items 11 and 15).

Examples from the RMI

Questions are phrased 'Do you . . .?', not 'Can you . . .?' For example:

1 Turning over in bed

Do you turn over from your back to your side without help?

3 Sitting balance

Do you sit on the edge of the bed without holding on for 10 seconds?

5 Standing unsupported

Observe standing for 10 seconds without any aid.

11 Picking up off the floor

If you drop something on the floor, do you manage to walk 5 metres, pick it up and then walk back?

15 Running

Do you run 10 metres without limping in 4 seconds (fast walk is acceptable)?

Validity and reliability

Collen *et al.* (1991) tested the scale for reliability and validity among stroke patients. They obtained good results for the Fundamental (RMI-F) scale which contains 14 items ranging from turning over in bed to bathing, and one direct observation (standing for 10 sec). Poor results were obtained for the Elective (RMI-E) scale, which contains nine items on shopping, gardening, etc., which people may choose or choose not, to do, hence the name 'elective' (e.g. questions on 'Do you get in and out of a car/taxi?'; 'Do you do your own shopping?'; Do you cross roads?'). The correlation between the Barthel Index and the RMI was lower ($r = 0.39$) for elective ADL items. The authors decided, therefore, not to continue with the Elective part of the scale, and concentrate instead only on the Fundamental scale, which they described as a simple method of measuring mobility.

There are few other data on the scale's reliability, but more on validity. A correlation of 0.91 was obtained between the RMI and the Barthel Index for the 15 fundamental ADL questions, and correlations of between 0.63 and 0.89 were noted between the scale and other indexes of mobility, including gait speed, balance and the 6 min distance test (Collen *et al.* 1991). The scale was reported to be sensitive to diagnosis in a small study of 20 mixed neurological patients.

The authors are currently testing the scale for sensitivity, although they caution that it may be limited, and recommend further testing for reliability and validity. Wade (1992) reports finding the scale very useful with out-patients.

Disease-specific measures of quality of life: stroke

As can be seen from the above review, most studies have concentrated on physical functioning and mental state. The TyPE Scale for Acute Stroke is the most comprehensive scale developed for use with these patients, and even it does not include every relevant domain. As an alternative, researchers have resorted to using batteries of independent scales to measure broader quality of life.

HEALTH OUTCOMES INSTITUTE TyPE SCALES (HOI-TyPE) – ACUTE STROKE

This is a tool for the assessment of outcome of acute stroke, defined by the authors as a sudden or stepwise onset of focal neurological deficit that lasts more than 24 h, for which there is no evidence of a non-vascular aetiology.

The Stroke TyPE (Technology of Patient Experience) tool was developed in the USA for the Health Outcomes Institute (HOI) (previously Interstudy) by David Matchar and his colleagues at Duke University. The HOI is also one of several organizations that act as a registration body for the use of a version of the SF-36. The HOI has compiled a battery of outcome indicators for a wide range of medical conditions, including stroke. The tools were constructed on the basis of analyses of longitudinal data on patients' experiences. The first principle that they applied to scale construction was to capture outcomes that are relevant to stroke and, second, to include data that provide estimates of stroke severity, on the basis that these are early predictors of stroke outcome. The third principle was to keep the form simple. The elements of the TyPE specification were derived from a complete review of the literature, and the benefit of expert opinion (from neurologists and health services researchers). They encourage users to supplement the Stroke TyPE Specification with other scales where required, as well as basic demographic information that might affect outcome (e.g. age, sex, marital status, socio-economic status). The tool is licensed, and for a small fee users are kept informed of any updates.

Content, administration and scoring

The Stroke TyPE Specification consists of four forms (the first two are for the doctor to complete). The SF-36 health status questionnaire is also included, with the recommendation that it is administered during the period of the acute hospitalization, and at 1 and 12 months post-stroke.

The pack includes: (1) a form for the assessment by the patient (or carer, if necessary) of pre-stroke function in relation to the degree of limitation in a range of activities (e.g. walking, writing, driving, speaking); (2) a form for the doctor to complete on the severity of the patient's disability after the stroke (e.g. walking, etc.), including items on confusion and depression, co-morbidity, level of consciousness, complications and level of care given; (3) a form about post-stroke function to be completed by the patient (similar to the pre-stroke function form); and (4) a form for the doctor to complete 12 months post-stroke on 'later outcomes', which concentrates on medical diagnoses.

The patient's form is interviewer-administered or can be self-completed where patients are able to do this.

The handbook indicates that the range of conditions pre-coded on the forms is limited deliberately, as research indicates that there are few neurological findings that can be reliably measured, or are predictive of patient outcome, beyond the patient's level of consciousness on admission. The handbook points out the problem of assessing people once they are in hospital and states that it is important to determine the pre-stroke level of function. Thus, the SF-36 should be administered with an instruction to patients that they should reply to the questions in relation to their pre-stroke health state (responses at 1 and 12 months relate to function at that time).

The scale items are variously scored (e.g. from 1 to 2 or from 1 to 4) and the scales are analysed separately.

Examples from the HOI Acute Stroke Form

Impact of current stroke

Completion by other

In the week following the stroke, did the patient experience difficulty with the following:

Use of hands/arms
Writing
Speaking
Remembering distant events

Never / mild / moderate / severe

Completion by patient

In the last 4 weeks, did the stroke limit you in these activities? If so, how much?

Use of hands/arms
Writing
Speaking
Remembering events from years ago

Yes, limited a lot / yes, limited a little / no, not limited at all

Completion by clinician

Stroke type and severity
2 What was the patient's level of consciousness on admission?

Alert / drowsy / unresponsive

3 Is the current stroke responsible for the patient's major functional disability?   Yes/no

Later outcomes

1 At 12 months (or any time thereafter) after the stroke, had the patient experienced any of the following conditions since discharge from the hospital?

(a) New stroke
(b) Pneumonia requiring hospitalization
(d) Heart failure
(f) Deep vein thrombosis
(i) Death

Yes/no

Validity and reliability

Details of the TyPE tools for a range of diseases and conditions are available from the Health Outcomes Institute (2001 Killebrew Drive, Suite 122, Bloomington, MN 55425, USA). The instruments have not been fully tested for reliability and validity, and this work has yet to be systematically undertaken (Health Outcomes Institute, pers. comm.).

The tools are extremely concise. Those who require a more detailed set of assessment tools relating to functional ability will prefer the set used by Wade and his colleagues (see below), although this TyPE tool has the advantage of being a broader measure of health status by virtue of inclusion of the SF-36. A measure of psychological morbidity may need to be included if this scale is used.

KUDOS BATTERY FOR STROKE PATIENTS

The amended (simplified) Barthel Index was used together with a battery of other tests for the North East Thames Stroke Outcome Study (Gompertz *et al.* 1993a, 1993b). The other instruments included were the Nottingham Extended Activities of Daily Living Questionnaire (Nouri and Lincoln 1987), the Nottingham Health Profile (Hunt *et al.* 1986), the Geriatric Depression Scale (Yesavage *et al.* 1983; Arden *et al.* 1989), the London Stroke Satisfaction Scale (Pound *et al.* 1993, in press), the Delighted–Terrible Faces Scale (Andrews and Withey 1976) and items about the use of services and cost to the patient. The satisfaction scales were developed by the authors, and included a scale for measuring carers' satisfaction with services (Pound *et al.* 1993). The Nottingham Health Profile is a well-known and tested broader health status scale, and works well with stroke patients (Ebrahim *et al.* 1986). The Geriatric Depression Scale is a less well tested index, as is the Nottingham Extended Activities of Daily Living Questionnaire (although the latter has been widely applied in stroke research). This pack was reported to be reliable when used with stroke patients by Gompertz *et al.* (1993a), and yielded a 91 per cent response rate. They reported good agreement between most of the different scale items ($\kappa = 0.20$–1.0, with most achieving kappa values of more than 0.40).

EPILEPSIES

Treatment for epilepsy may be medical or surgical, depending on type. Hauser (1987) pointed out that a small but sizeable number of people who develop epilepsy are considered to be medically intractable and eligible for consideration for surgical intervention. Surgery does not always stop seizures, nor can surgery necessarily reverse any existing pattern of disability, social difficulties or impaired performance. The question of whether patients are 'better' following epilepsy surgery has not been resolved, although many specialists report good results (Taylor 1987).

Standardized results from throughout the world reported at the first International Conference on Surgical Treatment of the Epilepsies in 1987, and reproduced by Spencer and Spencer (1991), show that results of resective procedures are widely discrepant. Between 26 and 80 per cent of patients were reported to be seizure-free after temporal lobectomy, 0–73 per cent after extratemporal resection, and 0–100 per cent after hemispherectomy. Figures for 'worthwhile' and 'no' improvement were similarly variable. On average, 55 per cent of patients were seizure-free after temporal lobectomy, 43 per cent after extratemporal resection and 77 per cent after hemispherectomy. These figures are a powerful reason for further studies of patient outcome following surgery. Vickrey *et al.* (1993) reviewed the literature which suggests that surgery controls seizures in two-thirds of selected patients, although they point to other literature that indicates that surgery may adversely affect quality of life for some patients because of imposing new problems, in particular of memory.

The assessment of outcome requires the assessment of the patients before and after the surgical intervention. As with other conditions, the retrospective collection of pre-surgical information after surgery has been performed may be unreliable due to recall bias, and may be influenced by the patients' and carers' expectations of the surgery. Follow-up periods in the literature vary tremendously, from 6 months to several years. Spencer and Spencer (1991) reported that some centres follow-up patients for as long as 10–15 years, although others have much shorter follow-ups.

THE DOMAINS OF MEASUREMENT

The relevant dimensions for inclusion in a health-related quality of life scale for epilepsy patients have been discussed at length by Vickrey et al. (1993). They suggest the following: physical symptoms; physical functioning (see previous section); role activities (e.g. ability to remain in employment, school or manage a household; driving); mental health; cognitive functioning (e.g. verbal memory deficits, IQ, controlling for effects of medication); social functioning (e.g. the ability to develop and maintain relationships with friends and kin); general health perceptions; life satisfaction; energy/fatigue; sleep and rest. All scales require further development in order to incorporate specific questions on patient expectations of, and satisfaction with, the outcome.

What instruments have been used?

Vickrey et al. (1993) have reviewed the international literature on assessing quality of life of epilepsy patients. Among the most commonly used disease-specific scales are the Washington Psychosocial Inventory (Dodrill 1978; Dodrill et al. 1980), and the Epilepsy Surgery Inventory (Vickrey et al. 1992b). In relation to psychological morbidity, the most popular scales include the Minnesota Multiphasic Personality Inventory (Dahlstrom et al. 1972; Hathaway and McKinley 1990), the Beck Depression Inventory (Beck et al.

1961) and the General Health Questionnaire (Goldberg 1978). The most commonly used generic measures of health-related quality of life are the Sickness Impact Profile (Bergner et al. 1981), the Quality of Well-Being Scale (Kaplan et al. 1976; Bush 1984), and the SF-36 (Ware and Sherbourne 1992). Some of these scales were referred to earlier. Instruments used with children include the Achenbach Child Behaviour Checklist, the Children's Depression Inventory and the Revised Children's Manifest Anxiety Scale (see Vickrey et al. 1993). The UK Clearing House for Information on the Assessment of Health Outcomes cites the Epilepsy Surgery Inventory as a major reference.

Seizure control and other physical measures

Outcome should be evaluated according to the aims of the intervention. At the most basic level, the aim of surgery is presumably seizure control (see above). The assessment of outcome thus necessitates the collection of data on pre-operative frequency of seizures and variations in seizure patterns, duration and severity. Self-reports can be subject to recall bias and subjectivity in assessments, although adult patients are still the best source of information about seizures, and it has been suggested that they should be encouraged to keep seizure diaries (Hays et al. 1993). An outcome classification relating pattern and type of seizures has been developed by the Temporal Lobe Club, and has been reproduced by Engel (1987): class I = seizure-free, class II = rare seizures, class III = worthwhile improvement, class IV = no worthwhile improvement. Hays et al. (1993) criticized the subjectivity involved in the last two categories.

Hays et al. (1993) reported that the assessment of seizure severity is difficult, although they refer to recent attempts to develop such scales as encouraging. One example is the Chalfont Seizure Severity Scale (Duncan and Sander 1991), which is based on observer ratings of open-ended interviews with patients, relatives and care-givers. Such procedures are inevitably time-consuming. Hays et al. (1993), in their review, also report on the promising development of a 16-item patient-based seizure severity scale, which includes items on perception of control (Baker et al. 1991; see below). These scales are reviewed by Hays et al. (1993) and Vickrey et al. (1993). The use of some such classification is essential, given that surgery does not always stop seizures, although greater development and assessment of existing measures is required.

Also to be included are pre- and post-treatment details of medication, co-morbidity, adverse effects and complications (Hauser 1987). Mortality is also a pertinent indicator.

Seizure frequency and type

Outcome measurement in epilepsy surgery has traditionally focused on changes in seizure frequency and type, although the ultimate goal of surgery is to improve quality of life (Vickrey et al. 1993). Collings (1990b) questioned 392 people with epilepsy in support groups and out-patient departments in the UK and Ireland, and reported an association between seizure frequency and type with emotional well-being, confirming the importance of measuring these domains.

Generic measures

Broader indexes of outcome in relation to health-related quality of life in epilepsy have tended to be domain-specific and have focused variously on independence in living, functional ability, personality, adjustment, psychiatric status, the quality of family and other close relationships, social activities, sexual adjustment and performance at work/ school. Hays et al. (1993) reviewed studies using these indicators. Social support networks, IQ, socio-economic status and level of education have been suggested as affecting outcome and may require inclusion in an assessment tool.

The broader health status measures have been used less often in neurology, although Jacoby (1992) did attempt to use the Nottingham Health Profile, together with other measures. In a study of 541 of the 1021 patients participating in the MRC anti-epileptic drug withdrawal study, Jacoby (1992) measured quality of life using a battery of measures: the Nottingham Health Profile (Hunt et al. 1986), Rosenberg's (1965) Self-Esteem Scale, Bradburn's (1969) five positive affect items (from the Affect-Balance Scale), three adapted stigma questions from Hyman's (1971) questionnaire for stroke patients ('felt social activities restricted by epilepsy', 'did not do certain things because of

epilepsy', and 'felt that epilepsy made it more difficult to get a job'), and Pearlin and Schooler's (1978) Mastery Scale. Jacoby reported that the Nottingham Health Profile was not suitable for use with people with epilepsy as it is such a severe scale resulting in a small number of respondents achieving a positive score on each of its six domains. Jacoby's (1992) work is evidence of the importance of comparing results with population norms – she reported employment to be an issue for people with epilepsy, but that population norms showed that employment levels for people with epilepsy were the same as for the normal population.

Better results have been reported using the SF-36 (Ware 1993) as a core instrument within epilepsy batteries (Vickrey et al. 1992b). This is discussed later (and see Chapter 8).

Domain-specific measures

Cognitive impairment, personality and psychological morbidity

Epilepsy has a slight adverse effect on mental abilities, apart from the underlying neurological disease (Dodrill and Wilensky 1990). Scales to measure, psychiatric disorder (e.g. psychosis) and suicidal tendency, intellectual impairment, social functioning, sexual problems and aggression may be required, particularly when evaluating the effects of surgical intervention (Taylor 1987; Dodrill and Wilensky 1990). Dimensions of social adjustment may be affected by surgery, e.g. ability to interact with others, employment, performance (at work or school, or as a parent), sexual function and driving.

Cognitive impairment

A review of the literature on intellectual impairment and epilepsy reported that few investigators have utilized any formal psychological assessments and most studies are retrospective (Dodrill and Wilensky 1990). In addition, the incidence of pre-operative psychosis was estimated by Jensen and Larsen (1979) to be 15 per cent, and almost all the patients they studied had evidence of some psychiatric disorder. It is not known how representative their findings are of other patients with epilepsy. Spencer and Spencer (1991) briefly reviewed the literature on outcome, and reported that there was a suggestion of some improvement in neurotic, aggressive and personality traits after resective procedures, although pre-operative psychoses were unchanged. They also reported that there appeared to be a high rate of post-operative suicide, and of significant post-operative psychosis in 5–15 per cent of patients after temporal lobectomy. Each of these dimensions requires measurement.

The most commonly used IQ test is the Wechsler Intelligence Scale (Matazzo 1972; Wechsler 1986). American and British adaptations are available from the distributors. Just because scales are well known and widely used does not always imply that they are to be recommended. For example, the Wechsler Memory Scale will not necessarily distinguish between people with brain damage and those with non-psychotic functional disorders (see review by Dye 1982).

Personality

Personality is a relatively stable variable, but can have a modifying influence on adjustment to the condition. Personality assessment has usually involved the Minnesota Multiphasic Personality Inventory in the USA (Welsh and Dahlstrom 1956; Dahlstrom et al. 1972; Hathaway and McKinley 1990), or the Eysenck Personality Questionnaire in the UK (Eysenck and Eysenck 1985). Personality should be measured cautiously, given its stability, depending on the aims of the study.

Psychiatric status, including anxiety and depression

The most commonly used scales of psychiatric status include the Present State Examination (Wing et al. 1974) and, in the case of depression, the Hamilton Depression Scale (Hamilton 1967) and the Beck Depression Inventory (Beck et al. 1961). An attempt to develop a scale to permit a comprehensive assessment of general psychosocial problems among people with epilepsy is the Washington Psychosocial Inventory (Dodrill 1978; Dodrill et al. 1980).

Adaptation and coping

Important modifying variables include adaptation to, and coping with, the condition. If these are not represented by items and sub-scales in the disease-specific quality of life scale used, then the investigator may wish to use a specific scale. The Vineland Adaptive Behaviour Scales is a measure of adaptive behaviour (Sparrow et al. 1984a, 1984b, 1985; Volkmar et al. 1987). It includes the assessment of social sufficiency and is often used with epileptic patients. Another measure of adjustment is the Katz Adjustment Scale, which has been adapted for use with patients with epilepsy (Vickrey et al. 1992a). Spencer and her colleagues (pers. comm.) are considering the utility of including suitable scales of adaptive behaviour in the assessment of outcome, such as the Vineland Adaptive Behaviour Scales.

Social support

Improvements in social relationships and activities might also be included as an outcome measure, although social support is also a modifying variable (Taylor and Falconer 1968). Some of these scales have been reviewed by Bowling (1991; see also Sherbourne and Stewart 1991).

Functional ability

Functional ability, or disability, may require measurement because of associated disorders, or as a consequence of seizure (e.g. falls leading to fractures). However, Vickrey et al. (1993) reported that most patients who are considered for temporal lobectomy are independent in activities of daily living, although they argue that measures tapping the latter should be included in case of any disability resulting from surgical complications. The range of functional ability scales has been reviewed by Bowling (1991); the Rand SF–36 (Ware et al. 1993) contains some items which tap this dimension and form a sub-scale (see Chapter 8). Wade (1992) notes that 'the major effects of epilepsy are probably at the level of handicap . . . there are no good measures for use at this level with epilepsy'.

Other domains

The other relevant domains of measurement, as with other disease conditions, include self-esteem and self-concept, stigma and life satisfaction. Investigators should ensure that instruments include items on the effects of the condition on social roles and activities, as well as items on patient satisfaction. Interested readers are referred to Bowling

(1991) for examples of the measures on self-esteem and life satisfaction (and see Chapter 1 for literature on patient satisfaction).

MEASUREMENT SCALES

A SEVERITY MEASUREMENT SCALE

SEIZURE SEVERITY SCALE

This 16-item, patient-based scale was developed by Baker *et al.* (1991). It is a self-report scale, developed on the grounds that previous research had shown that patients' perceptions of the severity of their seizure disorders may be more important than seizure frequency in determining the psychological and social well-being of those with poorly controlled epilepsy. Originally a 19-item scale, the authors reduced the number of items to 16 when 3 items were not found to have any discriminative ability.

Content

The scale comprises two sub-scales: perception of control and ictal/post-ictal effects. The six perception of control items assess whether seizures occurred upon awakening, at any particular time of day, at random, whether an aura was present, and whether the patient could predict the seizure. The 10 ictal and post-ictal items assess loss of consciousness and duration, incontinence, falls, tongue biting, other injury, perceived severity and interference of seizures with normal activities. For each type of seizure, respondents report their experiences over the previous 4 weeks on a 4-point severity scale, from least to most severe. A carers' version has also been designed, as well as an adverse drugs event scale and an impact of epilepsy scale, with good results initially for reliability and validity (Jacoby *et al.* 1993).

Administration and scoring

Respondents complete the questionnaire themselves after instruction by an investigator. Responses are rated on a 4-point scale (1 = least severe, 4 = most severe), and the scores are summed. A weighting system was developed from principal components analysis but discarded as it was reported to be complex and gave no clear benefit.

Examples from the Seizure Severity Scale

Question 3

My attacks are:

(a) always when I am asleep
(b) usually when I am asleep
(c) sometimes when I am asleep
(d) never when I am asleep

My attacks:

(a) stop me doing all of the things I want to do
(b) stop me doing a lot of the things I want to do
(c) stop me doing a few of the things I want to do
(d) don't stop me doing anything I want to do at all

When I recover from my attacks:

(a) I always find that I have bitten my tongue
(b) I usually find that I have bitten my tongue
(c) I sometimes find that I have bitten my tongue
(d) I never find that I have bitten my tongue

When I have my attacks I can usually return to what I am doing:

(a) in less than a minute
(b) in between 1–5 minutes
(c) in between 6 minutes – 1 hour
(d) in over 1 hour

Validity

The authors tested the scale on 159 patients with seizures. Construct validity was supported by comparisons with relatives' and care-givers' responses to four of the items ($r = 0.64$–0.77). The ictal/post-ictal sub-scale was sensitive to type of seizure (Baker *et al.* 1991). Seizure severity was also associated with low self-esteem and external locus of control and greater anxiety in a sample of 100 patients (Smith *et al.* 1991).

Reliability

Test–retest correlations were found to be 0.80 and 0.79 for the two sub-scales. The Cronbach alpha was 0.85 for the ictal/post-ictal scale and 0.69 for the perception scale. Inter-rater reliability correlations ranged from 0.64 to 0.73. Test–retest reliability coefficients at 2–3 weeks were 0.79 for the perception of control sub-scale and 0.80 for the ictal/post-ictal sub-scale in a sample of 35 patients. Internal consistency reliability was 0.69 and 0.85 for the perception and ictal/post-ictal sub-scales, respectively, in a sample of 159 patients.

Disease-specific quality of life scales: epilepsy

WASHINGTON PSYCHOSOCIAL INVENTORY

Probably the most popular measure used to assess health-related quality of life in the treatment of epilepsy is the Washington Psychosocial Inventory (Dodrill 1978; Dodrill *et al*. 1980). Dodrill *et al*. (1980) developed the scale, after initial pilot work, using 127 adult epileptic out-patients who completed the 132-item scale. The inventory provides some measure of epilepsy-specific psychological and social adjustment, and patient satisfaction (Dodrill 1978; Dodrill *et al*. 1980).

Content

The inventory covers eight broad areas: family background, emotional adjustment, interpersonal adjustment, vocational adjustment, financial status, adjustment to seizures, management of medication and patient satisfaction (medical management), and overall psychosocial functioning. It contains 132 'yes/no' items.

Administration and scoring

The scale is based on self-report methods. It is easy to administer and score, and the items are summed. It was reported by the authors to be acceptable to patients. It is suitable for people aged 16 and over, and takes 15–20 min to complete.

Examples from the Washington Psychosocial Inventory

Emotional adjustment

Are you generally free from depression?
Are you often tense and anxious?

Interpersonal adjustment

Do you have trouble meeting people?
Do you enjoy social gatherings?

Vocational adjustment

Are you satisfied with your employment situation?
Is transportation a problem?

Adjustment to seizures

Do you feel resentful that you have seizures?
Are you comfortable going out despite possible seizures?

Medicine and medical management

Do you feel your seizures are being controlled as well as they can be?
Do you frequently have trouble remembering to take your medication?

Validity

Testing was carried out by Dodrill *et al*. (1980) on 127 epileptic out-patients, and professionals' and significant others' assessments of patients' psychosocial functioning were also made. The validity correlations between the scale as completed by the patients and the professionals ranged from 0.52 to 0.75, and as completed by the patients and significant others from 0.11 to 0.69, indicating less consistency between patients' and significant others' perspectives rather than unreliability of the scale.

Reliability

The scale's test–retest reliability coefficients ranged from 0.66 to 0.85 for the sub-scales (and fell to 0.28–0.58 for additional validity items, e.g. lie checks). Split-half reliability coefficients ranged from 0.68 to 0.95 (and 0.37 to 0.75 for the additional validity items).

In sum, this scale is a fairly well-tested measure, although it does not cover all the major domains of health-related quality of life. Hays *et al*. (1993) pointed out that the scale does have important omissions, particularly in relation to cognitive distress, physical functioning, energy/fatigue and overall quality of life. However, Dodrill *et al*. (1980) stated that the scale was not intended to cover emotional problems in detail, and recommended that the scale be supplemented with the

Minnesota Multiphasic Personality Inventory (Dahlstrom *et al.* 1972) if this was required. They admit that the scale may not be sensitive to cultural differences. Vickrey *et al.* (1993) also point out that a limitation of this scale in longitudinal research is the inclusion of some items that would not be expected to change on retesting (e.g. the items asking whether something had ever occurred).

EPILEPSY SURGERY INVENTORY

An improvement on this scale is the Epilepsy Surgery Inventory (ESI-55), which testing has so far revealed to be reliable, valid and sensitive to differences in seizure status (Vickrey *et al.* 1992b). This is the measure of choice of Hays *et al.* (1993) and Vickrey *et al.* (1993), who were involved in its development. The historical development of the scale has already been described by Vickrey (1993).

Content

The scale is really a supplemented SF-36. It contains 55 items and taps 11 health concepts: health perceptions, energy/fatigue, overall quality of life, social functioning, emotional well-being, cognitive functioning, role limitations due to emotional problems, role limitations due to memory problems, role limitations due to physical health problems, physical functioning and pain; it also includes an item on perceived change in health. Its generic core is comprised of the original version of the SF-36; Vickrey *et al.* 1992b; Ware and Sherbourne 1992; Hays *et al.* 1993). The ESI-55 also contains five other items taken directly from the Rand Medical Outcomes Study (MOS) and eight adapted items from the MOS, one Dartmouth COOP Chart (Nelson *et al.* 1990), one item on patient preference (Hadhorn and Hays 1991) and four other items. Two items ask specifically about quality of life – one forms a visual analogue scale with six Delighted–Terrible Faces as anchors, with best possible quality of life at one end and worst possible quality of life at the other. The other is the Dartmouth COOP Chart ladder scale, in which respondents circle a number on the ladder (from 1 = very well, could hardly be better, to 5 = very bad, could hardly be worse). The epilepsy items include memory, speech/language and perceptions of epilepsy. Some items are disease-specific and some items were adapted to make them disease-specific.

Administration and scoring

The scale was designed for self-completion. Despite all the items contained in it, the completion time is just 15 min. The scale scoring varies according to the sub-scale, and is too lengthy to summarize here. The questionnaire and a scoring manual are available from the authors. The manual also includes details of reliability.

Examples from the Epilepsy Surgery Inventory

Overall, how would you rate your quality of life?

Circle one number on the scale below:

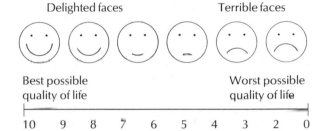

Compared with 1 year ago, how would you rate your health in general now?

Much better now than 1 year ago (1) / somewhat better now than 1 year ago? (2) / about the same (3) / somewhat worse now than 1 year ago (4) / much worse now than 1 year ago (5)

Have you worried about having another seizure?

Answer on a 6-point scale from 'all of the time' (1) to 'none of the time' (6)

I seem to get seizures a little easier than other people with epilepsy

Answer on a 5-point scale from 'definitely true' (1) to 'definitely false' (5)

Validity and factor structure

Construct validity was supported by correlations with instruments assessing mood (e.g. corresponding items on energy/fatigue correlated 0.64 and

−0.67 and emotional status/well-being items correlated 0.47 and −0.68). It was able to discriminate between patients who were seizure-free and those who continued to have seizures, and those having seizures without loss of consciousness (Vickrey *et al.* 1992b; Rand 1993). Multi-trait scaling supported item discrimination across scales. Factor analysis by the scale's authors confirmed mental and physical health factors, as well as a third factor defined by cognitive function and role limitations scales.

Reliability

In a study of 196–200 patients who had previously undergone surgery for epilepsy or who had been assessed for surgery, the alpha internal consistency reliability coefficients for the scales ranged from 0.68 to 0.88 (all but one scale satisfied the 0.70 reliability acceptance standard, the exception being the social function scale).

Because the recommended generic core instruments, SF-36 and other MOS scales are fast becoming widely used internationally, their use in disease-specific batteries provides a rich source of comparative data. The copyright is owned by Rand (for the SF-36 and MOS items which form the bulk of the battery) and Dartmouth College (for the Dartmouth COOP Chart Ladder).

KATZ ADJUSTMENT SCALES (REVISED FOR USE WITH EPILEPSY)

These scales were developed in the 1960s to measure the social adjustment and behaviour of people with schizophrenia discharged from hospital to the community (Katz and Lyerly 1963). They were revised for use with epilepsy patients by Vickrey *et al.* (1992a) using a sample of 328 epilepsy out-patients, and later cross-validating it in a postal survey of 193 adults with epilepsy.

Content, administration and scoring

The original Katz forms included ratings by the patient and a close friend or relative who assessed psychiatric symptoms, social behaviour and daily activities. The revised version for use with epilepsy patients used only the section for ratings by others (it was known as the KAS-R1). This was based on

the assumption that independent ratings are often required for people with neurological conditions when they are unable to respond due to disability or because their responses are potentially unreliable. This section contains 127 items.

For each of the 127 items in the scale, the relative/friend is asked to rate the patient according to 'how your relative or friend has looked to you during the past few weeks on these things'. There are four response choices for each item: almost never, sometimes, often and almost always. Items are summed. The examples below illustrate the limitation of this scale in that it is dependent on subjective judgements about aspects of another's personality.

Examples from the KAS-R1

Nervousness

16 Tries too hard
21 Jittery
83 Hands tremble

Dependency

17 Needs to do things very slowly to get them right
72 Needs a lot of attention
74 Acts helpless
93 Acts as if he or she can't make decisions

Oversensitivity/fearfulness

3 Cries easily
4 Feels lonely
15 Gets very sad/blue
125 Talks about suicide

Withdrawal

8 Just sits
69 Shy
70 Quiet
71 Prefers to be alone
102 Speaks very slowly

Social

39 Generous
46 Is cooperative
54 Friendly
58 Gets along well with people

Disorientation

85 Loses track of day, month or year
88 Acts as if he or she doesn't know where he or she is
89 Remembers important things (reverse coded)

Acting out

28 Gets angry and breaks things
33 Has temper tantrums
45 Gets into fights with people
51 Deliberately upsets routine

Irritability

42 Bossy
44 Argues
55 Gets annoyed easily
127 Gives advice without being asked

Validity

The original relatives' forms were able to distinguish between patients judged by clinicians to be well or poorly adjusted. Psychometric analyses by Katz and Lyerly (1963) suggested 13 factors. Vickrey *et al.* (1992a) evaluated the original 126 items (omitting the 127th – 'moves about very slowly' – in error), analysing their results using multi-trait scaling analysis. They finally accepted 113 items in 14 sub-scales: oversensitivity/fearfulness (18 items), social (10 items), irritability (9 items), dependency (15 items), acting out (12 items), paranoia (5 items), abnormal thought processes (5 items), withdrawal (11 items), emotional stability (6 items), nervousness (5 items), sociopathy (4 items), bizarreness (4 items), hyperactivity (4 items) and disorientation (5 items). The revised version improved the scaling successes and reduced scaling failures. The revised scale was able to discriminate between seizure-free patients and those having full seizures. The most sensitive sub-scales were: nervousness, dependency, oversensitivity/fearfulness and withdrawal.

Reliability

The original internal consistency reliability coefficients were less than 0.70 for 6 of the 11 sub-scales, which is not always regarded as acceptable (Nunnally 1978). The internal consistency reliability coefficients of the scales ranged from 0.57 to 0.89 upon first testing and from 0.66 to 0.88 after their revision (Vickery *et al.* 1992a).

Other

HEALTH-RELATED QUALITY OF LIFE MODEL

The authors of the Seizure Severity Scale (Baker *et al.* 1991) have recently extended their interest in measurement issues to the development of a health-related Quality of Life Model. This is a measure of health-related quality of life which is based explicitly on a definition of quality of life as encompassing social, psychological and physical domains.

Content

The model includes a battery of previously validated measures of anxiety, depression, happiness, overall mood, self-esteem, mastery, social satisfaction and general health, as well as the Seizure Severity Scale. The scales included in the battery are the Nottingham Health Profile (Hunt *et al.* 1986), the Social Problems Questionnaire (Corney and Clare 1985), Rosenberg's (1965) Self-Esteem Scale, the Hospital Anxiety and Depression Scale (Zigmond and Snaith 1983), the Affect–Balance Scale (Bradburn 1969), the Profile of Mood States (McNair *et al.* 1971), a mastery scale developed by the authors (Smith *et al.* 1991), the Seizure Severity Scale (Baker *et al.* 1991) and questions on activities of daily living (Brown and Thomlinson 1984).

All the scales can be self-administered, and each has its own independent scoring system. As each of the scales is an existing battery of generic and domain-specific scales, examples are not reproduced here. Readers are referred to the source references of the scales for further details, and reviews of the scales can be found in Chapter 3 and in Bowling (1991).

Validity and reliability

Each scale in the battery was shown to have good psychometric properties with 33 male and 47 female epilepsy patients in relation to internal consistency ($\alpha = 0.69–0.85$), with the exception of the Social Problems Questionnaire ($\alpha = 0.35$). Construct (convergent) validity of the battery was supported by its ability to discriminate between patients in relation to psychosocial function. Treatment effects were detected by the Seizure Severity

Scale, and the happiness and mastery scales (Baker *et al.* 1993). Total seizure count correlated with the battery of psychosocial scales (between 0.11 for depression and 0.49 for mood), and with the two scales within the Seizure Severity Scale (0.01–0.12) (Smith *et al.* 1993). The authors felt that most of the scales made a contribution to the assessment of outcomes. The battery needs further testing to assess its appropriateness and sensitivity with this patient group.

GENERAL TESTS OF NEUROPHYSIOLOGICAL FUNCTIONING

This is not the place for a detailed and comprehensive review of these scales, but as they are so essential in the assessment of specific groups of patients, and because mental impairments can have a severe impact on quality of life, brief reviews of well-known scales are included. There is no simple and coherent model of cognitive function, which makes the systematic assessment of appropriate measurements difficult. The measurement of cognitive impairments is the task of psychologists, although a number of scales have been developed for use by trained interviewers. Wade (1992) has described the relevant concepts and domains of cognitive impairments in relation to neurological rehabilitation, and referred to useful sources for the measurement of a range of domains such as memory (attention and learning), orientation, aphasia, perception, apraxia and intelligence. A small selection of the most popular scales is reviewed here.

TRAIL-MAKING TEST

The Trail-Making Test – which measures attention, perceptual speed, cognitive flexibility and visual memory – differentiates normally functioning individuals from those with brain damage. It is a two-part (A and B) instrument for the assessment of visual–motor speed and integration (Armitage 1946; Reitan 1958).

Content, administration and scoring

The tests are administered by a trained interviewer. Trail-Making A involves the subject drawing a line connecting (in sequence) 25 circles numbered 1–25. The circles are randomly arranged on one page. Trail-Making B also has 25 circles, of which 13 are numbered 1–13 and 12 are labelled A–L. It is a test of the time taken to join letters and numbers in sequence. It has frequently been used in studies of clinical outcome; for example, it has been reported to be sensitive to treatment and intervention in cardiovascular and circulatory disease (Jenkins *et al.* 1983b; Croog *et al.* 1986, 1990).

The score is based on the total time (in seconds) required to accomplish the task of connecting images by drawing lines (Reitan 1958). The procedure for the conversion of seconds to scores is given in the manual.

Validity and reliability

Reitan (1955) studied the results of 54 patients, half of whom were brain-damaged, and reported that 83 per cent had been correctly classified. Reitan and Tarsches (1959) reported that the scale was able to distinguish between patients with different types of brain damage. A vast amount of data on population and sub-group norms, and on correct classification rates, have been published. Many of the data on reliability and validity are contained in the manual, but are fairly dated.

WECHSLER SCALES

The Wechsler Scales include memory, intelligence and depression batteries. The 28-item depression battery is used less frequently and is not reviewed here (Wechsler *et al.* 1963)

WECHSLER MEMORY SCALE (WMS)

The WMS is frequently used across disciplines for use with a wide variety of population groups (Wechsler 1945; Wechsler and Stone 1973). It was developed to measure short- and long-term memory deficits and should only be administered by those who have received the appropriate training (Wechsler 1945, 1988). Scales suitable for use with both adults and children have been developed. There are several batteries, and short form versions are available. Extensive revisions have been made to the WMS over time (Russell 1982; Heiby 1984;

Wechsler 1988). The final revised version can be found in Wechsler (1988).

The WMS is used as a diagnostic and screening tool, in conjunction with a general neuropsychological examination or other clinical examination for the assessment of memory function.

Content, administration and scoring

The original version had seven components, forming three factors (Skilbeck and Woods 1980):

- *Orientation:* personal information, orientation.
- *Attention/concentration:* mental control (e.g. counting backwards), digit span.
- *Memory/learning factor:* logical memory (e.g. paragraph recall), visual reproduction (e.g. assessment of neurological function on the basis of reproduction of drawings); paired associates: (learning word pairs).

The logical memory component correlates well with behaviour (Sunderland *et al.* 1983).

The new revised version contains 12 sub-tests, grouped under five separate memory scores:

- *Sub-test I: Verbal memory:* includes sub-tests logical memory I and verbal paired associates I.
- *Sub-test II: Visual memory:* figural memory, visual paired associates I, visual reproduction I.
- *Sub-test III: General memory:* verbal memory plus visual memory.
- *Sub-test IV: Attention/concentration:* digit span, visual memory span.
- *Sub-test V: Delayed recall:* logical memory II, verbal paired associates II, visual paired associates II, visual reproduction II.

A preliminary sub-test – information and orientation – is scored separately and does not contribute to the memory scores.

Not all memory functions are tapped in the revised version. Long-term memory is not included, although an indication of long-term memory is obtained from the information sub-test of the scale. Olfactory memory, tactile memory and memory for previously learned skills (e.g. bicycling) are omitted.

The test takes 45–60 min to administer. A short form of the test can be administered by omitting the tests in sub-test V, which takes about 30 min.

Full details of its administration, scoring and scoring decisions, and psychometric properties are contained in the manual.

Validity, factor structure and reliability

The Wechsler Memory Scale, and the revised version, have been tested extensively for reliability, validity and sensitivity, and a manual is available (Wechsler 1987). Holden (1988) concludes his review with the statement that the revised WMS is the best available test for the major domains of verbal and visual memory. However, it may not be appropriate for use with elderly people (Kane and Kane 1988).

The population norms were updated with a large stratified sample of people. The psychometric properties of the scale were extensively retested for the revised version. Factor analysis yielded a two-factor solution: factor I appeared to be a general memory and learning factor (corresponding with the general memory index), and factor II resembled an attention–concentration factor, corresponding with the attention/concentration index. These factors are similar to those reported for the old version of the WMS. Based on a sample of 306 people, test–retest coefficients across age groups ranged from 0.41 to 0.90, with a median of 0.74. The inter-rater reliability coefficients were 0.99 and 0.97 for logical memory and visual reproduction, respectively. Reliability was highest with the oldest age groups.

WECHSLER ADULT INTELLIGENCE SCALE (WAIS)

The best-known test of mental performance is the IQ test, and the WAIS (Wechsler 1958, 1981a, 1981b) is the standard test for intelligence (Matazzo 1972). It consists of questions, problems and tasks constituting six verbal and five performance sub-tests. A short form is sometimes used comprising four of the sub-tests: vocabulary, comprehension, block design and object assembly. It was originally tested on 1700 randomly sampled American adults, for whom norms were provided by age group.

Content

The complete test takes 60 min to administer by a trained interviewer. The scale was revised by

Wechsler (1981b, 1986) and culturally biased and obsolete items were removed (known as the WAIS-R) (for a review, see Spruill 1984); about 80 per cent of the items are the same or have only been modified slightly. The old and revised versions of the scale both cover two domains, verbal intelligence and performance. The six verbal sub-scales are information (general knowledge, e.g. the naming of presidents), comprehension (e.g. the meaning of common sayings or what to do in common situations), arithmetic (reasoning rather than computation), similarities (e.g. between objects, items asking for an abstraction relating two common things), digit span (repeating of strings of digits presented orally), and vocabulary (meaning of words of increasing difficulty). The five performance sub-tests are digit–symbol (a simple written speed test of substituting one series of symbols for another), picture completion (line drawings of common things with something missing), block design (reproducing printed designs with one-inch blocks with different coloured sides), picture arrangement (a series of pictures which tell a story when arranged correctly), and object assembly (a very simple jigsaw puzzle) (for a review, see Matazzo 1972).

The commonly used digit–symbol test can be used independently. It takes 90 sec to complete and is easily scored. It assesses the speed of processing information. It is a paper and pencil test, which as Wade (1992) points out, is difficult to administer in cases of major motor impairments. However, it is a simple and sensitive test. The block design and digit symbol tests are also commonly used measures of visual–motor coordination and visual perception of abstract stimuli.

A version for children of similar format (WISC) was developed, which has since been revised (WISC-R).

The scores derived from the test represent verbal IQ, a performance IQ and a full scale IQ. The scoring details, and population norms for comparison, can be found in the manual.

Validity and reliability

The scales were developed and tested with large samples of adults in the USA, and with smaller sub-groups of the same population. Studies of validity in the USA have shown that students with

lower WAIS scores are less likely to graduate from high school (Matazzo 1972). Factor analyses generally show 3–5 factors, two of which usually relate to the verbal and performance scales (Krauskopf 1984). Convergent validity was supported by correlations with other tests ($r = 0.60–0.80$) among population sub-groups (82 brain-damaged adults, 52 reformatory inmates). A review of the major studies has been published by Botwinick (1977). Split-half reliability scores for the sub-tests ranged from 0.60 to 0.96, varying with age group. The reliability of the full scale and of the verbal and performance scales was better than for individual sub-tests. Test–retest coefficients of between 0.84 and 0.97 for intervals of several weeks were also reported (Wechsler 1958, 1981a).

There have been fewer studies of the reliability and validity of the revised version, though they would be expected to be similar to those of the original version given their similarities. The short form of the WAIS and the WMS (Wechsler 1945, 1948) are both popular among clinicians, and have been used in many follow-up studies, for example in cardiology and neurology. In a study of the outcome of 318 coronary artery bypass surgery patients, Jenkins et al. (1983b) reported that the logical memory sub-test of the WMS significantly improved post-surgery, supporting the inference that CABG was not associated with long-term adverse psychoneurological effects. Sengupta et al. (1975) administered the scales to 32 patients with ruptured aneurysms of the anterior communicating artery, 26 of whom had brain surgery. The authors were able to report that there was no evidence of post-operative intellectual impairment, although there were changes in psychological state, with loss of interest, initiative and energy. Population norms are available, based on national samples of the public in the USA. Norms are available for each age group.

SCALES FOR CHILDREN

Intelligence and memory scales

The Wechsler Intelligence and Memory Scales for Children (and revised versions) are the best known and most widely used tests for children, and with good results (Wechsler 1967, 1974, 1987). However, some researchers have criticized the choice of test designs in the Intelligence Scale (see Vernon

1984). Despite concluding that the scales have excellent psychometric properties and are probably the best available, Elbert and Holden (1985) question whether the scale measures identical cognitive processes at different ages, making longitudinal assessments difficult to compare.

Other developmental scales

Such tests are not reviewed here, but it is important to make some reference to developmental scales. Several other developmental – as opposed to intelligence – scales for children exist (e.g. Griffiths 1970). They enable the assessment of coordination, performance, locomotor development, personal social skills, speech and hearing. For children up to 17 years of age, cognitive development can be assessed by a short form IQ scale from the British Ability Scales (BAS: Elliot 1983). This includes measures of verbal and non-verbal reasoning ability, speed of information processing, short-term memory and language skills. There are also various school attainment tests available, which cover arithmetic, reading and spelling (Richman and Graham 1971). Such scales are inevitably culture-specific, and this is not the place for a comprehensive review. For younger children, behaviour can be assessed using the Richman Behaviour Scales (Richman and Graham 1971), and for children aged up to 17 years of age, with the Rutter A scales (Rutter et al. 1970). These scales have all been used with paediatric patients being treated for heart and lung disease. For example, in the UK, Wray et al. (1992) used them to assess perceived self-esteem and quality of life among children (n = 28), undergoing heart or heart–lung transplantation, in comparison with 28 controls. Few differences between the groups were reported, except a higher incidence of problem behaviour at home among the transplant group. Good selections of the many developmental scales for children have been reviewed in Keyser and Sweetland's (1984, 1985b, 1988) Test Critiques. Other source texts include Sattler (1982).

TESTS FOR COGNITIVE IMPAIRMENT IN ELDERLY PEOPLE

The most widely used instruments for the diagnosis of cognitive impairment are the Mini-Mental State Examination (MMSE: Folstein et al. 1975) and the Abbreviated Mental Test Score (AMTS: Hodkinson 1972; Qureshi and Hodkinson 1974), of which the latter is an adapted version of a scale developed by Blessed et al. (1968). For the diagnosis of dementia in epidemiological surveys and studies of outcome, the most widely used instrument is the Geriatric Mental State (GMS: Copeland et al. 1976), which is accompanied by a computerized algorithm for producing a standardized psychiatric diagnosis (AGECAT: Copeland et al. 1986), and the shorter version (CARE) is for use in the community (which also has a SHORT-CARE, which covers only dementia, depression and disability) (Gurland et al. 1984).

A number of scales have been omitted from this selective review, for example the Cambridge Mental Disorders of the Elderly Examination (CAMDEX: Roth et al. 1986, 1988). Scales also exist (but are not reviewed here) which have been developed for use with elderly people living in institutions, and which are administered to a staff member (e.g. the Crichton Royal Scales, which were developed by Wilkin and Jolley 1979). Examples of other, newer and 'user-friendly' tests include the Clock Drawing Test for early dementia (Sunderland et al. 1989), which involves the drawing of a clock face, the hands (hours and minutes) and spacing of numbers: 'First, draw a clock with all the numbers on it. Second, put hands on the clock to make it read 2.45.' Another new development is the Guy's Advanced Dementia Schedule, which presents a series of objects to respondents in order to elicit their response (to naming and using). Examples of some of the objects are a pencil and paper, a baby's rattle, a comb and a whistle (Ward et al. 1993). Mental status scales for use with the elderly have been reviewed by Copeland and Wilson (1989), and scales for Alzheimer's disease and related disorders have been reviewed by Jorm (1990).

ABBREVIATED MENTAL TEST SCORE (AMTS)

The AMTS was developed by Hodkinson (1972) and Qureshi and Hodkinson (1974), and has been used successfully to discriminate between patients with organic and functional psychiatric illness. The AMTS was derived from the Roth-Hopkins Test, which correlates well with pathological brain changes at autopsy (Blessed *et al.* 1968). They took the most discriminating items to form the AMTS.

Content, administration and scoring

The scale requires an interviewer to administer it. It is simple to administer and is composed of ten test questions covering such things as age, date, place, person recognition, etc. Each correct item scores 1 and the items are totalled. The maximum score is 10; the cut-offs for scoring (normal/abnormal) have varied between studies. Jitapunkul *et al.* (1991) briefly reviewed the literature and reported that investigators have used cut-offs in the range of <6 to <10 (a score of 10 = cognitively normal). They carried out a study of 168 acutely ill patients admitted to a ward for the care of the elderly and validated the AMTS (tested on admission and 1 week later) against clinical diagnoses plus medical records (based on DSM-III-R criteria) and reported that the best cut-off was 8.

The ten items of the AMTS

Age
Time (nearest hour)
Year
Name of place
Recognition of two persons
Date and month of birth
Date of First World War
Queen's name
Count 20–1 backwards
5 min recall: full street address

Validity

Vardon and Blessed (1986) tested the AMTS against clinical assessments of dementia among 99 residents in homes for elderly people. They reported that over 80 per cent of residents diagnosed with dementia scored 55 per cent or less correct answers on the AMTS. Correlations with longer mental status scales are generally over $r = 0.87$ (Qureshi and Hodkinson 1974; Thompson and Blessed 1987). The AMTS, in its original form, was described by Wade (1992) as the most well-established test to be validated against neuropathological evidence.

Reliability

Its performance has been assessed in institutional and community settings, with good results for inter-observer reliability and repeatability (Qureshi and Hodkinson 1974; Vardon and Blessed 1986; Little *et al.* 1987; Thompson and Blessed (1987). Thompson and Blessed (1987) reported that the 10-item test was better accepted by psychogeriatric patients than the original 37-item Roth-Hopkins Test.

Short version

Jitapunkul *et al.* (1991) developed a short version of the AMTS, the AMT7. Its validity, internal consistency and coverage of the relevant domains was comparable to the AMTS but it had a slightly higher sensitivity (81 per cent, with acceptable specificity of 85 per cent) than the full AMTS. Cronbach's alpha, based on the internal consistency of the AMT7, was 0.85 (it was 0.89 for the full version). The proportion of patients correctly classified was 89.9 per cent (91.1 per cent for the 10-item test).

The AMT7

Time (orientation)
Recall of address (attention/recent memory)
Hospital (orientation)
Persons (orientation)
Date of birth (remote memory)
Monarch (general knowledge and memory)
Count 20 to 1 backwards (attention)

The items excluded from the full AMTS are age (remote memory), year (orientation) and date of First World War (memory).

Examples of the AMT7

1 What is the date today?
3 What place is this?
5 What is your date of birth?

MINI-MENTAL STATE EXAMINATION (MMSE)

The MMSE is a brief test of cognitive mental state developed by Folstein *et al.* (1975), which is able to distinguish between patients with organic and functional psychiatric illness. It was developed for use with neurogeriatric patients.

Content, administration and scoring

The MMSE assesses a wide range of conditions, including the types of deficits that can be found in Alzheimer's disease and the dementias. It has been used extensively in the USA, and increasingly so in the UK and Europe. The MMSE was selected as the sole cognitive component of the Diagnostic Interview Schedule (Robins *et al.* 1981) and the CAMDEX (Roth *et al.* 1986) also incorporates it. It takes 5–10 min to administer.

The scale has two parts, verbal and performance. Four verbal sub-tests have a maximum score of 21 and evaluate orientation in time, memory and attention. One section contains two performance sub-tests having a maximum score of 9, and which involve naming objects, execution of written or spoken instructions, writing and copying a complex polygon. The test covers orientation (10 items), registration (1 item), attention and calculation (1 item), recall (1 item) and language (8 items). It is administered by an interviewer. The items are scored between 3 and 9, and the total score is 30 (lower scores represent cognitive impairment). The cut-off score is 23–24, and most non-dementing elderly people rarely score below 24. It has a broader range of scores for patient groups than the AMTS (Roth *et al.* 1986; Anderson 1990). The reading and writing involved may be difficult for respondents with visual problems.

Examples from the MMSE

Orientation

What is the (year) (season) (date) (day) (month)? (max. score 5)
Where are we (state) (county) (town) (hospital) (floor)? (max. score 5)

Language

Name a pencil and watch (2 points)
Repeat the following 'No ifs, ands or buts' (1 point)
Follow a three-stage command:

'Take a paper in your right hand, fold it in half, and put it on the floor' (3 points)

Read and obey the following:

Close your eyes (1 point)
Write a sentence (1 point)
Copy design (1 point)

(max. score 9)

Validity

Nelson *et al.* (1986) reviewed 11 validation studies of the scale, most of which reported correlations of sub-scale scores with clinical descriptions using DSM-III diagnoses and radiological investigations. Validation against clinical assessments has also been reported by Anthony *et al.* (1982) and Roth *et al.* (1986). It can separate patients with and without cognitive disturbance, and it correlates with clinical judgements.

On the basis of 69 elderly people who had affective disorders with or without cognitive impairment or who had dementia, and a group of normal controls, Folstein *et al.* (1975) reported that the scale was sensitive to changes in condition over time. Concurrent validity was tested against the Wechsler Adult Intelligence Scale, and the product–moment correlations were 0.78 for the verbal scale and 0.66 for the performance scale.

Reliability

Folstein *et al.* (1975) tested the scale initially on two groups of patients: the 69 elderly people reported above and a second group of 137 elderly people consecutively admitted to hospital with a variety of psychiatric illnesses. The inter-rater and test–retest reliabilities were satisfactory. The test–retest product–moment correlations 28 days apart were 0.83–0.98 (with the same and different raters).

The MMSE has been reported to be preferable to the AMTS, although the results can be influenced by respondents' sociodemographic background (Dick *et al.* 1984; Jorm *et al.* 1988; Brayne and Calloway 1990). Because of this bias, Jagger *et al.* (1992) suggested that the CAPE 10 sub-test, which measures information/orientation (Pattie and Gilleard 1979), is preferable to the MMSE, although it is less sensitive in relation to milder forms of dementia than the MMSE (Brayne and Calloway, 1990; Jagger *et al.* 1992).

The CAPE has been subjected to criticism over

its insensitivity (Black *et al.* 1990), and it is used less frequently than in the past.

MENTAL STATUS QUESTIONNAIRE (MSQ)

This is a measure of orientation and memory, derived partly from existing standard mental-status examinations. Pfeiffer (1975a, 1975b) modified it, and reduced it from 31 to 9 items. It has been widely used in a variety of settings and has been judged to be useful in community settings (Cornoni-Huntley *et al.* 1985) and institutional settings (Wilson and Brass 1973; Ebmeier *et al.* 1988).

Content, administration and scoring

This is a 9-item memory test involving date, place, time, birth date and name of the prime minister. It is simple to administer by an interviewer. Although these questions which test memory (in all these types of tests) can make an interviewer embarrassed and worry about losing rapport with the respondent, he or she needs to be encouraged to ask the questions during the interview (different items at different places if necessary) without making it obvious that the respondent is being tested (e.g. checks on the date, date of birth respondent's full name and address can easily be carried out in this way). The other, more obvious questions (e.g. on the name of the prime minister) will have to be prefaced by an honest explanation. Wilson and Brass (1973) reported that the following format rarely caused embarrassment: 'How is your memory, I would like to test it?' Correct replies are scored 1 and the responses are summed.

There are many variations on this test, and it is

The nine items of the MSQ

Address/name of place
Today's date (error of 3 days either side of correct date allowed)
Month
Year
Age
Year of birth
Month of birth
Name of prime minister
Name of previous prime minister

---

similar to the AMTS (Hodkinson 1972). Wilson and Brass (1973) reported that an initial first item (name of town) could be excluded, as it contributes little to the discriminative ability of the scale.

Validity and reliability

In a study of 1066 people in institutions, the MSQ was highly correlated with psychiatrists' assessments of the presence of chronic brain syndrome (Kahn *et al.* 1960b). Kahn *et al.* (1960a) reported reliability to be satisfactory. The test–retest coefficient was reported to be 0.80. Split-half reliability was reported to be $r = 0.68$ (Wilson and Brass, 1973). Wilson *et al.* (1973) repeated the MSQ four times at 3-week intervals with 55 people whose condition was expected to remain stable. They reported that three-quarters of the scores changed by 1 or less (Wilson *et al.* 1973).

As with all self-administered scales, the questions have to be written down for people with hearing difficulties, and they cannot be used with people who are dysphasic (Wilson and Brass 1973).

OLDER AMERICANS' RESOURCES AND SERVICES SCHEDULE (OARS) MENTAL HEALTH MEASURES

The Older American Resources and Services (OARS) instrument was developed at Duke University in the 1970s. It consists of two sections: the Multidimensional Functional Assessment Questionnaire, which assesses physical, psychological and social functioning, and the Service Assessment Questionnaire, which assesses service use. It has been employed in over 100 research studies (George and Fillenbaum 1985). There is extensive evidence of its reliability, validity and sensitivity (Fillenbaum and Smyer 1981; George and Fillenbaum 1985).

The OARS mental health sub-scales do not identify pathology in any precise way. When used with the full OARS multidimensional battery, it forms part of the database for global mental health ratings. Used alone, the questions are simply a fairly crude screen.

Content, administration and scoring

The OARS mental health sub-section aims to assess cognitive functioning, psychiatric status (but not diagnosis) and self-evaluation. It is administered by an interviewer (George and Fillenbaum 1985). It comprises four groups of items on mental health (Fillenbaum 1978): life satisfaction (3 items); self-assessment items on mental health (now and 5 years ago) (2 items); the Short Portable Mental Status Questionnaire (SPMSQ), a 10-item test of intellectual impairment or cognitive deficit (Pfeiffer, 1975a), which is based on other well-known scales of memory and mental status, and which is also used (in modified format) in the Wechsler Memory Scale (Wechsler 1945), and the Short Psychiatric Evaluation Schedule (15 items) (Pfeiffer 1975b).

No instructions for interpreting responses are given. However, Pfeiffer (1975a) suggests the following scoring for the SPMSQ: 0–2 errors = intact intellectual functioning; 3–4 errors = mild intellectual impairment; 5–7 errors = moderate intellectual impairment; 8–10 errors = severe intellectual impairment.

Examples from the OARS

Short Psychiatric Evaluation Schedule (Pfeiffer 1975b)

Life satisfaction
Satisfied with life
Daily life is uninteresting

e.g. Is your daily life full of things that keep you interested?

Psychosomatic symptomatology
Do not wake up rested
Sleep is disturbed
Heart pounding and shortness of breath

e.g. Do you wake up fresh and rested most mornings?

Alienation
Wants to leave home
No one understands

e.g. Have you at times very much wanted to leave home?

Short Portable Mental Status Questionnaire (Pfeiffer 1975a)

Examples: Cognitive deficit
 1 What is the date today?   (month, day, year)
 5 How old are you?
 6 When were you born?
10 Subtract 3 from 20 and keep subtracting 3 from each new number you get, all the way down

Total number of errors:

Validity and factor structure

The full OARS scales (and short version) have been tested extensively for reliability and validity, with excellent results (Fillenbaum 1978; Fillenbaum and Smyer 1981; Cairl *et al.* 1983). The full scales were reviewed by Bowling (1991). In a study of 997 community residents and 141 out-patients aged 65 and over, Pfeiffer (1975a) reported that the SPMSQ correlated highly with clinical diagnoses. There was a high level of agreement (88 per cent) between the clinical diagnoses of organic brain syndrome and the questionnaire scores, which indicated moderate or severe organic impairment.

Fillenbaum (1980) reported that the SPMSQ was highly correlated with the MSQ (Kahn *et al.* 1960a, 1960b). When compared with psychiatric assessments, however, a true positive rate of 55 per cent and a true negative rate of 96 per cent was achieved. The MSQ performed similarly. Such crude tests are inevitably subject to error.

The analysis of mental health items for the OARS batteries has been marked by diversity, with different investigators selecting different items for inclusion; there is clearly little consensus over which items should be included (see review by Liang *et al.* 1989). Because of this confusion, Liang *et al.* (1989) evaluated several measurement specifications of the OARS mental health items – a pool of 20 self-report items, including the 15-item Short Psychiatric Evaluation Schedule, five life satisfaction and self-rated mental health items and a summary score of cognitive functioning. They point to other factor analytic studies of the mental health measures, but note that these were largely descriptive. They tested the scale on two large community samples in the USA ($n = 1834$ and 2146). They reported that, in addition to the second-order construct of mental health, there were four first-order dimensions: life satisfaction, psychosomatic symptomatology, alienation and cognitive deficit. They examined the model for different sociodemographic mixes of the population under study and reported that the model fitted well, but that a model with cognitive deficit separate from the other factors fitted best.

Reliability

On the basis of a study of 997 people, test–retest correlations were found to be 0.82–0.83 at 4 weeks among two groups of people aged 65+ (*n* = 59) (Pfeiffer 1975a). These OARS sub-scales have been regarded as useful in surveys of older people in the USA, although their limitations have been acknowledged (Kane and Kane 1988).

BRIEF COGNITIVE FUNCTIONING SCALE (SIP SUB-SCALE)

This is an adaptation of the 6-item self-report 'alertness behaviour' sub-scale of the Sickness Impact Profile (SIP: Bergner *et al.* 1976a, 1976b, 1981; Gilson *et al.* 1979) by Sherbourne *et al.* (1992) for the Rand MOS. It can be used independently of the main health status instrument within which it is embedded.

Content, administration and scoring

The scale includes problems with concentration, memory, reasoning, attention, psychomotor ability, and confusion during the past month. The SIP scales were designed for self-administration or administration by an interviewer. Self-report cannot be undertaken by respondents with more severe levels of cognitive impairment, and an interviewer will need to administer the instrument. Interviewer administration is advisable in most instances. The responses are summed. An instruction manual is available.

Examples from the SIP sub-scale

2 I have more minor accidents; for example, drop things, trip and fall, bump into things
6 I sometimes behave as if I were confused or disoriented in place or time; for example, where I am, who is around, directions, what day it is
10 I have difficulty doing activities involving concentration and thinking

(Respondents are asked only to tick statements that describe them 'today' and which are related to their state of health)

Validity and reliability

The full SIP has been rigorously tested with impressive results for reliability and validity (Bergner *et al.* 1981; see review by Bowling 1991).

The few data that exist on the psychometric properties of this sub-scale when it is used alone suggest that the scale is reliable ($\alpha = 0.87$), and is correlated with, measures of emotional status (Sherbourne *et al.* 1992; Stewart and Ware 1992). Its reliance on self-repost is its weakness.

GERIATRIC MENTAL STATE (GMS) and COMPREHENSIVE ASSESSMENT AND REFERRAL EVALUATION (CARE)

The Geriatric Mental State (GMS) is a standardized diagnostic instrument for use with elderly people. It was developed by Copeland *et al.* (1976) from standardized instruments in the USA and UK – the Psychiatric (or Mental) Status Schedule (Spitzer *et al.* 1970) and the Present State Examination (Wing *et al.* 1974). They developed the schedule so that it would be appropriate in community settings in international studies, and used it within a broader semi-structured interview called the Comprehensive Assessment and Referral Evaluation (CARE) interview (Copeland *et al.* 1978, 1987; Gurland *et al.* 1983). The GMS was developed by a British research team working on a large study of psychiatric disorders in the elderly in New York and London, and the CARE was developed by the American team. It is regarded as the measure of choice in national and international epidemiological studies (Copeland 1990) and has been translated into several languages.

Content, administration and scoring

The CARE interview is broad and covers psychiatric, medical, nutritional, economic and social problems. The CARE takes most of the psychiatric content of the GMS and adds items on medical and social problems (Gurland *et al.* 1977). It is longer than the GMS at 1500 items. It takes about 90 min to administer. The interviewer draws information from several sources: self-reports from the respondent, test performance, observations and interviewer judgements. It can be administered by lay as well as clinical interviewers, although training is required (about 1 month for a lay interviewer). Shorter versions of the CARE have been developed – the CORE-CARE (314 items, and the SHORT-CARE (143 items). The CORE-CARE was derived after psychometric analysis, and also covers psychiatric, medical and social domains like the main CARE. The SHORT-CARE covers only three areas: dementia, depression and disability. It takes just over 30 min to complete.

Details of the rating, coding and scoring can be found in the manual, which is available from the authors. The psychiatric diagnosis which is derived from the GMS has since been standardized by a computer program called AGECAT (Dewey and Copeland 1986).

Examples from the GMS

Memory

23 Have you had any difficulty with your memory?

In rater's opinion, interviewee has difficulty with his or her memory (code 0, 1, 2)
If no apparent difficulty, skip to question 25.

24 What kinds of things do you forget? (Names of your family or close friends?) (Where you have put things?)

Forgets names of family or friends, or misnames them. (Do not include transient mistakes) (codes 0, 1, 2)
Forgets where he or she has placed things (code 0, 1, 2)

27 What is the name of the prime minister?

Does not recall name of prime minister (code 0, 1)

28 Who was the last prime minister?

Does not recall name of previous prime minister (code 0, 1)

Tension

34 Do you get worn out (exhausted)? If no: what about towards the evening?

Gets worn out or exhausted during daytime or evening (code 0, 1, 2)

35 Do you have difficulty in relaxing (resting)?

Difficulty in relaxing (code 0, 1, 2)

Autonomic symptoms

47 Have you felt your heart pound or felt yourself trembling, in the last month? (when this was not due to exercise?) What was happening at the time?

Palpitations (i.e. the patient is conscious of his or her heartbeat) (code 0, 1, 2)
Trembling or tremulous feeling (code 0, 1, 2).

Insight

Observation

122 Interviewee has not adequately admitted to or explained his or her emotional or physical problems

If interviewee has . . . skip to question 124

123 Do you think there is anything the matter with you? (Any emotional, mental or physical illness?) (Any problem you need help for?) (What do you think [a symptom] is due to?)

Denies he or she has been either physically or psychiatrically sick despite the evidence
Denies or doubts his or her symptoms have had psychiatric significance despite the evidence
Denies or doubts important symptoms, disabilities or problems observed by rater

Interviewee has obvious psychological problems which he or she denies or unreasonably regards as medical or social in nature

Code: 1 = minimizing; 2 = complete denial

Validity and reliability

The GMS and CARE are two instruments that are both highly reliable and valid, and they have been tested in collaborative centres throughout the world (Henderson *et al.* 1983). Claims have been made for face validity on the basis of expert review. To take examples, the full CARE interview has been tested against psychiatric assessments with high levels of agreement. In a study of 396 subjects in London, agreement on depression and dementia was 88 per cent (Cohen's kappa for overall agreement was 0.7), and AGECAT was found to provide a reasonable diagnosis (Copeland *et al.* 1986). Another study reported the agreement between psychiatrists' assessments and CARE to be 0.73 ($\kappa = 0.46$) (Toner *et al.* 1988).

The GMS has been shown to be reliable with trained psychiatric interviewers (Copeland and Gurland 1978). Reliability studies of the short versions were carried out by the scale's developers and their collaborators. Inter-rater reliability was reported to range from low to high (0.48–0.85), with one at 0.38 (Gurland *et al.* 1977; Copeland and Gurland 1978; Henderson *et al.* (1983).

CONCLUSION

In conclusion, it is worthwhile re-emphasizing that the outcome of intervention and rehabilitation, particularly in relation to stroke patients, can no longer be viewed solely in terms of morbidity and mortality, particularly given the debate about whether to survive in a vegetative state is no better than death, or even worse (Jennett 1976). One important dimension of health that ought to be measured is broader health status, or health-related quality of life.

In relation to epilepsy, investigators have tended to use batteries of domain-specific scales to measure health-related quality of life. A promising disease-specific quality of life scale for use with people with epilepsy is the Washington Psychosocial Inventory (Dodrill 1978), although it is not sufficiently broad in scope. An improvement on this scale is the Epilepsy Surgery Inventory (Vickrey et al. 1992b), which uses the original Rand SF-36 as the core instrument. More work on the appropriateness of the SF-36 with people with epilepsy is required. Its appropriateness for people with stroke is also worth investigating, given its inclusion as the core instrument in the TyPE batteries, although its physical functioning subscale is unlikely to be sufficiently sensitive.

In relation to tests of neurophysiological functioning, the most popular scales across specialities are the Trail-Making Test (Armitage 1946; Reitan 1958) and the Wechsler Intelligence and Memory Scales for both adults and children (Wechsler 1981a, 1981b, 1988). In relation to elderly people, the Abbreviated Mental Test Score (Hodkinson 1972), the Mini–Mental State Examination (Folstein et al. 1975) and the Mental Status Questionnaire (Pfeiffer 1975a, 1975b) are probably the most popular brief scales, although the longer Geriatric Mental State and CARE (Copeland et al. 1976; Copeland and Gurland 1978, Copeland et al. 1987; Gurland et al. 1983) instruments are believed to be the most reliable and valid measures developed to date.

6

RHEUMATOLOGICAL CONDITIONS

QUALITY OF LIFE IN PEOPLE WITH JOINT DISORDERS

Joint disorders, particularly osteoarthritis, are common, increase with age, and are a leading cause of disability, second only to heart disease (National Center for Health Statistics 1971; Martin *et al.* 1988; Verbrugge 1992).

Rheumatoid arthritis (RA) affects quality of life by limiting activities because of pain and disability. It is not directly associated with any effect on mental functioning and is not life-threatening, although disability can be severe. The pain and disability also affects social contacts (Weinberger *et al.* 1987). Research on osteoarthritis and rheumatoid arthritis has stressed the experience of loss of independence, being a burden on others, the difficulties involved in asking for help and consequently, the importance of being able to maintain independence and normal social roles, minimize pain and appear 'normal' (Weiner, 1975; Reisine *et al.* 1987; Williams 1987; Fitzpatrick *et al.* 1988; Williams and Wood 1988). These issues support the importance of measuring broader quality of life, rather than just physical functioning levels.

THE DOMAINS OF MEASUREMENT

Disease-specific indexes of functioning and other clinical indicators

It is generally recognized in rheumatology that outcome of treatment is multidimensional, a factor which also creates measurement difficulties (see Spector and Hochberg 1992). Rheumatologists frequently use self-report measures of functional ability, supplemented with clinical indicators, because it is felt that measures of functioning are unable to portray accurately ability at the extreme ends of a spectrum ('floor' and 'ceiling' effects), and they may not be sufficiently sensitive to outcome (Liang and Katz 1992). Disease-specific clinical measures of functional outcome for conditions of the hip, for example, would include pain, functional ability (particularly climbing stairs, transportation, sitting, putting on shoes and socks), range of motion (flexion, abduction, external rotation in extension, internal rotation in extension, adduction, extension) and absence of deformity (Harris 1969). Self-report scales of functioning tend to be less specific (see later). Pain is an essential dimension to measure, and there is evidence (Bombardier *et al.* 1986) that a 10 cm VAS is as sensitive and efficient at measuring pain in patients with rheumatoid arthritis as longer pain scales (Melzack 1975).

It is not the intention of this review to include diagnostic or clinical criteria, but some of these measures are briefly mentioned as they are among the items that should be included in disease-specific outcome batteries. Clinical measures of disease in RA include joint counts (in which joints are scored for tenderness or pain on motion, e.g. Ritchie *et al.* 1968), erythrocyte sedimentation rate (ESR), the

Arthritis Association Scale (Steinbrocker *et al.* 1949) and, depending on the site of the problem, grip strength (inflating a blood pressure cuff to 30 mmHg and asking the respondent to squeeze it as hard as possible), walking speed and the multivariate index of disease activity (Mallya and Mace 1981). The latter assesses disease activity with ESR, haemaglobin levels, grip strength, an articular index, period of morning stiffness, tenderness using the Ritchie Articular Index (Ritchie *et al.* 1968) and a visual analogue scale for pain. This index is scored to produce a 4-point scale of severity of disease. Other site-specific function tests may be included, for example a button test involving doing up and undoing buttons (a 'button board' may be used for this task). The range of 'quantitative' measures of outcome, from joint counts to radiography, have been reviewed by Pincus and Callahan (1992). Interviews and questionnaires are useful for collecting information about symptoms (e.g. pain, swellings, stiffness, timing and duration) and adverse effects of treatments, including skin conditions, gastrointestinal disturbances, and headaches.

Recommended scales of functioning and other clinical indicators

Deyo (1993) suggested that the older scales and classifications of functioning – for example, the American Rheumatology Association Scale (Steinbrocker *et al.* 1949), the Katz Activities of Daily Living (ADL) Scale (Katz and Akpom 1976a, 1976b), and the Barthel Index (Mahoney and Barthel 1965) – should be abandoned in favour of one of the more recently developed scales of functional status, such as the Health Assessment Questionnaire (Fries *et al.* 1980) or the Arthritis Impact Measurement Scales (Meenan *et al.* 1980; Meenan and Mason 1990) both of which are disease-specific, and the generic Sickness Impact Profile (Bergner *et al.* 1981) for the assessment of broader health status and functional ability (not disease-specific). The wide range of scales of functioning appropriate for use in rheumatology has been summarized by Liang and Katz (1992), and the most popular scales of functioning are reviewed later.

Some of the older scales had relatively good sensitivity, albeit within a narrow range. For example the Katz ADL Scale was shown to predict the long-term course and social adaptation of patients with a number of conditions including hip fractures, and was used to evaluate out-patient treatment for rheumatoid arthritis (Katz *et al.* 1963, 1966, 1968). It was also shown to predict mortality (Brorsson and Asberg 1984), although it was reported to underestimate dysfunction in community populations (Spector *et al.* 1987). Such concise indices tend to be insensitive to small changes in disease severity and to focus on a narrow range of physical performance measures.

The American College of Rheumatology has recommended the following core set of disease activity and functional ability measures for clinical trials in rheumatoid arthritis: tender joint count and swollen joint count (Cooperating Clinics Committee of the American Rheumatism Association 1965); patient's assessment of current pain (using a 10 cm VAS or Likert scale: Langley and Sheppard 1984); patient's assessment of his or her overall progress (e.g. the Arthritis Impact Measurement Scale's VAS rating on 'how well you are doing' or similar Likert scale) and doctor's assessment (VAS or Likert item) of disease activity; patient's assessment of physical functioning, using either the Arthritis Impact Measurement Scale (Meenan *et al.* 1980; Meenan and Mason 1990), the Stanford Health Assessment Questionnaire (Fries *et al.* 1982), the McMaster Health Index Questionnaire (Chambers *et al.* 1982) or the MACTAR (Tugwell *et al.* 1987, 1990); and laboratory evaluation of one acute-phase reactant (Westergren erythrocyte sedimentation rate or a C-reactive protein level) (Felson *et al.* 1993). These measures were selected on the basis of literature reviews and panel consensus as providing the best coverage of the broad range of improvement in RA, and are at least moderately sensitive to change.

Measurement considerations: Functional status

Although the WHO (1980) made a distinction between physical status (impairment), physical functioning (disability) and social functioning (handicap) most activities of daily living and health status measures incorporate aspects of all three dimensions, and not all of them clearly distinguish between them (e.g. by separation of sub-scale scores). Investigators need to clarify whether they aim to measure impairment, disability and/or handicap. They should also clarify whether they wish to measure ability or performance, and select scales accordingly.

It is also important to draw a distinction between the measurement of activities of daily living (ADL) and instrumental activities of daily living (IADL) (Lawton and Brody 1969; Suurmeijer and Kempen 1990). Most scales do not allow for split-scale scores within the functioning sub-scale; most ADL scales permit separate analysis of the individual items. ADL items would include eating/drinking, washing self, using the toilet, rising from a chair, getting in/out of bed, moving around indoors, dressing, walking outdoors. IADL would include preparing meals, bed-making, laundry/ironing, shopping and heavy housework. A scale with these distinctions suitable for people with chronic illnesses has been developed by Suurmeijer and Kempen (1990) for international use – the Groningen Activity Restriction Scale – but is in its early stages of testing. They argue that their instrument gives a better insight into people's needs and increases the range of measurement regarding functional outcomes (disability), and early results indicate strong psychometric properties. Investigators should also ensure that instruments measuring functional ability also include items on the effects of the condition on social roles and activities.

Peculiarities to the condition also need to be taken into account when administering measurement scales, for example the cyclical nature of rheumatoid arthritis (Isacson et al. 1987).

Generic measures

While measures of physical functioning and limitations on activity are of obvious value in measuring the outcome of joint disorders, they do not necessarily provide a sufficiently detailed assessment of functioning in everyday social roles (Gilson et al. 1975). The inclusion of health status and health-related quality of life items is now seen as desirable in outcomes research (Bendtsen and Hornquist, 1992). However, generic scales always require supplementation with disease-specific items (Bell et al. 1990).

Several of the popular generic health-related quality of life scales (also called health status scales) have been used to assess outcome in rheumatology.

Among the most popular have been the Sickness Impact Profile (Bergner et al. 1981) and the Nottingham Health Profile (Hunt et al. 1986). Other scales that have been used in rheumatology include the McMaster Health Index Questionnaire (Chambers et al. 1982) and the Index of Well-Being (IWB), also known as the Quality of Well-Being Instrument (Kaplan et al. 1976).

Sickness Impact Profile/Functional Limitations Profile
One of the most popular instruments to be developed in the USA is the Sickness Impact Profile (SIP: Bergner et al. 1981). The Anglicized version is known as the Functional Limitations Profile (FLP: Patrick 1982a, 1982b; Charlton et al. 1983). The SIP was developed as a measure of perceived health status, for use as an outcome measure for health care evaluation across a wide range of health problems and diseases. It was originally developed for use with patients undergoing treatment for arthritis, hyperthyroidism and hip replacement. The items are not disease-specific and therefore it is suitable for use with other populations.

In a cross-sectional longitudinal study of 99 women with RA, the SIP was reported to be sensitive to 1 year pre- and post-treatment changes showing both improvement and deterioration (Sullivan et al. 1990). Liang et al. (1990) used the SIP, the Health Assessment Questionnaire (HAQ: Fries et al. 1982), the Arthritis Impact Measurement Scale (AIMS: Meenan et al. 1980) and the Functional Status Index (Jette 1987) with 38 end-stage arthritis patients 2 weeks before hip or knee arthroplasty, and at 3 and 12–15 months follow-up. They reported that the instruments detected large responses in global health, pain and mobility at 3 months, and smaller changes at later follow-up, although social function showed smaller changes at successive follow-ups.

The disadvantage of both the SIP and the FLP is their length – both 136 items. Fitzpatrick et al. (1988) compared the FLP with the HAQ and concluded that they are both valid measures of function in rheumatoid arthritis. They pointed out that the physical scale of the FLP and the HAQ are comparable and produce similar results (the advantage of the FLP is that it covers a broader range of dimensions). However, as they pointed out, the literature relating to studies of medical and surgical out-patients, and patients with back pain, confirms their own research, which shows that the SIP/FLP is less sensitive to improvement than to deterioration (Deyo and Diehl 1983; Mackenzie *et al.* 1986).

Nottingham Health Profile

A generic health status instrument that has been popular in outcome studies in several clinical areas is the Nottingham Health Profile (NHP: Hunt *et al.* 1986). The popularity of the NHP is in part due to its brevity; its psychometric properties are also excellent. Its popularity has waned somewhat due to the highly skewed nature of responses. Its negative orientation also means that small improvements in health are not necessarily detected (its insensitivity to small improvements is enhanced by the dichotomous, rather than scaled, response formats).

Fitzpatrick *et al.* (1992) used the NHP with 73 RA patients, 26 of whom were in-patients at first interview. They compared its performance with the Arthritis Impact Measurement Scales (AIMS: Meenan *et al.* 1980). Other measures included the Ritchie Articular Index to assess joint tenderness (Ritchie *et al.* 1968), grip strength, a visual analogue scale for pain, an item on duration of morning stiffness and the Beck Depression Inventory (BDI), the latter after removing two items which assessed symptoms that might have been due to physical rather than psychological morbidity (Beck *et al.* 1961). They reported that on both the AIMS and the NHP, it is the physical mobility and pain dimensions which correlate most closely with the four clinical measures of disease activity ($r = 0.32$–0.50 for the NHP, $r = 0.26$–0.66 for AIMS), but the social scales of both the NHP and the AIMS did not agree at all. The energy sub-scale of the NHP also correlated significantly with the clinical measures ($r = 0.37$–0.43). The emotions scales of both instruments correlated with the BDI ($r = 0.54$ for the NHP, $r = 0.53$ for the AIMS). There were also significant correlations between the NHP and the AIMS for pain, mobility and emotions, but not for social functioning. With the exception of the social dimension of the NHP, the scales showed stability at repeat interview 3 months after the first ($r = 0.41$–0.89 for the NHP, $r = 0.61$–0.81 for the AIMS). The correlation coefficient for the social dimension of the NHP over time was weak at 0.18 and appeared unstable.

The Short Form 36-item Health Status Questionnaire (SF-36)

The SF-36 was developed by the Rand Corporation in the USA for use in the Health Insurance Study Experiment/Medical Outcomes Study (Ware *et al.* 1993). It is a concise 36-item health status questionnaire, which is less skewed than the Nottingham Health Profile. It is rapidly becoming the scale of choice for international use across a wide range of specialities.

The Medical Outcomes Institute in the USA has developed a range of disease-specific batteries for joint conditions, which include the Rand SF-36 as the core generic quality of life scale. This mirrors developments in other specialities (e.g. oncology, neurology). The SF-36 is reviewed in Chapter 8; its functional ability scale focuses mainly on mobility and, as such, it is unlikely to be sufficiently sensitive as an outcome measure in rheumatology unless it is supplemented with another scale of functioning (such as the AIMS or HAQ).

Batteries of generic and domain-specific measures

Several investigators have chosen to use batteries of several measures. For example, in a related study of outcome of hip fracture, Todd *et al.* (1991) included a general measure of health status, the NHP (Hunt *et al.* 1986), in addition to disease-specific indicators (Borgquist *et al.* 1992), measures of psychological functioning and well-being, the Mini-Mental State Examination (Folstein *et al.* 1975), the Hospital Anxiety and Depression Scale (Zigmond and Snaith 1983), the Life Satisfaction Scale A (Neugarten *et al.* 1961), a self-esteem scale (Pearlin *et al.* 1981), as well as questions on patient satisfaction with the treatment. The authors regarded these instruments as useful, and the comprehensiveness of such batteries can yield a vast amount of valuable data on broader outcomes.

However, too many batteries, particularly if they are long, can be tiring and irritating (i.e. they often have overlapping items) for respondents. An example of the inclusion of too many multiple scales is Bombardier and co-workers' (1986) randomized controlled trial of auranofin therapy and quality of life. They studied 154 patients and 149 controls, and used a wide battery of well-tested measures: clinical indicators (tender joints, swollen joints, 50 foot walk time, duration of morning stiffness, grip strength); four measures of functioning, including the Health Assessment Questionnaire (Fries *et al.* 1982) and the Quality of Well-Being Questionnaire (Bush *et al.* 1973; Kaplan *et al.* 1976; 1978; 1979; Anderson *et al.* 1989); three measures of pain – the McGill Pain Questionnaire, the Pain Ladder Scale and a pain VAS (Melzack 1987; Melzack and Torgerson 1971; Scott and Huskisson 1976; Dickson and Bird 1981); the National Institute of Mental Health (NIMH) Depression Scale (Husaini *et al.* 1979); the Rand General Health Perceptions Scale and the Rand Current Health Assessment (Brook *et al.* 1979a, 1979c), utility measurements and various other clinical health assessment items. The researchers reported that not all scales were equally sensitive to outcome up to 6 months. A brief pain VAS was as sensitive as the longer McGill Pain Scale; the NIMH Depression Scale and the Rand measures were not sensitive to outcome; the functional status measures were all sensitive to outcome. These were important findings in view of the simplicity and brevity of the HAQ and the length and complexity of the Quality of Well-Being Questionnaire, implying that the shorter HAQ is the measure of choice. However, until experts in rheumatology agree on an appropriate package, researchers will continue to experiment with measures that may be unsuitable.

Domain-specific measures

Anxiety and depression

Apart from physical functioning, a particularly important dimension is psychological well-being. Instead of being regarded as part of a 'rheumatoid personality', depression is now also regarded as a consequence of the disability suffered by patients with rheumatoid arthritis (Creed and Ash 1992), although the measurement of mood after years of experience of disabling chronic illness is complex and causality is difficult to assess.

Popularly used scales of anxiety and/or depression in rheumatology include the Beck Depression Inventory (Beck *et al.* 1961) and the Hospital Anxiety and Depression Scale (Zigmond and Snaith 1983). Most such scales also assess both anxiety and depression, and few studies have attempted to separate the two (Creed *et al.* 1989).

Beck Depression Inventory (BDI)

The Beck Depression Inventory (or Index) has been used with more success than the MMPI with RA patients, as the somatic items on the BDI have been found to correlate well with total BDI depression scores rather than being correlated with RA activity (Bishop *et al.* 1987). These authors also reported increased depression at times of acute flare-ups leading to hospital admission.

Hospital Anxiety and Depression (HAD) Scale

The Hospital Anxiety and Depression Scale was designed by Zigmond and Snaith (1983) specifically to exclude somatic items. Chandarana *et al.* (1987) used the HAD and Goldberg's (1972) General Health Questionnaire successfully with RA patients, and reported that depression scores were positively associated with pain, duration of morning stiffness and functional ability. Murphy *et al.* (1988) also reported that grip strength and HAQ score were significantly associated with depression using criteria similar to DSM-III. Creed and Ash (1992) recommended the use of the HAD in diagnostic assessments of RA patients.

Personality

Personality assessments should probably be avoided in outcome assessments, although personality can influence response to illness. A large body of data of questionable relevance and interpretation have been collected in relation to people with joint conditions. Personality is frequently measured in outcome studies in rheumatology in the USA. The lengthy Minnesota Multiphasic Personality Index (Hathaway and McKinley 1990) has most frequently been used. It is questionable whether this measure is appropriate in view of its length and the irrelevance of many of the items and domains. Some of the criticisms of the scale are referred to below. If personality is to be assessed, the instrument of choice in the UK is Eysenck's Personality Questionnaire (Eysenck and Eysenck 1985).

Minnesota Multiphasic Personality Index (MMPI)

There has been widespread use in the USA of the Minnesota Multiphasic Personality Index in relation to RA patients (e.g. Pincus *et al.* 1986), and results show that people with RA are more likely to score positively on such statements than 'normal controls'. However, as Creed and Ash (1992) have pointed out, the MMPI includes several items which rheumatologists commonly attribute to arthritis rather than to change in psychological status, for example 'I have few or no pains'. These items are scored on the MMPI as indicators of depression and hypochondriasis, but they can be attributable to arthritis. Thus, several doubts have been raised about the use of the MMPI with patients with chronic disease such as rheumatoid arthritis, because their elevated scores on some dimensions (hypochondriasis, depression and hysteria) may reflect the disease rather than psychopathology (Pincus *et al.* 1986). A number of investigators have used the DSM-III or similar diagnostic assessment criteria (see Chapter 3), but these still contain somatic items which may artificially inflate scores (Frank *et al.* 1988; Murphy *et al.* 1988; Creed *et al.* 1989).

Adjustment and coping

Adjustment and coping ability are relevant modifying variables to be considered in the assessment of health outcomes. Ability to cope has been reported to be associated with personality, although the direction of relationships is unclear (Crown and Crown 1973). There is a significant sociological and psychological literature on coping abilities among people with chronic illnesses, including attempts to cover up one's condition and acting as though one is physically normal (Davis 1973; Weiner 1975). A disease-specific coping scale (the Arthritis Helplessness Index) for use with RA patients was developed by Nicassio *et al.* (1985). This is presented on pp. 231–2.

Social support

Social support is both a modifying and outcome variable: the availability of support can buffer the individual from deleterious effects of stress (e.g. illness), while illness can also reduce the individual's capacity to maintain social contacts and activities. Fitzpatrick *et al.* (1988) reported a reduction in the availability of a wider social network (friends and neighbours) among people with RA, but not among close family members. This was associated with functional ability. The implication is that, due to its disabling nature, the condition prevents people from actively maintaining wider social contacts. Measures of social network and support were reviewed by Bowling (1991), and an additional measure of support, which appears promising, is the Rand Medical Outcomes Study Social Support Questionnaire (Sherbourne and Stewart 1991).

Other domains

Investigators interested in other aspects of emotional well-being as outcome indicators may wish to include scales of life satisfaction and morale or self-esteem. A review of these scales can be found in Bowling (1991). Patient satisfaction and expectations are also important; references for patient satisfaction measures can be found in Chapter 1.

THE MEASUREMENT SCALES

DISEASE SEVERITY AND FUNCTIONAL CLASSIFICATIONS

Several classifications of severity of the disease and level of functioning have been developed by clinicians. For example, the New York Criteria for the diagnosis of RA grades patients according to severity for diagnostic purposes (Bennet and Wood 1968). The American Rheumatology Association

---

American Rheumatology Association Diagnostic Criteria

- joint stiffness in the morning, persisting for more than 1 hour
- pain on motion and/or tenderness in at least one joint
- swelling of soft tissues of at least one joint, persisting 6 weeks
- swelling of at least one other joint within 3 months
- swelling of the same joint on both sides of the body
- nodular growths under the skin over bony prominence
- X-ray changes typical of rheumatoid arthritis
- positive blood test for rheumatic factor
- poor mucin precipitate from synovial fluid
- characteristic microscopic picture of the synovium
- characteristic microscopic picture of rheumatoid nodules

(ARA) has also developed 11 diagnostic criteria for RA (Ropes *et al.* 1958). The presence or absence of clusters of these criteria determine whether arthritis is 'possible', 'probable' or 'definite'.

The ARA also developed an early functional scale in four classes (Steinbrocker *et al.* 1949), although it correlates weakly with clinical measures (e.g. grip strength, ESR, X-ray) and with the Sickness Impact Profile (Deyo *et al.* 1983). The authors do not recommend that this classification is used alone in studies of outcome.

American Rheumatology Association Functional Classification

1 Complete functional capacity with ability to carry on all usual duties without handicaps
2 Functional capacity adequate to conduct normal activities despite handicap or discomfort or limited mobility of one or more joints
3 Functional capacity adequate to perform only little or none of the duties of usual occupation or self-care
4 Largely or wholly indicated, with patient bedridden or confined to wheelchair, permitting little or no self-care

---

The criteria developed by Steinbrocker *et al.* (1949) for the classification of global functional status in RA was revised by the American College of Rheumatology (Hochberg *et al.* 1990):

I   Complete ability to perform all usual activities
II Able to perform all usual self-care and vocational activities but limited in avocational activities
III Able to perform all usual self-care activities but limited in vocational and avocational activities
IV Unable to perform all usual self-care activities

Functional classifications are crude and of questionable value in research. More useful are the broader scales of physical functioning, particularly the more recently developed scales.

DISEASE-SPECIFIC SCALES: PHYSICAL FUNCTIONING

Several investigators have noted that an instrument has yet to be developed which assesses a comprehensive range of dimensions relevant to health status in rheumatology (Liang *et al.* 1982; Fitzpatrick *et al.* 1992). Scales of physical functioning have tended to be described as health-related quality of life measures, often with an implicit assumption that they encompass all the relevant domains of quality of life.

Popular scales of physical functioning have included the Karnofsky Performance Index (Karnofsky *et al.* 1948), the Katz Activities of Daily Living Scale (Katz and Akpom 1976a, 1976b) and the Barthel Index (Mahoney and Barthel 1965). However, these scales are being superseded by newer disease-specific functional ability scales, including the Functional Status Index (FSI: Jette 1980a), the Arthritis Impact Measurement Scales (AIMS: Meenan *et al.* 1980; Meenan and Mason 1990) and the Health Assessment Questionnaire (HAQ: Fries *et al.* 1980). The older scales also tend to be fairly limited and insensitive in relation to the finer degrees of information needed about functional disability. Popular scales of functioning are reviewed below, followed by broader disease-specific quality of life scales.

STANFORD ARTHRITIS CENTER HEALTH ASSESSMENT QUESTIONNAIRE (HAQ)

The HAQ is an arthritis-specific scale that measures difficulties in performing activities of daily living (ADL), the need for equipment and physical assistance to perform tasks. The HAQ is suitable for use in community settings and has been administered to patients with rheumatoid and osteoarthritis, systemic lupus and ankylosing spondylitis. Fries *et al.* (1980) developed the HAQ on the basis that outcome should be measured in terms of the patient's value system, i.e. functional ability (the ability to walk) is a component of this but sedimentation rate is not. The framework used for the development of the HAQ was based on the belief that a patient desires to be alive, free of pain, functioning normally, experiencing minimal treatment toxicity, and financially solvent.

In the process of developing this questionnaire, 62 potential questions were selected from questionnaires in use in the rheumatic diseases and elsewhere, including the Uniform Database for Rheumatic Diseases (Fries *et al.* 1974; Convery *et al.* 1977), the Barthel Index (Mahoney and Barthel 1965) and the Activities of Daily Living Index (Katz *et al*. 1963). Testing the instrument for reliability and validity with patients with RA reduced the number of questions to 21, grouped into nine components, and graded in ordinal fashion from 0 to 3. Individual items with correlations of 0.85 or higher were eliminated, on the assumption that this suggested redundancy between components. Correlations of remaining items ranged between 0.35 and 0.65 (Fries *et al*. 1980).

Content

The full HAQ questionnaire measures functional ability as well as items on other symptoms, medication, services used, medical care costs and arthritis status. Most investigators only use the disability index, and sometimes the arthritis status index. Functional ability is measured by nine components: dressing and grooming, rising, eating, walking, hygiene, reach, grip, outside activity and sexual activity. Each of these components consists of one or more relevant questions. Pain, discomfort, drug toxicity and financial costs are also assessed.

Administration and scoring

The HAQ is self-administered and takes 5–10 min to complete. In relation to functional ability, the ordinal scoring of 1–3 is based on the following scale: without difficulty = 0, with difficulty = 1, with some help from another person = 2 and unable to do = 3. The highest score on any question within a component is taken as the score for that component. The index is calculated by summing the scores and then dividing the score by the total number of components answered. The authors reported reluctance among patients to report sexual activity (Fries *et al*. 1980), and thus some investigators omit this item (Fitzpatrick *et al*. 1988). The scale scores for pain and drug toxicity range from 0 = 'none' to 3 = severe adverse pain or side-effects. The scale for discomfort comprises better = 1, the same = 2 or worse = 3. The scoring procedures are similar to those for the functional scale.

In the personal cost section (applicable to private health care systems), medical and surgical costs are calculated for the past year. The number and type of medications, X-rays, surgeries, physician and paramedical visits, appliances, number of laboratory tests and hospitalizations are detailed. The average cost in the area covered by the research team (Stanford, CA) was determined and used for the computation of the dollar values. Social costs are calculated by determining changes in employment, income, the need to employ domestic help, the cost of transport for medical care and all arthritis-related costs over the previous 12 months (Fries *et al*. 1980).

Examples from the Stanford HAQ

In this section we are interested in learning how your illness affects your ability to function in daily life . . . Please check (tick) the one response which best describes your usual abilities over the past week. Are you able to:

1 Dressing and grooming

Dress yourself, including tying shoelaces and doing buttons?

7 Grip

Open jars which have previously been opened?
Turn taps on and off?

8 Activities

Get in and out of a car?
Do chores such as vacuuming, housework or light gardening?

Without any difficulty/with some difficulty/with much difficulty/unable to do

Arthritis status

1 Are you stiff in the morning?   Yes/no

If yes, about how long does this stiffness usually last?

2 Are any of your joints tender?   Yes/no

If yes, please circle the tender joints:

Knuckles, wrists, elbows, shoulders, hips, knees, ankles, toes

3 Are any of your joints swollen?   Yes/no

If yes, please circle the swollen joints:

Knuckles, wrists, elbows, shoulders, hips, knees, ankles, toes

Validity and factor structure

The scale has been extensively validated. Correlations of the HAQ against observed patient performance ranged from fair to high ($r = 0.47$–0.88) (Fries *et al*. 1980, 1982; Fries 1983; Kirwan and Reeback 1983). Several studies have tested the validity of the HAQ, in particular by correlation of the results of the HAQ with the Arthritis Impact Measurement Scale 6 (AIMS-6) (Fries *et al*. 1982; Brown *et al*. 1984). The two instruments were shown to measure the same dimensions of disability; the correlation coefficient reported by Fries *et al*. (1982) was $r = 0.91$. Interrcorrelations between the three parts of each instrument relating to physical disability, psychological state and pain were high and those across these three dimensions were weak. Patient self-assessed global arthritis scores were also strongly associated with disability score and less strongly with pain. Liang *et al*. (1985) have also reported good correlations between the HAQ and other scales of health status and functional ability, including the Sickness Impact Profile (Bergner *et al*. 1981) and the Functional Status Index (Denniston and Jette 1980; Jette 1980a).

In a recent study of 105 arthritis patients in the UK, Fitzpatrick *et al*. (1988) reported high correlations between the HAQ, the Functional Limitation Profile (FLP: Charlton *et al*. 1983), observations of grip strength and the articular index (e.g. the correlations between grip strength and the HAQ on two occasions were $r = -0.73$ and $r = -0.68$). The HAQ appears to be a valid measure of function in RA. Fitzpatrick *et al*. also reported that the complex scoring system of the FLP did not lead to greater precision when compared with the simpler ordinal assumptions of the HAQ. The HAQ performed better than the FLP in relation to specificity and sensitivity (detection of change over time). The large standard deviations in the scores of both measures indicated the presence of many 'false-cases' for improvement and deterioration. The HAQ was reported in early studies to be sensitive to change (Fries 1983), and it has been reported to be sensitive to change after treatment (Bombardier *et al*. 1986). However, this sensitivity may only be moderately good (Fitzpatrick *et al*. 1988).

Initial tests for the validity and reliability of the drug toxicity scale revealed weak results, and this component requires further testing (Fries *et al*. 1980). The cost questions have yet to be tested satisfactorily; initial tests for validity suffered from poor patient recall.

Principal components analysis has shown factor loadings along the first 'disability' component, explaining 65 per cent of the variance, and a second component with positive loadings for fine activities of the upper extremity and negative loadings for weight-bearing actions of the lower extremity, explaining an additional 10 per cent of the variance (Fries *et al*. 1980, 1982). From this, it was inferred that the resulting disability index (an equal weight sum) is well-focused and appropriate for measuring overall arthritis severity.

Bombardier and co-workers' (1986) study reported the HAQ to be the measure of choice because it was superior or equal to other measures in relation to its sensitivity to treatment, and because of its brevity and ease of administration and scoring.

Reliability

Fries *et al*. (1980) reported early tests for reliability, which were based on just 20 patient volunteers attending an RA clinic. The correlations for individual items for self-administration *vs* interviewer-administered HAQ ranged from average (or 'respectable') to excellent (0.56–0.85). The corresponding correlation for the disability score was 0.85, indicating good reliability for this component. The inter-item correlations ranged from 0.47 to 0.88. The weaker items (e.g. reach) were subsequently reworded to minimize variability in responses. For example, the question on 'reach' originally read 'reach and get down heavy objects'. The respondents' ideas of 'heavy' varied widely and so a standardized item was constructed: 'reach and get down a 5 lb bag of sugar which is above your head'. The authors also compared overall questionnaire and evaluator agreement; these agreed exactly in 59 per cent of cases and were within one point in 93 per cent of cases (the weighted kappa statistic result, using rank disagreement rates, was 0.52, implying 'moderate' agreement).

Fries *et al*. (1982) reported a test–retest correlation of 0.98, based on 331 people. The mean values showed stability on repeat testing. The responses are similar whether the instrument is self-administered or administered by a nurse or doctor.

The HAQ is a good measure of function, and has been extensively tested for reliability and validity. It is concise, sensitive to change, can be self- or interviewer-administered, and is suitable for use in the community. It has been used extensively among clinicians in the USA and Europe.

ARTHRITIS IMPACT MEASUREMENT SCALES (AIMS)

The AIMS is a slightly broader scale than the HAQ and other 'ADL' scales in common use. The content of AIMS overlaps by about two-thirds with the Health Assessment Questionnaire (HAQ). The scale was revised in 1990, and the new version is called AIMS-2.

The original version, AIMS-1, and the second revised version, AIMS-2, were developed by Meenan et al. (1980) and Meenan and Mason (1990). AIMS was partly adapted from Katz's Index of Daily Living, the Rand and Bush scales (Patrick et al. 1973; Brook et al. 1979a, 1979b; Ware et al 1979; Bush 1984). This measure aims to assess patient outcome in arthritis and other chronic diseases. It covers physical, social and emotional well-being.

Content

AIMS-1

The original AIMS-1 had 45 multiple-choice items, with nine sub-scales. It assessed nine dimensions of health and functional ability: mobility, physical activity (walking, bending, lifting), activities of daily living, dexterity, household activities (management of money, medication, housekeeping), pain, social activity, depression and anxiety. An additional 19 items covered general health, health perceptions and demographic details (e.g. a visual analogue item that assessed the respondent's overall health rating; perceived susceptibility to illness; other diseases present and treatment).

A shortened version of AIMS-1 was produced, which appears to have retained adequate internal consistency, test–retest reliability and concurrent and predictive validity, similar to those achieved with the longer version (Wallston et al. 1989).

AIMS-2

The revised instrument, AIMS-2, is a 78-item questionnaire; some new items have been added and others have been deleted. The first 57 items

form 12 scales: mobility level, walking and bending, hand and finger function, arm function, self-care tasks, household tasks, social activity, social support, pain from arthritis, work, level of tension and mood. The remaining items relate to satisfaction with health status in each of the areas of functioning measured, functional problems due to arthritis, prioritization of the three areas in which the respondent would most like to see improvement, general health perceptions, overall impact of arthritis in each of the areas of functioning measured, type and duration of arthritis, medication usage, co-morbidity and sociodemographic characteristics (Meenan and Mason 1990). Most questions refer to problems experienced within the last month.

Administration and scoring

The AIMS-2, like AIMS-1, is self-administered, and takes approximately 20 min to complete. The items are listed in Guttman scale order, so that a respondent who indicates a disability on one item will also indicate disability on section items falling below it. Unlike AIMS-1, which had a combination of dichotomous 'yes/no' and scale response categories, AIMS-2 has mainly scaled response choices. Scale scores are summed, the range of scores depending on the number of items in the sub-scale. No item weights are used. A 'normalization procedure' converts scores into the range 0–10, with 0 representing good 'health status' and 10 representing poor 'health status' (AIMS-1 and AIMS-2). The scale is ordinal in type and has been described as superior to other applications of Guttman scaling (McDowell and Newell 1987).

Examples from AIMS-2

During the past month:

5 How often were you in a bed or chair for most or all of the day?
6 Did you have trouble doing vigorous activities such as running, lifting heavy objects, or participating in strenuous sports?
12 Could you easily button a shirt or blouse?
29 How often did you get together with friends or relatives?
39 How often did you have severe pain from your arthritis?

44 How often were you unable to do any paid work, housework or schoolwork?

All days (1) / most days (2) / some days (3) / few days (4) / no days (5)

48 How often have you felt tense or strung up?

54 How often have you been in low or very low spirits?

Always (1) / very often (2) / sometimes (3) / almost never (4) / never (5)

Validity and factor structure

While the scaling properties, validity and reliability of AIMS-2 have been reported to be satisfactory with initial tests, most information on the psychometric properties of AIMS comes from the extensive work carried out on AIMS-1 (Meenan and Mason 1990). Given that items have been revised, deleted and some new items have been added, and given that most responses are now scaled, it is uncertain to what extent the results from AIMS-1 apply to AIMS-2. The results for AIMS-1 are reported below.

AIMS-1 was tested extensively for reliability and validity (Meenan et al. 1980, 1982, 1984; Meenan 1982, 1985; Brown et al. 1984). AIMS-1 was tested for validity on a sample of 625 English-speaking patients with various rheumatic diseases, drawn from 15 different clinical establishments in ten US states. No major problems with the administration occurred. All nine of the AIMS-1 scales were weakly to moderately (all significant) correlated with two physician-derived general standards of health status – the American Rheumatism Association Function Scale ($r = 0.24–0.52$) and disease status ($r = 0.14–0.52$). The AIMS-1 scales were also correlated with clinical rheumatology standards: walking time, grip strength, joint count, range of motion. The items measuring physical well-being (mobility, physical activity, dexterity, household activities, activities of daily living) were more highly correlated with these physical standards than were the AIMS psychological and social scales (e.g. dexterity correlated highly with grip strength; mobility and physical activity were most strongly related to walking time).

The authors reported that single scale factor analyses demonstrated that each set of AIMS-1 items except household activities loaded strongly on a single factor. This indicated that the group items represented a coherent scale. The nine AIMS-1 items were grouped into three discrete factors in relation to health status: physical function, psychological function and pain. More recent developments by its authors include a 4-factor and a 5-factor model, developed from studies of 360 RA patients, on the grounds that these are more likely to reflect the major dimensions of health status and represent a fuller assessment of health status. In the 5-factor model, the physical dimension of AIMS-1 exhibits separate upper extremity and lower extremity components. The fourth factor, primarily represented by the pain scale, reflects the added arthritis symptom measure (Mason et al. 1988).

The sensitivity of AIMS-1 was assessed by comparing it with standard clinical outcome measures (joint counts for tenderness and swelling, grip strength, physician assessments of disease activity and functional class) in a double-blind, multi-centre clinical drug trial based on 161 patients (Meenan et al. 1984). Using AIMS, differences between treatments were found for physical activity, anxiety, depression, pain and the overall impact using the visual analogue scale item. The findings were consistent with other studies of the same treatments and demonstrated that AIMS is sensitive enough to detect clinically meaningful differences in treatment outcomes. It was as sensitive as traditional clinical measures, and also indicated additional differences not detected by standard approaches.

AIMS-1 was used by Weinberger et al. (1990) in a study of 439 patients with osteoarthritis, and they reported a strong association between poor self-esteem and a poor AIMS-1 score. A study administering the HAQ and the AIMS-1 to patients with RA demonstrated that the scales measured similar dimensions of health status. The instruments were highly correlated, providing further support for the convergent validity of the scale. These analyses supported the existence of three relatively discrete components of health status: pain, physical disability and psychological status (Brown et al. 1984).

Reliability

AIMS-1 was tested for reliability on a sample of 625 English-speaking patients with various rheumatic diseases, drawn from 15 different clinical establishments in ten US states. No major problems with AIMS emerged with comprehension or administration. Coefficients of scalability and reliability on all nine of the AIMS-1 scales exceeded 0.60 and 0.90 respectively for all but the household activity scale (this had a reproducibility coefficient of 0.88). The test–retest correlation across all nine scale items was 0.87. These results indicate good internal consistency, strong hierarchical scale properties and test–retest stability. The tests for reliability and validity were repeated on a variety of subjects in different demographic, functional and diagnostic categories (AIMS-1). Most reliability coefficients were reported as meeting or exceeding accepted criteria. The pattern of validity correlations was maintained (Meenan *et al.* 1980, 1982; Meenan 1982; Brown *et al.* 1984).

While cross-cultural results for reliability and validity are generally supportive of AIMS, its original social activity and activities of daily living (ADL) sub-scales, unlike the remaining sub-scales, did not achieve satisfactory levels of reliability and validity in a study of Hispanics, whites of Eastern European origin and Blacks in the USA (Coulton *et al.* 1989).

AIMS-1 has been adapted and used to measure and compare health status across chronic disease groups, although its sub-scales were not all able to distinguish between these groups (Brown *et al.* 1984; Meenan 1985). Since its initial development, the three-component model of AIMS-1 has been used in many studies (Kazis *et al.* 1983, 1988; Meenan *et al.* 1984; Mason *et al.* 1988). It has been applied predominantly in clinical settings (with arthritis and rheumatism patients) as an assessment of outcome after therapy.

In sum, AIMS has good measurement properties, has been extensively tested for validity, and the identified dimensions explain the majority of illness impact estimated by patients. AIMS-2 promises to be a superior instrument. The AIMS scales are strictly copyrighted.

FUNCTIONAL STATUS INDEX (FSI)

This scale assesses the degree of dependence, pain and difficulty of arthritis sufferers living in the community. The scale's authors were critical of existing measures which emphasized (in)dependence at the expense of other domains (e.g. pain and degree of difficulty), and used broad categories when several complex activities were involved (Deniston and Jette 1980).

Content

The FSI comprises 135 questions on functioning, although a more commonly used short version is available (see below). For the assessment of dependency, the respondent is asked in relation to each item 'How much help did you use, on the average, during the past week to . . .'; for pain, the respondent is asked to use a ladder scale to rate 'the amount of pain you experienced when doing each activity on the average, last week'; for difficulty, the respondent is asked to 'make a check on the rung of the ladder which best represents the degree of ease or difficulty you experienced when performing each activity, on the average during the past seven days'.

A long 45-item and a short 18-item version are available, each containing three dimensions (i.e. 135 and 54 questions in total, respectively). The long version comprises 45 questions on each activity in relation to dependence, pain and difficulties, and fixed-choice responses with 4-point scales for pain and difficulty items, and a 5-point response scale for the dependency dimension.

Short form

The more commonly used short version measures the same three dimensions – dependency, pain and difficulties – in 18 activities of daily living grouped under five headings: mobility (3 items), hand activities (3 items), personal care (4 items), home chores (4 items) and interpersonal activities (4 items) (Jette and Deniston 1978; Deniston and Jette 1980; Jette 1980a). The questions are again repeated three times in relation to each of the three domains. For the 18-item version, 4-point scales are used for dependency (used no help, used equipment, used human assistance, used equipment and human assistance), and the pain and level of difficulty dimensions use either a 0–7 or 0–13 ladder scale.

Administration and scoring

The FSI is administered by an interviewer. The

longer 45-item version is less often used as it takes 60–90 min to complete (Jette 1980a, 1980b); the shorter 18-item version takes only 20–30 min to administer. The authors do not recommend computing an overall score for all dimensions and activities, but advise the analysis of sub-scale scores. One rating score is computed within each dimension (dependence, difficulty, pain) for each group of activities. The three sub-scale scores are computed by adding the scores for each activity within that domain.

Examples from the 18-Item FSI

Mobility

Walking inside
Climbing stairs
Chair transfer

Personal care

Washing all parts of body
Putting on pants
Putting on shirt
Buttoning shirt

Hand range

Opening containers
Writing
Dialling a telephone

Home tasks

Laundry
Reaching into low cupboards
Yardwork
Vacuuming a rug

Social activities

Driving a car
Visiting family/friends
Going to meetings
Work

Response codes

Assistance: 1 = independent, 2 = uses devices, 3 = uses human assistance, 4 = uses devices and human assistance, 5 = unable or unsafe to do activity

Pain: 1 = no pain, 2 = mild pain, 3 = moderate pain, 4 = severe pain

Difficulty: 1 = no difficulty, 2 = mild difficulty, 3 = moderate difficulty, 4 = severe difficulty

Validity

Liang *et al.* (1985, 1990) administered five health status measurements to 50 patients with arthritis before and after total joint arthroplasty: the FSI, the Health Assessment Questionnaire (HAQ: Fries *et al.* 1980), the Arthritis Impact Measurement Scale (AIMS: Meenan *et al.* 1980, 1982), the Quality of Well-Being Questionnaire (Kaplan *et al.* 1976) and part of the Sickness Impact Profile (SIP: Bergner *et al.* 1976a). Each instrument detected statistically significant improvements in *mobility* post-surgical intervention, with the AIMS, the FSI and the SIP being most sensitive. In relation to *pain*, the AIMS, HAQ and FSI measured this and all were sensitive to post-surgical improvements. The FSI performed best, with the AIMS performing almost as well, and the HAQ had the lowest efficiency. All the instruments except the AIMS detected improvements in *social functioning*, with the most efficient being the FSI. All the measurement scales had finely graded measurements for *global functioning*, and all registered post-surgical improvements. The FSI and HAQ, however, were less sensitive than the SIP, AIMS or Quality of Well-Being Questionnaire, possibly due to their failure to include a pain measure within the global indexes. The FSI, while being efficient for most dimensions, was weaker on the global rating. Validity correlations between the FSI and patient and staff ratings have been reported to be low (Deniston and Jette 1980). Jette (1980a) carried out a factor analysis and reported five factors: mobility, transfer, home chores, kitchen chores and personal care.

Reliability

Studies with RA patients show a high level of inter-observer reliability (Jette 1980a). Inter-rater agreement among nine raters was acceptable with intra-class correlations averaging 0.72–0.78 for dependency, 0.61–0.75 for difficulty and 0.75–0.78 for pain. Test–retest reliability coefficients for the three dimensions ranged from 0.69 to 0.77 (Jette and Deniston 1978; Liang and Jette 1981). Internal consistency reliability coefficients ranged from 0.70 to over 0.90 (Jette 1980b). The tests for the reliability and the validity of the 18-item version showed adequate results, although the internal consistency of hand activity items was weak (Jette 1980a; Harris *et al.* 1986).

The authors have also developed the Functional Status Questionnaire (FSQ), based on the FSI, the SIP and the Rand Functional Status Indexes (Jette and Cleary 1987). The similarity of their names and domains has created some confusion between the two. The distinction in aims is that the FSQ was designed for use with ambulatory patients in primary care settings, although evidence of its psychometric properties is still limited (Jette *et al.* 1986).

WESTERN ONTARIO AND McMASTER UNIVERSITIES ARTHRITIS INDEX (WOMAC)

The Western Ontario and McMaster Universities Arthritis Index (WOMAC: Bellamy 1988) assesses osteoarthritis-related disability in the hip and knee only. The scale was developed on the basis of a search of the literature, and on the views of 100 patients about relevant dimensions The original version also included social and emotional components. However, these were not retained after testing due to poor results.

Content

The scale consists of three sub-scales: pain (5 items: walking, stair climbing, nocturnal, rest, weight-bearing), stiffness (2 items: morning stiffness, stiffness occurring later in the day) and physical function (17 items: descending stairs, ascending stairs, rising from sitting, standing, bending to floor, walking on flat, getting in/out of car, going shopping, putting on socks, rising from bed, taking off socks, lying in bed, getting in/out of bath, sitting, getting on/off toilet, heavy domestic duties, light domestic duties).

The responses to the items on functioning are in the form of 5-point Likert scales where 0 = none, 1 = mild, 2 = moderate, 3 = severe and 4 = extreme. Some investigators have used a VAS for the responses.

Administration and scoring

The scale is self-administered and the item responses within each sub-scale are summed to give three separate scores.

Examples from the WOMAC

Section A

The following questions concern the amount of pain you are currently experiencing due to arthritis in your hips and/or knees. For each situation please enter the amount of pain recently experienced. (Please mark your answers with an 'X')

How much pain do you have:

1 Walking on a flat surface?
5 Standing upright?

None / mild / moderate / severe / extreme

Section B

The following questions concern the amount of joint stiffness (not pain) you are currently experiencing in your hips and/or knees. Stiffness is a sensation of restriction or slowness in the ease with which you move your joints. (Please mark your answers with an 'X')

2 How severe is your stiffness after sitting, lying or resting later in the day?

None / mild / moderate / severe / extreme

Section C

The following questions concern your physical function. By this we mean your ability to move around and to look after yourself. For each of the following activities, please indicate the degree of difficulty you are currently experiencing due to arthritis in your hips and/or knees. (Please mark your answers with an 'X')

What degree of difficulty do you have with:

5 Bending to floor?
8 Going shopping?
9 Pulling on socks/stockings?
15 Getting on/off the toilet?
17 Light domestic duties?

None / mild / moderate / severe / extreme

Validity and reliability

Research in Toronto among 254 patients following hip replacement and 88 patients following knee replacement by Young *et al.* (1994) indicated that five of the items in the WOMAC scale were of questionable value in terms of the homogeneity of the scale and the hierarchical ordering of items in terms of difficulty. Once these were removed, the scale was able to discriminate between the two types of patients in relation to functioning. The WOMAC was more sensitive to improvements following surgery than the Rand SF-36 physical functioning sub-scale, which was also used (Ware et al. 1993). Research is continuing on the validity of the scale and the relative responsiveness of the VAS and Likert scales used (Bellamy et al. 1988). The scale was tested for reliability on 57 patients with symptomatic osteoarthritis of the hip or knee. The final version of the scale has adequate test–retest reliability and good internal consistency ($\alpha = 0.85$ or over, except for pain where $\alpha = 0.73$). For example, the internal consistency of the physical functioning scale was 0.95, and that of seven items which used VAS scales 0.89–0.91. Test–retest reliability coefficients at 1 week for the stiffness scale was 0.48 on the Likert scale and 0.61 on the VAS. Test–retest reliability for the physical functioning sub-scale was 0.68 on the Likert Scale and 0.72 on the VAS scale.

OFFICE OF POPULATION CENSUSES AND SURVEYS (OPCS) DISABILITY SCALE

This scale was designed by Martin et al. (1988) for the national OPCS disability survey in the UK. The survey aimed to cover the disabilities in WHO's (1980) International Classification of Impairments, Disabilities and Handicaps. The main concept for the study was disability, although some information was also collected about the extent of handicap resulting from the disability (particularly financial), and impairment as a consequence of disease or disorder was included (operationalized as pain and suffering, such as anxiety and depression).

The questionnaire used to generate the scales was a household questionnaire (including institutions), and therefore the questions are phrased in relation to any household member (e.g. 'Does anyone in your household have the following difficulties . . .?').

Postal Screening Disability Questionnaire

This Questionnaire included difficulties in abilities (e.g. reaching and stretching, hearing, bending and

straightening) (12 questions); health problems and disabilities which limit activities (6 questions); long-term health problems or disabilities (8 questions); service use/special care/help (3 questions) and dependency (3 questions); child health and disabilities (5 questions); other difficulties (1 question with filter items).

This instrument was designed to screen people with low disability levels for the purposes of the survey, in order to avoid excluding anyone who was sufficiently disabled and should have been included. The questions were designed to include people with disabilities that were likely to have a significant effect on their ability to carry out normal everyday activities. Anyone with any of these problems was eligible for inclusion in the sampling frame for the second assessment by personal interview in order to obtain information about the cause of their disabilities, and to check on the accuracy of replies to the postal screen.

Severity scale

A severity scale of disability was constructed, defined as the extent to which a person's performance of activities is limited by impairments. This was quite complex and innovatory. The construction of the questionnaire was carefully carried out, based on literature reviews, and tested on OPCS staff, Department of Health staff, doctors, physiotherapists, occupational therapists, psychologists, etc., and also involved panels of judges to establish scales of severity of disability (professional survey researchers, members of relevant voluntary bodies and sufferers and their carers).

The severity scale includes a number of subscales, each with severity scores (see p. 224): locomotion (13 points on the scale, with severity scores of 0.5–11.5), reaching and stretching (10 points, with severity scores of 1.0–9.5), dexterity (11 points, with severity scores of 0.5–10.5), personal care (6 points, with severity scores of 1.0–11.0), continence (11 points, with severity scores of 1.0–11.5), seeing (9 points, with severity scores of 0.5–12.0), hearing (8 points, with severity scores of 0.5–11.0), communication (5 points, with severity scores of 1.0–12.0), behaviour (8 points, with severity scores of 0.5–10.5), intellectual functioning (11 points, with severity scores of 1.0–13.0), consciousness (14 points, with severity scores of 0.5–13.8), eating, drinking and digestion (1 point, with a severity score of 0.5) and disfigurement (1 point, with a severity score of 0.5).

Examples of the OPCS severity scales

Locomotion (severity score in brackets)

L1 Cannot walk at all (11.5)
L2 Can only walk a few steps without stopping or severe discomfort/cannot walk up and down one step (9.5)
L3 Has fallen 12 or more times in the last year (7.5)
L4 Always needs to hold on to something to keep balance (7.0)
L5 Cannot walk up and down a flight of 12 stairs (6.5)
L6 Cannot walk 50 yards without stopping or severe discomfort (5.5)
L7 Cannot bend down far enough to touch knees and straighten up again (4.5)
L8 Cannot bend down and pick something up from the floor and straighten up again (4.0)
L9 Cannot walk 200 yards without stopping or severe discomfort/can only walk up and down a flight of 12 stairs if holds on and takes a rest/often needs to hold on to something to keep balance/has fallen 3 or more times in the last year (3.0)
L10 Can only walk up and down a flight of 12 stairs if holds on (doesn't need a rest) (2.5)
L11 Cannot bend down to sweep up something from the floor and straighten up again (2.0)
L12 Can only walk up and down a flight of stairs if goes sideways or one step at a time (1.5)
L13 Cannot walk 100 yards without stopping or severe discomfort (0.5)

Intellectual functioning

The severity score is calculated by adding up the number of reported problems that correspond to the list below:

	Severity score	Number of problems
I1	13.0	11
I2	12.0	10
I3	10.5	9
I4	9.5	8
I5	8.0	7
I6	7.0	6
I7	6.0	5
I8	4.5	4
I9	3.5	3
I10	2.0	2
I11	1.0	1

Number of problems from the following

Often forgets what was supposed to be doing in the middle of something
Often loses track of what is being said in the middle of a conversation
Thoughts tend to be muddled or slow
Often gets confused about what time of day it is
Cannot watch a 30 min tv programme all the way through and tell someone what it was about
Cannot remember and pass on a message correctly
Often forgets to turn things off such as fires, cookers or taps
Often forgets the names of people in the family or friends seen regularly
Cannot read a short article in newspaper
Cannot write a short letter to someone without help
Cannot count well enough to handle money

The screening postal and interview questionnaires were not intended to be used by other researchers; their function was to generate the scales which other researchers can use in their interview questionnaires, prefaced by the appropriate question – for example, Can you do . . . (then go down the scale until the appropriate point for them is located)?

No permission is needed to use the questions, as OPCS regards them as public access, although intending users can contact them for advice. While the measures were carefully and ingeniously designed, there is no published information about their reliability, validity and sensitivity to change. OPCS still hope to carry out more testing in the future.

RHEUMATOID ARTHRITIS (RA) IMPACT ON THE HOMEMAKER QUESTIONNAIRE

Certain social roles have been ignored by most scale developers. Perhaps the most important omission is the measurement of the impact on the nurturant and instrumental care of children, probably because most scales were developed with older adults in mind; also, the care of other dependents has been neglected (e.g. older parents or spouses). Reisine *et al.* (1987) attempted to correct this imbalance for RA sufferers by developing the RA Impact on the Homemaker Scale.

Content, administration and scoring

This is a 13-item scale, with a range of response formats (including 'yes/no' answers, scales of 0–10 and categorical frequency ratings). It asks respondents if their condition affects the amount of time they take over various domestic tasks, the amount of childcare they undertake, and their satisfaction with their ability to care for their children. The nurturant dimension of the 'homemaker' role assesses how the respondents' condition affects, and their satisfaction with, their abilities in relation to listening/comforting and helping people solve their problems; making arrangements for others/taking them to places; maintaining social ties; any teaching or instructing; and with visiting or caring for sick people. Satisfaction ratings were not included for the last two items so as to limit the length of the questionnaire. The questionnaire also asks whether the disease has affected the respondents' sexual drive, activities, hobbies and personal interests. The scale's authors used items from the HAQ for the assessment of physical functioning. The questionnaire was designed for administration by an interviewer, and the items are summed within each scale. The scoring has not been fully clarified or tested.

Examples from the Homemaker Questionnaire

Instrumental dimension

1 Has arthritis caused changes in the amount of cooking (cleaning, shopping and errands) you do?

1 = Yes, more now / 2 = Yes, less now / 3 = No, about the same

2 Has arthritis changed the amount of time you spend cooking (cleaning, doing shopping and errands)?

1 = Yes, more now / 2 = Yes, less now / 3 = No, about the same

5 On a scale of 0–10, where 0 = not at all satisfied and 10 = completely satisfied, how satisfied are you that you are now able to do the amount of cooking (cleaning, shopping and errands) that you feel you ought to?

Nurturant dimension

1 Thinking about the way parents take care of children, supervising them and tending to their needs, has your arthritis changed the amount of time that you spend taking care of your children or changed the amount of child care that you do?   Yes/no

4 On a scale of 0–10, how satisfied are you that you are able to take care of your children the way you feel you ought?

5 Has arthritis affected the amount of time you spend comforting, listening or helping other people solve their problems (making arrangements, maintaining ties with others)?

1 = Yes, much less now / 2 = Yes, somewhat less / 3 = No, it's about the same / 4 = Somewhat more now / 5 = Much more now

Validity and reliability

Reisine *et al.* (1987) administered the scale to 142 women who were living with their spouse and/or dependent children and attending an arthritis outpatient clinic. While frequency distributions for the questionnaire have been presented by the authors, it has not been fully tested for its psychometric properties. This is a pity given their thoughtful approach to measurement.

BROADER DISEASE-SPECIFIC QUALITY OF LIFE SCALES

MACTAR (McMASTER–TORONTO ARTHRITIS) PATIENT FUNCTION PREFERENCE QUESTIONNAIRE

This questionnaire was developed by Tugwell and his colleagues in Canada. It is an individualized measure, which aims to address whether improvement has occurred in the leading physical disabilities that interfere most with activities of daily living, as well as the effects that the individual patient would most like to see improved by therapy (Tugwell *et al.* 1987, 1990). It is a patient preference disability questionnaire.

The questionnaire was developed with 50 consecutive rheumatology out-patient attenders who had strictly defined RA. Tugwell *et al.* (1990) used the McMaster Health Questionnaire, MACTAR and standard clinical measures (grip strength, walking time, etc.) in a double-blind, randomized drug trial of rheumatoid arthritis with 95 patients for the intervention and 94 patients for the placebo.

Tugwell *et al.* (1987) noted that there was considerable variation in the activities described by patients and their relative importance in relation to the impact of arthritis, many of which do not appear in conventional ADL questionnaires.

Content, administration and scoring

The scale is administered by an interviewer. Patients are asked to identify activities related to mobility, self-care, work, and social and leisure activity. Patients are then asked to rank these activities in the order in which they would most prefer to have them improved. They are then asked at the end of the study if there has been any improvement in these ranked disabilities. The response format is category scaling.

The MACTAR is scored by awarding +1 for improvement, 0 for no change and −1 for deterioration for each item. The scores are then standardized to index values ranging from 0.0 (worst function) to 1.0 (optimal function).

Examples from MACTAR

Baseline

2 Does your arthritis limit:
   (a) Any other activities around the house, such as getting around, cooking, housework, dressing, etc.?
   (d) Any (other) social activities, such as visiting, playing cards, going to church, etc.

3 Which of these activities would you most like to be able to do without the pain or discomfort of your arthritis?

Follow-up

Each of the disabilities identified at baseline is reviewed as follows:

Since the first interview 8 weeks ago have you noticed any change in your ability to _____?   No/yes
If yes, has your ability to _____ improved or become worse?

Validity and reliability

The MACTAR correlated with the McMaster Health Index Questionnaire physical function sub-section ($r = 0.53$), the emotional sub-section ($r =$ 0.39) and the social sub-section ($r = 0.35$). The correlations with the other outcome measures used (e.g. joint pain/tenderness count, joint swelling, grip strength, doctors' assessments of disease activity and disease-specific functional ability questions) ranged from $r = -0.33$ to 0.52 (Tugwell *et al.* 1990). The low correlations suggest that the measures are tapping different dimensions and cannot be substituted for each other.

The questionnaire was responsive to change and able to detect clinically important changes (more responsive than some of the clinical end-points used) probably because of the emphasis on 'transition' rather than being based on 'single state' questions. A relative efficiency analysis indicated that both the McMaster Health Index and the MACTAR were as (or more) efficient at achieving statistical significance than some of the clinical end-points used. The authors concluded that their results supported the suggestion that patient preference questionnaires have an important place in determining treatment outcomes (Feinstein *et al.* 1986). There is little information about its reliability to date. It is in the early stages of testing.

Tugwell *et al.* (1987) suggested that the MACTAR should be regarded as a complementary scale to conventional ADL questionnaires, and combined with them rather than substituted for them. As the MACTAR focuses primarily on physical and social functioning, it should also be complemented with a broader health-related quality of life scale, or with independent scales which measure missing but required domains (e.g. psychological functioning and emotional well-being, social support, coping and adjustment). Psychometric testing of the MACTAR is continuing, and a self-completion version is being developed. The advantage of the MACTAR is that the results relate to individual patients' values and has applications in individual patient care, as well as in research studies.

HÖRNQUIST'S QUALITY OF LIFE STATUS AND CHANGE SCALE

This scale was developed for use with a variety of conditions, including diabetes (see Chapter 8; Hörnquist and Elton 1983; Akerlind *et al.* 1987; Hörnquist 1989; Hörnquist *et al.* 1990, 1992; Hanestad *et al.* 1991), but has been successfully tailored for use with patients with rheumatoid arthritis (Bendtsen and Hörnquist 1992). It is derived from a model of quality of life based on perceived needs and satisfaction within six domains: somatic, psychological, social, behavioural/activity, structural and material.

Content

The version adapted for use as a disease-specific scale with rheumatoid arthritis patients contains the following items: somatic (RA symptoms, 1 item); general health (2 items); psychological (well-being, 1 item); cognition (2 items); social (social contacts in general, 1 item); family life (2 items); sex life (3 items); behavioural/activity (ability to live an active life, 1 item); capacity for self-care (2 items); work capacity (3 items); basic habits (4 items); structural (position in society, 1 item); ability to live a meaningful life (2 items); life satisfaction (3 items); material (material assets, 1 item); residence (2 items); capacity for self-support (3 items).

Administration and scoring

The scale can be self-administered. An overall quality of life index is calculated from the means of sub-scale scores (grand mean score). The disease-specific symptom item (on joint pain and swelling) is analysed separately. Sub-scale scores vary from −3 (very bad/deteriorated), through 0 (neither nor/unchanged) to +3 (very good/much improved), except for change in the somatic section where scores range from 0 to −3. Respondents are asked to rate their quality of life currently, and then dynamically (in order to measure, retrospectively, the intrusion of RA on their quality of life). Two questionnaires are given to respondents for the static and dynamic perspectives.

Examples from Hörnquist's Scale

My bodily health is:

greatly improved
clearly improved
somewhat improved
unaffected
somewhat worse
clearly worse
greatly worse

Now, my bodily health is:

very good
good
rather good
neither good nor bad
rather bad
bad
very bad

Validity

Bendtsen and Hörnquist (1992) tested the scale on over 200 patients with possible, probable and definite RA in Sweden. Inter-item correlations on physical, psychological and social well-being ranged from around 0.45 to 0.48. The greatest effects of RA on quality of life were, as would be expected, on physical functioning, and behavioural and activity domains. Patients' spouses were also asked to complete the questionnaire on the patients' behalf. The Pearson correlations between spouses' and patients' assessments on each dimension ranged from 0.47 to 0.63. Patients' ratings of their quality of life were consistently higher than their quality of life as perceived by their spouses. Their psychological dysfunction, as assessed by the scale, was not as great as suggested by previous studies using other scales (e.g. the SIP used by Sullivan *et al.* 1986). It is possible that the Hörnquist Scale is insufficiently sensitive, perhaps due to its brevity.

The original scale score, which was a measure of well-being, was tested for various groups of respondents against external raters' judgements of well-being, with low to moderate correlations between the respondent and the rater of between −0.2 to 0.59 (Hörnquist 1989).

Reliability

The internal consistency alphas for the well-being sub-scales ranged from 0.39 to 0.90; split-half reliability ranged widely from 0.10 to 0.90; inter-item correlations for the well-being sub-scales ranged from −0.00 to 0.73 (Hörnquist 1989).

The scale still requires extensive testing with disease-specific patient populations (Hörnquist and Elton 1983; Akerlind *et al.* 1987; Hörnquist 1989; Hörnquist *et al.* 1990; 1992; Hanestad *et al.* 1991).

SCHEDULE FOR THE EVALUATION OF INDIVIDUAL QUALITY OF LIFE (SEIQoL)

SEIQoL was devised from human judgement analysis to measure patients' health-related quality of life in five self-nominated areas of life (O'Boyle *et al*. 1992). SEIQoL is a relatively new method which quantifies the quality of life of an individual. SEIQoL, while not a disease-specific measure, can be applied to specific conditions such that it will produce disease-specific results. It requires supplementing with disease-specific items on symptoms and level of functioning. It has been used successfully with patients undergoing hip replacement, along with the McMaster Health Index Questionnaire (Chambers *et al*. 1982) and a disease-specific measure of functioning, the AIMS (Meenan *et al*. 1980).

In research on hip replacement, social/leisure activities and family were nominated most frequently by both patients and controls; happiness, religion, independence and finances were also nominated. Health was nominated more frequently by controls than patients (O'Boyle *et al*. 1992). Among a healthy population, relationships, health, family and finances were the most frequently nominated (by over 50 per cent), and among gastrointestinal clinic attenders, family, work, social and leisure activities, and health were the most frequently nominated domains (McGee *et al*. 1991).

Content, administration and scoring

Respondents are asked to list the five areas of life ('elicited cues') that they judge to be most important to their overall quality of life. Open-ended questions are used to elicit the relevant cues. Respondents rate their current status on each cue against a vertical visual analogue scale labelled at either end with 'as good as could possibly be' and 'as bad as could possibly be'. These ratings are then tabulated by the interviewer on five vertical bars. Respondents are then asked to rate their global quality of life on a single VAS, similarly labelled. The authors of the scale have developed a disc with which respondents weight each elicited cue. A scoring procedure for deriving overall quality of life for each respondent has been devised (O'Boyle *et al*. 1993). The scoring instructions are available

from the authors, and a computer program is also available for the analysis.

Examples from the SEIQoL

1 What are the five most important areas of your life at present – the things which make your life a relatively happy or sad one at the moment . . . the things that you feel determine the quality of your life?
2 Now that you have named the five most important areas in your life, I am going to ask you to rate how each of these areas are for you at the moment. First, I will show you an example of how the rating is done . . .

Validity and reliability

The scale was applied by O'Boyle *et al*. (1992) in a prospective intervention study of 20 patients undergoing unilateral total hip replacement surgery, with a 6 month follow-up. Comparisons were made with matched, non-patient controls. The scale showed improvements in scores after surgery.

The judgement reliability of the scale ranges from moderate to high (but is usually reported to be above 0.53) (McGee *et al*. 1991). A strong case could be made for the use of this scale as the core component of disease-specific measures, although more work is required on its acceptability to people in view of its potential complexity. A manual, which also summarizes the results of further tests of reliability and validity, has been produced, and is available from the authors.

HEALTH OUTCOMES INSTITUTE TyPE SCALES (HOI-TyPE) – JOINT CONDITIONS

TyPE condition-specific questionnaires have been developed for rheumatoid arthritis, hip fracture, hip replacement and osteoarthritis of the knee. They were developed by experts in the field who are well known for the development of rheumatology health status and functional ability measures. They still await the results of psychometric testing.

Each condition-specific set of measurements includes a questionnaire for patients and a form(s) for the clinicians to complete. The patients' forms are supplemented in each case with the Rand SF-36 health status scale (Ware *et al.* 1993). The forms are designed for repeated application (at follow-ups), unless otherwise stated and another follow-up form provided. The scales are self-administered. The scoring varies by question.

The Health Outcomes Institute, previously Interstudy (2001 Killebrew Drive, Suite 122, Bloomington, MN 55425, USA), has published the scales.

Rheumatoid arthritis

The rheumatoid arthritis form for patients has ten questions on two sides. They cover functional status (4 items), pain (2 items), limitation on activities (3 items), activity of the arthritis (1 item) and self-assessment of how well the patient is doing (1 item).

The clinician completes two forms – one for the initial examination and one at follow-up (total four sides) – covering diagnosis, symptoms, clinical indicators, medication and complications (drug toxicity).

Examples from the HOI-TyPE – Joint Conditions

Rheumatoid arthritis

Patients' form

4 Can you easily button articles of clothing?   Yes/no
7 During the past month, how often have you had severe pain from your arthritis?

Always / very often / fairly often / sometimes / almost never / never

8 At the present time, how much does your arthritis:

 (b) limit you from getting around the community?

No limitation / slightly limits me / moderately limits me / greatly limits me / totally limits me

---

Hip fracture

The baseline and post-fracture forms for patients are identical. They contain four questions on two sides. It covers limitation on activities (5 items), pain (1 item) and background details (place of residence, 1 item). The clinician's form (two sides) covers the type and severity of the fracture, cause, other conditions and treatment, including treatment effects. The clinician also completes one question at 12 months after the hip fracture on complications since discharge (e.g. hip joint or wound infection, non-union, etc.).

Examples from the HOI-TyPE – Joint Conditions

Hip fracture

Patients' form: baseline

2 During the 4 weeks immediately prior to the fracture, how frequently did the hip that was fractured cause you difficulty with the following activities?

 (a) Stooping or bending
 (c) Sitting in a chair
 (e) Walking while outdoors

Never / rarely / sometimes / often / always

Hip replacement

The patients' baseline questionnaire has 16 questions on three sides. They cover limitation of activities due to hip pain (1 item) and stiffness (1 item), physical limitations (1 item), limitations on sexual activity (1 item), limitations on work (1 item), pain (2 items), limitations on relationships (1 item) and other limitations on activities of daily living and type (8 items). The follow-up questionnaire is identical, except with the addition of two

---

Examples from the HOI-TyPE – Joint Conditions

Hip replacement

Patients' form

2 How often does hip pain limit your activities?

Never / once a month or less / 2–3 times a month / about once a week / several days a week / daily

7 How much pain do you have in your hips?

None / mild / moderate / severe

10 How difficult is it for you to put on your shoes and socks?

No trouble / able but difficult / unable

---

questions asking 'How much has your hip pain changed as a result of your hip surgery?' (A lot to A lot worse) and 'To what extent have you resumed your usual activities following your hip replacement?' (A lot to Not at all).

The clinician has to complete one pre-surgical form (two sides) on diagnosis, medication, history, complications, range of motion and leg lengths, and a post-operative form about complications, type of hip replacement, medications and range of motion.

Osteoarthritis of the knee

The patients' questionnaire contains 11 disease-specific questions on two sides, covering functional status (4 questions), knee pain (2) and its interference with sleep (1), medication (1), use of walking aids (1), activity of knee arthritis (1) and a self-assessment on how well the patient has been doing (1). The items are intended to supplement the AIMS.

The clinician has one form to complete (one side) on diagnosis, disease severity, clinical indicators and range of motion. The same form can be used for follow-up evaluations.

Examples from the HOI-TyPE – Joint Conditions

Osteoarthritis of the knee

3 Are you in bed or chair for most or all of the day because of your knee arthritis?   Yes/no
8 During the past month, how often has your knee arthritis pain interfered with your sleeping?

Always / very often / fairly often / sometimes / almost never / never

11 During the past month, how active has your knee arthritis been?

Very active / moderately active / mildly active / not at all active

---

RAND JOINT PROBLEMS BATTERY

The Rand Health Insurance Study (HIS) (sometimes also called the Rand Health Insurance Experiment) involved a large-scale social experiment with 8000 participants in six sites in the USA (assigned to one of 16 different health insurance plans) followed up from 3 to 5 years. It was designed to assess how variations in the cost of patients' health insurance schemes affected use of services, quality of care, satisfaction and health status. The evaluation of patient outcomes is known as the Rand Medical Outcomes Study (MOS). The Rand HIS designed a Medical History (screening) Questionnaire for the more common conditions: gout, rheumatoid arthritis, osteoarthritis, bursitis and tendinitis (Scott *et al*. 1981) entitled the Joint Problems Battery. The questionnaire detects those symptoms and duration periods common to all conditions and those more likely to be condition-specific (Scott *et al*. 1981).

The HIS respondents also underwent a medical examination. Due to the potential unreliability of individual physician assessments of range, swellings, etc., the Rand researchers adopted the common practice of using simple standardized physical assessments for grip strength (e.g. lifting, writing, opening doors, holding on to a stair railing), walking speed and joint size. A common method of assessing grip strength is squeezing a cuff as hard as possible (and the best of three tries is recorded), but the Rand team felt this to be an unreliable and crude method of assessing function of the arm and hands, and rejected this technique.

Content, administration and scoring

The Rand Joint Problems Battery is self-administered. It comprises 15 questions, one of which contains five items. Five questions cover symptoms (pain, swelling, stiffness), one question with five items covering functional ability, five questions cover diagnosis, treatment and medical consultations, and four questions cover disease impact.

The disease impact questions form a standard set of questions used in all the Rand disease-specific batteries. These questions deal with the amount of pain that the condition may have caused, the amount of worry or concern experienced, the amount of time a person's activities have been restricted because of the problem, and the number of days spent in bed attributable to the condition. The first three items refer to the previous 3 months and the last to the previous 30 days.

Responses to the pain, worry and limitations questions range from 'none' to 'a great deal' (or similar wording, depending on the item). A composite item called 'any impact' was constructed, composed of positive responses to the disease impact items. More detailed disease-specific questions are also included in the battery.

Examples from the Rand Joint Problems Battery

64 During the past 12 months, have you had any pain, aching, swelling or stiffness in your joints, for example your fingers, hip or knee? (Do not count problems caused by an injury)   Yes/no

64-D Have you had stiffness in joints or muscles when first getting out of bed, which lasted as long as 15 minutes?   Yes/no

70 During the past 3 months, how much pain has the trouble with your joints or muscles caused you?

A great deal of pain / some pain / a little pain / no pain at all.

71 During the past 3 months, how much has the trouble with your joints or muscles worried or concerned you?

A great deal / somewhat / a little / not at all

72 During the past 3 months, how much of the time has the trouble with your joints or muscles kept you from doing the kinds of things other people your age do?

All of the time / most of the time / some of the time / a little of the time / none of the time

73 During the past 30 days, how many days has the trouble with your joints or muscles kept you in bed all day or most of the day?

Validity and reliability

The researchers compared the scale's performance against clinical examination and tests. For example, the uric acid levels of people classified by the questionnaire as having gout were, as expected, higher than those not suffering from gout. Also, X-rays, grip strength, rheumatoid factor measurements and walking speed, for example, were found to be more abnormal and to occur more often among people classified by the questionnaire as having a joint disorder than among those with no such disorders. Joint swelling was also only associated with the more severe joint disorders. In addition, 75 per cent of respondents who reported a joint problem in the questionnaire also reported a joint problem at clinical examination. This suggests that people are more likely, or willing, to report symptoms on a self-administered questionnaire than to a doctor. The authors suggested that they may have been deterred in the latter situation by the prospect of facing an additional screening test. The 'non-reporters to the doctor' were also those who had acute rather than chronic disorders. A random sample of 8–10 per cent of respondents were retested for the assessment of reliability in relation to the standard measures used at examination (e.g. grip strength, etc.), with good results, but the self-report questionnaire was not re-administered. Fuller psychometric testing is still needed.

The questionnaire is short, and certainly not multidimensional, but the Rand battery impact of disease items are attractive because of their brevity and the fact that they can be used with other scales. The population norms are based on large numbers of people, and the questions were adapted for use across a wide range of disease types, making comparisons possible.

SUMMARIES OF OTHER SCALES

ARTHRITIS HELPLESSNESS INDEX (AHI)

This is a disease-specific coping scale, developed by Nicassio *et al.* (1985) in a postal survey of 219 patients with rheumatoid arthritis. The scale consists of 15 items which aim to measure patients' perceptions of their abilities (9 items) and inabilities (6 items) to control their arthritis. The response choices are on 4-point scales: 'strongly agree', 'agree', 'disagree', 'strongly disagree'. The scoring for the nine items indicating perceived control is reversed. Scale scores range from 15 to 60, with high scores indicating greater helplessness.

Examples from the AHI

1 Arthritis is controlling my life
3 I can reduce my pain by staying calm and relaxed
6 I can do a lot of things myself to cope with my arthritis
12 No matter what I do, or how hard I try, I just can't seem to get relief from my pain
13 I am coping effectively with my arthritis

Validity and factor structure

Nicassio et al. (1985) reported that the scale was sensitive to changes in functional ability over a 12-month period. The scale has been tested against a number of other scales of socio-psychological and physical functioning (Rosenberg 1965; Dupuy 1978; Wallston et al. 1978; Fries et al. 1980). Greater helplessness was associated with increasing age, lower self-esteem, lower internal locus of control, higher anxiety and depression, and impaired ability as assessed with the Stanford Health Assessment Questionnaire (Fries et al. 1980). The correlations of change between the AHI and the other scales ranged from –0.02 (locus of control) to 0.52 (difficulties with physical functioning). Although these were weak to moderate, they were in the expected direction.

Fitzpatrick et al. (1990) further tested the scale on a sample of 137 patients with rheumatoid arthritis, together with other scales including the English version of the Sickness Impact Profile (Bergner et al. 1981), known as the Functional Limitations Profile (FLP: Charlton et al. 1983), the Minnesota Multiphasic Personality Inventory (Hathaway and McKinley 1990), the Beck Depression Inventory (BDI: Beck et al. 1961), the Health Locus of Control Scale (Wallston et al. 1978) and the Rosenberg Self-Esteem Scale (Rosenberg 1965), as well as clinical measurements. Measures were repeated at 15 months. Fitzpatrick et al. (1990) reported that all items except one correlated significantly with the scale score at both times (the one exception was 'I want to learn as much as I can about arthritis' at time 2) (correlation coefficient not given).

Fitzpatrick et al. (1990) entered the data into a principal components factor analysis and could find no principal factors, although Stein et al. (1988) had previously reported a two-factor solution. They reported weak to moderate correlations between the scale and clinical indicators (e.g. grip strength, stiffness, pain, blood tests, etc.) of between -0.14 and 0.47. The correlations between the AHI and the FLP on both occasions were 0.55–0.59 (physical scale) and 0.44–0.46 (psychosocial scale), and between the AHI and BDI 0.32–0.35; with the Self-Esteem Scale they were 0.39–0.46 and with the Locus of Control sub-scales they were 0.19 to -0.49. These correlations were weak to moderate, but would be expected to be stronger. They give some support to the construct validity of the scale.

Reliability

Nicassio et al. (1985) reported the internal consistency of the scale to be $\alpha = 0.69$; they suggested that predictability might form a distinct component of the scale, explaining this value. Test–retest reliability testing was carried out over 12 months with 60 of the patients, with a correlation of $r = 0.53$. This modest correlation may reflect the long test–retest interval.

Fitzpatrick et al. (1990) reported the internal consistency reliability coefficient (Cronbach's alpha) to be 0.72 both initially and after 15 months. Their results were similar to those reported in previous studies (Nicassio et al. 1985; Affleck et al. 1987; Callahan et al. (1988). The scale appears promising but is in need of further development to strengthen its psychometric properties. Generic coping scales are reviewed in Chapter 3.

EURIDISS (EUROPEAN RESEARCH ON INCAPACITATING DISEASES AND SOCIAL SUPPORT)

Finally, brief mention should be made of efforts being made in Europe to produce standardized disease-specific scales. Participants from 11 universities in nine European countries are participating in a longitudinal research project called EURIDISS – European Research on Incapacitating Diseases and Social Support – which aims to identify the factors which contribute to the course of the disease and to the quality of life of people with a chronic illness. Two hundred and fifty patients will be followed up and a number of measurement scales are being designed and tested. These relate to activities of daily living (ADL) and instrumental activities of daily living (IADL), socio-psychological well-being, social support and subjective health status (EURIDISS, 1990). Some preliminary testing of these measures has been carried out, but they are yet to be extensively tested for reliability, validity and sensitivity.

CONCLUSION

Quality of life assessment in rheumatology has traditionally concentrated on physical functioning, and has sometimes been extended to include psychological morbidity. Where broader quality of life has been measured, most investigators have used generic health-related quality of life scales. Hörnquist *et al.* (1990, 1992) have developed a Quality of Life Status and Change Scale, which has been adopted for use with people with joint problems, but its sensitivity has yet to be con-firmed. A more exciting, although relatively com-plex, measure is the SEIQoL (O'Boyle *et al.* 1992), which has been used with patients undergoing hip replacement. It is not disease-specific and requires supplementation with scales of functional ability, such as the Health Assessment Questionnaire (Fries *et al.* 1982) or the Arthritis Impact Measurement Scales (Meenan *et al.* 1980), and symptoms. How-ever, it is based on patient-generated quality of life domains. Progress in developing disease-specific quality of life scales in rheumatology has been slow.

7

CARDIOVASCULAR
DISEASES

TRENDS IN MEASURING QUALITY OF LIFE IN PEOPLE WITH HEART DISEASE

Physical and mental functioning, the performance of social roles and psychological well-being can all be affected by cardiovascular diseases and their therapies (Walter *et al.* 1992). It is becoming apparent to many clinicians that a broad perspective of functioning is required. However, disease-specific quality of life scales have been poorly developed in relation to cardiovascular diseases (Mayou 1990).

The cardiovascular diseases cover a wide range of conditions and treatment, including chronic congestive heart failure, acute myocardial infarction, angina pectoris and hypertension (hypertension will be reviewed later), and can involve both medical and surgical interventions (e.g. from medication to coronary artery bypass surgery, depending on type of disease and severity).

Congestive heart failure is a chronic and progressively debilitating condition. The heart's failure to maintain adequate output leads to diminished blood flow to the tissues and leads to congestion in the pulmonary lung and/or the systemic circulations. This leads to shortness of breath upon exertion or lying down (e.g. during sleep), and swollen ankles (Rosenthal *et al.* 1981),

with inevitable effects on activities of daily life. Acute myocardial infarction, in contrast, is often a sudden event in a previously well individual, or a patient known to have cardiac disease whose condition is stable. Angina pectoris is characterized by short-term episodic chest pain that is caused by an imbalance of the oxygen supply and demand, thus resulting in the heart muscle being deprived of oxygen. Activity and excitement usually bring on chest pain, or it sometimes occurs with minimal stimulation (Rosenthal *et al.* 1981). These different conditions require the careful selection of outcome measures in order to ensure that they are sensitive to changes, and that they contain items that are relevant to the impact of the condition and its treatment on patients' lives.

In relation to surgery, the measurement of quality of life is particularly important in that outcome assessment incorporates a trade-off assessment between surgical risks and potential benefits. The potential risks include the short-term physical and psychological consequences of surgery, the operative risk, the need for further surgery, and economic implications versus the long-term broader health gains (Wenger *et al.* 1984). Research on coronary artery bypass grafting (CABG) has provided important data on outcomes, indicating that surgical intervention is superior to medical therapy in relieving the signs and symptoms of ischaemic heart disease (European Coronary Surgery Study Group 1982; Coronary Artery Surgery Study (CASS) 1983; Guyatt *et al.*

1985b; Folks *et al.* 1986; Peduzzi *et al.* 1987). More recently, data have been published on the high level of psychological impairment pre-operatively, which improved after CABG (Magni *et al.* 1987). However, not all patients experience an improvement in activity levels and return to work (Bolli 1987), and research findings are not always straightforward to interpret.

MOST AND LEAST FREQUENTLY USED INDICATORS

Unfortunately, most investigators in cardiology still frequently design a 'quality of life' study, but limit its operationalization to symptoms, measures of depression and crude items on level of functioning, and perhaps items on sex life and sleep (e.g. Engblom *et al.* 1992). Return to work is a popular outcome measure among clinicians, but this is more often influenced by economic, social and personal factors, and employment opportunities, than by the patient's motivation or ability (Croog and Levine 1977; Wilson-Barnett 1981). Moreover, it is rarely analysed meaningfully in relation to comparisons with population norms on employment (Wilson-Barnett 1981). Work capability has itself been subject to crude measurement (see Westaby *et al.* 1979). An average of 45 per cent of patients from all studies reviewed by Mai (1993) returned to full-time employment. Gortner *et al.* (1985) have reported that return to work is not a high expectation among patients undergoing coronary artery bypass surgery (CABS), even among those who were previously working.

Wilson-Barnett (1981) has reviewed the literature on the criteria used to evaluate outcome and recovery among cardiac patients. The most frequently used measures related to mortality rates/length of survival, followed by morbidity/serious complication, physical condition (exercise testing, cardiac function, angiography), patency of grafts, symptoms/pain, dyspnoea and return to work. Rarely used criteria were activity levels (other than work), adherence to medical advice, social activities/hobbies, financial status, sexual activity, satisfaction with operation. Exceptionally used criteria were family response, psychological status (affect, adjustment, self-esteem), perception of health status, resumption of normal life, 'minor' problems, satisfaction with advice, and patients' understanding of treatment.

Faris and Stotts (1990) later confirmed Wilson-Barnett's (1981) findings with an updated review (e.g. CASS 1983; Holmes *et al.* 1984; Raft *et al.* 1985; Sergeant *et al.* 1986; Peduzzi *et al.* 1987; Scheidt 1987; Taylor 1987; Danchin *et al.* 1988; Klonoff *et al.* 1989). While crude indicators of quality of life still abound, there has been a gradual shift towards using more sophisticated and sensitive measurements.

WHAT SHOULD BE MEASURED?

Apart from symptoms and disease-specific toxicities, the measurement of quality of life in cardiovascular disease needs to encompass broader physical, social and psychological domains. Wenger *et al.* (1984) stated that the components of quality of life, in relation to the assessment of outcome of cardiovascular diseases and therapies, include:

- *Physical capabilities:* including mobility, ability to care for self and perform activities of daily living.
- *Emotional status:* including mood changes, anger, guilt, hostility, depression, helplessness, sick-role behaviour and expectations about the future.
- *Social interactions:* including participation in social activities, family relationships, sexual functioning and marital satisfaction.
- *Intellectual functioning:* including memory, alertness and judgement.
- *Economic status:* including the ability to maintain standard of living, income, employment and in the USA, an ability to maintain insurance.
- *Self-perceived health status:* including evaluation of disease severity and level of impairment by the patient.

Fletcher *et al.* (1987) suggested a similar list of domains which merit measurement when assessing the outcome of cardiovascular disease or treatment, together with symptom and toxicity levels, and satisfaction with the results of treatment. Faris and Stotts (1990) developed an almost identical list, and also included the congruence between expected and realized benefits of treatment. Williams *et al.* (1984)

devised a list with similar domains that should be measured, specifically in the case of patients with acute myocardial infarction. Oberman *et al.* (1984) also produced a list of such domains in relation to the evaluation of CABG in relation to quality of life. They added adherence to medical advice (on lifestyle, diet and medication) and patient satisfaction with the outcome.

Other domains that are important include various types of social disruptions, pain, patients' fears, denial, coping and impaired sleep (Tyroler *et al.* (1984; Buxton *et al.* 1985; Wallwork and Caine 1985). In particular, care should be taken to measure *short-term*, as well as longer-term changes, for example, there may be short-term memory and concentration disturbances, particularly after CABG (Breuer *et al.* 1981; Smith *et al.* 1983; Shaw 1986). The selected outcome measures, however, must bear relevance to the effects of the intervention and the questionnaire must incorporate the impact of the symptoms and toxic/disadvantageous effects of therapy as perceived by the patient.

THE DOMAINS OF MEASUREMENT

Symptoms

Diagnostic criteria and medical tests have been described by Rosenthal *et al.* (1981). An important symptom to measure is dyspnoea (difficult or laboured breathing) and orthopnoea (difficulty breathing except when sitting or standing upright). Dyspnoea can be diagnosed by questionnaire using the scale which was first developed by Fletcher *et al.* (1959), and which was then adapted by the Medical Research Council in Britain and the World Health Organization (Rose and Blackburn 1968).

Generic measures of quality of life

Progress in the development of disease-specific quality of life scales has been slow in cardiovascular disease. Investigators of quality of life have been content to use existing generic scales or batteries of scales.

Nottingham Health Profile (NHP)
The Nottingham Health Profile (NHP: Hunt *et al.*

1986) is one of the most commonly used measures of broader health status among patients with angina (Vandenburg 1993) and other patients with cardiovascular disease. The NHP is sensitive to changes following dramatic treatment interventions, although its performance with less dramatic treatments is less certain. For example, Wallwork and Caine (1985) used the NHP together with other general quality of life questions (on work, finance, symptoms, lifestyle and expectations) to compare the quality of life of 84 CABG patients and 61 transplant patients. They also asked patients to rank the extent of any improvement (e.g. completely better, definitely improved, etc.). The NHP was able to discriminate between these two groups at the pre-intervention stage, but was less sensitive to differences between the groups 1 year after intervention.

Caine *et al.* (1991) also used the NHP to study the quality of life of 100 males aged under 60 before and after CABG. The NHP was sensitive to improvements in health following the procedure (at 3 months and 1 year later). The same research team (Caine *et al.* 1990) used the NHP to determine the quality of life of 196 heart transplant patients at Papworth Hospital, England, as part of a cost–benefit study (Buxton *et al.* 1985). The NHP was sensitive to deterioration in patients' condition prior to transplant and to post-transplant improvement. It was able to predict outcome in relation to length of hospital stay, return to work and leisure activity 3 months post-transplantation. O'Brien *et al.* (1987) used the NHP to measure the effectiveness of heart transplantation programmes at the Harefield and Papworth Hospitals. They concluded that the NHP related closely to the clinical categorization of patients, and that the scale was a useful indicator of prognosis for post-transplant survival. Van Agt *et al.* (1993) also used the NHP in a study of heart disease patients and people suffering from other chronic diseases; they reported that the NHP was sensitive to disease type. Finally, Permanyer-Miralda *et al.* (1991) reported that the NHP correlated strongly with exercise testing among stable coronary in-patients, thus supporting its validity.

Sickness Impact Profile (SIP)
Researchers in the USA have preferred the Sickness Impact Profile (SIP: Bergner *et al.* 1981), one of the

most commonly used generic health status measures among patients with angina (Vandenburg 1993). Ott *et al.* (1983) used the SIP to measure outcome of rehabilitation after myocardial infarction in a randomized controlled trial of 258 patients, and reported the SIP to be sensitive to type of rehabilitation given. The SIP has been reported to be sensitive to changes following treatment for myocardial infarction (Ott *et al.* 1983), and to be able to distinguish between potential survivors and non-survivors of cardiac arrest (Bergner *et al.* 1985). Not all investigators have used the full-length SIP (136 items). For example, Cleary *et al.* (1991) used the sub-sections relating to ability to perform household chores, recreation and work functioning (with modifications) in 1200 patients enlisted in a randomized controlled trial of percutaneous transluminal coronary angioplasty.

Recommended generic scales

There are several other generic scales that have been used with coronary patients. Fletcher *et al.* (1987) suggested that the Quality of Well-Being Scale (Kaplan and Bush 1982; Bush 1984), the SIP (Bergner *et al.* 1981) and the NHP (Hunt *et al.* 1986) are all of use in assessing outcome of cardiovascular disease and therapy. Their recommendations overlap with those of Wenger *et al.* (1984). Among the scales they selected were the Quality of Well-Being Scale, the SIP, the NHP, the McMaster Health Index Questionnaire (Chambers 1984) and the Psychological General Well-Being Schedule (Dupuy 1984; and see Stewart *et al.* 1992b). However, Visser *et al.* (1994) reported that the Quality of Well-Being Scale performed poorly in comparison with NHP and SIP in assessing the outcome of treatment for people with angina.

However, these scales are different in length and content. While the NHP and the SIP are similar in the domains covered, the SIP has 136 items while the NHP has only 38 (Part I). McMaster's Questionnaire covers more positive aspects of health, and is less negative than the NHP. The Quality of Well-Being Scale produces a single score, and thus cannot provide a comprehensive multidimensional profile of outcome nor inform the investigator which aspect of functioning has improved or deteriorated. The Psychological General Well-being Index is a measure of subjective feelings of well-being and distress only.

More promising is the Short Form-36, which was developed from the Rand Health Insurance Study (HIS) and Medical Outcomes Study (MOS) batteries (Ware *et al.* 1993). Its advantage is that it is short, with good psychometric properties (see Chapter 8). It is recommended for use as a disease-specific core in several other specialities. It has yet to be fully tested for its appropriateness with people with cardiovascular diseases.

Domain-specific measures of quality of life

Functional ability

Functional capacity and ability are essential domains to assess. Most activities of daily living (ADL) scales were developed for use with elderly people, stroke patients or people with arthritis or rheumatism. Deyo (1984b) reviewed the most widely used ADL scales in clinical trials – the Katz Index (Katz and Akpom 1976a, 1976b), the Barthel Index (Mahoney and Barthel 1965) and the Pulses Scale (Granger *et al.* 1979a) – and concluded that while their reliability was generally good, strong evidence of their sensitivity to change was lacking. A popular scale is the Karnofsky Performance Status Scale (Karnofsky *et al.* 1948), although in view of its questionable psychometric properties it appears to be uncritically accepted and used. These are all fairly old scales, and newer, more appropriate scales for use with cardiovascular patients are needed.

It was mentioned earlier that return to work and work performance are popular measures of outcome. One scale that is better developed, and covers more dimensions than most, is the Work Performance and Satisfaction Scale. This is a series of seven questions covering the ability to keep pace with the job, on-the-job fatigue, problems of concentration and job satisfaction. The items are scored on a 7-point scale, and scores range from 7 (high) to 49 (low). It was developed by Croog *et al.* (1986) from the initial work of House (1981). It was found to be sensitive to differences in medication therapy among 626 men with mild to moderate hypertension.

Sexual functioning is another important domain of well-being to measure. However. most investigators appear to have devised their own questions (e.g. Strauss *et al.* 1992). Engblom *et al.* (1992), for example, asked single-item questions on satisfaction with sexual life after CABS, and whether there were any differences compared with pre-surgery.

Psychological morbidity

While cardiovascular disease has been one of the major topics within psychosomatic medicine, research has been relatively narrowly focused (Mayou 1990; Strauss *et al.* 1992). The psychological consequences of myocardial infarction and life-saving interventions are well documented (Mayou *et al.* 1976; Croog and Levine 1982; Radley 1988; Bunzel *et al.* 1992). In particular, heart transplantation has attracted psychologists as a field of study, given the anxiety and depression, stress, changed body image, and fears experienced by the patient (Castelnuovo-Tedesco 1973; Lesko and Hawkins 1983; Watts *et al.* 1984; Kuhn *et al.* 1988, 1990; Mai 1993)

Popular scales of anxiety and depression

Popular scales of anxiety and depression with cardiovascular disease sufferers include the Beck Depression Inventory (BDI: Beck *et al.* 1961), the General Health Questionnaire (Goldberg 1972), The Zung Depression Scale (Zung 1965), the Hospital Anxiety and Depression Scale (Zigmond and Snaith 1983), the General Well-Being Schedule (Dupuy 1978; and see Stewart and Ware, 1992), the Brief Symptom Inventory (Derogatis and Spencer 1984) and the State–Trait Anxiety Inventory (STAI: Spielberger *et al.* 1973, 1983). The STAI is particularly popular, and it has been reported to be sensitive to improvements in cardiovascular condition following treatment or surgery (Jenkins *et al.* 1983a, 1983b; Shaw *et al.* 1986; Pim and Jude 1989; Faris and Stotts 1990), and correlates well with other depression scales used with heart disease patients (Erdman *et al.* 1993). Good examples of the use of some of the other depression scales with cardiovascular disease patients can be found in Mann (1977, 1984), Croog *et al.* (1986), Laerum *et al.* (1991) and Engblom *et al.* (1992).

Some broader scales of psychological functioning also tap anxiety, e.g. the Illness Behaviour Questionnaire, designed by Pilowsky *et al.* (1979).

There is increasing interest in the Profile of Mood States (POMS) as an index of mood (including depressed mood). Bulpitt and Fletcher (1990) have used the Symptom Rating Test (Kellner and Sheffield 1973; Kellner 1983) as well as the POMS in order to make comparisons between the scales (ongoing). As they point out, the limitation of the Symptom Rating Test is that it is symptom-based, and thus there is uncertainty about whether admission of a symptom, for example dizziness, is a treatment side-effect or an index of anxiety.

Personality

Personality is generally constant, and not regarded as a potential predictor of outcome. However, conditions or treatments which affect the brain might be expected to influence personality. It is unwise to include a measure of personality in outcome batteries unless such effects are expected. Personality, on the other hand, can be regarded as a modifying variable and an influence on the process of recovery (Pilowsky *et al.* 1979; Wilson–Barnett 1981).

In the UK, the Eysenck Personality Questionnaire (Eysenck and Eysenck 1985) is the personality measure of choice used by psychologists, although personality assessment in studies of outcome in the UK is rare, partly because it is not always appropriate. In the USA, the Minnesota Multiphasic Personality Inventory (MMPI: Hathaway and McKinley 1990) and the Cattell 16 Personality Factor (PF) Questionnaire (Cattell and Eber 1962) have frequently been included in outcome batteries used by clinicians. The latter provides a comprehensive personality measurement in broad areas of functioning (Cattell and Eber 1962). It has been popular among a number of investigators in the USA, and it has been reported to detect improvements in mood after CABG (Kornfeld *et al.* 1984). The MMPI requires some further discussion (or caution) in view of its wide use but questionable appropriateness.

The Minnesota Multiphasic Personality Inventory (MMPI)

The MMPI is included here because of its wide use in the USA. British psychologists regard it as an inappropriate measure, partly because of the length of time it takes to administer and score (it can take

2 h to administer, although the handbook indicates that the average time is much shorter). It contains several items and domains that are unlikely to be sensitive to change in condition. Full personality assessment, while of relevance in studies of predisposing factors to disease, is less appropriate in studies of outcome.

The MMPI (Hathaway and McKinley 1940a, 1940b, 1942a, 1942b, 1990; Dahlstrom et al. 1972); has frequently been used in the USA with cardiovascular disease patients. It is a 556-item inventory that measures emotional distress and personality disturbance. It was used by Lindal (1990) in 60 patients undergoing a CABG in order to measure psychological morbidity (e.g. depression, hysteria, schizophrenia, anxiety). He reported that over half of the patients had significant and ongoing depression. There do exist, however, more appropriate, specific measures for the measurement of anxiety and depression. It is not recommended here that investigators use the MMPI for this. The Cook-Medley Hostility sub-scale of the MMPI has been used to measure hostility in studies of coronary disease risk factors (Scherwitz et al. 1992; Siegler et al. 1992). The study of risk factors for disease is not, of course, the same as measuring outcome of a disease or treatment, and caution is needed before including personality measures in outcome batteries.

Shorter versions of the MMPI have been published, but none are in common use (Newark and Faschingbauer, 1978). There is a version for adults and for adolescents and children (Welsh and Dahlstrom 1956; Dahlstrom et al. 1972; Hathaway and McKinley 1990). Varying levels of validity have been reported (see Dahlstrom and Welsh 1960). Factor analyses of the scores have been somewhat inconsistent on the number of dimensions identified (2–4) (Dahlstrom et al. 1972). Several studies of reliability have been reported by Buros (1978), which generally indicate good results. It has been used in many studies of medical outcome, although it appears to be a useful measure of outcome only if personality issues are prominent (Green 1993). Otherwise, many of the items and domains are of questionable relevance. There is some doubt over its use with chronic conditions, where high scores on some domains may reflect the physical condition rather than psychological status (Pincus et al. 1986; Creed and Ash 1992).

Other

A wide range of scales measuring other relevant dimensions of psychological and social status have been used by investigators in relation to the cardiovascular diseases. For example, measures of Type A behaviour have been popular (Jenkins et al. 1967), but are currently less fashionable and the global concept of Type A personality has been disputed (Syme 1986). Again, such measures are not to be regarded as appropriate in the assessment of outcome, as their main use has been in the study of predisposing factors.

Cognitive impairment

Strauss et al. (1992) reported that a quarter of heart transplant recipients have a high level of neuropsychological impairment. Fletcher et al. (1987) suggested that it is important to include cognitive tests in assessments, in order to assess short-term memory impairment and drug therapy. There are numerous instruments for assessing cognitive function.

Measures which have been used in trials of hypertension and cognitive impairment among cardiac surgery patients include the Trail-Making Test (Reitan 1958) and some of the Wechsler Memory Tests (Wechsler and Stone 1973) – for example, the studies of Croog et al. (1986), Fays-Dunne and Willner (1989) and Willner (1989). Several similar scales are in use (Fays-Dunne and Willner 1989; Willner 1989). A practical limitation of these tests is that they do require administration by a trained interviewer, although computer-aided methods are being developed.

Trail-Making Test

The Trail-Making Test measures attention, perceptual speed, cognitive flexibility and visual memory (Reitan, 1958). Croog et al. (1986) used the scale, together with several others, to assess the effects of anti-hypertensive therapy on quality of life among 626 men with mild to moderate hypertension in a random controlled trial of alternative drug treatments. The results confirmed the scale's sensitivity to type of medication. Croog et al. (1990) also used this measure in a study of ethnic status and effects of hypertension treatment. Jenkins et al. (1983b) also used it in a study of outcome of CABG in 318 patients, and reported that average performance times on the test significantly improved post-surgery.

Wechsler Memory Scales (WMS)

The Wechsler Memory Scales are popular neuropsychological tests. Jenkins et al. (1983b) used the WMS in a study of outcome of CABG among 318 patients, and reported that visual reproduction scores from the WMS were unchanged post-surgery, but the logical memory sub-test of the WMS significantly improved post-surgery, supporting the inference that CABG is not associated with long-term adverse neuropsychological effects.

Brief scales of cognitive function

Several brief tests of cognitive function have been used in cardiology. One popular measure is the Mini-Mental State (Folstein et al. 1975). It has been suggested that it is appropriate for use with patients with acute myocardial infarction (Williams et al. 1984). The cognitive functioning sub-scale of the Sickness Impact Profile has also been used (Bergner et al. 1981). These scales are reviewed in Chapter 5.

Coping and adjustment

Coping ability is an important modifying variable in response to illness which is worth measuring independently if it is not represented in the scale chosen. Coping is defined as 'any response to external life-strains that serves to prevent, avoid, or control emotional distress' (Pearlin and Schooler 1978). This definition has been criticized by Radley (1988) as achieving too simple a distinction between the 'coping self' and 'external strain'. Other studies have emphasized the importance of patients trying to appear normal, despite their condition, as a common coping behaviour (Davis 1963; Strauss 1975). Clinical studies have reported that coping styles do contribute to differences in how patients adjust to their illness, although different illnesses are apparently not met with different coping styles (Radley 1988). Felton et al. (1984) reported that individuals whose coping style was emotion-based (involving avoidance or perceptual distortions of reality), had poorer adjustment than those whose coping style involved a cognitive restructuring of the problem.

The Ways of Coping Scale, a widely used measure of coping, is popular with cardiovascular disease patients (Folkman and Lazarus 1980; Meyerowitz et al. 1989). Redeker (1992) used this scale and reported that the most frequent coping strategy at 1 and 6 weeks after CABG was seeking social support, followed by problem-focused coping and the emotion-focused coping strategies of blaming self, wishful thinking and avoidance.

Adjustment to the condition is a related concept that is important to measure in outcome studies, and several brief scales have been developed (Weissman and Bothwell 1976; Cooper et al. 1982). Other popular adjustment scales include the Structured and Scaled Interview to assess maladjustment (Gurland et al. 1972a), and the Katz Adjustment Scales (Katz et al. 1963). These are reviewed in Chapter 3.

Self-esteem

Self-esteem, self-concept and body image have rarely been included within quality of life measures for people with cardiovascular disease, and appears to be a neglected domain in this field. Some appropriate scales of self-esteem are reviewed by Bowling (1991).

Life satisfaction

Several studies have analysed satisfaction with life and quality of life in relation to myocardial infarction, heart transplantation and elderly people in cardiac rehabilitation groups (Julian 1987; Lough et al. 1987; Herlitz et al. 1988; Packa 1989). Investigators have often selected single items from life satisfaction scales. For example, items from various scales, including the Rand Medical Outcome Study Batteries (Stewart and Ware 1992), Andrews and Withey's (1974) life satisfaction ladder scale and Ruberman and co-workers' (1984) life events scale, were selected for use by Wiklund et al. (1992) in their assessment of quality of life in a cardiac arrhythmia suppression trial. The reliability and validity of these instruments were reported to be acceptable.

Neugarten's Life Satisfaction (Index A) Scale

Neugarten and co-workers' (1961) Life Satisfaction (Index A) scale has been used in studies of recovery after myocardial infarction (e.g. Fridlund *et al.* 1991). The scale was sensitive to improvement at 6 months in those patients participating in a rehabilitation programme ($n = 53$) in Sweden, compared with less improvement in controls ($n = 63$).

Andrews and Withey's Ladder Scale

Andrews and Withey's (1974) Life Satisfaction scale has also been used with people with cardiovascular diseases. Respondents rate which of ten rungs they consider themselves to be on (e.g. this can be in relation to now, before the illness episode and 1 year on). The tenth rung indicates the best possible quality of life and the first indicates the worst. This measure was used by Unden *et al.* (1993) in a controlled study of the effects of increased nurse support on 103 male patients after acute myocardial infarction. They reported that increased nurse support was associated with increased expectations about future quality of life.

Social support

Family and social support are frequently reported in the literature to affect recovery from heart attack (Croog and Levine 1977). An index of social activities is also worth including. Part 2 of the Personal Resource Questionnaire is often used to measure perceived social support with cardiovascular disease patients (Weinert and Brandt 1987). It is a 25-item, 7-point Likert scale with items that assess provision for attachment/ intimacy, social integration, opportunity for nurturant behaviour, reassurance of worth as an individual and in role accomplishments, and the availability of information, emotional and material help. Weinert and Brandt (1987) reported adequate internal consistency (Cronbach's alpha $r = 0.89$) and test–retest reliability ($r = 0.72$). Conn *et al.* (1991) also used it for their study of gender differences in social and psychological circumstances and physical health status 1–2 years after myocardial infarction.

Health behaviour

Health behaviour, and changes in behaviour, are modifying variables in recovery, and may be required in some outcome studies in relation to cardiovascular disease. Many investigators include measures of smoking, exercise, alcohol intake and dietary habits in their questionnaires on outcomes, given their importance in the recovery process. These areas of questioning are highly prone to social desirability bias. Questions on diet are also notoriously difficult to construct so that they are reliable and valid (for guidelines, see Kemm and Booth 1992). Rather than indulge in a long health behaviour questionnaire, however, most investigators ask fairly brief questions about whether the behaviour in question has increased, decreased or is unchanged (e.g. Unden *et al.* 1993). Standard questions on smoking and drinking behaviour suitable for face-to-face interviews, can be found in the annual General Household Survey and Annual Health Survey questionnaires in Britain (Breeze *et al.* 1994, Thomas *et al.* 1994); standard questions measuring exercise and dietary intake, suitable for face-to-face interviews, can be found in the questionnaires for the British National Health and Lifestyle Survey questionnaires (Cox *et al.* 1987). In the USA, the Rand organization included the soundest questions on smoking behaviour (i.e. those attracting least 'socially desirable' response bias) for inclusion in the Health Insurance Study (HIS). Their selected questions were reported to have a 12 month stability coefficient of $r = 0.90$ (Ware *et al.* 1987). These will not be replicated here. Other psychological determinants of health behaviour may be required, depending on the aims of the study. Health locus of control scales can be found in Chapter 3.

Patient satisfaction

Despite its importance, patient satisfaction is notoriously difficult to measure accurately, and most patient satisfaction scales are fairly superficial, obtaining mainly positive responses. Unden *et al.* (1993), in their controlled study of the effects of increased nurse support after myocardial infarction among 103 patients, used satisfaction with care as an outcome measure: satisfaction with care during the hospital stay, with staff contact, with care after discharge and with staff contact after discharge. As with most satisfaction measures, these were fairly insensitive, with most patients in both groups reporting satisfaction, although the study group were more satisfied with post-discharge care and contact with staff.

As in other chapters, a caution is given here that any one study attempting to measure adequately each domain will become unwieldy and suffer from high non-response rates. Investigators should ensure that they have an instrument, or battery, that reflects the broad domains of quality of life, and supplement it with domains of particular interest, rather than attempt to measure everything.

THE MEASUREMENT SCALES

CATEGORIZATIONS AND MEASURES OF PHYSICAL ACTIVITY

Several systems have been developed to categorize the degree of cardiovascular disability. Category scales should not be confused with functional ability scales, the former are simply crude graded ratings of disability made by professionals for classification purposes (not necessarily for research). They are negative in orientation, defining health negatively at one end of a continuum in relation to absence of symptoms, rather than positively. They give no indication of the effects of the condition on specific domains of mental, social and physical functioning, producing one score (the category allocated).

The most often used system is the New York Heart Association Functional Classification Scale, although data on its reliability and validity are limited. More detailed criteria were later proposed by the Canadian Cardiovascular Society, which have been adopted in several studies. Again, data on its reliability and validity are limited. Such category scales, completed usually by physicians, are popular in cardiology research because they are short and easy for busy clinicians to complete. Their results should be interpreted with caution, and they should not be regarded as substitutes for functional ability scales rated by the patient (and carer where necessary). They are regarded as useful severity scales, with the interpretation being that if a patient experiences an improvement after treatment, then the medical intervention is regarded as clinically successful.

NEW YORK HEART ASSOCIATION FUNCTIONAL CLASSIFICATION SCALE

The Criteria Committee of the New York Heart Association (NYHA) 1964 gradings represent a functional and therapeutic classification in the prescription of physical activity for cardiac patients. Patients are graded I–IV, according to the degree of their impairment. Doctors generally make the gradings (Harvey *et al.* 1974; Goldman *et al.* 1982; Olsson *et al.* 1986). The measure is widely used in clinical trials of congestive heart failure.

NYHA Functional Classification Scale

Class I: No limitation on activities; suffers from no symptoms from (performance of) ordinary activities. Patients with cardiac disease but without resulting limitations on physical activities. Ordinary physical activity does not cause undue fatigue, palpitation, dyspnoea or anginal pain

Class II: Slight limitation on activities; comfortable at rest or mild exertion. Patients with cardiac disease resulting in slight limitation on physical activities. They are comfortable at rest. Ordinary physical activity results in fatigue, palpitation, dyspnoea or anginal pain

Class III: Marked limitation on activities; comfortable only at rest. Patients with cardiac disease resulting in marked limitation on physical activities. They are comfortable at rest. Less than ordinary physical activity causes fatigue, palpitation, dyspnoea or anginal pain

Class IV: Discomfort with any physical activity; should be completely rested or confined to bed. Patients with cardiac disease resulting in an inability to carry on any physical activity without discomfort. Symptoms of cardiac insufficiency or of the anginal syndrome may be present even at rest. If any physical activity is undertaken, discomfort is increased

Validity and reliability

The NYHA classification correlates poorly with exercise testing, indicating poor discriminative ability; it also has high inter-observer variability (Goldman *et al.* 1981; Wiklund *et al.* 1987, 1992). Goldman *et al.* (1981) tested the NYHA and Canadian Cardiovascular Society criteria and reported that the NYHA criteria, using estimates of two physicians, had a reproducibility rate of only 56 per cent, and only 51 per cent of the estimates agreed with treadmill exercise performance. It has been blamed in part, together with other poorly validated measures, by Fletcher *et al.* (1987) for the discrepancies in the results of clinical trials. Moreover, while current clinical classifications such as exercise testing or the NYHA measurements may point to important clinical changes, they do not necessarily reflect how a patient feels about his or her day-to-day level of functioning.

OLSSON RANKING SCALE

The Olsson Ranking Scale is based on the NYHA categories (Olsson *et al.* 1986) and was originally developed for use in a trial of metoprolol. This scale classifies patients according to seven mutually exclusive categories of health state (from worst state to best state).

Olsson Ranking Scale

1 Dead
2 Alive — but has sustained non-fatal atherosclerotic complications such as reinfarction, cerebrovascular event, coronary artery bypass surgery, leg amputation
3 Alive and in NYHA Class IV without atherosclerotic complications
4 As in 3 but in functional NYHA Class III without atherosclerotic complications
5 NYHA Class II without atherosclerotic complications
6 NYHA Class I and side-effects of treatment, without atherosclerotic complications
7 NYHA Class I without side-effects of treatment or atherosclerotic complications

CANADIAN CARDIOVASCULAR SOCIETY FUNCTIONAL CLASSIFICATION FOR ANGINA PECTORIS

This was developed as a more detailed scale than the NYHA criteria (Campeau 1976). It is a four-group classification of angina developed by the Canadian Cardiovascular Society (CCS) to measure changes in the severity of chest pain (Coronary Artery Surgery Study: CASS 1983).

CCS Functional Classification for Angina Pectoris

Class I: Ordinary physical activity, such as walking and climbing stairs, does not cause angina. Angina with strenuous or rapid or prolonged exertion at work or recreation

Class II: Slight limitation on ordinary activity. Walking or climbing stairs rapidly, walking uphill, walking or stair climbing after meals, or in cold, or in wind, or under emotional stress, or only during the few hours after awakening. Walking more than two blocks on the level and climbing more than one flight of ordinary stairs at a normal pace and in normal conditions

Class III: Marked limitation on ordinary physical activity. Walking one or two blocks on the level and climbing one flight of stairs in normal conditions and at normal pace

Class IV: Inability to carry on any physical activity without discomfort – anginal syndrome may be present at rest

Validity and reliability

The measure appeared to be only sensitive to fairly dramatic improvements in chest pain (Coronary Artery Surgery Study: CASS 1983). Engblom *et al.* (1992) also used this classification with their trial of rehabilitation after CABG and reported it to be sensitive to recovery. Faris and Stotts (1990) carried out a small study of 20 patients before and after elective treatment with percutaneous transluminal coronary angioplasty (PTCA). They used the Quality of Life Index (Ferrans and Powers 1985), Spielberger and co-workers' (1983) State–Trait Anxiety Inventory (STAI) and a modified physical functioning questionnaire which provided the basis for classifying patients according to the Canadian Cardiovascular Society Classification for Angina Pectoris (Campeau 1976). Their results showed that the scales were sensitive to improvements in physical condition, higher quality of life scores, improved levels of physical functioning, and diminished state–trait anxiety levels after successful PTCA. There are few data on the reliability of the classification. Goldman *et al.* (1981) tested the NYHA and CCS criteria and reported the CCS criteria to be more reproducible (73 per cent) than the NYHA criteria, but not significantly more valid (59 per cent of the estimates agreed with treadmill testing). Further psychometric testing is required.

SPECIFIC ACTIVITY SCALE (SAS)

The Specific Activity Scale (SAS) was designed to

broaden the NYHA Functional Classification Scale, by including more functional measures. It assesses cardiac functional class based on the metabolic demands of a variety of daily activities (Goldman *et al.* 1981).

Content

The SAS is an ordinal scale, four-class physical functioning instrument (best = I to worst = IV). It is based on the metabolic expenditures of various personal care tasks, housework, occupational and recreational activities (e.g. carrying heavy objects, mopping floors).

Examples from the SAS

(RESPONSES LIMITED TO YES/NO)

met = metabolic equivalents of activity

1 Can you walk down a flight of steps without stopping (4.5–5.2 mets)   Yes = go to q. 2; no = go to q. 4

2 Can you carry anything up a flight of 8 steps without stopping (5–5.5 mets) or can you:

   (a) have sexual intercourse without stopping (5–5.5 mets)
   (b) garden, rake, weed (5–6 mets)
   (c) roller skate, dance foxtrot (5–6 mets)
   (d) walk at a 4 miles per hour rate on level ground (5–6 mets)

(any yes go to q. 3; no = class III)

3 Can you carry at least 24 pounds up 8 steps (10 mets) or can you:

   (a) carry objects that are at least 80 pounds (8 mets)
   (b) do outdoor work – shovel snow, spade soil (7 mets)
   (c) do recreational activities such as skiing, basketball, touch football, squash, handball (7–10 mets)
   (d) jog/walk 5 miles per hour (9 mets)

(any yes = class I; no = class II)

4 Can you shower without stopping (3.6–4.2 mets) or can you:

   (a) strip and make a bed (3.9–5 mets)
   (b) mop floors (4.2 mets)
   (c) hang washed clothes (4.4 mets)
   (d) clean windows (3.7 mets)

   (e) walk 2.5 miles per hour (3–3.5 mets)
   (f) bowl (3–4.4 mets)
   (g) play golf (walk and carry clubs) (4.5 mets)
   (h) push power lawn mower (4 mets)

(any yes = class III; no = go to q. 5)

5 Can you dress without stopping because of symptoms (2–2.3 mets)

(yes = class III; no = class IV)

Validity and reliability

The scale has good psychometric properties (Lee *et al.* 1988). It has been reported to be sensitive to age differences in people aged over 50 undergoing major, elective, non-cardiac surgery, and correlated moderately to well with most of the Rand SF-36 (Ware *et al.* 1993) sub-scales used with these patients ($r = -0.30$ to -0.66, except with mental health (SF-36) $r = -0.19$) (Mangione *et al.* 1993).

Cleary *et al.* (1991) used the scale in a randomized controlled trial of 1200 patients in relation to percutaneous transluminal coronary angioplasty. They modified the scale to enable them to ask, in telephone interviews, about ability rather than performance. They also found some items less salient or too sensitive for a telephone interview and so excluded them (e.g. 'Can you have sexual intercourse without stopping?'; 'Can you carry objects that are at least 80 pounds?').

In contrast to the low or variable reproducibility of the other functional classification scales reviewed, Goldman *et al.* (1981) reported the reproducibility of the SAS to be 73 per cent using two physicians, and 68 per cent of the estimates agreed with treadmill testing. Both the NYHA and the CCS systems were reported by Goldman *et al.* to underestimate performance. Correlations relating to inter-observer reliability were also higher than those obtained for the NYHA. Like the commonly used scales of physical functioning, these scales are only sensitive to treatments that produce substantial change (Guyatt *et al.* 1985a).

While the SAS performed better than the NYHA and CCS scales, as Goldman *et al.* (1981) pointed out, its 73 per cent reproducibility and 68 per cent validity rates indicate that no cardiovascular functional classification system based on medical history can be perfectly reproducible or valid. They reported that variability in the way that the questions were asked and contradictory answers from patients were apparent in their study.

RANKIN HANDICAP SCALE

This is a similar functional classificatory scale to the NYHA and CCS (see above). Although it has been used in research on cardiovascular disease, it is strictly a grading for stroke patients (Rankin 1957). It is reviewed in Chapter 5.

SYMPTOM QUESTIONNAIRES

Symptoms and comprehensive checklists of all known side-effects of drugs and other treatments and interventions need to be incorporated into disease-specific quality of life scales for heart failure, angina and hypertension. The most widely used symptom questionnaires in cardiology are for dyspnoea. A broader range of dyspnoea scales and tests were reviewed in Chapter 4. In relation to cardiovascular disease, these have been simply described by the World Health Organization (1993).

Dyspnoea scales

FLETCHER QUESTIONNAIRE AND THE ROSE (WHO) QUESTIONNAIRES: THE LONDON SCHOOL OF HYGIENE DYSPNOEA QUESTIONNAIRE AND CARDIOVASCULAR QUESTIONNAIRE (ANGINA OF EFFORT)

1 Dyspnoea Questionnaire

Fletcher *et al.* (1959) developed a dyspnoea questionnaire in the 1950s, which has been adapted for use by the Medical Research Council in Britain and the World Health Organization (Rose and Blackburn 1968; Rose *et al.* 1982). Rose and Blackburn (1968) suggested a 5-point scale of severity (with 0 corresponding to no shortness of breath and 4 to severe, clinically significant, shortness of breath). It attempts to relate shortness of breath to the kinds of physical activities that provoke it. A slightly modified version has also been used by Rand in their Health Insurance Study/Medical Outcomes Study (Rosenthal *et al.* 1981). The Rand Shortness of

Breath Battery, known as the Dyspnoea Severity Scale, was an improvement on the Rose Dyspnoea Scale. It was developed by Rand in order to assess the prevalence of congestive heart failure in the Health Insurance Study (Rosenthal *et al.* 1981).

Content

Apart from questions about the patient's knowledge of any diagnosed heart disease, the core of the current version of the questionnaire contains four questions which ask respondents whether they have been troubled, over the past 3 months, by shortness of breath when hurrying or walking uphill, when walking with persons of own age on level ground, when walking at own pace on level ground, when bathing or dressing self. Additional items that were added to the original Fletcher Questionnaire ask whether, in the past 3 months, the respondents woke up at night so short of breath that they had to sit on the side of the bed or get up for relief, slept on more than one pillow because of a problem with shortness of breath, whether their ankles swelled, whether they had pain, worried about the condition and whether there was any restriction on their usual activities. The four core questions on shortness of breath are similar to those on the original questionnaire (with the addition of the time period). Replies are dichotomous (yes/no) and only those with positive responses on an item proceed to the next question. They are computed to form a severity score, with good psychometric properties. It can be self-administered.

Examples from the Rose Dyspnoea Questionnaire

1 Are you troubled by shortness of breath when hurrying on level ground, or walking up a slight hill?   Yes/no
2 Do you get short of breath walking with other people of your own age on level ground?   Yes/no
3 Do you have to stop for breath when walking at your own pace on level ground?   Yes/no

---

Variations

The UK's health survey, conducted by OPCS (White *et al.* 1993; Breeze *et al.* 1994), used the scale with some modifications. For example, the survey questionnaire omits washing and dressing, and adds questions on shortness of breath at night and wheeziness, shortness of breath at rest, chest tightness at rest and for no reasons, and various other symptom questions for those with positive responses (e.g. dizziness or light-headedness, pins and needles). Cleary *et al.* (1991) also used it in a randomized controlled trial of 1200 patients in relation to percutaneous transluminal coronary angioplasty, although they did adapt the wording for use in the USA and they also added questions to determine whether patients had difficulty walking for reasons unrelated to their heart condition.

The Rose Dyspnoea Grades

Grade 1: not troubled by breathlessness, except on strenuous exertion

Grade 2: short of breath when hurrying on the level or walking up slight hill

Grade 3: patient walks slower than most people on the level

Grade 4: patient has to stop for breath after walking about 100 yards on the level

Grade 5: too breathless to leave home, or breathless after undressing

Validity

There is limited evidence of the scale's reliability and validity. Further tests for validity, using medical diagnosis as a gold standard, are continuing. Initial, crude tests against a single physician diagnosis question on the medical battery from the Rand Health Insurance Study showed that half of those with this crude diagnosis would have been classifiable on the Congestive Heart Failure Questionnaire, of which the dyspnoea items form part (although the diagnostic question only identified 41 per cent of those with congestive heart failure according to the study criteria). The modified Rand version showed high repeatability and correlated well with walking tests (Mahler *et al.* 1984). It has been reported to be sensitive to surgical intervention (e.g. CABS: Jenkins *et al.* 1983a, 1983b).

Reliability

The Rand version of the scale was reported to have good consistency of responses. Of the 73 people

who, at screening examination, would eventually be classified as at risk of possible or probable congestive heart failure according to the screening questionnaire, 53 (74 per cent) answered 'yes' to the question about shortness of breath and/or heart failure (Rosenthal *et al.* 1981).

The scale is a popular measure among clinicians for the assessment of outcomes. It is widely used across the world, and is also commonly used in prevalence studies (Smith *et al.* 1990; White *et al.* 1993; Breeze *et al.* 1994).

2 Cardiovascular Questionnaire (Angina of Effort)

The Rose Questionnaire, also known as the London School of Hygiene Chest Pain (Cardiovascular) Questionnaire, attempts to identify angina of effort (Rose *et al.* 1977).

Content

The questionnaire contains three parts, A, B and C. Part A consists of seven questions on chest pain, including a diagram on which respondents are asked to mark the site of their pain. Part B contains one question on the site of the pain and length of time it lasts. Part C contains eight questions relating to pain in the legs and situations in which it occurs. The response categories are either dichotomous 'yes/no' codes or 2-point or 3-point choices.

Examples from the Rose Cardiovascular Questionnaire

Part A

(a) Have you ever had any pain or discomfort in your chest? Yes/no

(e) Does it go away when you stand still? Yes/no

Part C

(a) Do you get pain in either leg on walking? Yes/no

(d) Do you get it when you walk uphill or hurry? Yes/no

(h) What happens to it if you stand still?

Usually continues more than 10 minutes / usually disappears in 10 minutes or less

Validity

The Rose Questionnaire (angina) has been tested for reliability and validity, although validation is still incomplete (Garber *et al.* 1992). However, it is generally regarded as a reliable and valid method of identifying classical or typical angina in men aged over 35 (Rose 1962, 1965, 1968, 1971; Zeiner-Henriksen 1972; Rhoads *et al.* 1975). For example, it correlated highly with physician diagnoses of angina: questionnaire results agreed 100 per cent with unanimous angina-negative diagnoses by doctors and with 14 of 17 non-unanimous angina-positive cases (Rose 1962).

Berman *et al.* (1981) used the Rose Questionnaire, with a slightly modified scoring method, in the Rand Health Insurance Study. Their scoring method was 1 = angina not present, 2 = angina probably present, 3 = angina present with mild impairment, and 4 = angina present with moderate impairment. An algorithm was developed to derive these scores. A score of 3 or 4 corresponded to Rose's grades 1 or 2 (mild or moderate), respectively (for details see Berman *et al.* 1981). The results on prevalence were similar to those reported by Rose. They further tested the validity of the Rose Questionnaire against clinical examination. Thirty-four of the 1291 participants aged over 35 who had been randomly assigned for medical screening and ECG were considered to have angina according to the Rose Questionnaire and, of these, 10 (29 per cent) had ischaemic ECG changes. Of the 1257 people without angina according to the Rose Questionnaire, 1045 (83 per cent) had no ECG changes indicating ischaemia. These results are similar to the early results reported by Rose (1965).

Further tests and validity checks on initially misclassified persons led Berman *et al.* (1981) to conclude that the Rose questions are a satisfactorily valid method of classifying people who exhibit classic signs and symptoms of angina, although they did add that additional information may be needed to make a valid judgement about those who seem to have variant forms of angina.

More disturbing results on its validity have been presented recently by Garber *et al.* (1992). They compared its performance against exercise thallium 201 myocardial scintigraphy (an objective measure of myocardial ischaemia in patients with chest pain referred for clinical exercise testing) in 147 male and 97 female patients with chest pain. Their results indicated a poor relationship between the Rose Questionnaire and the tests. The specificity of the Rose Questionnaire was 77 per cent in males and even lower at 56 per cent in females. The specificity values reflected the higher prevalence of false-positive Rose Questionnaire results in females (75 per cent), compared with males (27 per cent). In addition, males had a greater number of false-negative results (53 per cent, compared with 29 per cent for females). The accuracy of the Rose Questionnaire for myocardial ischaemia was 0.19 in females, 0.48 in males and 0.29 for males and females combined.

Reliability

The Rose Cardiovascular Questionnaire was also used in the Rand Health Insurance Study to screen for angina pectoris in men and women (Berman *et al.* 1981), and in a large population prevalence study in Scotland (Smith *et al.* 1990). Cleary *et al.* (1991) also used it, although they only used the items necessary for scoring the severity of angina and classified patients into three groups:

1 Those who experienced no chest pain.
2 Those who experienced chest pain with substantial activity (i.e. walking uphill or hurrying).
3 Those who experienced chest pain without substantial activity (i.e. walking at an ordinary pace on level ground).

Cleary *et al.* (1991) reported that 'patients who reported that they experienced chest pain, discomfort, pressure, or heaviness that was not provoked even by substantial activity were not classified since these reports were difficult to interpret without additional clinical data'.

Despite these problems, the questionnaire is popular and is frequently used in epidemiological and outcomes research. For example, the National Health Survey in Britain carried out by the Office of Population Censuses and Surveys (White *et al.* 1993; Breeze *et al.* 1994), included Parts A and B of the Rose Cardiovascular Questionnaire.

Other scales

FEINSTEIN'S INDEX OF DYSPNOEA

Feinstein *et al.* (1989) developed a clinical index of

dyspnoea and fatigue specifically for people with congestive heart failure. The three components are: magnitude of the task that causes the shortness of breath, magnitude of the pace or effort that evokes the problem, and functional impairment. Each dimension is rated on a 5-point rating scale. The scores are summed to form a composite score. The authors describe it as an index of quality of life for people with heart failure, although it is really simply a dyspnoea index. It has been shown to be sensitive to improvement with medical treatment (see also Chapter 4).

RATIO PROPERTY SCALE

This scale was designed by Borg (1982a, 1982b) to measure self-perceived physical exertion in general and chest pain. Symptoms are rated between 0 and 10 ('nothing at all' to 'maximal'). It has been used in studies of recovery after myocardial infarction (e.g. Fridlund et al. 1991). The scale was sensitive to improvement at 5 weeks and 6 months among patients participating in a rehabilitation programme ($n = 53$) in Sweden, compared with less improvement in controls ($n = 63$) (Fridlund et al. 1991; see Chapter 4).

DISEASE-SPECIFIC QUALITY OF LIFE SCALES: HEART DISEASE

This section reviews the most well-known scales, although a small number of other scales have been developed which await further testing for their psychometric properties. While many of these are fairly crude, and are simply lists of symptoms, two of the better ones include the Minnesota Living with Heart Failure Questionnaire (Rector et al. 1993), and the Quality of Life Questionnaire in Severe Heart Failure (Wiklund et al. 1987). Interested readers are referred to the scale sources for further details.

HEALTH OUTCOMES INSTITUTE TyPE SCALES (HOI-TyPE) – ANGINA

The Health Outcomes Institute (HOI), previously known as Interstudy (2001 Killebrew Drive, Suite 122, Bloomington, MN 55425, USA) has also produced condition-specific specifications (TyPE)

for angina. They await results of testing. In the case of angina, they advise that the forms should be supplemented with the SF-36 in an attempt to produce a broad quality of life profile, with a generic core and disease-specific items. The forms are designed for repeated application (at follow-ups), unless otherwise stated.

Angina form

This includes the physical functioning sub-scale of the SF-36, as well as questions on symptoms, diet and smoking (to be completed by the patient), and the NYHA Functional Classification (to be completed by the physician). Clinicians have two forms to complete (total of four sides) and the patients a baseline and a follow-up questionnaire. The patient's baseline form is a four-sided questionnaire, covering work status (1 item), diagnosis and related medication (3), smoking (3), the SF-36 physical functioning sub-scale (10 items), family history (2), medical history of heart disease (5), hospital use (1) and chest discomfort (1). The

---

Examples from the HOI-TyPE Scales

Patient's form: Baseline

A11 Have you ever had a heart attack?   Yes (date)/no

Patient's form: Follow-up

B3 How has your chest discomfort changed over the last few weeks?

Getting much better / getting a little better / no change / getting a little worse / getting much worse / no chest discomfort

Clinician's forms

1 Does the patient have chest pain?

Yes (typical / atypical / non-anginal / frequency and course) / no

2 Does the patient have symptoms of congestive heart failure?   (NYHA severity classification)
3 Other patient diseases . . .
5 ECG findings

Procedures . . .

Complications . . .

---

patient's follow-up form covers three sides, and comprises nine questions (some multi-item). It covers chest discomfort in the last week (1 item), changes in chest discomfort (1 item), medication (1 item), smoking (1 item), diet (1 item), medication (2 items), hospital use (2 items), and the SF-36 (10 items).

HOI recommends that this form should be supplemented with the SF-36 and socio-demographic information.

RAND CONGESTIVE HEART FAILURE (SHORTNESS OF BREATH/ENLARGED HEART/ HEART FAILURE) BATTERY AND RAND CHEST PAIN (ANGINA) BATTERY

Measurement of the prevalence and adverse effects of congestive heart failure and angina pectoris were used in the Rand Health Insurance Study (HIS) to investigate the effect of different levels of insurance on health status and quality of care. Heart Disease was selected for study because of its widespread prevalence, ease of measurement, and associations with morbidity and mortality.

1 Rand Congestive Heart Failure (Shortness of Breath/ Enlarged Heart/Heart Failure) Battery

The Congestive Heart Failure Questionnaire uses the Rand Shortness of Breath/Enlarged Heart/ Heart Failure Battery (adapted from the Rose Questionnaire, see above). It comprises 19 questions, 12 of which cover symptoms, 1 medical consultations, 2 relate to treatment and 4 relate to the impact of the disease on the respondent's life.

Content, administration and scoring

The questions on the impact of the disease form a standard set of questions used in all the disease batteries from the Health Insurance Study (Rosenthal et al. 1981). The questions deal with the amount of pain that the condition may have caused, the amount of worry or concern experienced, the amount of time the person has restricted his or her activities because of the problem, and the number of days spent in bed attributable to the condition. The first three items refer to the previous 3 months and the last to the previous 30 days.

The questionnaire can be self-administered. Responses to the pain, worry and limitations

questions range from 'none' to 'a great deal' (or similar wording, depending on the item). A composite item called 'any impact' was constructed, composed of positive responses to the disease impact items. Other items in the battery require a 'yes/no' response, or offer 3-point to 5-point response scales.

Examples from the Rand Shortness of Breath Battery

76A During the past 3 months, have you been troubled by shortness of breath when you hurried or walked uphill?   Yes/no

76F During the past 3 months, did you ever sleep on more than one pillow because of a problem with shortness of breath?   Yes/no

77 Thinking of the past 3 months, did your ankles ever swell during the day enough to make your shoes feel tight?   Yes/no

80 During the past 3 months, how much pain has your shortness of breath, enlarged heart, or heart failure caused you?

A great deal of pain / some pain / a little pain / no pain at all

81 During the past 3 months, how much has your shortness of breath, enlarged heart, or heart failure worried or concerned you?

A great deal / somewhat / a little / not at all

82 During the past 3 months, how much of the time has your shortness of breath, enlarged heart, or heart failure kept you from doing the kinds of things other people your age do?

All of the time / most of the time / some of the time / a little of the time / none of the time

83 During the past 30 days, how many days has your shortness of breath, enlarged heart, or heart failure kept you in bed all day or most of the day?   (If none, write '0').

Validity and reliability

The validity and reliability of the shortness of breath items were discussed earlier; testing is ongoing at Rand. In support of the Rand scale's construct validity, the disease impact questions were able to distinguish between respondents who were considered by HIS criteria as possibly or probably having congestive heart failure and those who did not have it. Among sufferers, the problem experienced most frequently was worry or concern about the condition, followed by pain and restriction of activities.

The questionnaire is short, and not multidimensional, but the Rand impact of disease items are attractive because of their brevity and the fact that they can be used with other scales. They are also attractive given the population norms that are available, based on large numbers of people.

2 Rand Chest Pain (Angina) Battery

This battery is based on the Rose Cardiovascular (Chest Pain) Questionnaire, supplemented with questions on medical history and impact on quality of life (Berman *et al.* 1981).

Content, administration and scoring

The angina battery comprises 19 questions, ten of which relate to symptoms, one to medical consultions, two to diagnosis, two to treatment, and four to disease impact. The disease impact questions form a standard set of questions used in all the Rand disease batteries (pain, worry or concern, restrictions, and bed days).

The questionnaire can be self-administered. Responses to the pain, worry and limitations questions range from 'none' to 'a great deal' (or similar wording, depending on the item). Other items in the battery require a 'yes/no' response, or offer 3-point to 6-point response scales. A composite item called 'any impact' was constructed, composed of positive responses to the disease impact items.

In the Health Insurance Study, a respondent was considered to have angina if scored as such on the Rose Cardiovascular Questionnaire and if aged 35 or older; or if the respondent reported a medical diagnosis of angina and at least a probable score on the Rose Questionnaire; or if the respondent had filed at least three insurance claim forms listing a diagnosis of angina pectoris.

Examples from the Rand Chest Pain Battery

99A Have you had any discomfort, heaviness or pressure in your chest during the past 12 months (not caused by a cold or by an accident or injury)? Yes/no

101 Do you get this feeling when you walk uphill or hurry?   Yes/no

101B What do you usually do when you get this feeling in your chest while walking?

Stop for a while / slow down / continue at same pace

107 During the past 3 months, how much pain has your chest pain or heart trouble caused you?

A great deal of pain / some pain / a little pain / no pain at all

108 During the past 3 months, how much has your chest pain or heart trouble worried or concerned you?

A great deal / somewhat / a little / not at all

109 During the past 3 months, how much of the time has your chest pain or heart trouble kept you from doing the kinds of things other people your age do?

All of the time / most of the time / some of the time / a little of the time / none of the time

110 During the past 30 days, how many days has your chest pain or heart trouble kept you in bed all day or most of the day?

Validity and reliability

The validity and reliability of the Rose questionnaires was discussed earlier, and some data are given by the Rand investigators (Berman *et al.* 1981). Those with a fairly definite diagnosis of angina in the HIS reported pain and worry about angina more often than restrictions on one's activity or days in bed. The questions on impact on quality of life were able to discriminate between respondents with and without probable angina. Respondents with angina had significantly more pain, worry and restricted activity than those without angina. These findings support the scale's construct validity. There are few other data on reliability and validity.

GUYATT'S CHRONIC HEART FAILURE QUESTIONNAIRE (CHQ)

The CHQ was developed as a measure of subjective health status for people with heart failure by Guyatt *et al.* (1988, 1989a). The authors aimed to include both physical and emotional health, and areas of functioning of importance to patients. Scale items were generated from a literature review, consultations with health professionals and interviews with patients. Eighty-eight patients with heart failure were asked about the impact of their condition on their lives, and then asked to rate 123 items relating to physical and emotional functioning. Items were scored according to their importance on a 5-point Likert scale. The most frequently selected and important items were included in the final 16-item version of the questionnaire.

Content, administration and scoring

The final version covers dyspnoea during daily activities, fatigue and emotional function. The questionnaire is administered by an interviewer. It is based on the 19-question/20-item Guyatt's McMaster Chronic Disease Questionnaire (CRQ: Guyatt *et al.* 1987a, 1987b, 1987c, 1991; see Chapter 4). The 16 items of the CHQ are identical to 16 of the 20 items of the CRQ, which were tested on patients with respiratory disease with good results.

Response choices for the fixed choice items are on 7-point scales of frequency (e.g. 'all of the time' to 'none of the time') or severity (e.g. 'extremely short of breath' to 'not at all short of breath'). Scores are summed within the dimensions to yield sub-scale scores for dyspnoea, fatigue and emotional functioning.

Examples from the CHQ

1 I would like you to think of the activities that you have done during the last 2 weeks that have made you feel short of breath. These should be activities which you do frequently and which are important in your day-to-day life. Please list as many activities as you can that you have done during the last 2 weeks that have made you feel short of breath.

2 I will now read a list of activities that make some people with lung problems feel short of breath. I will pause after each item long enough for you to tell me if you have felt short of breath doing that activity during the last 2 weeks. If you haven't done the activity during the last 2 weeks, just answer 'no'. The activities are . . .

   1 Being angry or upset
   5 Dressing
   6 Eating
   7 Going for a walk
  10 Lying flat

  15 Playing sports
  16 Reaching over your head
  19 Talking
  20 Vacuuming
  23 Walking upstairs
  26 Trying to sleep

6 What about fatigue? How tired have you felt over the last 2 weeks?

7 How often during the past 2 weeks have you felt inadequate, worthless, or as if you were a burden on others?

13 How often during the last 2 weeks have you felt worn out or sluggish?

Validity and reliability

The CHQ was tested in a small-scale, controlled trial of digoxin in patients with heart failure. It was reported to be able to distinguish between patients who improved and those who did not. It correlated moderately with patients' global ratings of dyspnoea, fatigue and emotional functioning (change scores, $r = 0.34$–0.65), 6 min walking test scores ($r = 0.60$) and clinical classifications of heart failure ($r = 0.42$). Correlations between the CHQ and patients' global ratings of change in shortness of breath, change in walking test score and change in heart failure classification score ranged between 0.42 and 0.65, and were higher than the correlations between these change scores and the NYHA Functional Classification and the Specific Activity Scale. The authors reported that it was reproducible with 25 patients. The results require confirmation by other investigators, but appear promising.

FERRANS AND POWERS' QUALITY OF LIFE INDEX (CARDIAC)

This is a well-known but relatively little used scale (Ferrans and Powers 1985). It was developed and used by Faris and Stotts (1990) in a small-scale study of 20 patients on the effect of percutaneous transluminal coronary angioplasty on quality of life.

Validity and reliability

Faris and Stotts reported that it was sensitive to improvements in health. They also reported a

Examples from Quality of Life Index (CARDIAC)

Part I: Domain satisfaction

How satisfied are you with the amount of chest pain you still have?

How satisfied are you with your physical independence (ability to do things for yourself, get around)?

How satisfied are you with your potential to live a long time?

Very dissatisfied/moderately dissatisfied/slightly dissatisfied/slightly satisfied/moderately satisfied/very satisfied

Part II: Domain importance

How important is it to you to be completely free of chest pain?

How important is your physical independence (ability to do things for yourself, get around) to you?

How important is living a long time to you?

---

test–retest correlation of $r = 0.87$, and a Cronbach's alpha of $r = 0.93$. There are few other data on its psychometric properties.

REHABILITATION QUESTIONNAIRE

This questionnaire was designed by Stocksmeier (1979) and modified by Fridlund *et al.* (1991). It is based on WHO criteria for the rehabilitation of myocardial infarction patients (see WHO 1993). The questions include subjective items on health behaviour, diet, exercise, smoking, sex, self-reported physical and psychological problems, and items on family, leisure, relationships, society and work situation. Ratings are based on a Likert scale ranging from 1 to 5 ('not at all' to 'a great extent') or dichotomous answers ('yes/no') or 'better' – 'unchanged' – 'worse'/'improved' – 'unaltered' – 'deteriorated'. Items are analysed separately in relation to the presence or absence of the problem, the extent of problems and perceived changes (Fridlund *et al.* 1991).

Examples from the Rehabilitation Questionnaire

Anger
Anxiety
Breathlessness
Chestpain
Depression
Fear
Irritation
Nervousness
Sleeplessness

The Rehabilitation Questionnaire has been used – and sometimes modified – in studies of recovery after myocardial infarction (MI, e.g. Fridlund *et al.* 1991). The scale was sensitive to improvement at 6 and 12 months in those patients participating in a rehabilitation programme ($n = 53$) in Sweden, compared with less improvement in controls ($n = 63$) (Fridlund *et al.* 1991).

CIRCULATORY DISEASE

TRENDS IN MEASURING QUALITY OF LIFE IN PEOPLE WITH CIRCULATORY DISEASE: HYPERTENSION

The treatment of hypertension is long term and the aim is to reduce risk of morbidity and mortality (e.g. from stroke and heart disease). Individuals with hypertension may have no overt manifestations of illness, but intervention with a therapeutic agent, while having long-term protective effects (e.g. against strokes), raises interest in quality of life assessments in clinical trials of new drugs. This is made more important by the 'labelling effect' and adoption of the sick role by people given a diagnosis of hypertension, who previously perceived themselves as well (Sackett *et al.* 1983).

In addition to taking clinical measurements (e.g. recording blood pressure levels), most outcome studies of hypertension have focused on symptom reporting, including psychological symptoms such as depression. People with hypertension may be symptom-free before diagnosis, or they may, depending on severity, report symptoms which include uneasiness, heavy headedness, memory impairment and blurred vision, with a reduction in work capacity and limitations on leisure activities. The symptoms and side-effects reported by people receiving the older therapeutic agents include anxiety, depression, fatigue, blurred

vision, nausea, diarrhoea, dry mouth, poor appetite, male impotence, gout, dizziness and headaches. These sometimes caused patients to
discontinue treatment (Medical Research Council:
MRC 1981). A number of investigators, using
activity and psychiatric symptom instruments (e.g.
for depression) have reported adverse effects of
hypertension or its treatment on quality of life (e.g.
Curb *et al*. 1985; Avorn *et al*. 1986). Research
during the 1970s reported sexual dysfunction to be
a significant problem in males treated for hypertension, regardless of the type of medication, in
comparison with controls (Hogan *et al*. 1980). The
newer agents apparently produce fewer side-
effects, but they are not free of effects (Fletcher and
Bulpitt 1993). The implication of the latter is the
need for the constant updating and testing of
symptom checklists.

Increasingly, studies have attempted to measure
quality of life among hypertensive patients in
relation to, for example, well-being, physical
symptoms, work performance, cognitive function
and life satisfaction (Croog *et al*. 1986; Fletcher and
Bulpitt 1989; Herrick *et al*. 1989), and have reported greater patient acceptability of newer drugs
for the treatment of hypertension, in comparison to
more established drugs. Levine and Croog's (1984,
1989; Croog *et al*. 1986) study of the quality of life
of hypertensive patients was based on five major
dimensions: the performance of social roles
(spouse, parent, worker, friend and community
citizen); physiological state; emotional state; intellectual or cognitive functioning; and general well-
being and life satisfaction. They used the Rand HIS
22-item General Well-Being Scale, which is based
on Dupuy's (1978) Psychological General Well-
Being Schedule (Brook *et al*. 1979a, 1979b); and a
series of sub-scales from the 53-item Brief Symptom Inventory for the assessment of psychological
symptom patterns (Derogatis and Spencer 1982);
the visual reproduction test of the Wechsler Memory Scale, which assesses neuropsychological function (Wechsler 1945; Wechsler and Stone 1973) and
the Trail-Making Test, which measures visual
motor speed and integration, both for assessing
intellectual and cognitive functioning. The authors
admitted that compiling quality of life measures
was not easy, as these scales were not disease-
specific and required modification and the inclusion of new measures (Levine and Croog 1989).

They constructed a Physical Symptoms Index
from questions in common use in clinical practice,
a Sexual Symptoms Distress Index, measures of life
satisfaction and work performance, based on previous scales. The measures were sensitive to type of
medication and their effects. In retrospect, Levine
and Croog (1989) reported that they would have
preferred to have selected fewer or shorter scales
and to have employed widely used standardized
measures. They would still include the Rand
General Well-Being Index. In sum, they would
have preferred a shorter version of the same
battery.

WHAT SHOULD BE MEASURED?

Wenger *et al*. (1984) argued that, in addition to
clinical indicators, quality of life assessment in
clinical trials of hypertensive therapy should include those areas in which the therapy affects the
quality of life of the patient: mental alertness,
sexual function, activity tolerance and performance
of activities of daily living (ADL), sleep disturbances and ultimately their life satisfaction. However, it would seem that most functional ability
scales are totally inappropriate, given their design
for use with elderly and ill populations, rather than
people affected by, for example, fatigue. The ADL
components of general health status measures are
more appropriate, e.g. the complete Rand Short
Form-36 (SF-36) (Stewart and Ware 1992).

Bulpitt and Fletcher (1990), however, have
warned against the use of general health status
measures, such as the Sickness Impact Profile and
the Nottingham Health Profile, given that hypertensive patients are free of other symptoms, and the
many items on loss of self-care ability and mobility
are inappropriate. They argued that a questionnaire
for hypertensive patients should cover physical
symptoms, psychological well-being and perception of the effects of the treatment on lifestyle, and
provide their own as an example. It purposely does
not include measures of positive well-being (e.g.
vitality) or social functioning (e.g. social participation, performance and satisfaction at work). The
authors do not include objective tests of cognitive
functioning, but argue that such tests should be
included if there is concern about the effects of
medication in this area. Bulpitt and Fletcher's

Hypertension Questionnaire has three sections, and was designed for self-administration. The authors report that it is acceptable to patients, and takes between 20 and 40 min to complete. It is described later.

Furberg *et al.* (1984) defined quality of life in relation to mild hypertension in terms of three broad components: functioning, perceptions and symptoms. *Functioning* includes personal care ability, physical activity, social activity, work and family, sexual functioning, emotional functioning (general well-being and the ability to cope with stress) and intellectual functioning (mental alertness and memory). Perceptions include life satisfaction and perceived health status. Symptoms include perceptions, such as pain, anxiety and fatigue, as well as the symptoms associated with hypertension and its treatment. They clarified the position in relation to emotional functioning and pointed out that diagnostic instruments such as the Diagnostic Interview Schedule (Robins *et al.* 1979) are not appropriate, and instead recommended symptom scales that relate to the most common problems, such as the General Well-Being Schedule (Dupuy 1973), the Rand HIS Mental Health Inventory (Veit and Ware 1983) or the Profile of Mood States (POMS: McNair *et al.* 1971), in addition to tests of cognitive and intellectual functioning. The authors also emphasize the importance of health perceptions among these patients, and suggested the Rand HIS General Health Rating Index as the most adequate measure of self-perceived health, health outlook and worry about health (Davies and Ware 1981).

DISEASE-SPECIFIC QUALITY OF LIFE SCALES: HYPERTENSION

PALMER'S SYMPTOM CHECKLIST AND BATTERY

Palmer *et al.* (1992) assessed the quality of life of 265 hypertensive adults treated with atenolol or captopril in a double-blind crossover trial. They used a set of condition-specific questions that included 30 symptoms and side-effects which they had drawn up for previous research (Bulpitt *et al.* 1974), and assessed psychiatric morbidity with the Symptom Rating Test (Kellner and Sheffield 1973) and the Profile of Mood States (McNair *et al.* 1971).

Content

The symptoms include: sleepiness, hours of sleep, weak limbs, slow walking pace, headache, blurred vision, depression, frequency of defecation, diarrhoea, nocturia, dry mouth, change of therapy, impotence, failure of ejaculation, frequency of sexual intercourse.

Administration and scoring

The checklist is self-administered, usually with an interviewer present. The items are analysed separately; they can also be summed to produce a total score. There is evidence that the psychometric properties of the instrument are limited.

Examples from Palmer's Symptom Checklist

The answers are yes/no, unless otherwise specified:

 8 Since your last visit have you often felt sleepy during the day?

11 Compared with other men/women your age, do you tend to walk slower / faster / about the same pace?

16 Have you, since your last visit, been depressed?

21 Do you suffer from a dry mouth?

22 How many times, on average, do you rise at night to pass urine?

0 / 1 / 2 / more than twice. (Please indicate number)

Supplementary questions for males

During sexual intercourse are you:

25 Troubled by failure to sustain an erection?

HEALTH OUTCOMES INSTITUTE TyPE SCALES (HOI-TyPE): HYPERTENSION

The Health Outcomes Institute (HOI), previously known as Interstudy (2001 Killebrew Drive, Suite 122, Bloomington, MN 55425, USA), has produced condition-specific specifications (TyPE) for hypertension. They await results of testing.

Content, administration and scoring

The hypertension questionnaire for patients has 11 questions, some of which are multi-item. The questions cover age at onset (1 item), smoking

(1 item), problems with sexual activity (6 items), medication (2 items) and symptoms (21 items). There is also a form for clinicians. The forms for hypertension are designed for repeated application (at follow-ups), and for self-completion. Each item is scored differently.

Examples from the HOI Hypertension/Lipid Form

Patient questionnaire

6 How much of a problem was each of the following during the past 4 weeks?

   (a) Lack of sexual interest
   (b) Unable to relax and enjoy sex
   (c) Difficulty in becoming sexually aroused

No problem / mild problem / moderate problem / severe problem

10 How often have you had the following symptoms during the past 4 weeks?

   (a) Shortness of breath with exercise or work
   (d) Feeling drowsy or sedated
   (f) Chest discomfort/pain brought on by activity
   (h) Headaches more than usual

Never / once or twice / a few times / fairly often / very often

11 Have you experienced any of the following in the past 6 months?

   (a) Unexpected sweating
   (d) Blurred vision
   (g) Nausea
   (k) Increased urination

Clinical questionnaire

10 Is there evidence that the patient currently has or has experienced any of the following?

   (a) Congestive heart failure
   (e) Stroke
   (f) Cardiac arrythmias

Yes/no

12 Is there evidence of cardiomegaly on chest X-ray? Yes/no

16 Has any form of secondary hypertension been diagnosed? Yes/no

Physical examination

2 Blood pressure (mm Hg): (a) systolic, (b) diastolic:

Pulse (beat/min)

Any laboratory measurements this visit?

BULPITT'S HYPERTENSION QUESTIONNAIRE AND BATTERIES

This questionnaire focuses on the symptoms associated with hypertension (Bulpitt 1982); it also measures the effects on everyday life and functioning by adapting Fanshel and Bush's (1970) Health Status Index.

Content

The first section of the questionnaire enquires about disease-specific symptoms – headache and nocturia (the two main symptoms associated with high blood pressure or its treatment), and a variety of other symptoms due to the side-effects of medication. The second section covers the effect of hypertension on daily life and functioning (e.g. work, hobbies, activities around the house). The effect of treatment on lifestyles and level of functioning is scored in this battery by a modified version of Fanshel and Bush's (1970) Health Status Index (Bulpitt 1982).

Fletcher *et al.* (1987) supplemented the scale with the Profile of Mood States (POMS: McNair *et al.* 1971) to measure psychological well-being (on an experimental basis, in order to assess its appropriateness). Bulpitt and Fletcher also used the Symptom Rating Test (Kellner and Sheffield 1973; Kellner 1983) for methodological testing.

Administration and scoring

The questionnaire and batteries can be self-administered. The response format to the hypertension symptoms section ranges from a dichotomous format, requiring 'yes/no' answers to an open response structure, whereby the respondents have to write in their answers. The responses can be analysed separately or summed to form a total score.

The disability section of the questionnaire scores disability as a health index on a continuum from 0 (dead) through to 1 (total well-being): total well-being, minor dissatisfaction, discomfort, minor disability, major disability, disabled, confined, bedridden, isolated, comatose, dead. The advantage of this is that patients who die or who default from the study can be given a rating and included in the analysis.

Examples from Bulpitt's Hypertension Questionnaire

Section 1: Symptoms

Response = yes/no

1   In the last month have you suffered from lightheaded-ness or faintness?
2   IF YES, does the lightheadedness or faintness occur only when you are standing?
4   In the last month have you often felt sleepy during the day?
5   How many hours per 24 do you usually sleep?
6   Have you in the last month noticed weakness in the limbs?
8   Do you get short of breath walking with people of your own age on level ground?
9   Are your ankles swollen at the end of the day?
15 In the last month have you suffered from a dry mouth?
25 Do your fingers go white in cold weather?
27 Have you, in the last month, suffered from head-aches?
35 Filter question, for men only:

During sexual intercourse are you troubled by failure to sustain an erection?

Section 2

37 If you ticked in paid employment:

How many days off work did you have due to ill health in the last month? Please write the number of days in the box, or write none if you had no days off due to ill health.

38 If you had days off work due to ill health, what was the reason?
39 During the last month have you been unable through ill-health to carry out your usual activities around the house and garden?   Yes/no
41 What were the reasons that you were unable to carry out your usual activities through ill health?

(Respondent writes in reply, no pre-codes)

44 Has your state of health interfered with these hobbies recently?   Yes/no
45 IF YES, in what way?

(Respondent writes in reply, no pre-codes)

Examples of the Modified Health Index scoring

Disablement

(i)   Score 0.625 when 'unemployed for medical reasons' (Q. 36)

Minor disability

(iii) Score 0.8 when high blood pressure or treatment interfered with hobbies (Q. 44) or life (Q. 46)

The score recorded is the lowest of the above scores. Please note, if patient has died, score 0; confined to bed, score 0.125; and confined to the house but not to bed, score 0.375

Validity

The symptom items were initially developed by Bulpitt *et al.* (1974, 1979) with good results for reliability, validity and sensitivity. Although the questionnaire itself is crude, it has been shown to distinguish between people with hypertension and those without, matching for age and sex in a community-based study (Battersby *et al.* 1989), and it is sensitive to differences in treatments (Bulpitt and Fletcher 1990).

Reliability

The responses to the questions about symptoms were highly repeatable in a follow-up survey at 10 months (Bulpitt *et al.* 1976), with repeatability scores ranging from 0.95 to 1.0 (1.0 being perfect agreement), and were found to be sensitive to differences in treatments (Bulpitt and Fletcher 1990). The questionnaire will have to be modified as new treatments, with new side-effects, are introduced.

QUALITY OF LIFE IMPAIRMENT SCALE: HYPERTENSION

The Quality of Life Impairment Scale (or the Relative's Questionnaire) was designed by Sengupta *et al.* (1975) for use in a study of quality of life after brain surgery. It has been adapted for use with hypertensive patients (Jachuck *et al.* 1982).

Content, administration and scoring

The scale asks a relative or close friend to evaluate adverse changes in the patient in 20 areas and yields a score of 0–32. The scale includes a sex interest item, which is not included in the overall scoring as it is not always completed (the respondent may not know). The scale can be self-administered. The items are scored 0, 1, 2 or 3, with high scores reflecting a more severe problem. The scores from the scale are divided into three groups representing mild, moderate and severe changes in quality of life. The scores are summed to form the three scales.

Examples from the QoH Impairment Scale: Hypertension

(b) Memory

Unchanged / less good / worse / very much worse

(g) Feeling

Rarely shows emotion now / emotion seems just ordinary / over-emotional, sometimes happy or sad

(i) Laughter

Never laughs / laughs more than before / laughs unnecessarily

(l) Initiative

Cannot make any decisions now / needs a lot of pushing to do things / seems to have lost a bit of initiative / gets on with things just as before

(s) Sex

Does not find an interest in sex any more / sexual interest is very much less than it was / no change in his sexual interest / much more interested in sex matters than before

---

Validity and reliability

There is little evidence of the scale's reliability and validity. It was used in a study of the effect of hypotensive drugs on the quality of life in 75 patients by Jachuck *et al.* (1982), and they reported it to have high internal reliability ($r = 0.87$). The authors also reported that the patients' general practitioners rated 100 per cent improvement, as the patients all had adequately controlled blood pressure, there had been no clinical deterioration since the onset of treatment and the patients had not complained to the doctors about problems. In contrast, less than half of the patients themselves said they felt they had improved and 8 per cent felt worse. Moreover, the relatives rated 25 per cent of the patients to have suffered negligible or mild

adverse changes (e.g. in energy, general activity, sexual activity and irritability), 33 per cent to have suffered moderate adverse changes and 30 per cent to have suffered severe impairment after receiving anti-hypertensive medication.

RAND HEALTH INSURANCE STUDY BLOOD PRESSURE BATTERY

Data on the prevalence and adverse effects of hypertension were used in the Rand Health Insurance Study (HIS) to investigate the effect of different levels of insurance on health status and quality of care. Hypertension was selected for study because of its widespread prevalence, ease of measurement, its association with considerable morbidity and mortality, and amenability to treatment or control (Brook *et al.* 1980b).

The investigators recognized that hypertension may be unsymptomatic generally but also lead to disabling and life-threatening events (e.g. stroke), and that people labelled as hypertensives may worry about their condition and be more inclined to adopt a sick role. They were concerned to reflect this anxiety in the questionnaire. Altogether, 821 of their 5453 respondents reported having a medical diagnosis of high blood pressure and completed the blood pressure battery (blood pressure was also measured at screening examination).

Content, administration and scoring

The hypertension battery is self-administered and comprises 17 questions, 8 of which relate to diagnosis and treatment, 4 to management (e.g. diet and salt intake), 1 to medical consultations and 4 to disease impact. Again, the four standard Rand disease impact questions are used (measuring pain, worry or concern, restriction and bed days).

As with the other Rand disease-specific batteries, the responses to the pain, worry and limitations questions range from 'none' to 'a great deal' (or similar wording, depending on the item). Over all the questions, item responses vary from dichotomous (e.g. 'Yes/no') replies to 4- or 5-point categorical scales. A composite item called 'any impact' was constructed, composed of positive responses to the disease impact items. More detailed disease-specific questions were also included in the battery. Items are analysed separately, apart from the composite score.

Examples from the Rand Blood Pressure Battery

86 Has a doctor ever said that you had high blood pressure?   Yes/no

89A Are you taking any pills or medicine now?

Yes, taking now / no, I decided to stop / no, doctor told me to stop / no, never took pills or medicine

91A How often do you add salt to your food at the table?

95 During the past 3 months, how much pain has your high blood pressure caused you?

A great deal of pain / some pain / a little pain / no pain at all

96 During the past 3 months, how much has your high blood pressure worried or concerned you?

A great deal / somewhat / a little / not at all

97 During the past 3 months, how much of the time has your high blood pressure kept you from doing the kinds of things other people your age do?

All of the time / most of the time / some of the time / a little of the time / none of the time

98 During the past 30 days, how many days has your high blood pressure kept you in bed all day or most of the day?   (If none, write in '0')

Validity and reliability

The battery distinguished between those classified as hypertensive and those classified as normotensive: the former reported more adverse effects and restrictions to activity, days in bed, worry and pain. This supports the validity of the battery.

Brook *et al.* (1980b) reported that the self-report hypertension items in the battery correlated well with findings at screening interview, although congruence was not perfect ($r = 0.65–0.71$). Apparently, about a third of the respondents who were diagnosed at examination as hypertensive did not indicate on the questionnaire that they were aware of, or had been informed about, their condition. While self-report questionnaires are not the ideal vehicle for obtaining medical history and diagnostic data in the case of sometimes asymptomatic conditions (as in hypertension), this battery can be used once patients have been medically diagnosed as having hypertension.

CONCLUSION

Quality of life assessment in coronary heart disease has largely been limited to single-domain measures of quality of life, ranging from crude indicators of return to work to more sophisticated studies of psychological morbidity. Where broader quality of life assessments have been attempted, investigators have usually relied on generic measures of health-related quality of life. In relation to heart failure, the most promising disease-specific quality of life measure is the Chronic Heart Failure Questionnaire (Guyatt *et al.* 1988). This is based on patient-generated domains of quality of life.

In relation to hypertension, there is strong debate about the appropriateness of generic health-related quality of life measures. These are probably too severe for use with a group who have a fairly normal lifestyle. Most disease-specific 'quality of life' scales are really extended symptom scales. These all require supplementation with broader quality of life domains. The 'impact of disease' scale from the Rand hypertension battery may suffice as a supplement (Brook *et al.* 1980b).

8

OTHER DISEASE-
AND
CONDITION-SPECIFIC
SCALES

OTHER DEVELOPMENTS IN THE MEASUREMENT OF DISEASE-SPECIFIC QUALITY OF LIFE

A number of specific quality of life indicators have been developed for use with conditions other than those reviewed in this book. The list is long and includes:

- anaemia (Scott *et al*. 1980);
- back pain (Ruta *et al*. 1994a, 1994b);
- diabetes (Brook *et al*. 1981; Diabetes Control and Complications Trial Research Group 1988; Bradley *et al*. 1990; Bradley 1991; Hanestead *et al*. 1991; Meadows 1991; Hammond and Aoki 1992; Hörnquist *et al*. 1993; McColl *et al*. 1993, 1995; the Health Outcomes Institute TyPE batteries);
- end-stage renal disease (Evans *et al*. 1985; Guyatt *et al*. 1986; Parfrey *et al*. 1989; Koch and Muthny, 1990; Wright *et al*. 1994);
- hay fever (Beck *et al*. 1981a);
- HIV and AIDS (Hays and Shapiro 1992; Lubeck and Fries 1992; Schag *et al*. 1992; Ganz *et al*. 1993; Holzemer *et al*. 1993);
- inflammatory bowel disease (Guyatt *et al*. 1989d; Kunsebeck *et al*. 1990);
- migraine (Santanello *et al*. 1994);
- minor surgical procedures such as haemorrhoids and varicose veins (Rubenstein *et al*. 1983; Garratt *et al*. 1993a);
- neurological conditions (other than those

included here) such as Parkinson's disease, multiple sclerosis (see Wade 1992);
- peptic ulcer (Zielske *et al*. 1982);
- skin diseases such as psoriasis (Fredriksson and Pettersson 1978; Finlay and Kelly 1987); onychomycosis (fungal infection of the nails) (Lubeck *et al*. 1993); eczema and acne (Brook *et al*. 1980a; Motley and Finlay, 1989);
- thyroid disease (Brook *et al*. 1982);
- vision impairment and hearing loss (Rubenstein *et al*. 1982; Beck *et al*. 1981b).

A selection of these measures is reviewed in this chapter. For many of these other conditions, e.g. Parkinson's disease, the quality of life measures are limited to disease-specific severity indexes, symptoms, psychological functioning, or general measures of functioning (Shindler *et al*. 1993). Some of the measures referenced here are brief outcome measures designed for use with the Rand Health Insurance Study/Medical Outcomes Study with common questions on the impact of the condition on the respondent's life and amount of worry caused by the condition, as well as disease-specific items.

There are also a number of areas which the reader will find conspicuously absent from this review. Liver disease and treatment (e.g. transplantation) is one example, because it is an area where little progress has been made in the development of a disease-specific quality of life scale. A computer based literature search (MEDLINE) from 1966 by

Roberts (1989) produced just 13 articles which dealt with quality of life assessment of survivors of liver transplantation. Investigators have used existing generic measures, such as the Nottingham Health Profile, supplemented with disease-specific items (e.g. van Agt *et al.* 1993). Others have adapted quality of life questionnaires developed for use with cancer patients, such as the EORTC quality of life questionnaire (Aaronson *et al.* 1986, 1993; Kober *et al.* 1990). Popular scales have included the Minnesota Multiphasic Personality Inventory (16 items) (Hathaway and McKinley, 1990) and standard intelligence scales (which are not necessarily appropriate), the Social Behaviour Assessment Schedule (Platt *et al.* 1980, 1983), the STAI-Anxiety Scale (Spielberger *et al.* 1970, 1973, 1983), and Bergner and co-workers' (1981) generic Sickness Impact Profile (e.g. Tartar *et al.* 1983, 1984, 1988). Roberts (1989) comments that impaired mental status makes it difficult to use subjective quality of life scales with these patients.

HEALTH OUTCOMES INSTITUTE TyPE DISEASE-SPECIFIC OUTCOME SCALES (HOI-TyPE)

The Health Outcomes Institute (HOI) in the USA has developed several condition-specific outcomes specifications, called TyPE: Technology of Patient Experience (TyPE) Specifications. They are available from the Health Outcomes Institute, 2001 Killebrew Drive, Suite 122, Bloomington, MN, 55425, USA, but they have not yet been fully tested for reliability or validity. The scales include back pain, heart disease and hypertension, respiratory disease, schizophrenia, depression and other psychiatric disorders, joint disorders, diabetes, alcohol use, sinusitis, cataracts, prostatism, and others are being continuously developed. Interested readers should consult the Health Outcomes Institute for details.

While little consensus exists as to which measures are most appropriate, it is encouraging that the HOI has made a start by commissioning experts in each area to design fairly brief outcomes instruments, taking social, physical and psychological indicators into account. Most of these scales have only one or two items covering important domains (e.g. restriction on social activities) because of the requirement for brevity. However,

these scales can easily be supplemented by broader health status measures. Many of them include the physical functioning sub-scale of the SF-36 and could easily be supplemented by the full instrument if necessary. The forms containing the disease-specific items on symptoms and treatments are of value. Another organization, the Medical Outcomes Trust in Boston, is also considering the development of disease-specific quality of life outcome measures (The Medical Outcomes Trust, P.O. Box 1917, Boston, MA, 02205, USA).

POPULAR GENERIC MEASURES USED TO SUPPLEMENT DISEASE-SPECIFIC SCALES

It was pointed out in the earlier chapters that in the USA, the Sickness Impact Profile (Bergner *et al.* 1981) has been one of the most popular generic measures used to supplement disease-specific indicators in outcome studies. Even when a wide range of disease-specific quality of life measures has been included in a battery, several investigators have supplemented them with Bergner and co-workers' (1981) Sickness Impact Profile (e.g. Salek 1993). The SIP has been widely used in studies of joint and orthopaedic conditions (see Chapter 6).

In Europe, the Nottingham Health Profile (Hunt *et al.* 1986) has been a popular measure of health status outcome in relation to health-related quality of life. It has been used to supplement disease-specific questions in outcome studies across many medical specialities (see Hunt *et al.* 1986 for reviews). More recently, it has been used in outcome assessment of cholecystectomy (Bardsley *et al.* 1992), hysterectomy (Clarke 1993), prostatectomy (Black *et al.* 1991, 1993) and urinary incontinence (Grimby *et al.* 1993).

The Short Form 36-item questionnaire (SF-36) (Ware *et al.* 1993) has become an increasingly popular measure with which to supplement disease-specific items in outcome studies, for example varicose veins, back pain and in hernia repair (Garratt *et al.* 1993a, 1993b; Ruta *et al.* 1994, in press; Lawrence *et al.* 1993). These generic measures still require supplementation with disease-specific items. For example, in Garratt and co-workers' (1993a) varicose vein study, items were added on the distribution of veins, pain, analgesia, ankle swelling, itching, discoloration, skin conditions etc). In Ruta and co-workers' back pain study (in press) it was supplemented with detailed questions on pain and sensation, functional ability and mobility.

While these measures have been among the most popular, several other generic measures have been used to supplement disease-specific items and single domain indicators of quality of life. Examples were given in the earlier chapters. Only the SF-36 (Ware *et al.* 1993) is reviewed in this chapter because it is a frequently recommended core instrument for disease-specific quality of life scales.

DISEASE-SPECIFIC MEASURES OF QUALITY OF LIFE

DIABETES

Diabetes has no known cure, and is a major cause of morbidity and mortality. Serious complications can include cardiovascular problems, hypertension, kidney failure, blindness and amputations. Outcome assessments involve biomedical assessments of control of symptoms (e.g. measures of glycaemic control such as fasting plasma glucose), rates of hospital admission with acute complications (e.g. hyperglycaemia and hypoglycaemia), or the incidence of chronic complications (e.g. chronic renal failure, limb amputation, retinopathy, blindness, vascular insufficiency) (Williams 1989). Such problems inevitably have a major impact on quality of life.

Measures of effects on quality of life as a result of clinical and patient-centred management include social support (which may be an important determinant of effective self-management rather than an outcome measure *per se*), disruption of work and social life (usually not severe), neuropsychological deficits (e.g. during glucose depletion, transitory impairments include speed of recall, verbal fluency and rate of decision making), well-being, depression and psychological stress (Holmes 1987; Goodall and Halford 1991), as well as patient satisfaction with treatment (Bradley and Lewis 1990) and perceived control of diabetes (Bradley *et al.* 1990). Despite the extensive work on the psychological well-being (e.g. depression) of diabetic patients by Bradley and Lewis (1990) and Bradley (1994), and scale development in relation to diabetic health profiles (Meadows *et al.* 1989;

Meadows 1991), there is still no generally recommended battery of well-tested quality of life measures for use with these patients.

A frequently used generic measure, supplemented with disease-specific items, is Bergner and co-workers' (1981) Sickness Impact Profile (e.g. see Rodin 1990; Tebbi *et al.* 1990). Popular measures of psychological well-being include the Rand version of the General Well-being Scale (Stewart and Ware 1992), the Beck Depression Inventory (Beck *et al.* 1961), and Goldberg's (1972) General Health Questionnaire (Wilkinson *et al.* 1988). Scales of perceived control, and locus of control and other relevant psychological domains to measure in relation to diabetes, have been reviewed by Bradley et al. (1990) and Bradley (1991).

OUTCOME MEASURES IN AMBULATORY CARE (ASTHMA AND DIABETES) (OMAC)

McColl *et al.* (1993) aimed to develop 'practical, condition-specific outcome measurement methodologies for routine application in judging the effectiveness of care in ambulatory settings (general practice and hospital outpatients)'. They reviewed over 500 measures of general health status and quality of life, and asthma- and diabetes- condition-specific measures.

The domains considered for inclusion in their final battery of measures were: clinical (clinical control, e.g. of symptoms, complications, iatrogenic problems, severity and co-morbidity); functional (ambulation/mobility, body care/activities of daily living, pain, sleep/energy); psychosocial ('quality of life', social function, role function, mental health, health and sickness perceptions).

Content, administration and scoring

The scales which were considered suitable *initially* were the Functional Limitations Profile (UK version of SIP) (Charlton *et al.* 1983), the SF-36 (Ware *et al.* 1993), the Duke 17-item Health Profile (Parkerson *et al.* 1990), the Dartmouth COOP Chart (Nelson *et al.* 1990) and the Euroqol (Euroqol Group 1990). The Hospital Anxiety and Depression Scale (Zigmond and Snaith 1983) was also selected to measure psychological morbidity. The condition-specific measures they selected for diabetes were the Diabetes Health Profile for insulin requiring diabetes (Meadows *et al.* 1988), and, following consensus reviews with specialists, a 36–40 item symptom questionnaire for non-insulin-requiring and insulin-requiring diabetics.

Each of these scales was designed for self completion, and are scored separately. Readers are referred to the source references for further details of each non–disease-specific scale.

DIABETES ITEMS

Examples

1 In the last month, on how many days have you had a headache?

Never–Every day

2 In the last month, on how many nights have you had to get up at least twice during the night to pass water?

Never–Every day

3 In the last month, on how many days have you felt abnormally thirsty?

Never–Every day

4 In the last month, on how many days have you had blurred vision?

Never–Every day

18 In the last month, on how many days have you had a feeling of pins and needles?

Never–Every day

15 In the last month, on how many days have you had cold hands and feet?

Never–Every day

Thinking about the doctor/practice nurse who looks after your diabetes, do you agree or disagree with the following statements:

My doctor/practice nurse has helped me to make my diabetes better
My doctor/practice nurse tells me everything I want to know about my diabetes

Strongly agree–Strongly disagree

Validity and reliability

Analyses of initial results from preliminary investigations showed that the Functional Limitations Profile had a high rate of item non-response and also ceiling effects, and so this was excluded from further study (in fact 95 of its 136 items were only completed by less than 10 per cent of the sample: McColl *et al.*, 1995); the Duke 17-item Health Profile was found to have poor internal consistency and convergent validity and was excluded; all other measures were judged to be psychometrically sound and included in the next stage of analysis. The remaining questionnaire battery was estimated to take about 15 min to complete. Given the need for brevity in clinical practice, the investigators are conducting further analysis aimed at item reduction. The SF-36 and the HAD explained much of the variance between groups, and factor analyses confirmed their reported factor structure. Factor analyses also confirmed the three-factor solution originally reported for the Diabetes Health Profile (Meadows *et al.* 1988).

For diabetic patients, the SF-36 (physical function and energy sub-scales), the HAD and condition-specific items explained 52 per cent of the variance in health perceptions among non-insulin-requiring diabetics and 72 per cent of the variance of insulin-requiring diabetics. As the research is currently ongoing and much of the psychometric data are in preparation for publication, further details can be obtained from the authors.

DIABETES IMPACT MEASUREMENT SCALES (DIMS)

This instrument is a measure of health status in type I and type II adult diabetic patients. The scales were developed after a literature review, and the authors drew heavily on existing scales in the construction of the DIMS, particularly the Rand batteries (see Stewart and Ware 1992), the SIP (Bergner *et al.* 1981) and the AIMS (Meenan *et al.* 1980). The questionnaire was developed using two groups of 130 and 52 patient-volunteers (Hammond and Aoki 1992).

Content, administration and scoring

The domains include symptoms, diabetes-related morale (attitude towards managing the disease), social role fulfilment and well-being. It was designed for self-administration and takes 15–20 min to complete. Items are scored according to the selected response, with high values representing less severe or less frequent symptoms, greater morale, greater social role fulfilment, and greater well-being. Item responses are simply summed. Perceptions of control of diabetes and health perceptions were measured using a 9 cm VAS.

Examples from DIMS

1 During the past month, have you felt optimistic about your diabetes?
9 Over the past month, how much energy have you had?
11 During the past month, how worried have you been about having an insulin reaction or a dangerously low blood sugar?
24 How often did you vomit after eating during the past month?

Validity, factor structure and reliability

Principal components analysis confirmed that a major factor was measured by all sub-scales, and also several minor factors. The scale requires strengthening. Correlations between sub-scale and total scale scores ranged from 0.46 to 0.97. Cronbach's alpha for the sub-scales and total score ranged from 0.60 to 0.94, and test–retest correlations for these ranged from 0.61 to 0.77. Further work on its psychometric properties is required (Hammond and Aoki 1992).

QUALITY OF LIFE, STATUS AND CHANGE (QLSC)

Hörnquist (1982, 1989), Hanestad et al. (1991) and Hörnquist et al. (1993) have developed a quality of life battery which can be used with diabetic patients. The scale was developed in Scandinavia. The authors defined quality of life as the extent to which needs are satisfied within the domains of illness (diabetic symptoms and regimen), physical, psychological, social activity/behaviour and habits (Wikby et al. 1993). Implicit in the quality of life model are the following assumptions: the inner state, determined by subjective experiences, is of greater significance for quality of life than exterior aspects; the entirety of the concept of quality of life is more important than its parts, although both should be considered in assessments; perceptions of quality of life are lasting and radical; and while quality of life studies are mainly descriptive, they can be normative (Hanestad et al. 1991).

It has been used with a number of different types of groups (e.g. alcohol abusers) as well as diabetics. It has been reported to be sensitive to treatment among diabetics in relation to an insulin pen. While generic, it is reported here because it has been tailored for use with people with diabetes (Hörnquist et al. 1990).

Content, administration and scoring

The battery has two components: life domain rating and well-being. The life domain ratings appear in a status as well as in a change questionnaire. The questionnaire comprises six self-rated life domains: somatic, psychological, social, behavioural/activity, material and structural. The somatic life domain covers overall bodily health and specific sickness impact; the psychological life domain covers satisfaction with life, well-being in general and intellectual functioning; the social life domain covers social contact in general and that specifically related to family and sexual life; the behavioural/activity life domain deals with mobility, working capacity and basic habits; the structural life domain includes religion; and the material life domain covers the respondent's economic situation (Hanestad et al. 1991).

The ratings focus on the respondent's current appraisal (mainly in terms of good/bad) within the domains; a parallel retrospective version with the same items addresses the changes that occur due to an intervention over a specified time period (mainly in terms of improved/deteriorated). Complementary to this life domain rating scale is a well-being rating scale, which contains ten statements to be matched to the rater's perceptions of him/herself and his/her life situation. Some items have a primarily emotional content (basic mood, security, resignation, loneliness, inferiority, anxiety and guilt, together with future-orientation); others, although overlapping, are labelled as behavioural (tension, obsessiveness and sociability) (Hanestad et al. 1991; Hörnquist et al. 1993). The content is disease-specific and general. The life domain ratings can also be administered to significant others.

The scales comprise ten separate statements which range from 0 to 10 points on each. For inferiority, loneliness, guilt, tension, anxiety, indolence and obsessive traits, an optimal score is towards 0; for sociability, basic mood, security and future orientation, an optimal score is towards 10.

Several versions of the scale of varying length have been developed: a mini version comprising 9 life domain items and 1 well-being item (resignation); a midi version comprising 18 life domain and 6 well-being items; and a maxi format comprising 37 life domain and 12 well-being items (Hörnquist *et al.* 1993).

Examples from the QLSC

A (self-rating). Which personal changes have you noticed as a consequence of your new insulin pen treatment/ since the time of last rating? How are you now?

My bodily health is:

Greatly improved / clearly improved / somewhat improved / unaffected / somewhat worse / clearly worse / greatly worse

Now, my bodily health is:

Very good / good / rather good / neither good or bad / rather bad / bad / very bad

Resignation scale

Examples:

I would like to be more involved
I lead quite an exciting life
I often feel tired, passive and out of sorts
I am usually full of energy and ideas
My life is often dull and drab

Validity and reliability

In a study of 247 people with insulin diabetes, Hanestad (1993) reported that the life domain ($r = 0.45$–0.64) and well-being ($r = -0.64$ to 0.56) scores correlated with a global life satisfaction score, supporting construct validity. Hanestad *et al.* (1991) reported no association between objective physical state (e.g. blood glucose levels) and self-assessed global life satisfaction, but they did report an association with metabolic control and subjective satisfaction within the somatic and behavioural/activity life domains. Well-regulated people felt, on average, less sociable and more

lonely than poorly regulated people, in support of the instrument's discriminative validity.

Hörnquist *et al.* (1993) reported the results of a study using an adapted form of the questionnaire, which was tailored for patients with insulin-dependent diabetes. It was used with 74 consecutive insulin-dependent diabetic out-patients in Sweden, all of whom had changed from syringe treatment to pen treatment. In relation to the well-being scales, Cronbach's alpha ranged from 0.71 to 0.82; split-half correlations ranged between 0.58 and 0.81, except for the anxiety scale which only achieved 0.45; test–retest correlations over 2 years ranged from 0.34 to 0.61. In relation to the life domain ratings, inter-item correlations ranged between 0.49 and 0.70, except for the 'behavioural/ activity' index which was lower at 0.34–0.43. The different types of life domain change measures correlated significantly ($r = 0.34$–0.60). The life domain self-ratings were also associated with corresponding ratings by a significant other ($r = 0.29$–0.70, with most around or above 0.50). Detailed results are presented in Hörnquist *et al.* (1993). On the whole, the well-being scales achieved a better level of reliability than the life domain ratings. Hanestad (1993) also reported similar ranges for reliability coefficients. It requires further testing, and testing in other languages, including English, before its use becomes more widespread.

HEALTH OUTCOMES INSTITUTE TyPE SCALES (HOI-TyPE) – DIABETES

The Health Outcomes Institute (HOI) TyPE outcome questionnaires have yet to be fully tested, but they include one for diabetes. The HOI, previously known as Interstudy (2001 Killebrew Drive, Suite 122, Bloomington, MN 55425, USA), has published the scales.

Content, administration and scoring

The patient's form covers two sheets, and has two questions (one of which is a 19-item symptom scale). The symptoms in the scale include constitutional symptoms that may be associated with hyperglycaemia (e.g. blurred vision, dizziness, urinary frequency, nocturia) or as a result of treatment, including hypoglycaemia (e.g. head-aches, adrenergic symptoms relieved by eating, hunger). A clinical questionnaire for completion by the doctor is included. The clinician's form in-cludes details of diet, medication, glycaemic con-trol, chronic complications and medical history, and use of medical services.

The forms can be self-administered and are designed for repeated application (at follow-ups). Each item is scored differently, and can be analysed separately. The batteries await psychometric test-ing. A manual is available from the HOI.

Examples from the HOI-TyPE Scale – Diabetes

Patient's form

2 How often have you had any of the following symp-toms during the past 4 weeks:

 (b) Nausea
 (c) Headaches or head pains
 (f) Feeling lightheaded or unsteady while on your feet
 (i) Shortness of breath when lying down flat
 (m) Pins and needles, pain, numbness or burning in your feet
 (n) Heart pounding or palpitation
 (p) Urinating more than usual
 (q) Skin irritations
 (s) Feeling unusually hungry before dinner

RAND DIABETES MELLITUS BATTERY

This disease-specific battery was devised, among others, for use in the Rand Health Insurance Study (HIS)/Medical Outcomes Study (MOS). Data were collected on the prevalence and outcome of diabetes, in relation to the type of insurance scheme respondents were randomized to for the duration of the study. Diabetes was selected for study because of its high prevalence (the HIS detected a 2.7 per cent prevalence), serious complications and amenability to control with insulin, weight loss and dietary regimens (Brook *et al*. 1981). All subjects were given a screening examination, where blood glucose tests were performed. The diabetes questionnaire was also administered to all participants.

Content, administration and scoring

The diabetes battery contains 14 questions, two of which contain five items each. The questions relate to diagnosis, treatment and management, and disease impact. The questionnaire assesses the impact of diabetes through four standard HIS questions on the amount of pain, worry, activity restrictions and days in bed due to the condition (the diabetes). The first three items refer to the previous 3 months and the last to the previous 30 days. More detailed disease-specific questions were also included in the battery, including questions on self-care activities, such as checking urine, watch-ing one's weight and following preventive measures.

The questionnaire is self-administered. Re-sponses to the pain, worry and limitations ques-tions range from 'none' to 'a great deal' (or similar wording, depending on the item). Item responses

Examples from the Rand Diabetes Mellitus Battery

181 Do you actually do any of these things for diabetes or pre-diabetes, whether or not a doctor told you to?

 (a) Keep your feet clean
 (b) Cut your toenails straight across and not too short
 (c) Do not walk barefoot
 (d) Do not wear tight hose supporters
 (e) Watch your weight because of diabetes or pre-diabetes

Yes/no

182 During the past 3 months, how much pain has your diabetes or pre-diabetes caused you?

A great deal of pain / some pain / a little pain / no pain at all

183 During the past 3 months, how much has your diabetes or pre-diabetes worried or concerned you?

A great deal / somewhat / a little / not at all

184 During the past 3 months, how much of the time has your diabetes or pre-diabetes kept you from doing the kinds of things that other people your age do?

All of the time / most of the time / some of the time / a little of the time / none of the time

185 During the past 30 days, how many days has your diabetes or pre-diabetes kept you in bed all or most of the day? (If none, write in '0').

vary from dichotomous 'yes/no' responses to 4- to 6-point frequency and severity scales. A composite item called 'any impact' was constructed, composed of positive responses to the disease impact items. Items are analysed separately, with the exception of the composite score.

Validity and reliability

Taking the screening examination as the gold standard, the sensitivity of the questionnaire was estimated to be only fair at 0.53. Of 74 people classified as diabetic by the screening examination, 39 responded as diabetic to the questionnaire. The specificity of the questionnaire was 0.98. Of the 3189 people who were considered not to be diabetic at screening examination, 3138 denied being diabetic on the questionnaire (Brook *et al.* 1981). Regarding sensitivity, the results indicate that screening cannot rely on questionnaires, but has to rely on blood glucose tests at examination. As Brook *et al.* (1981) pointed out, about half of respondents who were judged to be diabetic according to objective physiological evidence were apparently not aware of it (according to their questionnaire responses).

The responses to the question on days spent in bed corresponded fairly well to responses to a comparable question in the Health Interview Survey in the USA (for details, see Brook *et al.* 1981). Respondents with diabetes reported significantly more worry, activity restrictions and overall impact than respondents who were classified as normal with respect to diabetes at screening examination. The most common impact of diabetes on respondents' lives was worry. Too few respondents reported pain or days in bed for differences to be significant. These associations support the construct validity of this part of the battery. Further psychometric testing is still required.

The questionnaire is short, and not multidimensional, but the Rand battery impact of disease items are attractive because of their brevity and can be used with other scales. They are also attractive given the population norms based on large numbers of people that are available, and also because the questions were adapted for use across a wide range of disease types, making comparisons possible.

DIABETES QUALITY OF LIFE MEASURE (DQOL)

This is a measure of quality of life for use with people with insulin-dependent diabetes mellitus. It was designed by the multicentre, Diabetes Control and Complications Trial Research Group (1988). The questionnaire items were generated from the literature, clinical experience, and diabetic patients who reviewed drafts of the questionnaire.

Content, administration and scoring

The DQOL is a multiple-choice instrument, designed for use with adolescents and adults. It has four main scales: satisfaction, impact, worry about diabetes, and social/vocational worry. It has 46 core items for all respondents, and 16 additional questions that assess experience at school and family relationships where relevant. Respondents are asked to make their ratings in relation to current functioning. Responses are made on a 5-point Likert scale. Satisfaction is rated from 1 = very satisfied to 5 = very dissatisfied. The impact and worry scales are rated from 1 = no impact and never worried to 5 = always feels an impact and always worried. The items are summed for each sub-scale.

Examples from the DQOL

Satisfaction

  5 How satisfied are you with the flexibility you have in your diet?
  6 How satisfied are you with the burden your diabetes is placing on your family?
 13 How satisfied are you with the time you spend exercising?

Very satisfied–Very dissatisfied

Impact

  1 How often do you feel pain associated with the treatment for your diabetes?
  2 How often are you embarrassed by having to deal with your diabetes in public?
 15 How often do you find that your diabetes interrupts your leisure time activities?

No impact–Always feels an impact

Worry

Social/vocational

6 How often do you worry about whether you will miss work?

Diabetes-related

1 How often do you worry about whether you will pass out?

Never worried–Always worried

Validity and reliability

It was assessed by the Group for validity and reliability with 192 diabetic patients. It correlated moderately to well with measures of psychiatric symptoms, perceived well-being and adjustment to illness (the total scale correlations ranged from 0.38 to 0.81), supporting its convergent validity. The other measures used were the Symptom Checklist-90 (Derogatis *et al.* 1976), the Affect–Balance Scale (Bradburn 1969) and the Psycho-social Adjustment to Illness Scale (Derogatis and Lopez 1983). The scale was reported to have good internal consistency – Cronbach's alpha for the scales ranged from 0.66 to 0.92, and test–retest reliability at 9 days ranged from 0.78 to 0.92. However, Parkerson *et al.* (1993b) reported that the scale provided less information on health-related quality of life than generic health status and health perception indicators.

RENAL DISEASE

The development of scales to measure quality of life in these patients has been limited. The pertinent domains to measure (e.g. depression, denial, body image, self-esteem, social and vocational impact) have been reviewed by Lindsay *et al.* (1985) and McGee and Bradley (1994).

FUNCTIONAL CLASSIFICATION

The National Kidney Foundation (NKF) has developed a functional classification, part of which is shown below.

Part of the NKF Functional Classification

Class 1: capable of performing all usual types of physical activity

Class 2: unable to perform the most strenuous of usual physical activities

Class 3: unable to perform usual daily activities more than occasionally

Class 4: severe limitation of usual physical activity

This was used by Bonney *et al.* (1978), together with indicators of psychological status, sexual functioning, work status and a 64-item physical symptom questionnaire, in a study of the impact of long-term haemodialysis and renal transplantation on quality of life. Along with the other measures used, the instrument was sensitive to patient group (transplant or dialysis) and treatment type. There is little evidence of its reliability or validity.

THE USE OF GENERIC SCALES AND DOMAIN-SPECIFIC BATTERIES

Generic quality of life measures have often been used with patients with end stage renal disease (Evans *et al.* 1985; Guyatt *et al.* 1986; Churchill *et al.* 1991).

Wright *et al.* (1994) reviewed the literature on quality of life in end stage renal failure and reported that generic life satisfaction measures, dialysis-specific health-related quality of life scales, functional ability and health status measures (e.g. the Nottingham Health Profile: Hunt *et al.* 1986) were the most commonly used broader outcome indicators with renal patients. The disease-specific health-related quality of life scales they reported included just one *broad* scale – the Haemodialysis Quality of Life Questionnaire (Churchill *et al.* 1991) – and the others measured dimensions of psychological state (Lindsay *et al.* 1985; Parfrey *et al.* 1989; Simmons and Abress 1990).

The Short Form-36 (Ware *et al.* 1993) has also been used successfully as an outcome measure with end stage renal disease patients (Medical Outcomes Trust 1993a). Evans *et al.* (1985) used a range of indicators of life satisfaction, psychological well-being and also the Karnofsky Performance Index to compare the effectiveness of alternative dialysis methods for patients with end stage renal disease. While the functional status measure (the Karnofsky Index) was able to discriminate between treatment types, the subjective well-being and life satisfaction measures performed poorly. Simmons and Abress (1990) also used a battery of existing measures of psychological state, which encompassed Bradburn's (1969) item on happiness, Campbell and co-workers' (1976) Index of Well-Being, and various items on satisfaction with health, therapy, self-esteem, general affect and life satisfaction, physical and social well-being. The battery was sensitive to type of treatment among end stage renal patients.

HAEMODIALYSIS QUALITY OF LIFE QUESTIONNAIRE (HQLQ)

Churchill and co-workers' (1991) Haemodialysis Quality of Life Questionnaire (HQLQ) was developed from 79-item responses from 30 haemodialysis patients and 13 health care professionals, and tested with 45 haemodialysis patients who indicated whether a list of items was important to them. This procedure reduced the items to 61.

Content, administration and scoring

The current version contains 61 items which relate to five domains: haemodialysis-specific symptoms (15 items, e.g. thirst, itch), end stage renal disease-specific symptoms (23 items, e.g. easy bruising, dry mouth), mood (9 items, e.g. anxiety and depression), socio-vocational (10 items, e.g. work limitation, social limitation), and family/sexual (4 items, e.g. family adjustment, role limitation). Patients select items relevant to them. The scale can be self-administered. Full scoring details have not been published, probably because the scale is in its early stages of development.

Examples from the HQLQ

Examples of items the patient is given to select from

- *Haemodialysis symptoms:* general fatigue, boredom
- *End stage renal disease symptoms:* thirst, joint pains
- *Mood:* distressed by dependence, anger
- *Socio-vocational:* vacation limitation, frustration with medication
- *Family/sexual:* end state renal disease – burden on family, sexual desire decreased

---

Validity and reliability

The scale has yet to be fully tested, although initial results for reliability are encouraging. In a further study of 47 chronic haemodialysis patients, Churchill *et al.* (1991) reported test–retest intra-class correlations of more than 0.90 for all five domains. However, the questionnaire was not responsive to improvements in haemodialysis treatments.

LEICESTER URAEMIC SYMPTOM SCALE (LUSS)

Wright *et al.* (in press) have given careful thought to the scales that should be included in batteries assessing outcome. In a double-blind prospective study with patients starting CAPD treatment over 12 months, with a 12-month follow-up period, Wright *et al.* (in press) are using several scales measuring various psychological domains, including self-efficacy, life satisfaction and affect, adjustment to illness, activities of daily living, overall self-ratings of health and quality of life, a generic health status measure (the Nottingham Health Profile: Hunt *et al.* 1986), and a disease-specific symptom scale which they designed, the Leicester Uraemic Symptom Scale (LUSS: Wright *et al.* 1994).

Content

This is an 11-item symptom scale which scores the frequency and importance of symptoms. The item scores for frequency range from 0 to 3 (3 = every day to 0 = never) and the item scores for importance also range from 0 to 3 (0 = not at all to 3 = extremely important). The scale can be self-administered. Item composite scores are then summed to give a total score of 0–99 for the full 11-item scale, or 0–90 if just 10 of the 11 items are used (the eleventh item, restless legs, can be omitted). The other ten symptoms asked about are listed below.

Symptoms included in the LUSS

Itching
Sleep disturbance
Loss of appetite
Excessive tiredness
Pain in bones/joints

Poor concentration/mental alertness
Impotence/lack of sex drive
Loss of muscle strength/power
Shortness of breath
Muscle spasm/stiffness

Validity and reliability

These symptoms correlated moderately well with the Nottingham Health Profile sub-scale scores (r = 0.42–0.63) and with the other socio-psychological scales used (r = 0.39–0.79). The symptom items were able, on the whole, to discriminate between patients and controls, supporting the construct validity of the scale, and therefore its concurrent validity. The internal reliability of the scale (Cronbach's alpha) was 0.86. Further testing is ongoing. However, this is not a complete generic disease-specific scale, but a symptom scale to be used in conjunction with a battery of other scales.

QUALITY OF LIFE ASSESSMENT

Parfrey *et al.* (1989) developed a disease-specific questionnaire, the Quality of Life Assessment, for use with patients with end stage renal disease. It was tested on 107 dialysis patients and 119 transplant recipients, and further tested in a follow-up study of 63 stable dialysis patients, 67 stable transplant patients and 15 dialysis patients who were successfully transplanted during a 1-year period.

Content, administration and scoring

The questionnaire contains a mixture of new and existing batteries of measures. The questionnaire was intended to be brief, although this has the result of a restricted focus on quality of life. It can be self-administered. The instrument contains 24 symptom questions, with items on severity and the clinical features of each symptom. Patients are asked to rate each symptom on a scale of 1 (very severe) to 5 (absent) (maximum score = 60). An affect scale, which comprises 12 arbitrary emotions considered by the researchers to influence patients' well-being, includes two positive and nine negative emotions (the twelfth asks about 'other' emotions experienced). The emotions are graded 1 (very severe) to 5 (absent).

Subjective quality of life is measured using Campbell and co-workers' (1976) indexes of general affect (eight items on a scale of 1–7), well-being and life satisfaction (one item, with responses graded from 1 to 7, with 1 representing total dissatisfaction and 7 total satisfaction). The latter two components are combined as a total measure of well-being, with added weight given to life satisfaction. Spitzer and co-workers' (1981) quality of life visual analogue scales are also used. Functioning (called 'objective quality of life') is measured with the Karnofsky Performance Index (Karnofsky and Burchenal 1949). Further details of this instrument are available in the source references.

Examples from the Quality of Life Assessment

1 Symptoms

Tiredness
Headaches
Cramps
Stomach pain

Absent / mild / moderate / severe / very severe

2 Affect

Determination
Confused
Angry
Sad

3 Overall life satisfaction

Completely   1   2   3   4   5   6   7   Completely
dissatisfied   satisfied

4 General affect

Life is:

Miserable / empty / boring / lonely

Validity and reliability

The existing scales have been tested for their psychometric properties – the Spitzer and Karnofsky scales are reviewed in Chapter 2, and are not without their limitations. Parfrey *et al.* (1989) found the questionnaire to be partly sensitive to change and to have good construct validity. The scales were reproducible – the correlation co-efficients for inter-rater reliability (two inter-viewers) were reported to be 0.80 or above, except with the Spitzer subjective quality of life single scale ($t = 0.50$). Intra-observer reproducibility was good at 0.73 or above for most items; it was 0.45 for the Spitzer quality of life scales (5 VAS scales). The questionnaire is still in its early stages of testing, however, and there is still no comprehensive disease-specific quality of life scale in use with renal patients.

In sum, although initial test results are promising, the scale is restricted to symptoms and feelings of affect, life satisfaction and a VAS for rating subjective quality of life. It does not attempt to tap other major domains of quality of life.

BOWEL DISEASES

Bowel diseases are common in the western world, and thought to be associated with low-fibre diets. Although treatment and management can be problematic, few quality of life questionnaires have been designed to assess outcomes. Haemorrhoids are particularly common (around 5 per cent of populations) and can cause pain, bleeding, soreness, itching and soiling. As many as 88 per cent of people with haemorrhoids claim to have been bothered by them (National Center for Health Statistics 1974).

INFLAMMATORY BOWEL DISEASE QUESTIONNAIRE (IBDQ)

Guyatt *et al.* (1989d) developed this questionnaire in order to assess changes in disease-related dysfunction and subjective health status in clinical trials. They felt that other questionnaires failed to address the socio-psychological aspects of outcome.

The IBDQ was developed for use with people with ulcerative colitis or Crohn's disease. During its development, patients were recruited from gastroenterology out-patient clinics. The items on the questionnaire were selected on the basis of interviews with professionals and 77 patients with the disease. During further interviews, the number of items was reduced to include those mentioned most frequently and rated as most important by patients.

Content, administration and scoring

It consists of 32 questions in four sub-scales: gastrointestinal (bowel) symptoms, systemic symptoms, emotional dysfunction and social dysfunction. Administration takes 15–25 min at first administration, and 10–20 min for subsequent administrations. It requires a trained interviewer. Although it is a sensitive questionnaire, it is apparently acceptable to patients. Each question contains various 7-point response categories (e.g. relating to frequency, severity, satisfaction) with 7 = 'best function' and 1 = 'worst function'. Scores are summed to produce a score for each of the four sub-scales.

Examples from the IBDQ

Bowel symptoms

1 How frequent have your bowel movements been during the last 2 weeks?
13 How often during the last 2 weeks have you been troubled by pain in the abdomen?

Systemic symptoms

2 How often has the feeling of fatigue or of being tired and worn out been a problem for you during the last 2 weeks?
10 How often during the last 2 weeks have you felt generally unwell?

Emotional function

23 How much of the time during the past 2 weeks have you felt embarrassed as a result of your bowel problem?
32 How satisfied, happy or pleased have you been with your personal life during the past 2 weeks?

Social function

4 How often during the last 2 weeks have you been unable to attend school or work because of your bowel problems?
28 To what extent has your bowel problem limited sexual activity during the last 2 weeks?

Validity and reliability

The instrument's construct validity was supported by correlations with a number of global ratings by patients about whether their condition had improved or deteriorated at follow-up. In contrast, the Rand physical functioning scale was not able to detect changes. It was tested for reproducibility using retests with 61 patients at 1 month; the coefficient of variation (the standard deviation divided by the mean of the baseline and follow-up scores) for the sub-scales ranged from 0.06 to 0.15 (Guyatt *et al*. 1989d). Further testing of the scale's psychometric properties is still required.

RAND SURGICAL CONDITIONS BATTERY: HAEMORRHOIDS

The Rand Health Insurance Study (HIS)/Medical Outcomes Study (MOS) selected haemorrhoids as one of the conditions for inclusion in its surgical conditions battery, which also included hernia and varicose veins (Rubenstein *et al*. 1983). It was selected for study because of its high prevalence (in the HIS it was 15 per cent among adults aged 14–62 years) and the potential for surgical treatment.

Content, administration and scoring

The haemorrhoids battery contains 12 items: service use and treatments (8 items) and impact of disease (4 items). The disease impact questions are identical for all surgical conditions; they form a standard set of questions used in all the disease batteries from the HIS (pain, worry or concern, restriction and bed days).

Responses to the pain, worry and limitations questions range from 'none' to 'a great deal' (or similar wording, depending on the item). A composite item called 'any impact' was constructed, composed of positive responses to the disease impact items. More detailed disease-specific questions were also included in the battery.

Examples from the Rand Surgical Conditions Battery: Haemorrhoids

198 In the past 3 months, have you taken any rectal suppositories for your piles or haemorrhoids? Yes/no

200 During the past 3 months, how much pain have your piles or haemorrhoids caused you?

A great deal / some / a little / no pain at all

201 During the past 3 months, how much have your piles or haemorrhoids worried or concerned you?

A great deal / somewhat / a little / not at all

202 During the past 3 months, how much of the time have your piles or haemorrhoids kept you from doing the kinds of things people your age do?

All of the time / most of the time / some of the time / a little of the time / none of the time

203 During the past 30 days, how many days have your piles or haemorrhoids kept you in bed all day or most of the day? (If none, write in '0').

Validity and reliability

The results of Rubenstein *et al*. (1983) emphasized the amount of distress caused by the condition, and supported the validity of the questions. In the HIS, 64 per cent of respondents with self-reported haemorrhoids reported pain or distress, 46 per cent worry or concern, 11 per cent restriction of activity, and 1 per cent reported 1+ days in bed. Altogether, 68 per cent gave a positive response to at least one of the disease impact questions. These questions were sensitive to the use of haemorrhoidal treatments (rather than doctors' prescriptions of treatments). People who did not use treatments were less likely to report any disease impact. Those who were prescribed treatments reported greater levels of pain and worry than those who were not. These findings support the validity of the questions. No information is available about their reliability with this group.

HUMAN IMMUNODEFICIENCY VIRUS (HIV) AND ACQUIRED IMMUNE DEFICIENCY SYNDROME (AIDS)

Treatment for AIDS is only palliative, the disease is progressively debilitating and painful, and results in death. The measurement of health-related quality of life is important in relation to such conditions. Given the international interest in AIDS, and the favourable funding climate for AIDS-related research during the 1980s and early 1990s, disease-specific quality of life scales have been developed much more quickly than for other, longer established diseases. These instruments are being applied to people with asymptomatic and symptomatic HIV infection.

Measures relating to chronic disease from the Rand Health Insurance Study (HIS) and the Medical Outcomes Study (MOS) have also been used with good results with patients with HIV, as well as various measures of disability, depression, and changes in role, physical and social functioning (Wu *et al*. 1990, 1991; Wachtel *et al*. 1992; Burgess *et al*. 1993). Hays and Shapiro (1992) reviewed the Rand measures used in HIV research, together with a number of other potential measures. While the advantage of these measures is that they provide a thorough assessment of multiple quality of life concepts, they do not produce an overall score. The authors caution against using the popular SF-36 alone, as it omits cognitive function/distress, and requires supplementation.

Several other measures have been used with people with HIV, although most are limited to specific domains such as physical functioning. For example, the Karnofsky Performance Index (Karnofsky and Burchenal 1949) has been used in several studies, but it is really limited to physical functioning and is no substitute for patient self-assessments of quality of life and of scales of psychosocial and sexual aspects of life (Fischl *et al*. 1987, 1990). The Medical Outcomes Trust have also recently developed an instrument called the MOS-HIV 30-item Form, although this is not really disease-specific. It is a subset of the Rand MOS measures of generic health-related quality of life, which the authors selected for use with people with HIV infection (Wu *et al*. 1991). While promising measures have been developed for use with people with HIV (e.g. the HIV Overview of Problems–Evaluation System developed by Ganz *et al*. 1993), or adapted for use, there is still no consensus over which is the most suitable.

HIV OVERVIEW OF PROBLEMS–EVALUATION SYSTEM (HOPES)

The HIV Overview of Problems–Evaluation System, developed by Schag *et al*. (1992) and Ganz

et al. (1993), was essentially derived from a cancer-specific scale, the Cancer Rehabilitation Evaluation System (CARES: Ganz *et al*. 1990). CARES was adapted after interviews with health professionals and HIV patients, although it remains remarkably similar to CARES. It was piloted on 38 patients, before being tested on a further 318 patients with HIV.

Content, administration and scoring

It is a 165-item, self-administered scale which produces a global scale and five summary scales measuring physical, psychosocial, significant other, medical interaction and sexual functioning, as well as 35 sub-scales covering day-to-day functioning and problems (e.g. ambulation, pain, weight loss, difficulty working, body image, psychological distress, sexual interest, problems with chemotherapy). The scores range from 0 = not at all to 4 = very much. A global score can be calculated.

Examples from the HOPES

Physical

I have difficulty walking or moving around
I frequently have pain
I find that HIV infection or its treatments interfere with my
    ability to work

Medical interaction

I find that the medical team withholds information from
    me about the disease
I would like to have more control over what the doctors
    do to me

Psychosocial

I am concerned about my physical appearance
I feel that I cannot tell everyone I know about the HIV
    infection
I find that my friends or relatives avoid talking with me
    about the HIV infection
I have difficulty helping my children cope with my illness

Sexual

I am less active/interested in sex because I am afraid of
    infecting others
I have difficulty initiating new relationships

Significant others/partners

My partner(s) and I are not getting along as well as we
usually do
My partner(s) do not take care of me enough

Miscellaneous

I become nauseated during/before chemotherapy
I feel fatigued after my radiation treatments

Validity, factor structure and reliability

It was further tested on 318 HIV patients (symptomatic and asymptomatic, and AIDS patients with cancer). Correlations with other scales were in the predicted direction. The authors used it together with the Profile of Mood States (McNair *et al.* 1971), Karnofsky Performance Index (Karnofsky and Burchenal 1949), various laboratory data, single items, and global quality of life LASA ratings. The global scale score was significantly associated with the Karnofsky Index, suggesting convergent validity ($r = 0.48$). The instrument's overall score was moderately to strongly correlated with the other instruments used ($r = -0.57$ to 0.79) (Schag *et al.* 1992). The sub-scale scores were also sensitive to disease stage. Schag *et al.* (1992) reported a stable factor structure and good reliability for the scale. Internal consistency was good with an alpha coefficient of 0.82. Initial results are good, but it requires far more testing before any conclusions can be drawn.

AIDS HEALTH ASSESSMENT QUESTIONNAIRE

This is really an adapted battery of existing generic scales. The AIDS Health Assessment Questionnaire (Lubeck and Fries 1992) was developed from the Health Assessment Questionnaire (Fries *et al.* 1982), which is widely used to assess functional ability in rheumatology. The physical functioning component contains 27 items. Items were added on anxiety and depression, energy, social functioning, cognitive functioning, and the presence of HIV-specific symptoms. The adapted scale was based on the investigators' clinical experience, rather than discussions with patients. Other scales which were incorporated were taken from the Rand Medical Outcomes Study and comprised items on mental health, cognition, energy and health distress (Stewart and Ware 1992). Patients were also given a disease-specific symptom checklist (e.g. anaemia, night sweats, weight loss, numbness in extremities), and three additional items were included: social functioning, frequency and intensity of social activities, and interactions with friends.

It has been used in a study of 669 HIV-positive patients in the USA, although results for reliability and validity have not been given (Lubeck and Fries 1992).

VARICOSE VEINS

The prevalence of varicose veins has been put at 8–16 per cent, with women being most affected (Chant *et al.* 1972). Few disease-specific questionnaires have been developed for use with these patients, although a promising start has been made by Rubenstein *et al.* (1983) and Garratt *et al.* (1993a).

VARICOSE VEINS QUESTIONNAIRE

Garratt and co-workers' (1993a) Varicose Veins Questionnaire used the Rand SF-36 (Ware *et al.* 1993) as its core, with the addition of items on symptoms. The items were based on questions commonly used in the clinical assessment of patients with varicose veins, according to a review of the literature. The initial content validity of the questionnaire was confirmed by two specialists, and the questionnaire was pre-piloted with 12 patients. The measures were then tested on a combined sample ($n = 373$) of subjects reported by GPs to have varicose veins and patients who had been referred to surgical out-patient departments. These patients were compared with a random sample of 900 members of the general population identified from electoral registers. Items were retained if they had high item–total correlations, if they had face validity and if they contributed to the factor structure of the questionnaire.

Content

The core part of the questionnaire is the SF-36 (Ware *et al.* 1993), and the disease-specific symptoms questionnaire comprises 15 questions which cover the distribution of veins, pain, analgesia and other medication, ankle swelling, itching, discoloration and various skin conditions, use of support stockings, concern about the condition, influence on choice of clothing, interference with daily activities and leisure activities.

Administration and scoring

The questionnaire can be self-administered. Respondents are asked to mark their varicose veins on a diagram, and to tick a response box for the right leg and for the left leg. Responses to the subsequent items range from dichotomous 'yes/no' answers to 4- and 5-point response scales of frequency and severity. The total score ranges from $0 =$ no evidence of varicose veins to $100 =$ most severe varicose veins. Question 1, which involves the respondent indicating his or her varicose veins on an outline of a pair of legs (back and front), has a separate scoring format. The scoring for this is carried out by placing a grid over the diagram. The scores and their weights were derived from values assigned by two consultant surgeons. Scoring details are available from the authors.

Examples from the Varicose Veins Questionnaire

2 In the past 2 weeks, for how many days did your varicose veins cause you pain and ache?

Right:
Left:

None at all / between 1 and 5 days / between 6 and 10 days / for more than 10 days

5 In the past 2 weeks, how much ankle swelling have you had?

None at all / slight ankle swelling / moderate ankle swelling (for example, causing you to sit with your feet up whenever possible) / severe ankle swelling (for example, causing you difficulty putting on your shoes)

12 Does the appearance of your varicose veins cause you concern?

No / yes, slight concern / yes, moderate concern / yes, a great deal of concern

13 Does the appearance of your varicose veins influence your choice of clothing, including tights?

No / occasionally / often / always

15 During the past 2 weeks, have your varicose veins interfered with your leisure activities (including sport, hobbies and social life)?

Yes, my enjoyment has suffered to a slight extent / yes, my enjoyment has suffered to a moderate extent / yes, my veins have prevented me taking part in any leisure activities

Validity, factor structure and reliability

The questionnaire correlated highly with the SF-36, patients with varicose veins having poorer perceived health than members of the general population. The varicose vein severity scores among the patient population achieved significant correlations with all eight sub-scales of the SF-36, four of which exceeded $r = 0.40$ (physical functioning, pain, social functioning and role limitations attributable to emotional problems) and only one fell below 0.30 (general health perceptions) (Garratt et al. 1993b).

Factor analyses identified four important health factors: pain and dysfunction, cosmetic appearance, extent of varicosity and complications. Results showed that for the items finally selected, moderate item–total correlations (0.20–0.56) were obtained, supporting the internal consistency of the questionnaire. Cronbach's alpha for the final and definitive questionnaire was 0.72 (Garratt et al. 1993b)

RAND SURGICAL CONDITIONS BATTERY: VARICOSE VEINS

Varicose veins were included in the Rand Health Insurance Study (HIS)/Medical Outcomes Study (MOS) battery because of their high prevalence. Although they cause no major disability, apart from the occasional ulcer on the lower leg, over two-thirds of sufferers have been reported to be bothered by them (National Center for Health Statistics 1974). In the HIS, 13 per cent of adults reported having varicose veins, although this proportion increased at leg inspection (this was only randomly assigned for women: 24 per cent had varicosities, most of which were minimal or moderate, and another 41 per cent had spider angiomata). At screening examination, varicosity was defined as being present when a vein showed distension and tortuosity for at least 1 inch. The number of varicosities was the main criterion by which a respondent was classified into one of five severity categories (see below). A person was defined as having varicose veins if his or her worst leg met the criteria for categories 3, 4 or 5.

Categories of Severity of Varicose Veins

1 No varicose veins present
2 Spider angiomata only. Six or more full spider angiomata were scored as category 3
3 Minimal: one to three varicosities. If oedema (swelling), redness or hardening of the skin was present, the varicosities were scored as category 4
4 Moderate: four to six varicosities. If oedema, redness or hardening of the skin was present, the varicosities were scored as category 5
5 Severe: more than six varicosities, with or without additional abnormalities

Content, administration and scoring

The varicose vein battery, which was completed by sufferers, contains 12 questions: one relates to diagnosis, two relate to surgery, four relate to management, one relates to clothing restrictions (shorts) and four relate to impact of the condition.

The standard Rand disease impact questions were asked (pain, worry or concern, restriction and bed days). The scale can be self-administered. Responses to the pain, worry and limitations questions range from 'none' to 'a great deal' (or similar wording, depending on the item). Other response choices range from dichotomous 'yes/no' responses to 4-point frequency or treatment plan scales. A composite item called 'any impact' was constructed, composed of positive responses to the disease impact items. More detailed disease-specific questions were also included in the battery.

Examples from the Rand Surgical Conditions Battery: Varicose Veins

214 In the past 12 months, did you avoid wearing shorts because of varicose veins?   Yes/no
217 Do you currently keep your feet up during the day because of varicose veins?

Yes, most of the time / yes, sometimes / yes, a little of the time / no

220 During the past 3 months, how much pain have your varicose veins caused you?

A great deal of pain / some pain / a little pain / no pain at all

221 During the past 3 months, how much have your varicose veins worried or concerned you?

A great deal / most of the time / some of the time / a little of the time / none of the time

222 In the past 3 months, how much of the time have your varicose veins kept you from doing the kinds of things other people your age do?

All of the time / most of the time / some of the time / a little of the time / none of the time

223 During the past 30 days, how many days have your varicose veins kept you in bed all or most of the day?   (If none, write in '0')

Validity and reliability

The respondents' replies revealed that the impact of this disease is great, despite the common belief that it is trivial. Over a fifth of sufferers had avoided wearing shorts (frequently worn in the USA) because of the problem, 32 per cent reported pain, 39 per cent worry, and 8 per cent restricted activities; less than 1 per cent reported any bed days. Among the women, 49 per cent reported some impact. Those who were categorized as having severe varicosity reported the most adverse effects, supporting the validity of these impact questions.

The reliability of the varicose vein measurements used at screening examination was good. Of 120 women who received a repeat examination, 95 per cent received identical diagnoses at both examinations; of the other 5 per cent, they were differently classified at repeat examination by 1 to 2 severity levels. Regarding the validity of the self-reported varicose veins question, the respondents' replies were compared with clinical examination scores. These showed that, of the 930 women who had some signs of vein problems, 325 were aware of it according to their questionnaire reply; this gave a sensitivity of 33 per cent. Among the women with moderate to severe varicosities, sensitivity was 78 per cent, with a specificity of 82 per cent. As sensitivity improved, specificity declined (details are given by Rubenstein et al. (1983).

As with the other Rand disease-specific batteries, the questionnaire is short but it can be used in combination with other scales.

BACK PAIN

Back problems are the most common cause of days off work in many countries. They represent substantial costs to health services (Office of Health Economics 1985) and can lead to considerable distress among sufferers (Mechanic and Angel 1987), made worse by the relative lack of effective treatment. Given the considerable interest in treatment evaluation on the part of governments, and the disability and handicap caused by these conditions, it is surprising that so little work has been carried out on disease-specific quality of life scales.

In their review of the literature, Ruta et al. (in press a) pointed out that most outcome studies have used pain scales as their main measure. They found that of the 22 different pain scales reported in the literature, the McGill Pain Questionnaire was the most popular (Melzack 1983, 1987). They found only three measures of health status in patients with low back pain which were not simply restricted to impairment: the Oswestry Disability Score (Fairbank et al. 1980), the Waddell Disability Score (Waddell and Main 1984) and the Low Back Outcome Score (Greenough and Fraser 1992). As they pointed out, however, none of these measures has been subjected to rigorous testing of its psychometric properties. These reviewers then went on to develop their own scale.

CLINICAL BACK PAIN QUESTIONNAIRE

Ruta and co-workers' (1994a, 1994b) back pain questionnaire used the Rand SF-36 (Ware et al. 1993) as its core, supplemented with detailed questions on pain and sensation, functional ability and mobility. The disease-specific questions were based on a review of the literature. It was piloted on a small sample of patients with low back pain.

It was further tested on a combined sample (n = 568) of subjects reported by GPs to have low back pain and patients who had been referred to outpatient departments. These patients were compared with a random sample of 900 members of the general population taken from the electoral register. The patients were sent the questionnaire by post, together with the SF-36, and their GPs were asked to assess the severity of their condition on a 4-point symptom severity scale from 'none' to 'severe'. Questions were retained if they had a high response rate, if they helped to identify the main factors and if they had item–total correlations of >0.20. After testing, three items were discarded (Ruta et al., 1994a, 1994b).

Content, administration and scoring

This is a 20-question, multi-item questionnaire measuring type, frequency, treatments and handicap stemming from back pain. The questionnaire contains one question on the frequency of back pain, two questions on medication, eight questions on type of pain, one question on effects on sleep, one on ability to sit down, one on ability to stand, one on ability to walk, and one each on ability to perform work/housework, leisure activities, self-care, one on bed days and one on effects on sex life.

The questionnaire is self-administered. The questions are based on forced-choice response formats (requiring the respondent to tick one category) or are multiple-choice (requiring the respondents to tick all categories that apply). The possible responses to each forced choice are assigned a score (for example, the frequency score for pain ranges from none = 0 to more than 10 days = 3). For the multiple-choice questions, the responses are each assigned a score of 1 point. The responses are then summed and converted to percentages to produce a 'back pain severity score' of between 0 and 100 (with high scores indicating more severe levels of back pain).

Examples from the Clinical Back Pain Questionnaire

1 In the last 2 weeks, for how many days did you suffer pain in the back or legs?

None at all / between 1 and 5 days / between 6 and 10 days / for more than 10 days

5 In your left leg, do you have any pain in the following areas?

Pain in the buttock

Pain in the thigh
Pain in the shin/calf
Pain in the foot/ankle

15 In the last 2 weeks, did the pain prevent you from carrying out your work/housework and other daily activities?

No, not at all / I could continue with my work, but my work suffered / yes, for one day / yes, for 2–6 days / yes, for 7 days+

18 In the last 2 weeks, have your leisure activities been affected by your pain (including sports, hobbies and social life)?

Not affected by the pain / mildly affected by the pain / moderately affected by the pain / severely affected by the pain / pain prevents any social life at all

---

Validity, factor structure and reliability

Content validity was supported by a specialist in orthopaedic surgery, a rheumatologist and a physiotherapist. Construct validity was supported by results showing that referred patients had a higher back pain score than non-referred patients, and those taking analgesics had higher scores than those not taking them. There was also a significant correlation between scores and with analgesic strength, and with general practitioners' perceptions of severity.

Back pain patients had poorer health status than the general population. The questionnaire scores correlated moderately to highly with their scores on the SF-36, also supporting validity. The correlations with the eight sub-scales of the SF-36 ranged from 0.36 (general health perceptions) to 0.66 (social functioning) and 0.69 (pain). Four of the SF-36 scales – pain, social functioning, physical functioning and role limitations – together with age on leaving full-time education, explained over 60 per cent of the variance in low back pain scores.

Factor analysis yielded seven factors: functional disability, physical impairment or pain in the legs, physical impairment or pain around the hips, pain and disability relating to standing, pain and disability relating to sitting, pain on coughing or sneezing, and pain on lying down. Questions which did not contribute to this factor structure were removed. The final version achieved a Cronbach's alpha of 0.80. In the tests with 568 patients,

test–retest reliability was assessed at 2 weeks with a sub-sample of those who reported no change in health status. The correlation between the two administrations was $r = 0.94$ (the authors also reported acceptable confidence intervals).

In summary, this is a well-developed and well-tested questionnaire for measuring back pain and its impact. It is multi-domain in nature, but because several domains are included within one question (see examples), the results do not shed light on which precise aspect of life is affected. Thus, the implication is that investigators who are interested in, say, the effects of back pain on social relationships will need to supplement the scale with a social support scale. On the other hand, the brevity of the scale makes it attractive, and it certainly provides information on the effects of back pain in general areas of life.

Further developments on quality of life and back pain

These investigators also investigated people's own definitions of health-related quality of life, using a separate index called the 'Patient Generated Index' (Ruta 1992; Ruta *et al.* in press). This approach involves asking patients about the five most important areas or activities of their life that are affected by their condition. They are then asked to rate how badly each of these is affected using a scale of 0–100, where 0 = worst they can imagine for themselves and 100 = exactly as they would like to be. A sixth box is provided for other areas of life affected by their medical condition not previously mentioned. They are finally asked to imagine that they can improve some or all of the chosen areas of their life, and are given 60 points which they can 'spend' across one or more areas. The points they allocate to each area are taken to represent the relative importance of potential improvements in that area. By multiplying each of the six ratings by the proportion of points allocated to that area, and summing, the authors generated an index between 0 and 100. This method appears complex.

It was initially tested with 20 patients, and a checklist version of areas of life was generated for a postal questionnaire version. This was further tested in a postal survey of 20 more patients, who were subsequently interviewed, and the questionnaire later modified. A further postal survey of 74 people identified by general practitioners as suffering from low back pain resulted in 47 per cent being returned completed; 27 per cent were returned partly completed and 31 per cent were returned blank. The five most frequently mentioned areas of life were housework, gardening, sport, work and walking (these accounted for over 35 per cent of the areas mentioned). The index correlated well with the Rand SF–36 scales measuring pain, social functioning and role limitations attributable to physical problems, and with the clinical questionnaire used. The scores reflected general practitioners' assessments of severity.

CHILDREN

While numerous generic and disease-specific health-related quality of life measurement scales have been developed, most of them relate to adults. Children have been largely neglected, except in the area of educational and psychological assessments. A few scales have been developed for use with children undergoing bone marrow transplants, but these are in their early stages of psychometric testing (see Chapter 2).

Surveys of households have typically asked mothers to rate their children's health, and disease-based studies have relied on clinicians' and parents' judgements, sometimes supplemented with psychological, developmental and educational assessment batteries (see Chapter 5), as well as observer-rated functional assessments. There have been attempts to develop scales for children, for example Maylath's (1990) Children's Health Rating Scale, but these are still relatively underused. The Medical Outcomes Trust in the USA, together with the Children's Health and Quality of Life Project Team at the New England Medical Center in Boston, have recently developed Child Health Forms for age groups 5–15 (long and short forms available) and infant–pre-school, which are parent-completed, and middle childhood–adolescent, which are completed by the child (Medical Outcomes Trust 1993b). However, these are not disease-specific. The Rand Health Insurance Study team developed a battery for measuring health status in children aged under 14, as well as brief condition-specific symptom report batteries (e.g. convulsions, eczema, poisoning, etc.). They

depend on the parent completing the questionnaire on behalf of the child (Eisen *et al.* 1980).

Research has demonstrated variability in the congruence between parents' and children's assessments of children's physical, psychological and social health status, and the impact of medical care (Pantell and Lewis 1987). This indicates that both views must be measured. It is not known whether it is the child's cognitive limitations in handling abstract questions or real differences of perception and opinion within the family that lead to low parent–child concordance on some health status ratings (Pantell and Lewis 1987).

ELDERLY PEOPLE

Apart from any disease-specific measures which may be regarded as important, the domains which require measurement among older people include health problems which can cause handicap and which are potentially remediable (e.g. hearing, eyesight, feet and incontinence) (Carabellesse *et al.* 1993), mental health (cognitive functioning and memory, anxiety/depression), functional ability and broader health status, life satisfaction/morale/control and social support. Social support is particularly important in older age in facilitating independent living in the community (Waters *et al.* 1989). This multidimensional approach to assessment requires the separate (rather than aggregated) measurement and analysis of physical, mental and social health, self-esteem, life satisfaction and morale (Fletcher *et al.* 1992a). Measurement of these dimensions will enable needs to be assessed, progress monitored and outcome to be evaluated.

Recommended batteries

Among the appropriate measures of life satisfaction and self-esteem, Lawton's (1972, 1975) Philadelphia Geriatic Morale Scale is the most popular; of the brief mental status tests, the Abbreviated Mental Test (Hodkinson 1972) is frequently used. Other scales for the assessment of cognitive state in elderly people are reviewed in Chapter 5. In relation to measures of physical functioning, the functioning sub-section of the Older Americans' Resources and Services Schedule (OARS) is judged to be superior to most scales for use with elderly people (Fillenbaum 1978; Fillenbaum and Smyer 1981). A scale for measuring depression and anxiety which does not include somatic items, such as the Hospital Anxiety and Depression Scale (Zigmond and Snaith 1983), is also appropriate for use with older people. A range of scales appropriate for measuring inter-generational support was reviewed by Kane and Kane (1988), and another more recent scale for measuring supportive relationships generally is the Rand Medical Outcomes Study (MOS) Social Support Questionnaire (Sherbourne and Stewart 1991).

The generic OARS includes most relevant domains, and has good validity and reliability, although it is lengthy and complex in parts. A short version has been developed, called the Functional Assessment Inventory (Fillenbaum 1978). Pearlman (1987) selected the questions that were assessed as clinically essential by 20 clinicians in a delphi survey for further testing. Questions were also retained if they had discriminative and predictive validity and were sensitive to change in studies of community residents and nursing home patients. He organized these questions into a questionnaire, the Comprehensive Older Person's Evaluation.

A working group representing the British Geriatrics Society and the Royal College of Physicians identified a set of assessment scales for use with elderly patients which they recommended for the evaluation of their care and outcome of care (BGS/RCP 1992; Fletcher et al. 1992a). The battery they recommended for use in community settings included the broad Sickness Impact Profile (Bergner et al. 1981) – or its English version, the Functional Limitations Profile (Charlton et al. 1983) – and the Philadelphia Geriatric Center Morale Scale (Lawton 1972, 1975). As the working group pointed out, these scales will also need supplementing with a measure of cognitive function and memory and depression.

The Royal College of General Practitioners has developed a package of appropriate assessment scales for use by general practitioners in Britain in their annual health checks on patients aged 75 and over. Its national distribution is at the planning stage (Wallace 1994). The scales have to be concise for use in practice settings. The scales included in the pack include the Abbreviated Mental Test

(Hodkinson 1972), the Geriatric Depression Scale (Yesavage et al. 1983) and the Barthel Functional Assessment Scale (Mahoney and Barthel 1965).

Lack of consensus

There is no consensus on which packages are to be recommended, which is inevitable when there are so many scales to choose from (for a review, see Kane and Kane 1988). While international opinion agrees that the Philadelphia Geriatric Center Morale Scale is the instrument of choice for measuring life satisfaction and morale (its psychometric properties are slightly superior to other existing scales), there is disagreement over the other recommended scales.

A major disadvantage of the Sickness Impact Profile (SIP)/Functional Limitations Profile (FLP) is its length. A major study in the UK of outcomes of asthma and diabetes in general practice has discarded the FLP because of its ceiling effects and the high level of item non-response (95 of the 136 items were endorsed by less than 10 per cent of the respondents) (McColl et al. in press). Also, the use of such a long scale means that the researcher has little opportunity to add other batteries of interest. McColl and her colleagues believe that the length of the FLP limits researchers to the addition of just one other scale, whereas other, shorter scales, such as the SF-36, permit the addition of several other scales. The SF-36 requires further testing with elderly people as there are conflicting results on its appropriateness (Medical Outcomes Institute 1990; Brazier et al. 1992; Mangione et al. 1993; Wagner et al. 1993; Hill and Harries 1994).

A multi-centre standardized assessment of the elderly was carried out alongside the production of the BGS/RCP (1992) report. The assessments that were used included the Barthel Index (Mahoney and Barthel 1965; Collin et al. 1988), the Abbreviated Mental Test (Hodkinson 1972), the Geriatric Depression Scale (Yesavage et al. 1983), the Philadelphia Geriatric Center Morale Scale (Lawton 1972; 1975) and several questions on communication and social circumstances. However, the choice of such a battery is also open to debate. Several investigators have criticized the use of the Barthel Index in community settings (it is a severe and limited measure, appropriate to institutional settings; see Chapter 5). Others have suggested it can be used but with more appropriate adaptations for use in the community (Rodgers *et al.* 1993). It was mentioned before that the Abbreviated Mental Test is a popular instrument, although there are other similar, shorter scales to choose from (see Chapter 5). Other scales also exist for the measurement of depression in disease-specific and generic health status studies (for example, as was mentioned before, an increasingly popular short scale, with no somatic items, is the Hospital Anxiety and Depression Scale: Zigmond and Snaith 1983).

The unsatisfactory length of the SIP and the insensitivity of the Barthel Index when used in community settings and used generically (as opposed to disease-specific situations, e.g. stroke), illustrates the crude state of existing screening instruments for use with older people. Far more research is needed into the development and use of health status and functional ability scales for use with older people living at home.

Disease-specific and/or generic scales?

The assessment of older people requires the use of scales that are specific and are sensitive to the needs and problems of this age group (e.g. functional ability scales). It should not, however, be forgotten that the majority of the chronic diseases prevalent in Western society are the diseases of old age – for example, cancers, arthritis and rheumatism, stroke and heart disease – and disease-specific scales are also appropriate for use with older people. Only a small proportion of people over retirement age are severely disabled or in need of long-term care. A critique on ageism in medicine (e.g. in clinical oncology) and a plea for providing (rather than withholding) the *appropriate* treatment for elderly patients, with a view to enhancing quality of life, has been made by Fentiman *et al.* (1990).

This has been given weight by a Belgian study of 1371 patients aged 75 and over (mean age = 77 years) undergoing CABG, and 257 'neutral risk patients' undergoing CABG (mean age = 59 years), in a follow-up assessment at 5 years (Walter and Mohan 1994). These investigators included the Older Americans' Resources and Services Schedule (Fillenbaum 1978; Fillenbaum and Smyer 1981), the Rose Angina and Dyspnoea Scales (Rose and Blackburn 1968; Rose *et al.* 1977) and Andrews and Withey's (1976) Delighted–Terrible Faces Life

Satisfaction Scale in the assessments of outcome. While the operative mortality rate of the older group (7.2 per cent) was higher than for the younger group (0 per cent), and fewer were alive at follow-up (81.1 *vs* 91.8 per cent), the scores reported by both groups in relation to physical health, self-care, daily activities and life satisfaction led the authors to conclude that CABG is justified in very elderly people as the *quality* of their survival is as good as that of younger patients, and of age-adjusted populations. A more detailed analysis of the results does reveal a more complex picture, which will require consideration in future debates. The older patients did have worse scores than the younger group at follow-up in relation to confusion and depression, and were more likely to have undergone percutaneous cardiac catheterization, although they were more likely to be satisfied with the operation.

Disease-specific measures need to be supplemented with scales appropriate for older people, particularly functional ability. Functional ability and self-rated health status measures have been reported to be better predictors of service needs and use than traditional disease-oriented assessments (Waters *et al.* 1989). Assessments and interventions that focus on functional ability are often judged likely to improve outcomes (Almy 1988; Rubenstein *et al.* 1989a). However, such judgements have not been based on studies that have determined the effectiveness of functional status assessment in real-life clinical practice, partly due to the scarcity of data. A recent trial of functional disability screening in clinical practice showed no significant differences in outcome between experimental and control groups in relation to functional or health status (Neuhauser and Studer 1989; Rubenstein *et al.* 1989b).

In sum, although multidimensional measures are essential elements in any assessment of the elderly, disease-specific scales *are also* appropriate in relation to specific conditions. For example, elderly people, as well as those younger than them can suffer from breathlessness in various situations when suffering from coronary and respiratory disease, and they also suffer from the toxic effects of any treatments which they may receive (e.g. chemotherapy). It is just as desirable to measure these effects in order to assess the need for, and outcome of, care of elderly people, particularly with the increasing number of people in their 70s and 80s and the emphasis on positive ageing. Research on the values of elderly people is needed here (Browne *et al*. 1994).

Multiple pathology

One methodological difficulty is the existence of multiple pathology among very elderly people, and it may not be practical or desirable to apply several disease-specific scales to the same group of elderly patients. While a Cumulative Illness Rating Scale has been developed to measure impairment from multiple pathologies (Linn *et al*. 1968; for a review, see Kane and Kane 1988), there is no easy solution to this problem, and it needs to be considered in relation to the individual clinical problem or research issue. Readers interested in the broader scales of health status, physical and mental functioning, life satisfaction and social support are referred to Bowling (1991) and Mulder and Sluijs (1993) for a full review.

A POPULAR CORE (GENERIC) MEASURE FOR USE IN DISEASE-SPECIFIC STUDIES OF ADULTS: THE SHORT FORM-36 (SF-36)

The SF-36 is reviewed here because several medical organizations (see earlier chapters) recommend its inclusion as the generic core in disease-specific batteries of health-related quality of life. It is a short questionnaire that was derived from the Rand health batteries. The Rand Corporation's health batteries were designed for the Health Insurance Study (HIS), an experiment of health outcome following the random allocation of approximately 8000 adults aged 14–61 years to various insurance plans. The Medical Outcomes Study (MOS) involved the more detailed analysis of patient outcomes in different systems of medical care, and led to the further development of the batteries (Stewart and Ware 1992). The batteries were developed for use in population surveys. More specifically, the Rand HIS batteries were developed as an outcome measure to detect changes in health status that might be expected to occur as a result of health service use within a relatively short period of time.

There is increasing international interest in the Rand HIS and MOS batteries, particularly the Short Form-36 item version (SF-36) (Stewart *et al*. 1988; McHorney *et al*. 1992, 1993; Ware and Sherbourne 1992; Ware *et al*. 1993). The SF-36 was developed as an improvement to a previously developed 20-item version (Ware and Sherbourne 1992). The SF-36 is rapidly becoming the generic health status measure of choice; it has increased in popularity in the UK to the extent that researchers are beginning to use it in preference to the traditional UK measure, the Nottingham Health Profile (Hunt *et al*. 1986), in studies of outcome of medical interventions, partly because it is a less skewed measure (Brazier *et al*. 1992). There are similar trends internationally. Some of the Rand, HIS and MOS batteries on physical functioning and positive affect (see Stewart and Ware 1992), from which the SF-36 was derived, have been shown in longitudinal research to be sensitive to intervening illness among relatively healthy elderly people (Wagner *et al*. 1993).

In addition, it is frequently recommended as the generic core in disease-specific batteries. For example, the Cancer Control Research Committee of the Southwest Oncology Group (USA) has included the short-form Rand instrument (the 20-item version, which has now been overtaken by the 36-item version) in its list of preferred measurements (Moinpour *et al*. 1989). Many of the TyPE disease-specific batteries of the Health Outcomes Institute require the use of the SF-36 as the core instrument. The disease-specific batteries being developed at the University of Aberdeen also use the SF-36 as the core instrument (Garratt *et al*. 1993a; Ruta *et al*. 1994), and it is recommended as a core scale in the assessment of outcome of epilepsy (Vickrey *et al*. 1993).

Background

The Rand HIS batteries are based on a definition of health as multidimensional, incorporating physical, mental and social well-being. The batteries cover physical health, physiological health, mental health, social health and perceptions of health. The measures were intended to be sensitive to differences in health in general populations (Ware and Karmos 1976; Stewart *et al*. 1978, 1981, 1989; Brook *et al*. 1979b; Ware *et al*. 1979, 1980). The measures were developed on the basis of extensive reviews of the literature. Each section can be used independently. Their use has been largely confined to populations in the USA.

The authors of the SF-36 aimed to develop a short, generic measure of subjective health status that was psychometrically sound, and that could be applied in a wide range of settings. The two main short-form versions of the Rand instruments are known as the Short Form-20 (SF-20) and the Short Form-36 (SF-36). The 20-item version has been used in studies of clinical outcome and has been shown to be quite reliable (Stewart *et al.* 1988); however, the 'floor effects' on some of the scales have limited the responsiveness of the scores to changes in health status (Bindman *et al.* 1990; Hays and Hadhorn 1992).

The SF-20 comprised 17 items taken from the questionnaires used in the HIS and three new items (Ware *et al.* 1992), and was then used in the MOS. The authors decided to extend the scale to make it more comprehensive and to give it better psychometric properties. This led to the longer SF-36 version. Response rates to the scale in postal surveys in the UK have been high (Brazier *et al.* 1992; Jenkinson *et al.* 1993a, 1993b), except among elderly people (Brazier *et al.* 1992).

Content

The SF-36 comprises 36 of the 149 items from the above measures which loaded best on factor analyses. It was initially tested in the USA on over 22,000 patients as part of the Rand MOS. It is a self-administered questionnaire and takes 5–10 min to complete. The 36 items measure eight dimensions: physical functioning (10 items), social functioning (2 items), role limitations due to physical problems (4 items), role limitations due to emotional problems (3 items), mental health (5 items), energy/vitality (4 items), pain (2 items) and general health perception (5 items). There is also a single item about perceptions of health changes over the past 12 months. It claims to measure positive as well as negative health. Item scores for each of these dimensions are summed and transformed, using a scoring algorithm, into a scale from 0 per cent (poor health) to 100 per cent (good health). The coding format requires recoding before the sub-scales can be summed. Apart from the

SF-36, there is also the SF-36-D, which includes depression items (obtainable from the Health Outcomes Institute).

UK version

The SF-36 was modified slightly to make it more appropriate for UK populations (Brazier *et al.* 1992). The only changes to the original version include Anglicization of some of the language and a slight alteration of the positioning and coding of one of the social functioning items in order to facilitate reliability and ease of administration. The SF-36 questionnaire and description is available free of charge from the UK Clearing House for Information on the Assessment of Health Outcomes, Nuffield Institute for Health Service Studies. Population norms from some of the UK studies, together with the UK version of the questionnaire and scoring details, can be purchased from the Department of Public Health and Primary Care, University of Oxford (Jenkinson *et al.* 1993a).

Psychometric properties

The SF-36 is increasingly being used after recent testing in the USA and UK has shown good results; it is also being tested elsewhere in Europe. An International Quality of Life Assessment (IQOLA) Project is aiming to translate and adapt the SF-36 for use in 15 countries, and to validate and provide norms for the new translations, in order that they can be used in international studies of health outcomes (Aaronson *et al.* 1992). It is likely that this will be the international health status measure of the future, and it is constantly being refined (Stewart and Ware 1992; Ware and Sherbourne 1992). Population norms for the UK have now been published from a series of postal surveys (Brazier *et al.* 1992; Garratt *et al.* 1993b; Jenkinson *et al.* 1993b; Ware *et al.* 1993).

The literature on the testing of the SF-36 and its psychometric properties has been reviewed by Ware *et al.* (1993). The detailed results of the testing of the Rand HIS/MOS batteries have been published by Stewart and Ware (1992), together with the history of the development of the SF-36. This describes how the most predictive items from the fuller batteries were selected for inclusion in the SF-36. The five items on mental health have a particularly impressive validity, and correlated ($r =$ 0.92–0.95) with the full Mental Health Inventory from different samples from the HIS (Davies *et al.* 1988; Stewart and Ware 1992).

Examples from the SF-36

2 Compared with 1 year ago, how would you rate your health in general now?

Much better now than 1 year ago / somewhat better now than 1 year ago / about the same / somewhat worse now than 1 year ago / much worse now than one year ago

3 Does your health limit you in these activities? If so, how much?

(a) Vigorous activities, such as running, lifting heavy objects, participating in strenuous sports
(g) Walking more than a mile
(h) Walking half a mile

Yes, limited a lot / yes, limited a little / no, not limited at all

4 During the past 4 weeks, have you had any of the following problems with your work or other regular daily activities as a result of your physical health?

(a) Cut down on the amount of time you spent on work or other activities
(d) Had difficulty performing work or other activities (e.g. it took extra effort)

Yes/no

7 How much bodily pain have you had during the past 4 weeks?

None / very mild / mild / moderate / severe / very severe

Validity

On the basis of a postal survey in Sheffield in the UK, Brazier *et al.* (1992) reported that the SF-36 had good construct validity, and found it to be more sensitive to gradations in poor health than the Euroqol (Euroqol Group 1990) and the Nottingham Health Profile (NHP: Hunt *et al.* 1986). The authors cautioned that there was a higher rate of item non-response among older people, and the SF-36 may not be appropriate for postal surveys with this group (as opposed to interview surveys). Its applicability among older people requires further investigation (Hill and Harries 1994). However, a survey of the health of 3024 people living in eight counties in rural Oregon and Minnesota demonstrated the appropriateness of using the SF-36 with elderly people, and its sensitivity to service use (Health Outcomes Institute 1990). Mangione *et al.* (1993), carried out a study of 745 patients undergoing major elective, non-cardiac surgery in Boston. They reported that the SF-36 was able to discriminate between surgical groups, and between younger patients and patients who were aged 70 years and over in relation to role function, energy, fatigue and physical function (the older patients had poorer scores on these domains). It did not detect any differences in health perceptions between age groups. The data suggested that older people's health perceptions are determined by different factors which the battery of scales used did not detect. They reported that, in the total sample, the SF-36 health perception scale had the greatest correlation with the energy and fatigue scale ($r =$ 0.45), correlated moderately with mental health ($r = 0.35$), social function ($r = 0.32$) and physical function ($r = 0.33$), and correlated less well with pain ($r = 0.23$).

In the SF-36 manual, Ware *et al.* (1993) reported that in tests of validity the SF-36 was able to discriminate between groups with physical morbidities, but the physical functioning sub-scale performed best, and the mental health sub-scale discriminated between patients with mental health morbidities the best. Correlations between the SF-36 and the General Psychological Well-Being Scale (Dupuy 1984) ranged from 0.19 to 0.60, with a median of 0.36; the SF-36 and quality of life criteria (e.g. housing, neighbourhood, standard of living, family life and friendships) sub-scales were all significantly positively correlated, although few of the criteria items were correlated above 0.30. However, Ware *et al.* (1993) cites the correlations as evidence in support of the SF-36 as an indicator of quality of life. Ware *et al.* (1993) also collated the correlations between the SF-36 and other measures from the results of several studies, and with other MOS scales. The correlations for the sub-scales ranged from weak to strong, but strong correlations were reported between the physical functioning sub-scale and the equivalent sub-scales of the SIP, the AIMS and the NHP ($r = 0.52$–0.85). Strong correlations were reported between the mental health sub-scale and other psychological sub-scales ($r = 0.51$–0.82).

Ware *et al.* (1993) also reported the results of a factor analysis of the SF-36, which provided strong evidence for the conceptualization of health underlying the SF-36, and indicated that some scales principally measure physical health, some measure mental health and others measure both.

Not all results have been good, as Anderson *et al.* (1993) have pointed out. For example, the bodily pain scale has been reported to have poor convergent validity with severity of illness and independent pain scores in the case of knee conditions (McHorney *et al.* 1993). Other studies have reported 'floor' effects in the role functioning scales in severely ill patients, where 25–50 per cent of patients obtained the lowest score possible, with the implication that deterioration in condition will not be detected by the scale (Kurtin *et al.* 1992). The comparable percentage in an HIV population is 63 per cent (Watchel *et al.* 1992). Anderson *et al.* (1993) have also suggested that the item codes can be subject to 'ceiling' effects as they appear too crude to detect improvements. They, like several other investigators, criticize the physical functioning scale for focusing on mobility at the expense of performance of domestic chores where important changes may occur.

The questions are general in scope, and not suitable for a full assessment of disability; if used in the assessment of disability, it will require supplementation with a more specific and detailed functional disability scale. The instrument needs further testing for its discriminatory powers between different disease and treatment groups. Its sensitivity may vary with disease type. For example, Levine *et al.* (1988) reported that some of the Rand batteries (emotional and physical scales) had little discriminatory power in relation to women with stage II breast cancer who had either completed treatment or were still undergoing treatment. In a controlled trial of long- versus short-duration adjuvant chemotherapy for women with stage II breast cancer, Guyatt *et al.* (1989c) and Levine *et al.* (1988) reported that the longer Rand batteries of physical and emotional functioning were unable to distinguish between these two groups. There is some evidence on its discriminative ability (see Garratt *et al.* 1993b in next section).

Reliability

On the basis of the Sheffield survey, Brazier *et al.* (1992) reported that the short-form version has good internal consistency and test–retest reliability. They reported that the internal correlation coefficients for the eight scales ranged from 0.60 to 0.81, with a median of 0.76. High inter-item correlations were reported for the sub-scales (e.g. mental health). On the basis of a postal survey in Oxford, Jenkinson *et al.* (1993a) reported that it has high internal consistency between dimensions, with high Cronbach's alphas (0.76–0.90). Garratt *et al.* (1993b) carried out a postal survey in Grampian of patients with low back pain, menorrhagia, suspected peptic ulcer and varicose veins. They reported that the internal consistency between the items exceeded 0.80 (Cronbach's alpha) and that inter-item correlations ranged from 0.55 to 0.78. All items satisfied statistical criteria of acceptable levels. A factor analysis confirmed the distinct scale dimensions. Moreover, each medical condition achieved a distinct score profile, indicating that the SF-36 can discriminate between conditions (validity).

The SF-36 manual, published in the USA by Ware *et al.* (1993), provides full listings of studies using the SF-36, and collates the results of tests for reliability and validity across numerous studies. Fourteen studies in the USA have analysed the reliability of the SF-36. The reliability coefficients for internal consistency range from 0.62 to 0.94 for the sub-scales; for test–retest reliability, the coefficients range from 0.43 to 0.90; and for alternate form reliability the coefficient was 0.92. In relation to internal consistency, all but 11 coefficients reported in studies in the USA and UK exceeded the 0.70 standard suggested by Nunnally (1978).

Ware *et al.* (1993) reported that the level of reliability achieved by the SF-36 is lower than that achieved by the full-length versions of the MOS scales (e.g. mental health, health perceptions). The minimum reliability standards appear to have been most consistently met by the physical functioning sub-scale.

Copyright and registration

There are four versions of the SF-36. The first was the 'developmental' version (Ware and Sherbourne 1992), on which the UK version is based (with minor language modifications). Two more recent versions of the SF–36 were subsequently developed in the USA (more up to date than the one tested for use in the UK), which contain minor modifications, and the scoring is slightly different. The situation for registration in the USA is complicated by the existence of three centres for copyright and/or registration purposes. The recent versions of the SF–36 are separately available from either the Health Institute (Ware *et al*. 1993) or the Rand Corporation (Rand 1992).

Rand distribute their version free of charge – the Rand 36-item Health Survey 1.0 Questionnaire and Scoring Booklet. It can be obtained from Dr Ron Hays or Dr Cathy Sherbourne at Rand, 1700 Main Street, PO Box 2138, Santa Monica, CA 90407–2138, USA. New users are asked by Ware *et al*. (1993) to register with the Medical Outcomes Study (MOS) Trust of the Health Institute, New England Medical Center, NEMCH Box 345, 750 Washington Street, Boston, MA 02111, USA. They have recently produced a handbook for the SF–36, covering both the US and UK versions, which is available for purchase (Ware *et al*. 1993).

Past users have also been formally registered with the Health Outcomes Institute (previously known as Interstudy, then the Health Outcomes Trust) (2001 Killebrew Drive, Suite 122, Bloomington MN 55425, USA). Changes in copyright mean users who were registered with the Health Outcomes Institute are requested to call the questionnaire the Health Status Questionnaire (although it has the same content as the SF–36).

9

COMMENTS ON
MEASUREMENT
ISSUES AND
SOURCES OF
INFORMATION

The development of disease- and condition-specific measures has been uneven across specialities, which makes definitive recommendations about the use of particular scales difficult. However, there are several methodological guidelines which can be specified. Some of the most pertinent of these are outlined or referred to below.

STUDY DESIGN

Sampling issues

All research projects require sufficient numbers of respondents to satisfy power calculations for achieving statistical significance. Given the large numbers of patients that are often required in outcome studies (depending on the study aims), there is increasing interest in pooled data among clinical investigators and in meta-analysis (Spector and Thompson 1991). In addition, in any research which aims to generalize findings beyond the subjects studied, the sample of choice should be a representative random sample of the population of interest, and non-response minimized. While random sampling, based on population registers of community populations, is a commonly used method in cross-sectional (at one point in time) and longitudinal (followed up over a period of time) survey research (e.g. as in surveys of the general health status of a population), it is not a realistic or practical method when studying the effects of an intervention on a clinical population. Studies of

disease-specific outcome studies tend to depend on in-patient or out-patient populations in hospital or in general practice settings. Referred populations are inevitably subject to sampling bias, and even with multi-centre trials there is no guarantee that the patients studied are representative of all patients with the condition of interest. This is more of a problem in the case of non–life-threatening conditions. For example, in the case of mental illnesses, many people with these conditions do not seek medical help, and, of those that do, many are treated by their general practitioners and not referred to specialists (Goldberg and Huxley 1980).

However random or representative of the population of interest the initial sample may be at the outset of a study, this status is not necessarily maintained in longitudinal (follow-up) study designs, but it can be checked and bias estimated. For example, the exclusion of people who die or withdraw from trials is a major source of bias. Some investigators, when they report their post-intervention results exclude such groups, which makes the statistics showing an improvement in health status for the remaining study members misleading. As Fletcher et al. (1987) commented, a score needs to be incorporated for patients' health status at withdrawal from the study, and a score to indicate death (or health status if the scale is not completed due to illness).

Issues of sample size, statistical power, significance testing and study design (randomization) can be found in Pocock (1983).

Case series studies

Such studies involve the selection of a current group of patients with the condition of interest and a retrospective analysis of morbidity and treatment toxicities. The advantage of this design is the potential for studying a large number of patients, with a known outcome, although the disadvantages include selection bias in various forms and the varying quality and completeness of retrospectively collected data (whether from records or patient recall).

Cohort studies

People who are identified as sharing a predefined category form a cohort (e.g. people aged 18 and over with insulin-dependent diabetes). These respondents can be studied retrospectively (e.g. patients who are identified from medical records with diabetes can be followed up and questioned about their current and past health status and quality of life, and current and past medical history records can be analysed). These studies involve a great deal of effort in relation to tracing people who have moved or died, the sample can still suffer from selection bias, and all retrospective data can be of variable quality. In prospective cohort studies, the identified respondents are followed up over a period of time and the data collected relate to the present and recent past, and eventual outcome is assessed. It is important that the periods between interviews are not too far apart, otherwise the data suffer from all the disadvantages of retrospective studies. These studies are always expensive in terms of tracing respondents.

Intervention studies

The aim of such studies is to examine the effect of a therapy or intervention on the condition of interest. The ideal method is a randomized controlled trial, in which patients or subjects are randomly allocated to the intervention (e.g. treatment) of interest, to standard treatments and a placebo treatment (an inert preparation formulated to appear indistinguishable from the treatment(s) of interest). This method reduces potential for bias and facilitates comparisons. Double-blind trials are recommended wherever practical (where subjects,

health professionals and interviewers are unaware of the hypotheses to be tested and the treatment identities), although this is not always possible. Placebo treatments are not always practical or ethical, and the differing treatments cannot always be effectively concealed from the health professionals treating the patients.

Where randomized controlled trials are not practical or ethical, an alternative method for identifying factors which occur more (or less) often in the cases is the (non-randomized) case control study, which involves comparing the characteristics of people with a particular disease, or undergoing a particular intervention (i.e. the cases), with a group of people without the disease or the particular intervention (i.e. the controls). In the case of intervention studies, data can be collected about the cases before and after an intervention, and outcomes compared with a similar group of patients undergoing a different intervention and, if possible, a placebo group. It is usual practice to match cases and controls on age and sex. Other variables must be matched with caution in case the variable of importance is 'controlled out'. Again, the ideal method is a 'blind' study. The limitations of these studies are the potential for bias due to sampling, and the effect of confounding factors. Without random allocation of patients to intervention and non-intervention groups, it will never be known whether any observed changes occurred as a result of an intervention or whether they would have occurred anyway.

Some investigators, for ethical or practical reasons, take the patient as his or her own control, and collect data on respondents before and after an intervention. Many before–after studies have been published where no controls have been used. Such studies can only be viewed as generating hypotheses to be tested in future well-designed trials, due to the same limitations referred to above. It is easy to criticize the standard of research design on health outcomes; it is not so easy to design a trial that can *realistically* be carried out in real-life settings.

It should be cautioned that the detection of any improvement or deterioration in the condition of a group of patients as a result of an intervention, once confounding variables and any sampling biases have been ruled out, can always be due to regression to the mean. This problem occurs when subjects have been selected for study on the basis of an extreme measurement which contains a degree of random error. On subsequent measurements, this value will tend to return to normal. The implication is that, if a group of patients in a severe disease category at a particular point in time is selected for study, they may improve in the short term independently of any intervention simply because of the random variation inherent in the disease.

Further exploration of such methodological issues is outside the scope of this book, but investigators are encouraged to design studies on outcome according to valid scientific criteria, and to make explicit the ethical and practical limitations which prevent the ideals of study design being reached. Relevant methodological and statistical texts include those by Moser and Kalton (1971), Pocock (1983), Barker and Rose (1984) and Armitage and Berry (1987).

QUESTIONNAIRE FORMAT

When compiling a questionnaire, one should be careful that the wording of the questions and their order and format do not influence how subjects respond. For rules governing the design of questionnaires, readers are referred to textbooks on the topic (e.g. Oppenheim 1968; Sudman and Bradburn 1983).

An important question in quality of life assessment relates to whether to use a self-completion format or an interviewer-administered questionnaire. Self-completion scales were developed during the early part of this century for use in large-scale psychiatric screening programmes, during a period when there was a shortage of psychiatric interviewers (Woodworth 1918). They are used today because they are relatively economical and easy to analyse.

The method of choice will often be determined by practical considerations, such as the financial resources available for the research and the condition of the patient, as well as the likely length of the instrument. Methodological considerations may pose a paradox for the researcher. *Concise, self-report scales* are cheaper to administer and analyse, they can be sent by post or given to respondents to complete themselves in the presence of an interviewer, and they are less taxing for respondents. However, they may be insufficiently sensitive and informative to answer the research question. Short questionnaires inevitably lose sensitivity, and postal questionnaires have to be short and simple. *Long interview questionnaires or longer batteries of self-report scales* may sometimes be preferable, but they are expensive to administer and analyse, and longer batteries of self-report scales usually require an interviewer to administer them, or to at least explain their instructions. Interviewer-administered questionnaires, which may also include some self-report scales to be given to respondents to complete during the interview, usually result in better quality data, because ambiguities can be explained, assistance can be given where necessary (e.g. with reading), in-depth information can be collected and the good rapport between the interviewer and the interviewee usually leads to a better overall and item response rate.

RESPONSE FORMAT AND RESPONSE SCALES

Response format in health-related quality of life questionnaires (both generic and disease-specific) is commonly in the form of category rating scales with labelled tick boxes for response choices (i.e. one from several descriptions is chosen). Sometimes visual analogue scales (VAS) are also used.

Visual analogue scales

Visual analogue scales are also known as linear analogue scales. These scales require respondents to place a mark on a line on which opposing statements or descriptions are placed at either end of a (usually) 10 cm line. The point at which respondents make their mark represents where they perceive their answer to lie on this continuum. The distance between their mark and one end (or the mid-point) of the scale is recorded and coded. Visual analogue scales are horizontal (usually) or vertical, and have between 5 and 7 points if they are numbered (most are unnumbered), although they have been known to have a range of 0 to 100 (e.g. pain rating scales). Numbered scales are usually known as *numeric* scales.

The following is an example of a severity of pain scale:

Mild   Severe

Few studies have compared visual analogue scales with other methods, in relation to reliability and validity and ease of completion on the part of respondents. Fine discrimination is provided, in theory, by the VAS method, in contrast to the discrete categories of categorical scales. In theory, visual analogue scales, by providing a greater range of response choices, are more valid, reliable and sensitive than categorical scales. Visual analogue scales have been used successfully in the measurement of mood (Aitken 1969; Bond and Lader 1974) and in the classification of psychiatric patients (Remington *et al.* 1979). The latter authors reported that a visual analogue scale was not markedly superior to categorical scales in relation to reliability or validity. Overall, evidence to date has not conclusively shown visual analogue scales to have superior validity, and it has been reported that patients sometimes find them difficult to understand and complete, and they are more labour-intensive to analyse (Fayers and Jones 1983; Selby and Robertson 1987). On the other hand, they are apparently easy to administer to 5-year-old children (Scott *et al.* 1977). Insufficient research evidence exists to support a position on either side of this debate, although the Southwest Oncology Group in the USA recommended researchers to use categorical rather than visual analogue scales in their measures of quality of life (Moinpour *et al.* 1989).

Category scales

Category scales (also called categorical scales), in contrast to the continuous response format of visual analogue scales, provide discrete response categories in the form of a series of descriptive phrases. Category scales may order the response choices in a particular sequence (e.g. from 'best' to 'worst' state) or may be simply dichotomous (e.g. 'yes/no' response choices). The most common scaling method used with category scales is the Likert (see p. 290). For example, in their study of the treatment effects of women with breast cancer, Palmer *et al.* (1980) asked respondents: 'How much

did the full course of treatment interfere with your life?' The response categories provided were 'not at all', 'slightly', 'moderately' and 'severely'. The main advantage of category scales over visual analogue scales is their greater ease of administration (less detailed explanations are needed), coding and analysis (categorical scales are pre-coded and ready for analysis).

Some categorical scales involve coded visual displays, and ask respondents to select a picture (e.g. a face showing expressions) rather than a phrase for their response. Andrews and Crandall (1976) investigated the validity of measures of self-reported well-being with various response formats in home interviews with a non-random sample of 222 adults in Toledo, Ohio and with 1297 adults from a probability sample in 48 US states. With the smaller sample, they asked their respondents to rate six pre-defined aspects of well-being (e.g. 'your independence or freedom – the chance to do what you want'). They tested six types of response formats: a phrased Likert delighted–terrible scale; scales depicting faces in which respondents select a face to represent their feelings; circles containing numbers prefixed by '+' and '−' signs, depicting positive and negative feelings respectively, one of which respondents pick to depict their feelings; ladders, which are similar to visual analogue scales, and where respondents mark a labelled rung to depict their feelings; a scale in which respondents compared their lives with those of six people they knew well; and a scale in which named others completed a questionnaire about the respondent's quality of life. The second investigation also explored people's feelings about themselves, problems and accomplishments, their families and relationships and income. The authors reported the delighted–terrible scale, the faces scale and the circles scale to have the highest mean validity coefficients. The delighted–terrible and faces scales are popular in psychiatry.

One problem with categorical scales is the choice of categories offered. Too many categories may lead to difficulties in decision making, whereas the use of too few may have the effect of not providing enough choice and of thus forcing the respondent to choose falsely from adjacent categories less closely resembling their response. There is some inconsistency in the literature over the optimum

number of response choices with regard to reliability. On the whole it appears that a 4- or
5-point scale is appropriate (Fayers and Jones 1983).

Likert scale

A Likert scale (Likert 1952) is a rating system which
is subdivided numerically into a series of ordered
responses; for example, from 'never' through
'sometimes' to 'always', or 'strongly agree' and
'agree' through 'undecided' to 'disagree' and
'strongly disagree'. Thus the respondent is not
simply asked to agree or disagree with an item, but
to choose between several response categories,
indicating various strengths of agreement and
disagreement. Five categories are usually employed, although some have three or seven. The
categories are assigned scores and the respondent's
attitude is measured by the total score. It is not an
interval scale of measurement and no conclusions
can be drawn about the meaning of distances
between scale points. It is a reasonable ordinal
scale.

Other scales

Other types of response scaling include Guttman
scales, semantic-differential scales and Thurstone
scaling (the latter is usually used in scale development). Guttman scales (Guttman 1944) are cumulative and the respondent is required to endorse all
the items less extreme than the one with which he
or she agrees. Such scales are criticized for their
complexity, and there is no guarantee that all scale
items cover the concept of interest, and those that
are included tend to be narrow in content. The
Arthritis Impact Measurement Scales (Meenan *et
al.* 1980) is an example of Guttman scoring: for each
sub-scale, the items are listed so that a respondent
indicating disability on one item will also indicate
disability on section items falling below it (Guttman scoring is ignored in the final overall score
calculation). This scaling method attempts to attain
interval level measurement, although it is doubtful
if it achieves it.

The semantic-differential method (Osgood *et al.*
1957) is a popular attitude measurement technique
that asks respondents to rate an attitude object on a
number of adjective scales (e.g. good–bad, happy–
sad, strong–weak, easy–hard, fast–slow, old–

young). For example, subjects are asked to place a
cross or tick in one of the spaces on each scale
(good–bad, etc.) to indicate their rating of the
object's position with respect to the adjectives
involved. The positions are then assigned scores
(e.g. 1–7 for 7 spaces: good———————bad).

The Thurstone method (Thurstone 1927a,
1927b) involves choosing the attitude object to be
measured (e.g. euthanasia) and then collecting a
wide range of belief statements expressing favourable or unfavourable sentiments about this attitude
object (e.g. 'euthanasia is morally wrong under all
circumstances', 'euthanasia is a form of murder',
'euthanasia is every person's right'). Numerical
values (scale values) are derived by judges who sort
the statements into piles according to the degree of
favourable or unfavourable evaluation each one
expresses. Statements are narrowed down to a
smaller group that the judges agree have particular
locations on the evaluative continuum. This
method is sometimes used in scale development
and the calculation of item weights; for example,
Hunt *et al.* (1986), the developers of the Nottingham Health Profile, used this method. This
method attempts to attain interval level measurement, although it is again doubtful if it achieves it.

Middle scale values

Caution should be exercised if odd numbers are
used to label visual analogue or categorical scales,
thus providing a middle number, or if neutral
choices are offered in categorical scales. Many
respondents prefer not to commit themselves one
way or the other and opt for the middle or neutral
categories. In some cases, the researcher may wish
to measure this neutrality where it is a valid option.
In other instances, the researcher may wish to force
respondents to make a choice one way or the other,
and thus they omit the middle or neutral value. The
researcher should be aware of the dangers of
creating biased responses when forcing choices.

TYPES OF MEASUREMENTS

Single-item questions

Questionnaire formats may vary from single-item
questions, to batteries of single-item questions, to

complete measurement scales. These will incorporate the response formats described above (e.g. visual analogue scales, or verbal ratings in the form of category scales such as a Likert scale). A popular, single verbal rating item to measure health status is the well-known question, 'Would you describe your health (for your age) as "excellent", "good", "fair", or "poor"?' Some investigators add 'very good' in order to increase the sensitivity of this scale as responses tend to cluster towards the positive end (e.g. the Rand MOS Short Form Questionnaire, the SF-36: Stewart and Ware 1992). As around 50 per cent of a random sample of the population will rate their health as 'excellent' or 'good', and most of the remainder as 'fair', the sensitivity of the question is limited (Ware 1984b). On the other hand, it has been shown to be a valid predictor of crude outcomes (e.g. mortality) and satisfaction with health (Wright 1987; and see review by Idler 1992).

A more sophisticated example of a single-item question that is popularly used by social scientists and clinicians is a ladder scale, commonly labelled as a self-anchoring scale because the method allows the respondent to situate his or her response according to personal experience and expectations. Single ladder scale questions have been developed by Cantril (1965) and by Andrews and Withey (1976). For example:

> Here is a picture of a ladder. At the bottom of this ladder is the worst situation you might reasonably expect to have. At the top is the best you might expect to have. The other rungs are in between. Where on the ladder would you put your quality of life over the past four weeks? On which rung would you put it?'

> (Andrews and Withey 1976)

Single items in the form of a list of problems (e.g. symptom checklists) are also commonly used (e.g. see Forsberg and Bjorvell 1993), but need to be carefully constructed because they usually yield a high proportion of affirmative responses, because trivial problems are usually included in people's replies (see Dunnell and Cartwright 1972).

Single items are popular because they are brief, easy to administer and analyse, although it is doubtful whether single questions can effectively tap and measure a given domain, and it is difficult to fully assess their reliability (e.g. they cannot be split for multiple forms or split-half reliability testing). Several investigators have shown how single-item measures are more likely to fall short of the minimum level of precision needed when testing hypotheses because of their coarseness (Ware and Karmos 1976; Manning *et al.* 1982; and see Ware *et al.* 1993).

Multi-item scales

The superiority of multi-item scales over single-item questions has been demonstrated by Davies and Ware (1981) and Manning *et al.* (1982). The quality of data collection is improved by the use of standardized, well-tested scales, with good psychometric properties.

In addition, account must be taken of the type of scoring that the instrument is based on and whether it yields:

- *Nominal data*: numbers are used simply for classification (e.g. 'died', 'survived').
- *Ordinal scale data*: scale items stand in some kind of relation to each other (e.g. 'very difficult' through to 'not very difficult').
- *Interval scale data*: the characteristics of an ordinal scale but the distances between any two numbers on the scale are of a known size (e.g. temperature).
- *Ratio scale data*: the characteristics of an interval scale with the addition of a true – not arbitrary – zero point (e.g. weight).

The full definitions of these concepts can be found in most research methods textbooks (e.g. Blalock and Blalock 1971; Moser and Kalton 1971). Their consideration is crucial because different scales are suitable for answering different types of question. In addition, interval and ratio scales are required if powerful statistical analysis is envisaged.

RELIABILITY AND VALIDITY

Questionnaire design can be difficult and question wording is fraught with difficulties (Guyatt 1993). Scales need to be adequately tested for their reliability and validity. This is a lengthy and expensive process, and is one reason for using – or adapting – existing scales rather than creating new ones. All measures should satisfy the criteria for reliability and validity. Validity is the extent to which an instrument measures what is intended. Reliability is the extent to which measurements on the same respondent are similar on repeated applications of the measure at different times. Another important property of quality of life scales when used as outcome measures is their responsiveness to change, particularly clinically important changes. There is an unresolved debate about whether responsiveness is an aspect of validity (Hays and Hadhorn 1992). Several texts describe these concepts in more detail (e.g. Carmines and Zeller 1979; Kline 1986; Streiner and Norman 1990). They are described briefly in the next section.

Measuring the quality of life of patients is inevitably difficult. Questions about the sensitivity, reliability, validity and generalizability of data continue to be raised because of the complex nature of diseases, treatments (Smart and Yates 1987) and, of course, the concept itself.

Reliability

Reliability refers to the ability to produce consistent results, and consistent results on different occasions, when there is no evidence of change. This is tested by test–retest reliability (administration of the scale on different occasions to the same population), internal consistency (measurement of the same concept by different scale items), and inter- and intra-rater reliability (consistency of a measure when administered by different interviewers or the same interviewer on different occasions).

A few of the appropriate statistical techniques for assessing reliability are referred to below, in order to clarify the chapters in this volume where values are presented. Readers are referred to the references below and to appropriate methodological and statistical texts for further details, and for details of other tests as well as appropriate levels of statistical significance in relation to sample size (e.g. Pocock 1983; Armitage and Berry 1987).

Internal consistency involves testing for homogeneity. Tests assess the extent to which individual items are inter-correlated and the extent to which they correlate with overall scale scores. Internal scale consistency is usually tested with inter-item correlations and with Cronbach's alpha (Cronbach 1951), based on the average correlation among the items and the number of items in the instrument (values range from 0 to 1). Although some regard 0.70 as the minimally acceptable level for internal consistency reliability (Nunnally 1978), others accept the level >0.50 as an indicator of good internal consistency, as well as of test–retest reliability (Cronbach 1951; Cronbach et al. 1972; Ebel 1951; Helmstater 1964). If Cronbach's alpha is high (e.g. >0.80), the responses are consistent, and the sum of the item responses yields a score for the underlying dimensions that the item represents. If the items are adequately sampled from the quality of life domain, the sum of the responses should give a better indication of quality of life for the respondent than responses to any one item. A low coefficient alpha indicates that the item does not come from the same conceptual domain (Williams and Wood-Dauphinee 1989).

The items of the measure can also be split and the alphas for the alternative forms compared (the Spearman–Brown formula uses this correlation to estimate reliability after adjusting for the number of scale items); or the scale can be divided into two groups and coefficients can be computed for each half and compared. Comparable coefficients confirm the consistency of the responses (Zeller and Carmines 1980; Williams and Wood-Dauphinee 1989). It is also accepted practice to examine item–total correlations, and to reject scale items below $r = 0.20$ (Kline 1986).

Other tests of reliability include inter-rater agreements (the concordance, or reliability, of scores by different raters on a single occasion) and intra-rater agreement – the reliability of the rating by the same rater (of the same subjects) on different occasions (repeat testings). If the measure is categorical, then the most appropriate statistical method to employ is Cohen's (1968) kappa test of concordance. Kappa has a value of 0 if agreement is no better than chance, a negative value if worse than chance, and a value of unity (1.0) if agreement is perfect. Fleiss (1981b) suggested that less than 0.40 is poor agreement, 0.40–0.59 is fair agreement, 0.60–0.74 is good agreement, and 0.75–1.00 is excellent agreement. Spearman's rho and Kendall's tau may also be used. However, simple correlation analysis is less appropriate for studying concordance as it makes no allowance for chance agreement. Pearson's product–moment correlation is used for comparing quantitative scores.

Intra-class correlation coefficients compare the variance between subjects, the variance between raters and the variance between times with error variance (Fleiss 1986). An intra-class correlation coefficient of, for example, 0.80 or more indicates that the scale is highly reliable.

The stability of a measure over a period of time is measured by repeated administrations of the test on subjects and domains not expected to change in their scores over a carefully defined time period. Test–retest reliability is generally assessed by correlations of the measure administered on the different occasions. A high level of consistency in response is desired. The observed associations can sometimes be difficult to interpret – a low correlation may reflect a genuine change in health status, rather than poor reliability. Some investigators also feel that correlations are a weak measure of test–retest reliability, and recommend the use of confidence intervals to assess the size of the difference between the scores (Bland and Altman 1986; Ruta *et al*. 1994).

Validity

Validity refers to the extent to which the scale measures the underlying concept of interest, and is measured by testing for face validity (at face value, does it appear to be measuring what it is intended to measure? is it unambiguous and appropriate?), content validity (does the scale tap all relevant concepts of the attribute to be measured?) and criterion validity (the extent to which the measure correlates with a 'gold standard'). Validity is often difficult to assess because there is no objective 'gold-standard' measure of quality of life. Criterion validity encompasses concurrent validity (correlations with an existing measure of the same construct) and predictive validity (correlations against other measures to assess predictive powers). Quality of life scales are often reliant on predictive validity to demonstrate their psychometric properties. There is also construct validity where hypotheses are generated and the scale tested against a measure central to the hypothesis. Construct validity is usually divided into convergent validity (tests for correlations with other indicators intending to measure the same concept) and discriminant validity (lack of correlations with unrelated indicators) (see Campbell and Fiske 1959).

Hyland (1992a, 1993) has cautioned against reliance on claims for content validity by scale developers. He pointed out that quality of life comprises several connected constructs, and any questionnaire may reflect one or more of these constructs. In the absence of an agreed theoretical description of quality of life, validity can be difficult to assess.

FACTOR STRUCTURE

Questions that deliberately tap different dimensions within a scale cannot be expected to necessarily have high item–total or full item–item correlations. Therefore, factor analysis should be used to identify the separate factors within the scale. Factor analysis is a technique which defines a small number of underlying dimensions (factors that account for a high proportion of the common variance of the items), and in so doing it demonstrates whether the items in the scales group together in a consistent and coherent way. Exploratory factor analysis is usually used in scale development in order to identify and discard items that are not correlated with the items of interest. Factor analysis is also used to confirm that scale items principally load on to that factor and correlate weakly with other factors. While small samples may be used in analysis, ultimately a confirmatory factor analysis should include a larger sample, as well as comparisons with several other samples for consideration of stability (Comrey 1978; Loo 1983). A factor is considered important, and its items worthy of retention in the scale, if its eigenvalue (a measure of its power to explain variation between subjects) exceeds a certain value. Jollife and Morgan (1992) state that this value should be 1.1, although 1.5 appears to be commonly taken.

SOCIAL DESIRABILITY BIAS

Questions designed to measure human behaviour and subjective feelings are inevitably subject to several types of potential biases, which often need to be checked in an attempt to make the measurement process as rigorous as possible (e.g. social desirability bias, interviewer bias and the tendency of respondents to simply say 'yes' to items, irrespective of their content) (Oppenheim 1968). In the case of social desirability bias, people may describe the quality of life they think the interviewer or investigator wants to hear, rather than their actual quality of life (Hurny *et al*. 1987).

Breetvelt and van Dam (1991) reported a tendency for cancer patients to report a better quality of life on self-administered questionnaires compared with personal interview techniques. This is also known as desirability bias. Social desirability bias is known to exert a small but pervasive effect on reports of life satisfaction and mood (Klassen *et al*. 1975; Campbell *et al*. 1976). Social desirability bias can be checked with the various desirability and lie scales that exist, although few investigators wish to lengthen their batteries of instruments even further. Webb *et al*. (1966) argued for the use of multiple research methods given that interviews and questionnaires inevitably introduce a foreign element into the social setting they attempt to describe, and they are limited to those who are accessible and will cooperate (e.g. observation, analysis of public and private records). In health-related quality of life research this is less easy − observations of individuals in institutions (e.g. hospitals) can be carried out, but observations of people in their private homes cannot be carried out easily or unobtrusively. Quality of life data can be collected from records and recorded behaviour patterns at a crude global level (e.g. air pollution records, crime figures, employment patterns, etc.) and interpreted carefully, but the only method of assessing subjective health related to quality of life is to ask the person concerned and, in some cases, his or her significant others.

The potential for bias is present in all social research, but the problems can be minimized by using interviewers who have been properly trained, briefed to be as objective as possible, and by ensuring that they are not clinical or nursing staff − or other health professionals − whom the patient may wish to influence or subconsciously give desirable answers to. The extent of any social desirability response bias will require testing in any relatively new measure. There are several scales available which have been developed and used to check for this, ranging from specific social desirability scales to lie scales. These scales have been reviewed by Paulhus (1991).

CROSS-CULTURAL APPLICABILITY

Illness has a different meaning in different cultures, and even between cultures living within the same society. Ethnicity and culture can have significant effects on assessments of subjective experiences, for example, assessments of social handicap and health-related quality of life and its various sub-domains (e.g. pain). Some of the pertinent literature has been summarized by Kleinman (1986) and Bowling (1994b).

The more well-known health status scales have been translated into many languages for use across the world and within multicultural societies, and many of the newer, popular scales are currently undergoing the same process, which involves the technical process of translation, back-translation, review and modification. This is not always sufficient, given that health status scales, like all questionnaires, reflect the cultural norms of the society within which they are created. Some questionnaire items may not translate well, or at all; and items that were of importance to the study population for whom the questionnaire was designed, may appear trivial in a different culture (Guyatt 1993). Different cultural groups may have different norms for the restriction of activity when ill (Deyo 1984a).

Most health status scales are American in origin, and their applicability to other cultures has still to be carefully assessed before use. There is a need for a critical appraisal of the applicability in Europe of the many subjective health status measures which have been developed in North America, rather than accepting the imposition of American values on different cultures.

TIME REFERENCES

The interest in measuring health status has gained momentum over the last three decades through the burgeoning interest in assessing the outcome of medical treatments; that is, in assessing any resulting changes in health, rather than the assessment of (static) health status at one point in time. Given that the aim of most current research studies is to assess outcome of care, investigators and clinicians will need to agree over what types of changes will be expected (outcomes) over specific time periods.

For some conditions, the reference periods may be from admission to hospital to 3 months and 12 months after discharge. In the case of chronic conditions, it will be necessary to consider longer time periods (Bardsley and Coles 1992). It may be regarded as desirable to measure patient outcomes not just once, in comparison with baseline measures, but several times (e.g. at quarterly intervals), in order to document the speed of any progress or deterioration. However, repeated follow-ups are expensive.

The time period over which to ask patients to base their assessments of quality of life, symptoms, etc., is also problematic. General health status scales usually limit their time reference to 4 weeks. Disease-specific scales often restrict time period references further, due to concern over memory and confusion (i.e. to 24 hours, 1–7 days or 2 weeks). There are few research data on which to base decisions, although Hamilton (1970) has provided justification for using the 7-day referent for psychiatric assessment, on the grounds that the last 7 days usually contain the most relevant information about current clinical status. However, there is little information about the ideal time reference in other areas of life.

The time reference which is selected will be dependent on the aims of the study and the predicted effects of the treatment, and this will have to be balanced against problems of recall bias.

PLACE OF INTERVIEW AND THE INTERVIEWER

Good survey research practice for *supervised* self-completion questionnaires or interviewer-administered instruments, involves an interview with the patient in his or her own home, uninterrupted by others and in a personal and comfortable environment. This personal approach also maximizes response, and leads to more valid results (except on some highly sensitive issues) as ambiguities or difficulties can be clarified by the interviewers. Sometimes instruments can only be administered, for practical reasons, on wards or in clinics. The guidelines issued by the Quality of Life Committee of the Clinical Trials Group of the National Cancer Institute of Canada (Osoba 1992) discourage postal questionnaires, and discourage

researchers from giving patients the questionnaire to take home to complete. The reason given is the introduction into the study of unnecessary variables (i.e. the variability of home surroundings and times of completion). However, questionnaires administered in the home setting by independent interviewers unquestionably produce the best quality data on complex issues or detailed topics, although it is essential that interviewers are properly trained in order to reduce bias and the questions are structured in order to avoid ambiguity (Cartwright 1989).

CONTAMINATION OF RESULTS BY HOSPITAL SETTING

Some caution in the choice of scales is required with regard to the collection of baseline data after the patient has been admitted to hospital, as health status scores may be affected by admission and thus the results may be contaminated (Bardsley *et al.* 1992). The hospital setting itself may contaminate the results (e.g. as with questions about staying in bed, lying down, sleeping, etc., on the SIP and NHP) (Bardsley *et al.* 1992; Ziebland and Fitzpatrick 1992). As Ziebland and Fitzpatrick (1992) showed, research designs which involve at least one in-patient-based completion of a health status measure with a subsequent out-patient follow-up could show an improvement in scores because the respondent is no longer restricted by the hospital setting – the mobility domain contributes 56 per cent of the score on the FLP (SIP). The NHP did not appear to be affected by this contamination (Bardsley *et al.* 1992; Ziebland and Fitzpatrick 1992).

It is also important to identify any patient characteristics or items that may affect outcome (e.g. age, co-morbidity, etc.), as well as disease severity (Krischer 1979).

SCALE SELECTION AND USE

The following list includes some of the most important criteria to consider when selecting and administering a scale (Cella and Cherin 1987; Selby and Robertson 1987; Bellamy 1989; Fletcher *et al.* 1992b).

- Define quality of life and operationalize the concepts used.
- Specify the key variables before commencing the study and select a scale to accord with these. The scale instructions should clearly define which aspect of quality of life it covers.
- Decide whether the scale required is generic, disease- and/or domain-specific, and select appropriate scales accordingly.
- Assess which dimensions of quality of life the scales measure, and decide if they need to be supplemented.
- The scale should be multidimensional, or otherwise be supplemented with other scales to ensure that the resulting questionnaire reflects each major domain of health-related quality of life of relevance to the study objectives.
- An item on satisfaction with medical care and the outcome of the treatment should also be included (Aaronson 1986).
- Supplement existing scales with additional items rather than design a new scale.
- Ensure that the scale purporting to measure quality of life measures more than level of functioning and distress.
- Check whether patients have been a main source in generating the questionnaire items.
- There should be published evidence of acceptable levels of scale reliability, validity, factor structure and sensitivity to clinically significant changes and changes in quality of life.
- Ensure that the time reference periods of the scale items coincide with the study aims and are appropriate for the study (e.g. questions measuring depression may ask about feelings in the last week or the last 2 weeks).
- Check whether separate sub-scale scores can be computed as well as a global score; these are needed for assessing which domain of quality of life is affected.
- Assess the ease of administration and scoring. Keep weightings simple where possible; they can be unjustifiably complex and their advantages are largely untested.
- Ensure that the scale is appropriate for the statistical requirements of the study. The best data are provided by continuous scales (at least interval data) in relation to the applicability of parametric statistics (few scales achieve this).
- The measurement process must be ethical.

- Ensure that the measure is easy to understand by different groups of people, for example those from different educational and social backgrounds and those from different cultural groups.
- Ensure that the number of items does not lead to patient fatigue (e.g. limit them to 50 on any one occasion), and is acceptable to patients.
- The instrument should be appropriate for use with the particular study population (e.g. children, adolescents, adults and elderly people, as well as specific patient groups). For example, if the population is elderly, then a functional ability scale will be required to supplement scales of choice.
- The scale should be based on patient self-report, and supplemented only where necessary by the assessments of significant others and health professionals.
- If relatives, friends or others are used to supplement patient-reported data, the patient's permission must be given.
- Questionnaires should not be administered in open clinic or ward areas where the patient may feel inhibited.
- Quality of life is a dynamic not a static concept, and the study design should take account of this by ensuring questions cover changes and have a follow-up design.
- In before–after study designs, administer the questionnaire before the inception of treatment where possible and avoid repeating measures at times of transient changes in health status (unless the study aims to measure these).
- All subjects should complete the scale at premature exit (i.e. at any episodes of premature withdrawal from the study) in order that remaining sample bias can be assessed.

DATABASES, CLEARING HOUSES AND SCALE DISTRIBUTORS

In the UK, the UK Clearing House for Information on the Assessment of Health Outcomes (Long et al. 1992) will undertake computer searches of their database in relation to quality of life and health outcomes in specific areas. It also acts as the distributor of the Short Form-36 and scoring manual (Ware et al. 1993) in Europe. A quarterly newsletter is published that includes information on the results of outcome assessments, critical reviews of measurement instruments, and information on activities in the field.

The emphasis on health care outcomes and the lack of collated information that is available to health care purchasers in Britain, has also led the Department of Health (via the NHS Management Executive) to commission a series of epidemiologically based research reviews, which compile epidemiological information in relation to specified diseases and the effectiveness of services. Over 20 reviews have been completed to date (e.g. diabetes, hip and knee replacement surgery, stroke, mental illness, etc.) and these are distributed free from the Department to district health authorities.

In the USA, the Health Outcomes Institute, previously known as Interstudy, is attempting to provide outcome scales for international use. The condition-specific specifications (TyPE) have been produced for a range of conditions, and are commissioned from experts in the field. Most await psychometric testing. They are known collectively as the Outcomes Management System, which is a collection of several general and condition-specific measures of patient function, well-being and clinical status. Examples include hip fracture, stroke, heart conditions, rheumatological conditions, depression and substance abuse.

The Medical Outcomes Trust (MOT) in Boston, USA has the objective of providing patient-based health status survey instruments, and scoring documentation, free of charge to those who request them, to standardize their scoring and content for international use, and to act as a clearing house for information about generic and disease-specific health status instruments. It is funded by the Kaiser Family Foundation. The MOT publishes an information bulletin several times a year (*Medical Outcomes Trust Bulletin*), and the content to date has ranged from information about Ware and co-workers' (1993) Short Form-36 Health Survey and other scales that the MOT distributes, to the calculation of confidence intervals (MOT 1993a, 1993b, 1994).

The National Clearing House on Health Indexes (1993) in the USA provides a bibliography on health indexes, and has sponsored research on quality of life data collection, principally from the National Health Interview Survey. Finally, the World Health Organization Quality of Life Group (WHOQOL Group 1994b) has recently produced a very useful annotated bibliography on quality of life assessment. This was compiled as part of their attempt to promote international quality of life collaboration, and to develop cross-cultural quality of life assessments.

There are several commercial sources for useful scales and publication citations: NFER-Nelson publishes many of the psychological scales in Britain, and there are dozens of scale publishers in the USA covering a wide range of health-related disciplines (listed in Test Corporation of America's *Test Critiques*; see Keyser and Sweetland 1986). In the USA, Behavioral Measurement Database Services have produced a CD-ROM 'HaPI-CD', which is a multidisciplinary database of health and psychosocial measurement instruments. A two-year project at Burroughs Wellcome Company led to the identification and publication of a 'Quality of life bibliography and indexes' published in *Medical Care* (Spilker *et al.* 1990; see Tilson and Spilker 1990). In relation to the elderly, Kane and Kane (1988) reviewed many relevant assessment scales, and the Netherlands Institute of Primary Health Care (NIVEL) have published a bibliography of quality of life indicators (Mulder and Sluijs 1993). The Royal College of Physicians (RCP) in the UK initiated a workshop on 'Measures of the Quality of Life' in 1992 and promoted open discussion among invited experts in the field in relation to the appropriate domains to measure and pertinent scales (Hopkins 1992). A series of RCP-commissioned disease-specific workshops on quality of life has also been initiated.

APPENDIX:
A SELECTION OF
USEFUL SCALE
DISTRIBUTORS AND
ADDRESSES

Abbreviated Mental Test 7 Item (AMT-7) Professor S. Ebrahim, Department of Public Health, Royal Free Hospital Medical School, Rowland Hill Street, London NW3 2PF, UK

Aids Health Assessment Questionnaire Dr P.D. Lubeck and Dr M.A. Tauber, Department of Medicine, Division of Immunology, Stanford University, Stanford, CA 94305, USA, or ATHOS, Dr M.A. Tauber, 1000 Welch Road, Suite 203, Palo Alto, CA 94304, USA

Arthritis Impact Measurement Scales (AIMS-2) Dr R.F. Meenan, Arthritis Center, Boston University Medical Center, Conte Building, 80 East Concord Street, Boston, MA 02118, USA

Asthma Quality of Life Questionnaire Dr E.F. Juniper, Department of Clinical Epidemiology and Biostatistics, McMaster University Medical Centre, 1200 Main Street West, Hamilton, Ontario L8N 3Z5, Canada

Asthma Self-Efficacy Scale Dr D.L. Tobin and Dr T.L. Creer, Department of Psychology, Ohio University, 207 Research and Technology Center, Athens, OH, 45701–2979, USA

Asthma Severity Scale Dr Tim Booth, Joint Unit for Social Service Research, University of Sheffield, Sheffield S10 2TN, UK

Asthma Symptom Checklist Dr R. Kinsman, Division of Psychobiology, Nelson F. Jones Associates, 2343 East Evans Avenue, Denver, CO 80210, USA

Attitudes to Asthma Questionnaire Dr Bonnie Sibbald, Centre for Primary Care Research, Department of General Practice, University of Manchester, Rusholme Health Centre, Walmer Street, Manchester M14 5NP, UK

Barthel Index (Expanded) Dr S. Shah, Department of Occupational Therapy, University of Queensland, St Lucia, Queensland 4067, Australia

Barthel Index (Granger's Modified Version) Dr C.V. Granger, Center for Functional Assessment, Department of Rehabilitative Medicine, University of Buffalo, 232 Parker Hill, 3435 Main Street, Buffalo, NY 14214–3007, USA

Beck Depression Inventory (Revised) Psychological Corporation, 555 Academic Court, San Antonio, TX 78204–2498 USA

Brief Symptom Inventory (BSI) National Computer Systems Assessments, 5605 Green Circle Drive, Minnetonka, MN 55343, USA

Camberwell Assessment of Need Questionnaires, PRISM Institute of Psychiatry, De Crespigny Park, Denmark Hill, London SE5 8AF, UK

CAMDEX Cambridge University Press, The Pitt Building, Trumpington Street, Cambridge CB2 1RP, UK

Canadian Neurological Scale Dr R. Côté, Division of Neurology, Montreal General Hospital, 1650 Cedar Avenue, Montreal H3G 1A4, Canada

Cancer Inventory of Problem Situations Dr C. Schag, Psychiatry Services (116A3), Veterans Administration Medical Center, 16111 Plummer Street, Sepulveda, CA 91343, USA

Cancer Rehabilitation Evaluation System (CARES) Manual, First Edition CARES Consultants Ltd, 2210 Wilshire Boulevard, Suite 359, Santa Monica, CA 90403, USA

Center for Epidemiologic Studies Depression Scale (CES-D) Ms K.H. Bundra, Epidemiology and Psychopathology Research Branch, Division of Epidemiology and Services Research, Department of

Health and Human Services, National Institutes of Health, Bethesda, MD 20892, USA

Center for Epidemiologic Studies Depression Scale/Children's Scale Dr M.M. Weissman, Department of Psychiatry, College of Physicians and Surgeons of Columbia University, 722 West 168th Street, Box 14, New York, NY 10032, USA

Chronic Heart Failure Questionnaire Guyatt and Ms S. Troyan, Department of Clinical Epidemiology and Biostatistics, McMaster University Health Sciences Center, Room 3H7, 1200 Main Street West, Hamilton, Ontario L8N 3Z5, Canada

Chronic Respiratory Disease Questionnaire (GUYATT) Ms S. Troyan, Department of Clinical Epidemiology and Biostatistics, McMaster University Health Sciences Centre, Room 3H7, 1200 Main Street, Ontario L8N 3Z5, Canada

Client Satisfaction Questionnaire Dr C. Attkisson, Department of Psychiatry, University of California, San Francisco, CA 94143, USA

Clinical Back Pain Questionnaire (also known as the Aberdeen Back Scale) Dr Danny Ruta, Department of Public Health, Tayside Health Board, PO Box 75, Vernonholme, Riverside Drive, Dundee DD1 9NL, Scotland

Clinical Varicose Veins Questionnaire Mr Andrew Garratt, Health Services Research Unit, Department of Public Health, University of Aberdeen Medical School, Polwarth Building, Foresterhill, Aberdeen, AB9 2ZD, Scotland

COOP Charts Dr J.R. Wasson, Department of Community and Family Medicine, Dartmouth Medical School, HB 7265, Hanover, NH 03756, USA

Coopersmith Self-Esteem Inventories Consulting Psychologists Press, 557 College Avenue, Palo Alto, CA 014306, USA. Computer scoring packs are available from Self-Esteem Development, 669 Channing Avenue, Palo Alto, CA 94301, USA

COPE Dr C.S. Carver, Department of Psychology, PO Box 248185, University of Miami, Coral Gables, FL 33124, USA

Dartmouth COOP Project Dr Deborah Johnson, Dartmouth COOP Project, Dartmouth Medical School, Hinman Box 7265, Hanover, NH 03755–3862, USA

Diagnostic Interview Schedule (DIS) Dr L. Robins, Washington University School of Medicine, Department of Psychiatry, 4940 Audubon Avenue, St Louis, MO 63110, USA

Epilepsy Surgery Inventory Rand Health Sciences Program, Distribution Services, 1700 Main Street, PO Box 2138, Santa Monica, CA 90407–2138, USA

European Organisation for Research and Treatment in Cancer (EORTC QLQ-C30) Dr S. Serbouti, EORTC Data Centre, Avenue E, Mounier 83, Bte 11, 1200 Brussels, Belgium.

Functional Independence Measure Dr C.V. Granger, Center for Functional Assessment, Department of Rehabilitative Medicine, University of Buffalo, 232 Parker Hill, 3435 Main Street, Buffalo, NY 14214–3007, USA

Functional Status Index Dr A.M. Jette, Department of Social Medicine and Health Policy, Division on Aging, Harvard Medical School, 643 Huntington Avenue, Boston, MA 02115, USA

GAA Consumer Satisfaction Survey Questionnaire Group Health Association of America Inc., 1129 Twentieth Street, NW Suite 600, Washington DC 20036, USA

General Health Questionnaire NFER-Nelson, Darville House, 2 Oxford Road East, Windsor, Berks SL4 1DF, UK

General Satisfaction Questionnaire Dr P. Huxley, Department of Psychiatry, University of Manchester, Mathematics Tower, Oxford Road, Manchester M13 9PL, UK

Geriatric Mental State and CARE Professor J.R.M. Copeland, Department of Psychiatry, Royal Liverpool Hospital, Prescot Street, Liverpool L7 8XP, UK

Global Assessment/Global Assessment of Functioning Scale Dr J. Endicott, New York State Psychiatric Institute, 722 West 168th Street, New York, NY 10032, USA

Hamilton Depression Scale Professor M. Hamilton, Department of Psychiatry, University of Leeds, Woodhouse Lane, Leeds LS2 9JT, UK

HaPI-CD ROM Behavioural Measurement Database Services, PO Box 110287, Pittsburgh, PA 15232–0787, USA

Health and Daily Living Form, MIND GARDEN PO Box 10096, 3803 E. Bayshore Road, Palo Alto, CA 94303, USA

Health and Psychosocial Instruments (database) PO Box 110287, Pittsburg, PA 15232–0787, USA

Health Outcomes Institute TyPE – Condition-Specific Measures Health Outcomes Institute, 2001 Killebrew Drive, Suite 122, Bloomington, MN 55425, USA

Health Status Questionnaire 2 Dr Harry Wetzler, Health Outcomes Institute, 2001 Killebrew Drive, Suite 122, Bloomington, MN 55425, USA

Hemispheric Stroke Scale Dr R.J. Adams, Department of Neurology, BIW 338, Medical College of Georgia, 1125 15th Street, Augusta, GA 30912–2366, USA

HIV Overview of Problem Situations (HOPES) Dr P.A. Ganz, Division of Cancer Control, UCLA, 1100 Glendon Avenue, Suite 711, Los Angeles, CA 90024, USA

Hörnquist Quality of Life Status and Change (QLSC) Professor J.O. Hörnquist, Nordic School of Public Health, PO Box 12133, S–402 42, Göteborg, Sweden

Impact of Event Scale Elsevier Science Publishing Company Inc., 52 Vanderbilt Avenue, New York NY 10017, USA

Index of Health-Related Quality of Life Ms Rosalind Rabin, Department of Psychiatry, University College Medical School, Wolfson Building, Riding House Street, London W1N 8AA, UK

Inflammatory Bowel Disease Questionnaire (GUYATT) Alba Mitchell School of Nursing, McMaster University, Health Sciences Center, Room 2J27, 1200 Main Street West, Hamilton, Ontario L8N 3Z5, Canada

Katz Adjustment Scales Professor M.M. Katz, Montefiore Medical Center, University Hospital for the Albert Einstein College of Medicine, 111 East 210th Street, Bronx, NY 10467–2490, USA

Katz Adjustment Amended Scale (Epilepsy) Dr B.G. Vickrey, Department of Neurology, University of California, C-128, Reed Building, 710 Westwood Plaza, Los Angeles, CA 90024–1769, USA

Key Informant Survey Scales Dr M.S. Ridgely, Center for Mental Health Services Research, University of Maryland School of Medicine, 645 West Redwood Street, Baltimore, MD 21201–1549, USA

Kudos Battery for Stroke Patients Professor Shah Ebrahim, Department of Public Health, Royal Free Hospital Medical School, Rowland Hill Street, London NW3 2PF, UK

Lancashire Quality of Life Interview Mr J.P.J. Oliver or Professor P. Huxley, Department of Psychiatry, University of Manchester, Mathematics Tower, Oxford Road, Manchester M13 9PL, UK

Living with Asthma Questionnaire Dr M. Hyland, Department of Psychology, University of Plymouth, Plymouth PL8 4AA, UK

MACTAR Dr P. Tugwell, Room 2C16, Department of Clinical Epidemiology and Biostatistics, McMaster University Health Sciences Centre, 1200 Main Street West, Hamilton, Ontario L8N 3Z5, Canada

McGill Pain Questionnaire Professor R. Melzack, Department of Psychology, Stewart Biological Sciences Building, McGill University, 1205 Docteur Penfield Avenue, Montreal, Quebec H3A 1B1, Canada

McMaster Health Index Questionnaire Dr L. Chambers, Department of Clinical Epidemiology and Biostatistics, McMaster University Health Sciences Centre, 1200 Main Street West, Hamilton, Ontario L8N 3Z5, Canada

Medical Outcomes Trust (standardized health status instruments) PO Box 1917, Boston, MA 02205, USA

Minnesota Multiphasic Personality Inventory NFER-Nelson, Darville House, 2 Oxford Road East, Windsor, Berks SL4 1DF. UK

Minnesota Multiphasic Personality Inventory NCS Assessments, 27 Church Road, Hove, East Sussex BN3 2FA, UK

Multidimensional Health Locus of Control Scale Dr K. Wallston, School of Nursing, Vanderbilt University, Nashville, TN 37240, USA

National Clearing House on Health Indexes US Department of Health and Human Services, Public Health Service, 6525 Belcrest Road, Hyattsville, MD, 20782, USA

National Institute of Health Stroke Scale Dr T. Brott, Department of Neurology, Stroke Research Center, 4010 Medical Sciences Building, 231 Bethesda Avenue, Cincinnati, OH 45267–0525, USA

Needs for Care Assessment Professor C. Brewin, Department of Psychology, Royal Holloway and Bedford College, Egham Hill, Egham, Surrey TW20 0EX, UK

NHS Management Executive Quarry House, Quarry Hill, Leeds LS2 7UE, UK

Nottingham Health Profile Dr Sonia Hunt, Galen Research, Southern Hey, 137 Barlow Moor Road, West Didsbury, Manchester M20 8PW, UK

Oregon Quality of Life Questionnaire Professor B.H. McFarland, Department of Psychiatry, Oregon Health Sciences University, 3181 SW San Jackson Park Road, Portland, OR 97201–3098, USA

Older Americans' Resources and Services Schedule (OARS) Center for the Study of Aging and Human Development, Duke University Medical Center, Durham, NC 27710, USA

Oregon Quality of Life Questionnaire – Interviewer Rating Version Professor B.H. McFarland, Department of Psychiatry, Oregon Health Sciences University, 3181 SW San Jackson Park Road, Portland, OR 97201–3098, USA

Outcome Measures in Ambulatory Care (Asthma and Diabetes) (OMAC) Professor Allen Hutchinson, Department of Public Health Medicine, University of Hull, Hull HU6 7RX, UK

Padilla QL Index and Revisions Dr. G.V. Padilla, School of Nursing, Factor Building, Room 2–244, University of California, 10833 Le Conte Avenue, Los Angeles, CA 90024–1702, USA

Paediatric Functional Independence Measure Dr C.V. Granger, Center for Functional Assessment, Department of Rehabilitative Medicine, University of Buffalo, 232 Parker Hill, 3435 Main Street, Buffalo, NY 14214–3007, USA

Profile of Mood States (POMS) NFER-Nelson, Darville House, 2 Oxford Road East, Windsor, Berkshire SL4 1DF, UK

Profile of Mood States (POMS) EdITS/ Educational and Industrial Testing Service, Box 7234, San Diego, CA 92167, USA

Psychosocial Adjustment to Illness Scale (PAIS) Clinical Psychometric Research Inc., PO Box 619, Riderwood, MD 21139, USA

Quality of Life Index for Mental Health (QLI-MH) Dr M. Becker, Division of University Outreach, University of Wisconsin-Madison, Room 315, 610 Langdon Street, Madison WI 53703–1195, USA

Quality of Life Interview Dr A.F. Lehman, Department of Psychiatry, University of Maryland at Baltimore, Division of Rehabilitation Psychiatry, 645 West Redwood Street, Baltimore, MD 21201–1549, USA

Quality of Life Questionnaire (QLQL) Multi-Health Systems, 908 Niagara Falls Boulevard, North Tonawanda, NY 14120–2060, USA

Quality of Life Scale Professor W.T. Carpenter, Maryland Psychiatric Research Center, PO Box 21247, Baltimore, MD 21228, USA

Quality of Life Schedule (Crosby) Dr Charles Crosby, Health Services Research Unit, Department of Psychology, University College of North Wales, Bangor, Gwynedd LL57 2DG, Wales

Quality of Well–Being Scale (QWB) Professor R.M. Kaplan, Division of Health Care Science, School of Medicine, University of California, 9500 Gilman Drive, La Jolla, CA 92093–0622, USA

Rand 8-Item Depression Screener Rand Health Sciences Program, Distribution Services, 1700 Main Street, PO Box 2138, Santa Monica, CA 90407–2138, USA

Rand 36-Item Health Survey Dr Ron Hays/Dr Cathy Sherbourne, Rand Health Sciences Program, 1700 Main Street, PO Box 2138, Santa Monica, CA 90407–2138, USA

Rand MOS/HIS Outcome Batteries Rand Health Sciences Program, Distribution Services, 1700 Main Street, PO Box 2138, Santa Monica, CA 90407–2138, USA

REHAB Dr R. Baker, Vine Publishing Ltd, 10 Elgin Road, Talbot Woods, Bournemouth, BH4 9NL, UK

Research Diagnostic Criteria Dr R.L. Spitzer, Biometrics Research, New York State Psychiatric Institute, 722 W 168th Street, New York, NY 10032, USA

Rivermead Behavioural Memory Test Thames Valley Test Company, 7–9 The Green, Flempton, Bury St Edmunds, Suffolk IP28 6EL, UK

Rivermead Scales and Other UK Developed Neurological Functioning Tests Many of the stroke measures reviewed, including the nine hole peg test, are available for purchase from Dr D.T. Wade,

Rivermead Rehabilitation Centre, Abingdon Road, Oxford OX1 4XD, UK

Rotterdam Symptom Checklist Dr J.C.J.M. de Haes, Department of Medical Psychology, University Hospital (AMC), Meibergdreef 9, 1105 AZ Amsterdam, Netherlands

St George's Respiratory Questionnaire Dr Paul W. Jones, Division of Physiological Medicine, St George's Hospital Medical School, Cranmer Terrace, London SW17 0RE, UK

SCAN Dr N. Sartorius, Division of Mental Health, WHO, Avenue Appia, Geneva, Switzerland *or* Research Unit, Royal College of Psychiatrists, 17 Belgrave Square, London SW1X 8PG, UK

Schedule of Recent Experience Manual of the Schedule of Recent Experience. Seattle: University of Washington Press, PO Box 50096, Seattle, Washington 98145, USA

SEIQoL Professor C.A. O'Boyle, Department of Psychology, Medical School, Royal College of Surgeons in Ireland, Mercer Building, Mercer Street, Dublin 2, Ireland

Seizure Severity Scale Dr G.A. Baker, University Department of Neuroscience, Walton Centre for Neurology and Neurosurgery, Rice Lane, Liverpool L9 1AE, UK

SELBY Version of LASA Professor P. Selby, Institute of Cancer Research, Royal Marsden Hospital, Sutton, Surrey SM2 5PT, UK

SF-36 and Variants (SF-20, SF-36, SF-36-D) For technical queries, Dr John Ware, Health Institute, New England Medical Center Hospital, NEMCH Box 345, 750 Washington Street, Boston, MA 02111, USA and for the questionnaires, The Medical Outcomes Trust, PO Box 1917, Boston, MA 02205, USA

SF-36: UK Version Dr Andrew Long, UK Clearing House for Information on the Assessment of Health Outcomes, Nuffield Institute for Health, University of Leeds, Fairburn House, 71–75 Clarendon Road, Leeds LS2 9PL, UK

Sickness Impact Profile Health Policy and Management, School of Hygiene and Public Health, The Johns Hopkins University, 624 North Broadway, Baltimore, MD, 21205, USA

SmithKline Beecham QOL Scale Mr G.C. Dunbar, CNS Therapeutic Unit, Clinical Research and Development, SmithKline Beecham Pharmaceuticals, 47–49 London Road, Reigate, Surrey RH2 9YF, UK

Social Adjustment Scale/Social Adjustment Scale II Yale University Depression Unit, Connecticut Mental Health Center, 904 Howard Avenue, Suite 2A, New Haven, CT 06519, USA

Social Behaviour Schedule Department of Psychology, Institute of Psychiatry, De Crespigny Park, Denmark Hill, London SE5 8AF, UK

Social Dysfunction Rating Scale Dr M.W. Linn, Social Science Research, Veterans Administration Medical Center, 1201 Northwest 16th Street, Miami, FL 33125, USA

Social Functioning Schedule Dr P. Tyrer, Academic Unit of Psychiatry, St Charles' Hospital, London, W10 6DZ, UK

Social Role Performance Schedule Dr Til Wykes, Department of Psychology, Institute of Psychiatry, De Crespigny Park, Denmark Hill, London SE5 8AF, UK

Social Support Questionnaire (Medical Outcomes Survey) Dr C.D. Sherbourne, Rand, 1700 Main Street, Santa Monica, CA 90407–2138, USA

Stanford Arthritis Center Health Assessment Questionnaire (HAQ) Dr J.F. Fries, Department of Medicine, Room S-102B, Stanford University, School of Medicine, Stanford, CA 94305, USA

State–Trait Anxiety Inventory (STAI) NFER-Nelson, Darville House, 20 Oxford Road East, Windsor, Berkshire SL4 1DF, UK

State-Trait Anxiety Inventory (STAI) Psychological Assessment Resources Inc., PO Box 998, Odessa, FL 335556, USA

State-Trait Anxiety Inventory (Form Y and Children's Scale) NFER-Nelson, Darville House, 2 Oxford Road East, Windsor, Berkshire SL4 1DF, UK

Stroke TyPE Scale Health Outcomes Institute (previously Interstudy), 2001 Killebrew Drive, Suite 122, Bloomington, MN 55425, USA

Structured and Scaled Interview to Assess Maladjustment (SSIAM) Dr B.J. Gurland, Biometrics Research, New York State Department of Mental Hygiene, 722 W 168th Street, New York, NY 10032, USA

Structured Interview Version of the Hamilton Depression Rating Scale Dr M. Potts, Department of Social Work, California State University, 1250 Bellflower Boulevard, Long Beach, CA 90840–0902, USA

Symptom Check List-90 (SCL-90) Revised National Computer Systems Assessments, 5605 Green Circle Drive, Minnetonka, MN 55343, USA

Symptom Check List-90 (Revised) NCS Assessments, 27 Church Road, Hove, East Sussex, BN3 2FA, England, UK

Symptom Rating Test Dr B.F. Sheffield, Consultant Clinical Psychologist, 2 Bank Parade, Avenham, Preston PR1 3TA, UK

Team for the Assessment of Psychiatric Services (TAPS) Schedules Purchasable, if copyright permission obtained, from the TAPS Research Unit, Hampstead Road Group Practice Building, 69 Fleet Road, London NW3 2QU, UK

Tennessee Self-Concept Scale Western Psychological Services, Manson Western Corporation, 12031 Wilshire Boulevard, Los Angeles, CA 90025, USA

Trail-Making Tests Neuropsychology Laboratory, University of WI, University Hospitals, Madison, Wisconsin 53711, USA

TyPE Disease-Specific Scales Medical Outcomes Institute (previously Interstudy), 2001 Killebrew Drive, Suite 122, Bloomington, MN 55425, USA

UK Clearing House for Information on the Assessment of Health Outcomes Nuffield Institute for Health, University of Leeds, Fairburn House, 71–75 Clarendon Road, Leeds LS2 9PL, UK

Vineland Adaptive Behaviour Scales NFER-Nelson, Darville House, 20 Oxford Road East, Windsor, Berkshire SL4 1DF, UK

Vineland Adaptive Behaviour Scales American Guidance Service, 4201 Woodland Road, Circles Pines, MN 55014–1796, USA

Washington Psychosocial Seizure Inventory Dr C.B. Dodrill, Epilepsy Centre, Department of Neurological Surgery, University of Washington School of Medicine, Seattle, WA 98104, USA

Ways of Coping Scale MIND GARDEN, PO Box 10096, 3803 E. Bayshore Road, Palo Alto, CA 94303, USA

Wechsler Adult Intelligence Scales – Revised Psychological Corporation, 555 Academic Court, San Antonio, TX 78204, USA

Wechsler Memory and Intelligence Scales – Revised Psychological Corporation, Foots Cray High Street, Sidcup, Kent DA14 5HP, UK

Wechsler Memory Scale – Revised Psychological Corporation, 555 Academic Court, San Antonio, TX 78204, USA

Wechsler Pre-School and Primary Scale of Intelligence Psychological Corporation, 555 Academic Court, San Antonio, TX 78204, USA

WHO Psychiatric Disability Assessment Schedule (WHODAS) Division of Mental Health, World Health Organization, 1211 Geneva 27, Switzerland

WHOQOL The WHOQOL Group, Division of Mental Health, World Health Organization, 1211 Geneva 27, Switzerland

WOMAC Dr N. Bellamy, Suite 303, Colls. 3, WT Victoria Hospital, 375 South Street, London, Ontario, N6A 4G5, Canada

Wyke's Assessment of Need Questionnaire Dr T. Wykes, Department of Psychology, Institute of Psychiatry, De Crespigny Park, Denmark Hill, London SE5 8AF, UK

Zung Self-Rating Depression Scale DISTA Products, Eli Lilly Corporate Center, Indianapolis, IN 46285, USA

Scale distributors' addresses in North America are listed in Keyser and Sweetland (1988). Many distributors are also based in Europe. They are too numerous to list here, but one of the largest scale distributors in the UK is: NFER–Nelson, Darville House, 2 Oxford Road East, Windsor, Berks. SL4 1DF.

REFERENCES

Aaronson, N.K. (1986). Methodological issues in psychosocial oncology with special reference to clinical trials. In: V. Ventafridda, F.S.A.M. van Dam, R. Yancik and M. Tamburini (eds), *Assessment of Quality of Life and Cancer Treatment*. Amsterdam: Elsevier.

Aaronson, N.K. (1987). *EORTC Protocol 15861: Development of a Core Quality-of-Life Questionnaire for Use in Cancer Clinical Trials*. Brussels: EORTC Data Centre.

Aaronson, N.K. (1990). Quality of life research in cancer clinical trials: A need for common rules and language. *Oncology*, *4*: 59–66.

Aaronson, N.K. (1993). The EORTC QLQ-C30: A quality of life instrument for use in international clinical trials in oncology (Abstract). *Quality of Life Research*, *2*: 51.

Aaronson, N.K. and Beckmann, J.H. (eds) (1987). *The Quality of Life of the Cancer Patient*. New York: Raven Press.

Aaronson, N.K., Bakker, W., Stewart, A.L. *et al.* (1986). *A Multi-dimensional Approach to the Measurement of Quality of Life in Lung Cancer Clinical Trials*. EORTC Monograph Series: The Quality of Life of Cancer Patients. New York: Raven Press.

Aaronson, N.K., Bullinger, M. and Ahmedzai, S. (1988). A modular approach to quality of life assessment in cancer clinical trials. *Recent Results in Cancer Research*, *111*: 231–49.

Aaronson, N.K., Ahmedzai, S., Bullinger, M. *et al.* (1991a). The EORTC core quality of life questionnaire: Interim results of an international field study. In: D. Osoba (ed.), *Effect of Cancer on Quality of Life*. Boca Raton, CA: CRC Press.

Aaronson, N.K., Meyerowitz, B.E., Bard, M. *et al.* (1991b). Quality of life research in oncology: Past achievements and future priorities. *Cancer*, *67*: 839–43 (suppl.).

Aaronson, N.K., Acquadro, C., Alonso, J. *et al.* (1992). International quality of life assessment (IQOLA) project. *Quality of Life Research*, *1*: 349–51.

Aaronson, N.K., Ahmedzai, S., Bergman, B. *et al.* (1993). The European Organisation for Research and Treatment of Cancer QLQ-C30: A quality of life instrument for use in international clinical trials in oncology. *Journal of the National Cancer Institute*, *85*: 365–76.

Abrams, R. and Taylor, M.A. (1978). A rating scale for emotional blunting. *American Journal of Psychiatry*, *135*: 226–9.

Achard, S. and Zittoun, R. (1993). Determinants of quality of life (QOL) during intensive chemotherapy (IC) or bone marrow transplantation (BMT) (abstract). *Quality of Life Research*, *2*: 67.

Adair, F.L. (1984). Coopersmith Self-esteem Inventories. In: D. J. Keyser and R.C. Sweetland (eds), *Test Critiques*, Vol. I, Kansas City, MO: Test Corporation of America.

Adams, L., Chronos, N., Lane, R. and Guz, A. (1986). The measurement of breathlessness induced in normal individuals: Individual differences. *Clinical Science*, *70*: 131–40.

Adams, R.J., Meador, K.J., Sethi, K.D. *et al.* (1987). Graded neurologic scale for use in acute hemispheric stroke treatment protocols. *Stroke*, *18*: 665–9.

Addington-Hall, J.M., MacDonald, L.D., Anderson, H.R. (1990). Can the Spitzer Quality of Life Index help to reduce prognostic uncertainty in terminal cancer? *British Journal of Cancer*, *62*: 695–9.

Adshead, F., Day Cody, D. and Pitt, B. (1992). BAS-DEC: A novel screening instrument for depression in elderly medical in-patients. *British Medical Journal*, *305*: 397.

Advances in Nursing Science (1985). Special Issue: Quality of life, P.L. Chin (ed.). *Advances in Nursing Science*, *8*: 1–85.

Affleck, G., Pfeiffer, C., Tennen, H. and Fifield, J. (1987). Attributional processes in rheumatoid arthritis. *Arthritis and Rheumatism*, *30*: 927–31.

Affleck, J.W., Aitken, R.C.B., Hunter, J. *et al.* (1988). Rehabilitation status: A measure of medico-social dysfunction. *Lancet*, i: 230–33.

Agle, D.P. and Baum, G.L. (1977). Psychological aspects of chronic obstructive pulmonary disease. *Medical Clinics of North America*, *61*: 749–58.

Aitken, R.C. (1969). Measurement of feelings using visual analogue scales. *Proceedings of the Royal Society of Medicine*, *62*: 689–93.

Akerlind, I., Hörnquist, J.O. and Hansson, B. (1987). Loneliness correlates in advanced alcohol abusers: Social factors and needs. *Scandinavian Journal of Social Medicine*, *15*: 175–83.

Aldwin, C.M. and Revenson, T.A. (1987). Does coping help? A re-examination of the relation between coping and mental health. *Journal of Personality and Social Psychology*, *53*: 337–48.

Aldwin, C.M., Folkman, S., Shaefer, C. *et al.* (1980). Ways of Coping Checklist: A process measure. Paper presented to the *88th Annual Convention of the American Psychological Association*, Montreal, September.

Almy, T.P. (1988). Comprehensive functional assessment of elderly patients. *Annals of Internal Medicine*, *109*: 70–2.

Alonso, J., Anto, J.M., Gonzalez, M. *et al.* (1992). Measurement of a general health status of non-oxygen-dependent chronic obstructive pulmonary disease patients. *Medical Care*, *30*: 125–35 (suppl. 5).

American Lung Association (1975). *Report of the Task Force on Comprehensive and Continuing Care for Patients with Chronic Obstructive Pulmonary Disease*. New York: ALA.

American National Heart and Lung Institute (1971). *Proceedings of the First NHLI Epidemiology Workshop*. Washington, DC: NHLI.

American Psychiatric Association (1980). *Diagnostic and Statistical Manual of Mental Disorders*, 3rd edn. Washington, DC: APA.

American Psychiatric Association (1987). *Diagnostic and Statistical Manual of Mental Disorders*, 3rd revised edn. (Also includes the Global Assessment of Functioning Scale (GAF).) Washington, DC: APA.

American Psychiatric Association (1994). *Diagnostic and Statistical Manual of Mental Disorders*, 4th edn. Washington, DC: APA.

American Thoracic Society (1978). *Epidemiology Standardization Project*. Report to Division of Lung Diseases, National Heart, Lung and Blood Institute. Washington, DC: NHLBI.

American Thoracic Society, Medical Section of the American Lung Association (1987). Standardization of spirometry – 1987 update. *American Review of Respiratory Disease*, *136*: 1285–98.

Amster, L.E. and Krauss, H.H. (1974). The relationship between life crises and mental deterioration in old age. *International Journal of Aging and Human Development*, *5*: 51–5.

Amundson, M.E., Hart, C.A. and Holmes, T.H. (1981). *Manual for the Schedule of Recent Experience*. Seattle, WA: University of Washington Press.

Andersen, B.L. (1985). Sexual functioning morbidity among cancer survivors: Current status and future research directions. *Cancer*, *55*: 1835–42.

Anderson, J. (1990). The TAPS project. 1: Previous psychiatric diagnosis and current disability of long stay psychogeriatric patients – A pilot study. *British Journal of Psychiatry*, *156*: 661–6.

Anderson, J.P., Kaplan, R.M., Berry, C.C., Bush, J.W. and Rumbaut, R.G. (1989). Interday reliability of function assessment for a health status measure: The Quality of Well-Being Scale. *Medical Care*, *27*: 1076–83.

Anderson, J., Dayton, D., Wills, W. *et al.* (1993). The TAPS project. 13: Clinical and social outcomes of long stay psychiatric patients after one year in the community. *British Journal of Psychiatry*, *162*: 45–56 (suppl. 19).

Anderson, R. (1992) *The Aftermath of Stroke: The Experience of Patients and Their Families*. Cambridge: Cambridge University Press.

Anderson, R.T., Aaronson, N.K. and Wilkin, D. (1993). Critical review of the international assessments of health related quality of life. *Quality of Life Research*, *2*: 369–95.

Andreasen, N.C. (1979). Affective flattening and the criteria for schizophrenia. *American Journal of Psychiatry*, *136*: 944–7.

Andrews, F.M. (1973). *List of Social Concerns Common to Most OECD Countries*. Paris: OECD.

Andrews, F.M. (1974). Social indicators of perceived life quality. *Social Indicators Research*, *1*: 279–99.

Andrews, F.M. (1981). *Subjective Social Indicators, Objective Social Indicators and Social Accounting Systems*. New York: Academic Press.

Andrews, F.M. and Crandall, R. (1976). The validity of measures of self-reported well-being. *Social Indicators Research*, *3*: 1–19.

Andrews, F.M. and McKennell, A.C. (1980). Measures of self-reported well-being: Their affective, cognitive, and other components. *Social Indicators Research*, *8*: 127–55.

Andrews, F.M. and Robinson, J.P. (1991). Measures of

subjective well-being. In: J.P. Robinson, P.R. Shaver and L.S. Wrightsman (eds), *Measures of Personality and Social Psychological Attitudes*, Vol. 1. San Diego, CA: Academic Press.

Andrews, F.M. and Withey, S.B. (1974). Developing measures of perceived life quality: Results from several national surveys. *Social Indicators Research*, 1: 1–26.

Andrews, F.M. and Withey, S.B. (1976). *Social Indicators of Well-being: Americans' Perceptions of Life Quality*. New York: Plenum Press.

Andrykowski, M.A., Henslee, P.J. and Farrall, M.G. (1989). Physical and psychosocial functioning of adult survivors of allogenic BMT. *Bone Marrow Transplantation*, 4: 75–81.

Andrykowski, M.A., Altmaier, E.M., Barnett, R.L. *et al.* (1990). The quality of life in adult survivors of allogenic bone marrow transplantation. Correlates and comparison with matched renal transplant recipients. *Transplantation*, 5: 399–406.

Angold, A. (1989). Structured assessments of psychopathology in children and adolescents. In: C. Thompson (ed.), *The Instruments of Psychiatric Research*. Chichester: John Wiley.

Annas, G.J. (1990). Quality of life in the courts: Early spring in fantasyland. In: J.J. Walter and T.A. Shannon (eds), *Quality of Life: The New Medical Dilemma*. New York, Paulist Press.

Anthony, J.C., Le Resche, L. and Niaz, U. *et al.* (1982). Limits of the Mini-mental State as a screening test for dementia and delirium among hospital patients. *Psychological Medicine*, 12: 397–408.

Anthony, W. and Farkas, M. (1982). A client outcome planning model for assessing psychiatric rehabilitation interventions. *Schizophrenia Bulletin*, 8: 13–38.

Antonovsky, A. (1979). *Health, Stress and Coping*. San Francisco, CA: Jossey-Bass.

Antonovsky, A. (1993). The structure and properties of the Sense of Coherence Scale. *Social Science and Medicine*, 36: 725–33.

Apple, D. (1960). How laymen define illness. *Journal of Health and Human Behavior*, I: 219–55.

Arden, D., Austin, C. and Sturgeon, R.C. (1989). Correlation between the Geriatric Depression Scale long and short forms. *Journal of Gerontology*, 44: 124–5.

Argyle, M., Martin, M. and Crossland, J. (1989). Happiness as a function of personality and social encounters. In: J.P. Forgas and J.M. Innes (eds) *Recent Advances in Social Psychology*. North Holland: Elsevier.

Armitage, P. and Berry, G. (1987). *Statistical Methods in Medical Research*, 2nd edn. Oxford: Blackwell Scientific.

Armitage, S.G. (1946). An analysis of certain psychological tests used for evaluation of brain injury. *Psychological Monographs*, 60 (whole issue).

Ashton, J. (1992). *Healthy Cities*. Buckingham: Open University Press.

Avner, S.E. and Kinsman, R.A. (1987). Psychological factors affecting the management of allergic diseases. In: W. Bierman and D. Pearlman (eds) *Allergic diseases from infancy to adulthood*, 2nd edn. Philadelphia: W.B. Saunders & Co.

Avorn, J., Everitt, D.E. and Weiss, S. (1986). Increased anti-depressant use in patients prescribed beta-blockers. *Journal of the American Medical Association*, 255: 357–60.

Aylard, P.R., Gooding, J.H., McKenna, P.J. and Snaith, R.P. (1987). A validation study of three anxiety and depression self assessment scales. *Psychosomatic Research*, 31: 261–8.

Babiker, I.E. and Thorne, P. (1993). Do psychiatric patients know what is good for them? *Journal of the Royal Society of Medicine*, 86: 28–30.

Baker, F. and Intagliata, J. (1982). Quality of life in the evaluation of community support systems. *Evaluation and Program Planning*, 5: 69–79.

Baker, G.A., Smith, D.F., Dewey, M. *et al.* (1991). The development of a seizure severity scale as an outcome measure of epilepsy. *Epilepsy Research*, 8: 245–51.

Baker, G.A., Smith, D.F., Dewey, M. *et al.* (1993). The initial development of a health-related quality of life model as an outcome measure in epilepsy. *Epilepsy Research*, 16: 65–81.

Baker, R. (1986). *The Development of a Behavioural Assessment System for Psychiatric Patients*. Final Report to the Grampian Health Board. Aberdeen: Department of Psychology, Royal Cornhill Hospital.

Baker, R. and Hall, J. (1983). *Users' Manual for Rehabilitation Evaluation*. Bournemouth: Vine Publishing.

Baker, R. and Hall, J. (1988). REHAB: A new assessment instrument for chronic psychiatric patients. *Schizophrenia Bulletin*, 14: 97–111.

Bakker, A., van Oosterom, A.T., Aaronson, N.K. *et al.* (1986). Vindesine, cisplatin and bleomycin combination chemotherapy in non-small cell lung cancer: Survival and quality of life. *European Journal of Cancer and Clinical Oncology*, 22: 963–70.

Baltes, P.B. and Baltes, M.M. (1990). *Successful Aging: Perspectives from the Behavioural Sciences*. New York: Cambridge University Press.

Bamford, J., Sandercock, P., Dennis, M. *et al.* (1988). A prospective study of acute cerebrovascular disease in the community: The Oxfordshire Community Stroke Project 1981–1986. I. Methodology, demography and incidence of cases of first-ever stroke. *Journal of Neurology, Neurosurgery and Psychiatry*, 51: 1373–80.

Bamford, J.M., Sandercock, P.A.G., Warlow, C.P. and Slattery, J. (1989). Interobserver agreement for the assessment of handicap in stroke patients (letter). *Stroke*, 20: 828.

Bandura, A. (1986). *Social Foundations of Thought and Action: A Social Cognitive Theory.* Englewood Cliffs, NJ: Prentice-Hall.

Banks, M. (1983). Validation of the GHQ in a young community. *Psychological Medicine*, *3*: 349–54.

Bardelli, D. and Saracci, R. (1978). Measuring the quality of life in cancer clinical trials: Methods and impact of controlled therapeutic trials in cancer. Geneva: Union Internationale Control le Cancer, Technical Report Series 36: 75–94.

Bardsley, M.J. and Coles, J.M. (1992). Practical experiences in auditing patient outcomes. *Quality in Health Care*, *1*: 124–30.

Bardsley, M.J., Venables, C.W., Watson, J. *et al.* (1992). Evidence for validity of a health status measure in assessing short term outcomes of cholecystectomy. *Quality in Health Care*, *1*: 10–14.

Barker, D.J.P. and Rose, G.R. (1984). *Epidemiology in Medical Practice.* Edinburgh: Churchill Livingstone.

Barnes, D. and Benjamin, S. (1987). The Self Care Assessment Schedule, SCAS-I: The purpose and construction of a new assessment of self care behaviours. *Journal of Psychometric Research*, *31*: 191–202.

Barr, H. and Krasner, N. (1991). Prospective quality of life analysis after palliative photoablation for the treatment of malignant dysphagia. *Cancer*, *68*: 1660–4.

Barry, M.M. and Crosby, C. (1993). Community mental health care: Promoting a better quality of life for long term clients. In: D.R. Trent and C. Reed (eds), *Promotion of Mental Health.* Aldershot: Avebury.

Barschak, E. (1951). A study of happiness and unhappiness in the childhood and adolescence of girls in different cultures. *Journal of Psychology*, *32*: 173–215.

Barton, R. (1959). *Institutional Neurosis.* Bristol: John Wright.

Battersby, C., Hartley, K., Fletcher, A.E. *et al.* (1989). Cognitive function and quality of life in hypertension – a community based study. *Clinical Science*, *76*: 16 (suppl. 20).

Bauer, R.A. (1966a). Detection and anticipation of impact: The nature of the task. In: R. A. Bauer (ed.), *Social Indicators.* Cambridge, MA: MIT Press.

Bauer, R.A. (1966b). *Social Indicators.* Cambridge, MA: MIT Press.

Baum, M., Priestman, T., West, R.R. and Jones, E.M. (1980). A comparison of subjective responses in a trial comparing endocrine with cytotoxic treatment in advanced carcinoma of the breast. *European Journal of Cancer*, *16*: 223–6 (suppl. 1).

Baumann, B.O. (1961). Diversities in conceptions of health and physical fitness. *Journal of Health and Human Behavior*, *3*: 39–46.

Bebbington, P. (1992). Assessing the need for psychiatric treatment at the district level: The role of surveys. In:

G. Thornicroft, C.R. Brewin and J. Wing (eds), *Measuring Mental Health Needs.* London: Royal College of Psychiatrists.

Bech, P. (1981). Rating scales for affective disorder: Their validity and consistency. *Acta Psychiatrica Scandinavica*, suppl. 295: 1–101.

Bech, P. (1992). Measuring quality of life: The medical perspective. *Nordic Journal of Psychiatry*, *46*: 85–9.

Bech, P., Gram, L.F., Dein, E. *et al.* (1975). Quantitative rating of depressive states. *Acta Psychiatrica Scandinavica*, *51*: 161–70.

Beck, A.T. (1970). *Depression: Causes and treatment.* Philadelphia, PA: University of Pennsylvania Press.

Beck, A.T. and Beck, R.W. (1972). Screening depressed patients in family practice: A rapid technic. *Postgraduate Medicine*, *52*: 81–5.

Beck, A.T., Ward, C., Mendelson, M. *et al.* (1961). An inventory for measuring depression. *Archives of General Psychiatry*, *4*: 561–71.

Beck, A.T., Rial, W.Y. and Rickels, K. (1974a). Short form of depression inventory: Cross validation. *Psychological Reports*, *34*: 1184–6.

Beck, A.T., Weissman, A., Lester, D. *et al.* (1974b). The measurement of pessimism: The Hopelessness Scale. *Journal of Consulting and Clinical Psychologists*, *42*: 861–5.

Beck, A.T., Steer, R.A. and Garbin, M.G. (1988). Psychometric properties of the Beck Depression Inventory: Twenty-five years of evaluation. *Clinical Psychology Review*, *8*: 77–100.

Beck, S., Brook, R.H., Lohr, K.N. and Goldberg, G.A. (1981a). *Conceptualisation and Measurement of Health for Adults, Vol. 13: Hay Fever.* Santa Monica, CA: Rand Corporation.

Beck, S., Brook, R.H., Lohr, K.N. and Goldberg, G.A. (1981b). *Conceptualisation and Measurement of Health for Adults, Vol. 14: Hearing loss.* Santa Monica, CA: Rand Corporation.

Becker, M.H. (1974). The health belief model and personal behaviour. *Health Education Monographs*, *2*: 326–73.

Becker, M., Diamond, R. and Sainfort, F. (1993). A new patient focused index for measuring quality of life in persons with severe and persistent mental illness. *Quality of Life Research*, *2*: 239–51.

Beckmann, D. and Richter, H.E. (1972). *GieBen-Test (GT).* Bern: Verlag Hans Huber.

Bedford, A., Foulds, G.A. and Sheffield, B.F. (1976). A new personal disturbance scale (DSSI/SAD). *British Journal of Social and Clinical Psychology*, *15*: 387–94.

Bell, D.R., Tannock, I.F. and Boyd, N.F. (1985). Quality of life measurement in breast cancer patients. *British Journal of Cancer*, *51*: 577–80.

Bell, M.J., Bombardier, C. and Tugwell, P. (1990). Measurement of functional status, quality of life and utility in rheumatoid arthritis. *Arthritis and Rheumatism*, *33*: 591–601.

Bellamy, N. (1989). Critical review of clinical assessment techniques for rheumatoid arthritis trials: New developments. *Scandinavian Journal of Rheumatology*, suppl. 80: 3–16.

Bellamy, N., Buchanan, W.W., Goldsmith C.H. *et al.* (1988). Validation study of WOMAC: A health status instrument for measuring clinically important patient relevant outcomes to antirheumatic drug therapy in patients with osteoarthritis of the hip or knee. *Journal of Rheumatology*, *15*: 1833–40.

Bendtsen, P. and Hörnquist, J.O. (1992). Change and status in quality of life in patients with rheumatoid arthritis. *Quality of Life Research*, *1*: 297–305.

Bennet, P. and Wood, P. (1968). *Population Studies of the Rheumatic Diseases*. International Congress Series No. 148. Amsterdam: Excerpta Medica Foundation.

Bentham, J. (1834/1983). *Deonotology*. Oxford: Clarendon Press.

Berg, R.L., Hallauer, D.S. and Berk, N. (1976). Neglected aspects of quality of life. *Health Services Research*, *11*: 391–5.

Berger, P. and Luckmann, T. (1967). *The Social Construction of Reality: A Treatise in the Sociology of Knowledge*. Harmondsworth: Penguin.

Bergman, B., Sullivan, M. and Sorenson, S. (1991). Quality of life during chemotherapy for small cell lung cancer. I. An evaluation with generic health measures. *Acta Oncology*, *30*: 947–57.

Bergman, B., Sullivan, M. and Sorenson, S. (1992). Quality of life during chemotherapy for small cell lung cancer. II. A longitudinal study of the EORTC Core Quality of Life Questionnaire and comparison with the Sickness Impact Profile. *Acta Oncology*, *31*: 19–28.

Bergner, L., Hallstrom, A.P., Bergner, M. *et al.* (1985). Health status of survivors of cardiac arrest and of myocardial infarction controls. *American Journal of Public Health*, *75*: 1321–3.

Bergner, M. (1984). The Sickness Impact Profile. In: N.K. Wenger, M.E. Mattson, C.P. Furberg and J. Elinson (eds), *Assessment of Quality of Life in Clinical Trials of Cardiovascular Therapies*. New York: Le Jacq.

Bergner, M. (1988). Development, testing and use of the Sickness Impact Profile. In: S.R. Walker and R.M. Rosser (eds), *Quality of Life: Assessment and Application*. Lancaster: MTP Press.

Bergner, M. (1993). Development, testing and use of the Sickness Impact Profile. In: S.R. Walker and R.M. Rosser (eds), *Quality of Life Assessment: Key Issues in the 1990s*, 2nd edn. Dordrecht: Kluwer Academic.

Bergner, M., Bobbitt, R.A., Kressel, S. *et al.* (1976a). The Sickness Impact Profile: Conceptual formulation and methodology for the development of a health status measure. *International Journal of Health Services*, *6*: 393–415.

Bergner, M., Bobbitt, R.A., Pollard, W.E. *et al.* (1976b). The Sickness Impact Profile: Validation of a health status measure. *Medical Care*, *14*: 57–67.

Bergner, M., Bobbitt, R.A., Carter, W.B. *et al.* (1981). The Sickness Impact Profile: Development and final revision of a health status measure. *Medical Care*, *19*: 787–805.

Berkman, L.F. and Breslow, L. (1983). *Health and Ways of Living: The Alameda County Study*. New York: Oxford University Press.

Berman, D.M., Brook, R.H., Lohr, K.N. *et al.* (1981). *Conceptualisation and Measurement of Physiologic Health for Adults, Vol. 4: Angina Pectoris*. R-2262/4-HHS. Santa Monica, CA: Rand Corporation.

Bernheim, J.L. and Buyse, M. (1983). The Anamnestic Comparative Self Assessment for measuring the subjective quality of life of cancer patients. *Journal of Psychosocial Oncology*, *1*: 25–38.

Berwick, D.M., Budman, S., Damico-White, J. *et al.* (1987). Assessment of psychological morbidity in primary care: Explorations with the General Health Questionnaire. *Journal of Chronic Diseases*, *40*: 71S–79S.

Berwick, D.M., Murphy, J.M., Goldman, P.A. *et al.* (1991). Performance of a five-item mental health screening test. *Medical Care*, *29*: 169–76.

Bigelow, D.A., Brodsky, G., Steward, L. and Olson, M.M. (1982). The concept and measurement of quality of life as a dependent variable in evaluation of mental health services. In: G.J. Stahler and W.R. Tash (eds), *Innovative Approaches to Mental Health Evaluation*. New York: Academic Press.

Bigelow, D.A., Gareau, M.J. and Young, D.J. (1990). A quality of life interview. *Psychosocial Rehabilitation Journal*, *14*: 94–8.

Bigelow, D.A., McFarland, B.H. and Olson, M.M. (1991a). Quality of life of community mental health programme clients: Validating a measure. *Community Mental Health Journal*, *27*: 43–55.

Bigelow, D.A., Gareau, M.J. and Young, D.J. (1991b). *Quality of Life Questionnaire: Interviewer Rating Version. Semi-structured Interview Including Guidelines*. Portland, OR: Oregon Health Sciences University.

Bigelow, D.A., Olson, M.M., Smoyer, S. and Stewart, L. (1991c). *Quality of Life Questionnaire: Respondent Self-report Version. I: Guidelines; II: Interview schedule*. Portland, OR: Oregon Health Sciences University.

Bigelow, D.A., McFarland, B.H., Gareau, M.J. and Young, D.J. (1991d). Implementation and effectiveness of a bed reduction project. *Community Mental Health Journal*, *27*: 125–33.

Biggs, J.T., Wylie, L.T. and Ziegler, V.E. (1978). Validity of the Zung self-rating depression scale. *British Journal of Psychiatry*, *132*: 381–5.

Billings, A.G. and Moos, R.H. (1981). The role of coping responses and social resources in attenuating the stress of life events. *Journal of Behavioural Medicine*, 4: 139–57.

Billings, A.G. and Moos, R.H. (1984). Coping, stress, and social resources among adults with unipolar depression. *Journal of Personality and Social Psychology*, 46: 877–91.

Billings, A.G. and Moos, R.H. (1985). Psychosocial processes of remission in unipolar depression: Comparing depressed patients and matched community controls. *Journal of Consulting and Clinical Psychology*, 53: 314–25.

Bindman, A.B., Keane, D. and Lurie, N. (1990). Measuring health changes among severely ill patients: The floor phenomenon. *Medical Care*, 28: 1142–52.

Bishop, D., Green, A., Cantor, S. and Torresin, W. (1987). Depression, anxiety and rheumatoid arthritis activity. *Clinical and Experimental Rheumatology*, 5: 147–50.

Bjordal, K. and Kassa, S. (1992). Psychometric validation of the EORTC core quality of life questionnaire, 30-item version, and a diagnostic-specific module for head and neck cancer patients. *Acta Oncology*, 31: 311–21.

Black, N., Pettigrew, M., Ginzler, M. *et al.* (1991). Do doctors and patients agree? Views of the outcome of TURP. *International Journal of Technology Assessment in Health Care*, 7: 533–44.

Black, N., Pettigrew, M. and McPherson, K. (1993). Comparison of NHS private patients undergoing elective transurethral resection of the prostate for benign prostatic hypertrophy. *Quality in Health Care*, 2: 11–16.

Black, S.E., Blessed, G., Edwardson, J.A. and Kay, D.W.K. (1990). Prevalence rates of dementia in an ageing population: Are low rates due to the use of insensitive instruments? *Age and Ageing*, 19: 84–90.

Blackledge, G. and Lawton, F. (1992). The ethics and practical problems of phase I and II studies. In: C. J. Williams (ed.), *Introducing New Treatments for Cancer: Practical, Ethical and Legal Problems*. Chichester: John Wiley.

Blalock, H.M. and Blalock, A.B. (1971). *Methodology in Social Research*. London: McGraw-Hill.

Bland, J.M. and Altman, D.G. (1986). Statistical methods for assessing agreement between two methods of clinical measurement. *Lancet*, i: 307–10.

Blank, K. and Perry, S. (1984). Relationship of psychological processes during delirium to outcome. *American Journal of Psychiatry*, 141: 843–7.

Blascovich, J. and Tomaka, J. (1991). Measures of self esteem. In: J.P. Robinson, P.R. Shaver and L.S. Wrightsman (eds), *Measures of Personality and Social Psychological Attitudes*, Vol. 1. San Diego, CA: Academic Press.

Blaxter, M. (1976). *The Meaning of Disability*. London: Heinemann.

Blaxter, M. (1983). The causes of disease: women talking. *Social Science and Medicine*, 17: 59–67.

Blaxter, M. and Patterson, E. (1982). *Mothers and Daughters: A Three Generational Study of Health Attitudes and Behaviour*. London: Heinemann.

Blessed, G., Tomkinson, B.E. and Roth, M. (1968). The association between quantitative measures of dementia and of senile change in the central grey matter of elderly subjects. *British Journal of Psychiatry*, 114: 797–811.

Blischke, W.R., Bush, J.W. and Kaplan, R.M. (1975). Successive intervals analysis of preference measures in a health status index. *Health Services Research*, 10: 181–98.

Bloom, B.L. (1975). *Changing Patterns of Psychiatric Care*. New York: Human Sciences Press.

Bloom, B.L. (1978). Social indicators and health care policy. Paper presented to the *Second National Needs Assessment Conference*, Louisville, KY, March.

Blumenthal, M.D. (1975). Measuring depressive symptomatology in a general population. *Archives of General Psychiatry*, 32: 971–8.

Boevink, W., van Nieuwenhuizen, C., Schene, A.H. and Wolfe, J. (1994). The use of a bottom up and top down method to shed some light on the quality of life concept of the chronically mentally ill. Paper presented to the *Conference of the Association of European Psychiatrists: Psychiatric Epidemiology and Social Psychiatry*. Quality of Life and Disabilities – Mental Disorders. Vienna, April 7–9.

Bolli, R. (1987). Bypass surgery in patients with coronary artery disease: Indications based on the Multicentre Randomised Trials. *Chest*, 91: 760–64.

Bombardier, C., Ware, J., Russell, I.J. *et al.* (1986). Auranofin therapy and quality of life in patients with rheumatoid arthritis. *American Journal of Medicine*, 81: 565–77.

Bond, A. and Lader, M. (1974). The use of analogue scales in rating subjective feelings. *British Journal of Medical Psychology*, 47: 211–18.

Bond, M.R. (1979). Psychologic and psychiatric techniques for the relief of advanced cancer pain. In: J.J. Bonica and V. Ventafridda (eds), *Advances in Pain Research and Therapy*, Vol. 2. New York: Raven Press.

Bone, M.R. (1992). International efforts to measure health expectancy. *Journal of Epidemiology and Community Health*, 46: 555–8.

Bonica, J.J. (1985). Treatment of cancer pain: Current status and future needs. In: H.L. Fields, R. Dubner and F. Cervero (eds), *Advances in Pain Research and Therapy*, Vol. 9. New York: Raven Press.

Bonney, S., Finkelstein, F.O., Lytton, B. *et al.* (1978). Treatment of end-stage renal failure in a defined geographic area. *Archives of Internal Medicine*, *138*: 1510–13.

Booth, T. (1985). *Home Truths*. London: Gower.

Borg, G. (1970). Perceived exertion as an indicator of somatic stress. *Scandinavian Journal of Rehabilitation Medicine*, *2*: 92–8.

Borg, G. (1982a). Psychophysical bases of perceived exertion. *Medical Science Sports Exercise*, *14*: 377–81.

Borg, G. (1982b). A category scale with ratio properties for intermodal and interindividual comparisons. In: H.G. Geissler, and T. Petzoldt (eds), *Psychophysical Judgements and the Process of Perception*. Berlin: Deutscher Verlag.

Borgquist, L., Nilsson, L.T., Lindelow, G. *et al.* (1992). Perceived health in hip-fracture patients: A prospective follow-up of 100 patients. *Age and Ageing*, *21*: 109–16.

Botwinick, J. (1977). Intellectual abilities. In: J.E. Birren and K.W. Schaie (eds), *Handbook of the Psychology of Ageing*. New York: Van Nostránd Reinhold.

Bowling, A. (1990). The prevalence of psychiatric morbidity among people aged 85 and over living at home. *Social Psychiatry and Psychiatric Epidemiology*, *25*: 132–40.

Bowling, A. (1991). *Measuring Health: A Review of Quality of Life Measurement Scales*. Milton Keynes: Open University Press.

Bowling, A. (1992). In: General discussion. In: A. Hopkins (ed.), *Measures of the Quality of Life and the Uses to which Such Measures May be Put*. London: Royal College of Physicians.

Bowling, A. (1993). *What People Say About Prioritising Health Services*. London: King's Fund Centre.

Bowling, A. (1994a). Social networks and social support among older people and implications for emotional well-being and psychiatric morbidity. *International Review of Psychiatry*, *6*: 41–58.

Bowling, A. (1994b). Beliefs about illness causation among Turkish and White British people living in a deprived inner London district. *Health Education Research*, *9*: 355–64.

Bowling, A. and Browne, P. (1991). Social networks, health, and emotional well-being among the oldest old in London. *Journal of Gerontology*, *46*: S20–S32.

Bowling, A. and Farquhar, M. (1993). The health and well-being of Jewish people aged 65–85 years living at home in the east end of London. *Ageing and Society*, *13*: 213–44.

Bowling, A. and Normand, C. (in press). Definition and measurement of outcome. In: M. Swash and J. Wilden (eds), *Outcomes in Neurological and Neurosurgical Disorders*. Cambridge: Cambridge University Press.

Bowling, A. and Parkman, S. (1993). *Needs of Psychiatric Patients*. London: East London and the City District Health Authority.

Bowling, A., Farquhar, M. and Browne, P. (1991). Life satisfaction and associations with social network and support variables in three samples of elderly people. *International Journal of Geriatric Psychiatry*, *6*: 549–66.

Bowling, A., Farquhar, M., Grundy, E. and Formby, J. (1992). Psychiatric morbidity among people aged 85 + in 1987. A follow-up study at two and a half years: Associations with changes in psychiatric morbidity. *International Journal of Geriatric Psychiatry*, *7*: 307–21.

Bowling, A., Farquhar, M. and Grundy, E. (1994). Associations with changes in level of functional ability. *Ageing and Society*, *14*: 53–73.

Boysen, G. (1992). The Scandinavian Stroke Scale: Cerebrovascular diseases (abstract). *Second European Stroke Conference Issue*, *2*: 239–40.

Bradburn, N.M. (1969). *The Structure of Psychological Well-being*. Chicago, IL: Aldine.

Bradburn, N.M. and Caplowitz, D. (1965). *Reports on Happiness*. Chicago, IL: Aldine.

Bradley, C. (1991). Evaluating new technologies: Psychological issues in research design and measurement. In: C. Bradley, P. Home and M. Christie (eds), *The Technology of Diabetes Care: Converging Medical and Psychosocial Perspectives*. Reading: Harwood Academic.

Bradley, C. (ed.) (1994). *Handbook of Psychology and Diabetes: A guide to psychological measurement in diabetes research and practice*. Reading: Harwood Academic.

Bradley, C. and Lewis, K.S. (1990). Measures of psychological well-being and treatment satisfaction developed from the responses of people with tablet-treated diabetes. *Diabetic Medicine*, *7*: 445–51.

Bradley, C., Lewis, K.S., Jennings, A.M. and Ward, J.D. (1990). Scales to measure perceived control developed specifically for people with tablet-treated diabetes. *Diabetic Medicine*, *7*: 685–94.

Brayne, C. and Calloway, P. (1990). The case identification of dementia in the community: A comparison of methods. *International Journal of Geriatric Psychiatry*, *5*: 309–16.

Brazier, J., Harper, R., Jones, N.M.B. *et al.* (1992). Validating the SF-36 health survey questionnaire: New outcome measures for primary care. *British Medical Journal*, *305*: 160–4.

Brazier, J., Harper, R., Waterhouse, J. *et al.* (1993a). Comparison of outcome measures for patients with chronic obstructive pulmonary disease. Paper presented to the *Fifth European Health Services Research Conference*, Maastricht, December.

Brazier, J., Jones, N. and Kind, P. (1993b). Testing the validity of the Euroqol and comparing it with the SF-36 health survey questionnaire. *Quality of Life Research*, *2*: 169–80.

Breetvelt, I.S. and van Dam, F.S. (1991). Under-reporting by cancer patients: The case of response shift. *Social Science and Medicine, 32*: 981–7.

Breeze, E., Maidment, A., Bennett, N., Flatley, J. and Cairey, S. (1994). *Health Survey for England, 1992.* Compiled for Office of Population Censuses and Surveys. London: HMSO.

Brehmer, B. and Joyce, C.R.B. (eds) (1988). *Human Judgement Analysis: The Social Judgement Theory View.* Amsterdam: North-Holland.

Brenner, M.H. (1973). *Mental Health and the Economy.* Cambridge, MA: Harvard University Press.

Brenner, M.H. (1977). Health costs and benefits of health policy. *International Journal of Health Services,* 7: 581–623.

Breytspraak, L.M. and George, L.K. (1982). Self-concept and self-esteem. In: D.J. Mangen and W.A. Peterson (eds), *Research Instruments in Social Gerontology,* Vol. 1. Minneapolis, MN: University of Minnesota Press.

Breuer, A.C., Furlan, A.J., Hansen, M.R. *et al.* (1981). Neurologic complications of open heart surgery. *Cleve Clinic Quarterly, 48*: 205–6.

Brewin, C.R. (1992). Believing what patients tell us. *Journal of Mental Health, 1*: 83–4.

Brewin, C.R. and Wing, J.K. (1989). *MRC Needs for Care Assessment: Manual for Version 2.* London: MRC Social Psychiatry Unit, Institute of Psychiatry.

Brewin, C.R., Wing, J.K., Mangen, S.P. *et al.* (1987). Principles and practice of measuring needs in the long term mentally ill: The MRC Needs for Care Assessment. *Psychological Medicine, 17*: 971–81.

Brewin, C.R., Wing, J.K., Mangen, S.P. *et al.* (1988). Needs for care among the long term mentally ill: A report from the Camberwell High Contact Survey. *Psychological Medicine, 18*: 457–68.

Brewin, C.R., Veltro, F., Wing, J.K. *et al.* (1990). The assessment of psychiatric disability in the community: A comparison of clinical, staff and family interviews. *British Journal of Psychiatry, 157*: 671–4.

British Geriatrics Society/Royal College of Physicians (1992). *Standardised Clinical Instruments and Measurement Scales for Elderly Patients.* Working Party Report. London: RCP.

Brock, D. (1993). Quality of life measures in health care and medical ethics. In: M. Nussbaum and A. Sen (eds), *The Quality of Life.* Oxford: Clarendon Press.

Bromet, E.J., Dunn, L.O., Connell, M.M. *et al.* (1986). Long-term reliability of diagnosing lifetime major depression in a community sample. *Archives of General Psychiatry, 43*: 435–40.

Brook, R.H. (1990). Relationship between appropriateness and outcome. In: A. Hopkins and D. Costain (eds), *Measuring the Outcomes of Medical Care.* London: Royal College of Physicians.

Brook, R.H., Rogers, W.H., Williams, K.N. *et al.* (1979a). *Conceptualisation and Measurement of Health for Adults in the Health Insurance Study, Vol. III: Mental Health.* Santa Monica, CA: Rand Corporation.

Brook, R.H., Ware, J.E., Davies-Avery, A. *et al.* (1979b). *Conceptualisation and Measurement of Health for Adults in the Health Insurance Study, Vol. VIII: Overview.* Santa Monica, CA: Rand Corporation.

Brook, R.H., Ware, J.E., Davies-Avery, A. *et al.* (1979c). Overview of adult health status measures fielded in Rand's Health Insurance Study. *Medical Care, 17*: 1–131 (suppl.).

Brook, R.H., Lohr, K.N., Goldberg, G.A. *et al.* (1980a). *Conceptualisation and Measurement of Physiologic Health for Adults, Vol. 2: Acne.* Santa Monica, CA: Rand Corporation.

Brook, R.H., Berman, D.M., Lohr, K.N. *et al.* (1980b). *Conceptualisation and Measurement of Physiologic Health for Adults, Vol. 3: Hypertension.* Santa Monica, CA: Rand Corporation.

Brook, R.H., Lohr, K., Berman, D.M. *et al.* (1981). *Conceptualisation and Measurement of Health for Adults, Vol. 7: Diabetes Mellitus.* Santa Monica, CA: Rand Corporation.

Brook, R.H., Lohr, K.N. and Goldberg, G.A. (1982). *Conceptualisation and Measurement of Health for Adults, Vol. 9: Thyroid Disease.* Santa Monica, CA: Rand Corporation.

Brook, R.H., Ware, J.E., Rogers, W.H., Keeler, E.M. *et al.* (1983). Does free care improve adults' health? Results from a randomised controlled trial. *New England Journal of Medicine, 309*: 1426–34.

Brook, R.H., Kamberg, C.J., Lohr, K.N., Goldberg, G.A. *et al.* (1990). Quality of ambulatory care: Epidemiology by insurance status and income. *Medical Care, 28*: 392–433.

Brooks, C.M., Richards, J.M., Bailey, W.C. *et al.* (1989). Subjective symptomatology of asthma in an out-patient population. *Psychosomatic Medicine, 51*: 102–8.

Brooks, N. (1984). *Closed Head Injury: Psychological, Social and Family Consequences.* Oxford: Oxford University Press.

Brooks, S.M. (1982). Task group on surveillance for respiratory hazards in the occupational setting: Surveillance for respiratory hazards. *American Thoracic Society News, 8*: 12–16.

Brorsson, B. and Asberg, K.H. (1984). Katz Index of Independence in ADL: Reliability and validity in short-term care. *Scandinavian Journal of Rehabilitative Medicine, 16*: 125–32.

Brott, T. (1992). Utility of the NIH Stroke Scale: Cerebrovascular diseases (abstract). *Second European Stroke Conference Issue, 2*: 241–2.

Brott, T., Adams, H.P., Olinger, C.P. *et al.* (1989).

Measurements of acute cerebral infarction: A clinical examination scale. *Stroke, 20*: 864–70.

Brown, G.L. and Zung, W.W.K. (1972). Depression scales: Self or physician rating? A validation of certain clinically observable phenomena. *Comprehensive Psychiatry, 13*: 361–7.

Brown, G.W. (1974). Meaning, measurement and stress of life events. In: B.S. Dohrenwend and B.P. Dohrenwend (eds), *Stressful Life Events: Their Nature and Effects*. New York: John Wiley.

Brown, G.W. (1991). Aetiology of depression: Something of the future? In: P.E. Bebbington (ed.), *Social Psychiatry: Theory, Methodology and Practice*. London: Transaction Publishers.

Brown, G.W. and Birley, J.L.T. (1968). Crises and life changes and the onset of schizophrenia. *Journal of Health and Social Behaviour, 9*: 203–14.

Brown, G.W., Birley, J.L.T. and Wing, J.K. (1972). Influence of family life on the course of schizophrenic disorders: A replication. *British Journal of Psychiatry, 121*: 241–58.

Brown, G.W. and Harris, T.O. (1978). *Social Origins of Depression*. London: Tavistock.

Brown, G.W. and Harris, T. (1982). Fall off in the reporting of life events. *Social Psychiatry, 17*: 23–8.

Brown, G.W. and Rutter, M. (1966). The measurement of family activities and relationships: A methodological study. *Human Relations, 19*: 241–63.

Brown, G.W., Sklair, F., Harris, T.O. and Birley, J.L.T. (1973). Life events and psychiatric disorders. Part I. Some methodological issues. *Psychological Medicine, 3*: 74–87.

Brown, G.W., Bhrolchain, M.N. and Harris, T.O. (1975). Social class and psychiatric disturbance among women in an urban population. *Sociology, 9*: 225–54.

Brown, G.W., Davidson, S., Harris, T. *et al.* (1977). Psychiatric disorder in London and North Uist. *Social Science and Medicine, 11*: 367–77.

Brown, G.W., Andrews, B., Harris, T. *et al.* (1986). Social support, self-esteem and depression. *Psychological Medicine, 16*: 813–31.

Brown, H.N. and Kelly, M.J. (1976). Stages of bone marrow transplantation: A psychiatric perspective. *Psychosomatic Medicine, 38*: 439–46.

Brown, J.H., Lewis, M.D., Kazis, E. *et al.* (1984). The dimensions of health outcomes: A cross-validated examination of health status measurement. *American Journal of Public Health, 74*: 159–61.

Brown, M. (1985). Selecting an instrument to measure dyspnoea. *Oncology Nursing Forum, 12*: 98–100.

Brown, S.W. and Thomlinson, L.L. (1984). Anticonvulsant side-effects: A self report questionnaire for use in community surveys. *British Journal of Clinical Practice, 18*: 147–9 (suppl.).

Browne, J.P., O'Boyle, C. A., McGee, H.M. *et al.* (1994). Individual quality of life in the healthy elderly. *Quality of Life Research, 3*: 235–44.

Brugha, T.S. and Bebbington, P.E. (1992). A comparison of DSM-III R major depression and ICD 10-DCR depressive episode criteria using PSE9 clinical data. *International Journal of Methods in Psychiatric Research, 2*: 11–14.

Brundin, A. (1974). Physical training in severe COPD. *Scandinavian Journal of Respiratory Disease, 55*: 25–36.

Bubolz, M., Eicher, J.B., Evers, S.J. and Sontag, M.S. (1980). A human ecological approach to quality of life: Conceptual framework and results of a preliminary study. *Social Indicators Research, 7*: 103–36.

Buchanan, R.B., Flaney, R.W. and Durrant, K.R. (1986). A randomised comparison of tamoxifen with surgical oophorectomy in premenopausal patients with advanced breast cancer. *Journal of Clinical Oncology, 4*: 1326–30.

Bullinger, M. (1994). Concepts of generic quality of life assessment. Theoretical foundation and international application. Paper presented to the *Conference of the Association of European Psychiatrists: Psychiatric Epidemiology and Social Psychiatry*. Quality of Life and Disabilities – Mental Disorders. Vienna, April 7–9.

Bullinger, M., Anderson, R., Cella, D. and Aaronson, N. (1993). Developing and evaluating cross-cultural instruments from minimum requirements to optimal models. *Quality of Life Research, 2*: 451–9.

Bulpitt, C.J. (1982). Quality of life in hypertensive patients. In: A. Amery, R. Fagard, P. Lijnen and J. Staessen (eds), *Hypertensive Cardiovascular Disease: Pathophysiology and Treatment*. The Hague: Martinus Nijoff.

Bulpitt, C.J. and Fletcher, A.E. (1990). The measurement of quality of life in hypertensive patients: A practical approach. *British Journal of Clinical Pharmacology, 30*: 353–64.

Bulpitt, C.J., Dollery, C.T. and Carne, S. (1974). A symptom questionnaire for hypertensive patients. *Journal of Chronic Diseases, 27*: 309–23.

Bulpitt, C.J., Dollery, C.T. and Carne, S. (1976). Change in symptoms of hypertensive patients after referral to hospital clinic. *British Heart Journal, 2*: 121–8.

Bulpitt, C.J., Hoffbrand, B.I. and Dollery, C.T. (1979). Contribution of drug treatment to symptoms of hypertensive patients. In: F. Gross, and T. Strasser (eds), *Mild Hypertension: Natural History and Management*. Tunbridge Wells: Pitman Medical.

Bunge, M. (1975). What is a quality of life indicator? *Social Indicators Research, 2*: 65–79.

Bunzel, B., Wollenek, G. and Grundbock, A. (1992). Psychosocial problems of donor heart recipients adversely affecting quality of life. *Quality of Life Research, 1*: 307–13.

Burdon, J.G.W., Juniper, E.F., Killian, K.J. *et al.* (1982). The perception of breathlessness. *American Review of Respiratory Disease, 128*: 825–8.

Burge, P.S., Prankerd, T.A.J., Richards, D.M. *et al.* (1975). Quality and quantity of survival in acute myeloid leukaemia. *The Lancet*, October, pp. 621–5.

Burgess, A., Dayer, M., Catalan, J. *et al.* (1993). The reliability and validity of two HIV-specific health related Quality of Life measures: A preliminary analysis. *AIDS*, 7: 1001–8.

Burnam, M.A., Karno, M., Hough, R.L. *et al.* (1983). The Spanish Diagnostic Interview Schedule: Reliability and comparison with clinical diagnoses. *Archives of General Psychiatry, 40*: 1189–96.

Burnam, M.A., Wells, K.B., Leake, B. and Landsverk, J. (1988). Development of a brief screening instrument for detecting depressive disorders. *Medical Care, 26*: 775–89.

Buros, O.K. (1978). *The Eighth Mental Measurements Yearbook*. Highland Park, NJ: Gryphon Press.

Buschke, W.R., Bush, J.W. and Kaplan, R.M. (1985). Successive intervals analysis of preference measures in a health status index. *Health Services Research, 10*: 181.

Bush, J.W. (1984). General health policy model: Quality of well-being (QWB) scale. In: N.K. Wenger, M.E. Mattson, C.D. Furberg, and J. Elinson (eds), *Assessment of Quality of Life in Clinical Trials of Cardiovascular Therapies*. New York: Le Jacq.

Bush, J.W., Chen, M. and Patrick, D.L. (1973). Cost-effectiveness using a health status index: Analysis of the New York State PKU screening program. In: R. Berg (ed.), *Health Status Indexes*. Chicago, IL: Hospital Research and Educational Trust.

Butland, R.J.A., Pang, J., Gross, E.R. *et al.* (1982). Two, six, and twelve minute walking tests in respiratory disease. *British Medical Journal, 284*: 1604–8.

Butow, P., Coates, A., Dunn, S., Bernhard, J. and Hurny, C. (1991). On the receiving end IV: Validation of quality of life indicators. *Annals of Oncology, 2*: 597–603.

Butz, A.M., Eggleston, P., Alexander, C. and Rosenstein, B.J. (1991). Outcomes of emergency room treatment of children with asthma. *Journal of Asthma, 28*: 255–64.

Buxton, M., Acheson, R.M., Caine, N. *et al.* (1985). *Costs and Benefits of the Heart Transplant Programmes at Harefield and Papworth Hospitals*. London: HMSO.

Buyse, M.E., Staquet, M.J. and Sylvester, R.J. (eds) (1984). *Cancer Clinical Trials*. Oxford: Oxford University Press.

Byrne, M. (1992). Cancer chemotherapy and quality of life. *British Medical Journal, 304*: 1532–3.

Caine, N., Sharples, L.D., English, T.A.H. and Wallwork, J. (1990). Prospective study comparing quality of life before and after heart transplantation. *Transplantation Proceedings, 22*: 1437–9.

Caine, N., Harrison, S.C.W., Sharples, L.D. and Wallwork, J. (1991). Prospective study of quality of life before and after coronary artery bypass grafting. *British Medical Journal, 302*: 511–16.

Cairl, R.E., Pfeiffer, E., Keller, D.M. *et al.* (1983). An evaluation of the reliability and validity of the Functional Assessment Inventory. *Journal of the American Geriatric Society, 31*: 607–12.

Callahan, L., Brooks, R. and Pincus, T. (1988). Further analysis of learned helplessness in rheumatoid arthritis using a 'Rheumatology Attitudes Index'. *Journal of Rheumatology, 15*: 418–26.

Calman, K.C. (1984). Quality of life in cancer patients – a hypothesis. *Journal of Medical Ethics, 10*: 124–7.

Calnan, M. (1988). The health locus of control: An empirical test. *Health Promotion Journal, 2*: 323–30.

Campbell, A., Converse, P. and Rogers, W.L. (1976). *The quality of American life: Perceptions, Evaluations and Satisfactions*. New York: Russell Sage.

Campbell, D.T. and Fiske, D.W. (1959). Convergent and discriminant validation by the multitrait–multimethod matrix. *Psychological Bulletin, 56*: 81–105.

Campeau, L. (1976). Grading of angina pectoris. *Circulation, 54*: 522–3.

Cantril, H. (1965). *The Pattern of Human Concerns*. New Brunswick, NJ: Rutgers University Press.

Caplan, R.D., Abbey, A., Abramis, D.J. *et al.* (1984). *Tranquilizer Use and Well-being: A Longitudinal Study of Social and Psychological Effects*. Ann Arbor, MI: Institute for Social Research.

Carabellesse, C., Appollonio, I., Rozzini, R. *et al.* (1993). Sensory impairment and quality of life in a community elderly population. *Journal of the American Geriatric Society, 41*: 401–7.

Carlens, E., Dahlstrom, G. and Nou, E. (1970). Comparative measurements of quality of survival of lung cancer patients after diagnosis. *Scandinavian Journal of Respiratory Disease, 34*: 268–75.

Carmines, E.G. and Zeller, R.A. (1979). *Reliability and Validity Assessment*. Beverly Hills, CA: Sage.

Carnrike, C.L.M. and Carey, M.P. (1990). Assessing nausea and vomiting in adult chemotherapy patients: Review and recommendations. *Annals of Behavioural Medicine, 12*: 79–85.

Carr-Hill, R. (1989). Assumption of the QALY procedure. *Social Science and Medicine, 29*: 469–77.

Carr-Hill, R. (1992). A second opinion: Health related quality of life measurement – Euro style. *Health Policy, 20*: 321–8.

Carr-Hill, R.A. and Morris, J. (1991). Current practice in obtaining the 'Q' in QALYs – a cautionary note. *British Medical Journal, 303*: 699–701.

Carroll, B.J., Fielding, J.M. and Blash, T.G. (1973). Depression rating scales: A critical review. *Archives of General Psychiatry, 28*: 361–6.

Carter, R., Peavler, M., Zinkgraf, S. *et al.* (1987). Predicting maximal exercise ventilation in patients with chronic obstructive pulmonary disease. *Chest, 92*: 252–9.

Carter, W.B., Bobbitt, R.A., Bergner, M. and Gilson, B.S. (1976). The validation of an internal scaling: The Sickness Impact Profile. *Health Services Research, 11*: 516–28.

Cartwright, A. (1989). *User surveys in general practice. I. Some suggestions about how to do such surveys by post.* London: Institute for Social Studies in Medical Care.

Carver, C.S., Scheier, M.F. and Weintraub, J.K. (1989). Assessing coping strategies: A theoretically based approach. *Journal of Personality and Social Psychology, 56*: 267–83.

Casey, R.L., Masuda, M. and Holmes, T.H. (1967). Quantitative study of recall of life events. *Journal of Psychosomatic Research, 11*: 239–47.

Cassileth, B.R., Lusk, E.J., Brown, L.L. *et al.* (1985). Psychosocial status of cancer patients and next of kin: Normative data from the Profile of Mood States. *Journal of Clinical Oncology, 3*: 99–105.

Cassileth, B.R., Soloway, M.S., Vogelzang, N.J. *et al.* (1992). Quality of life and psychosocial status in stage D prostate cancer. *Quality of Life Research, 1*: 323–30.

Castelnuovo-Tedesco, P. (1973). Organ transplant, body image, psychosis. *Psychoanalysis Quarterly, 42*: 349–63.

Cattell, R.B. and Eber, H.W. (1962). *Handbook for the 16 PF Questionnaire.* Urbana, IL: Institute for Personality and Ability Testing.

Cavanaugh, S. (1983). The prevalence of emotional and cognitive dysfunction in a general medical population: Using the MMSE, GHQ and BDI. *General Hospital Psychiatry, 5*: 15–24.

Cella, D.F. and Cherin, E.A. (1987). Measuring quality of life in patients with cancer. In: *Proceedings of the Fifth National Conference on Human Values and Cancer. A Service and Rehabilitation Education Publication.* New York: American Cancer Society.

Cella, D.F. and Perry, S.W. (1986). Reliability and concurrent validity of three visual analogue mood scales. *Psychological Reports, 59*: 827–33.

Cella, D.F. and Tross, S. (1986). Psychological adjustment to survival from Hodgkin's disease. *Journal of Consulting and Clinical Psychology, 54*: 616–22.

Cella, D.F. and Tulsky, D.S. (1990). Measuring quality of life today: Methodological aspects. *Oncology, 4*: 29–38.

Cella, D.F., Orofiamma, B., Holland, J.C. *et al.* (1987). The relationship of psychological distress, extent of disease, and performance status in patients with lung cancer. *Cancer, 10*: 1661–7.

Cella, D.F., Tross, S., Orov, E.J. *et al.* (1989). Mood states of patients after the diagnosis of cancer. *Journal of Psychosocial Oncology, 7*: 45–53.

Cella, D.F., Tulsky, D.S., Bonomi, A. *et al.* (1990). The functional assessment of cancer therapy (FACT) scales: Incorporating disease specificity and subjectivity into quality of life (QL) assessment. *Proceedings of the Annual Meeting of the American Society for Oncology, 9*: A1190.

Chambers, L.W. (1982). *The McMaster Health Index Questionnaire (MHIQ): Methodologic Documentation and Report of Second Generation of Investigators.* Hamilton, Ontario: McMaster University, Department of Clinical Epidemiology and Biostatistics.

Chambers, L.W. (1984). The McMaster Health Index Questionnaire. In: N.K. Wenger, M.E. Mattson, C.D. Furberg and J. Elinson (eds), *Assessment of Quality of Life in Clinical Trials of Cardiovascular Therapies.* New York: Le Jacq.

Chambers, L.W. (1993). The McMaster Health Index Questionnaire: An update. In: S.R. Walker and R.M. Rosser (eds), *Quality of Life Assessment: Key Issues in the 1990s.* Dordrecht: Kluwer Academic.

Chambers, L.W., Sackett, D.L., Goldsmith, C.H. *et al.* (1976). Development and application of an index of social function. *Health Services Research, 11.* 430–41.

Chambers, L.W., McDonald, L.A., Tugwell, P. *et al.* (1982). The McMaster Health Index Questionnaire as a measure of quality of life for patients with rheumatoid arthritis. *Journal of Rheumatology, 9*: 780–4.

Chambers, L.W., Haight, M., Norman, G. *et al.* (1987). Sensitivity to change and the effect of mode of administration on health status measurement. *Medical Care, 25*: 470–9.

Chandarana, P.C., Eals, M., Steingart, A.B. *et al.* (1987). The detection of psychiatric morbidity and associated factors in patients with rheumatoid arthritis. *Canadian Journal of Psychology, 32*: 356–61.

Chang, A.E., Steinberg, S.M., Culnane, M. *et al.* (1989). Functional and psychosocial effects of multimodality limb sparing therapy in patients with soft tissue sarcomas. *Journal of Clinical Oncology, 7*: 12–17.

Chant, A.D.B., Jones, H.O. and Weddell, J.M. (1972). A comparison of surgery and injection–compression sclerotherapy. *Lancet, ii*: 1188–91.

Chaplin, W.F. (1984). State–trait anxiety inventory. In: D.J. Keyser and R.C. Sweetland (eds), *Test Critiques*, Vol. 1. Kansas City, MO: Test Corporation of America.

Charlesworth, A. and Wilkin, D. (1982). *Dependency Among Old People in Geriatric Wards, Psychogeriatric Wards, and Residential Homes.* Research Report No. 6.

Manchester: Departments of Psychiatry and Community Medicine, University of Manchester.

Charlton, J., Patrick, D. and Peach, H. (1983). Use of multivariate measures of disability in health surveys. *Journal of Epidemiology and Community Health, 37*: 296–304.

Charlton, J., Charlton, G., Broomfield, J. and Mullee, M.A. (1990). Evaluation of peak flow and symptoms only self-management plans for control of asthma in general practice. *British Medical Journal, 301*: 1355–9.

Charlton, J., Charlton, G., Broomfield, J. and Mullee, M.A. (1991). Audit of the effect of a nurse run asthma clinic on workload and patient morbidity in a general practice. *British Journal of General Practice, 41*; 227–31.

Charmaz, K. (1983). Loss of Self: A fundamental form of suffering in the chronically ill. *Sociology of Health and Illness, 5*: 168–93.

Chubon, R.A. (1987). Development of a quality of life rating scale for use in health care evaluation. *Evaluation and the Health Professions, 10*: 186–200.

Churchill, D.N., Wallace, J.E., Ludwin, D. *et al.* (1991). A comparison of evaluative indices of quality of life and cognitive function in hemodialysis patients. *Controlled Clinical Trials, 12*: 159S–167S.

Cicero, M.T. (44 B.C). *Cato-major – De Senectute*. Translated by J. Logan (1744). *Cato major; or, His discourse of old age*. Philadelphia, PA: Benjamin Franklin. (Reprinted by Arno Press, 1979.)

Clark, A. and Fallowfield, L.J. (1986). Quality of life measurements in patients with malignant disease: A review. *Journal of the Royal Society of Medicine, 79*: 165–9.

Clark, P. and Bowling, A. (1989). Observational study of quality of life in NHS nursing homes and a long stay ward for the elderly. *Ageing and Society, 9*: 123–48.

Clark, P. and Bowling, A. (1990). Quality of everyday life in long stay institutions for the elderly: An observational study of long stay hospital and nursing home care. *Social Science and Medicine, 30*: 1201–10.

Clarke, A. (1993). Does shorter length of stay affect outcome: An investigation into the medical, social, psychological and economic effects of shorter length of stay for elective abdominal hysterectomy. MD thesis, London School of Hygiene and Tropical Medicine, University of London.

Cleary, P.D., Epstein, A.M., Oster, G. *et al.* (1991). Health-related quality of life among patients undergoing percutaneous transluminal coronary angioplasty. *Medical Care, 29*: 939–50.

Clinical Trials Cooperative Group Program (1988). *Cancer Therapy Evaluation Program: Guidelines*. Bethesda, MD: National Cancer Institute.

Coates, A.S. and Simes, R.J. (1992). Patient assessment of adjuvant treatment in operable breast cancer. In: C.J. Williams (ed.), *Introducing New Treatments for Cancer: Practical, Ethical and Legal Problems*. Chichester: John Wiley.

Coates,. A.S., Fischer Dillenbeck, C., McNeil, D.R. *et al.* (1983). On the receiving end II. Linear analogue self assessment (LASA) in evaluation of aspects of quality of life in cancer patients receiving therapy. *European Journal of Cancer and Clinical Oncology, 19*: 1633–7.

Coates, A.S., Gebski, V., Bishop, J.F. *et al.* (1987). Improving the quality of life during chemotherapy for advanced breast cancer. *New England Journal of Medicine, 317*: 1490–5.

Coates, A.S., Glasziou, P. and McNeil, D. (1990). On the receiving end III. Measurement of quality of life during cancer chemotherapy. *Annals of Oncology, 1*: 213–17.

Coddington, R.D. (1972). The significance of life events as etiologic factors in diseases of children. I. A survey of professional workers. *Journal of Psychosomatic Research, 16*: 7–18.

Coddington, R.D. (1981a). *Life Events Scale – Children*. St. Clairsville, OH: Stress Research Company.

Coddington, R.D. (1981b). *Life Events Scale – Adolescents*. St. Clairsville, OH: Stress Research Company.

Cody, M., Nichols, S., Brennan, C., Armes, J. and Slevin, M. (1993). Psychiatric morbidity in patients with advanced lung cancer (abstract). *Quality of Life Research, 2*: 57.

Coelho, G., Hamburg, D. and Adams, J. (eds) (1974). *Coping and Adaptation*. New York: Basic Books.

Cohen, C. (1982). On the quality of life: Some philosophical reflections. *Circulation, 66*: 29–33 (suppl. III).

Cohen, C.B. (1990). Quality of life and the analogy with the Nazis. In: J.J. Walter and T.A. Shannon (eds), *Quality of Life: The New Medical Dilemma*. New York: Paulist Press.

Cohen, F. (1987). Measurement of coping. In: S.V. Kasl and C.L. Cooper (eds), *Stress and Health: Issues in Research Methodology*. Chichester: John Wiley.

Cohen, J. (1968). Weighted kappa: Nominal scale agreement with provision for scaled disagreement or partial credit. *Psychological Bulletin, 70*: 213–20.

Cohen, S. and Wills, T.A. (1985). Stress, social support and the buffering hypothesis. *Psychological Bulletin, 98*: 310–57.

Cohler, B., Grunebaum, H., Weiss, J. *et al.* (1974). Social role performance and psychopathology among recently hospitalised mothers. *Journal of Nervous Mental Disease, 159*: 81–90.

Collen, F.M., Wade, D.T. and Bradshaw, C.M. (1990). Mobility after stroke: Reliability of measures of impairment and disability. *International Disability Studies, 12*: 6–9.

Collen, F.M., Wade, D.T., Robb, G.F. and Bradshaw, C.M. (1991). The Rivermead Mobility Index: A further development of the Rivermead Motor Assessment. *International Disability Studies, 13*: 50–4.

Collin, C. and Wade, D.T. (1990). Assessing motor impairment after stroke: A pilot reliability study. *Journal of Neurology, Neurosurgery and Psychiatry, 53*: 567–9.

Collin, C., Wade, D.T., Davies, S. and Horne, V. (1988). The Barthel ADL Index: A reliability study. *International Disability Studies, 10*: 61–3.

Collings, J.A. (1990a). Epilepsy and well-being. *Social Science and Medicine, 31*: 165–70.

Collings, J.A. (1990b). Psychosocial well-being and epilepsy: An empirical study. *Epilepsia, 31*: 418–26.

Collins, D.L., Baum, A. and Singer, J.E. (1982). Coping with chronic stress at Three Mile Island: Psychological and biological evidence. *Health Psychology, 2*: 149–66.

Comrey, A.L. (1978). Common methodological problems in factor analytic studies. *Journal of Consulting and Clinical Psychology, 46*: 648–59.

Comstock, G.W. and Helsing, K. (1976). Symptoms of depression in two communities. *Psychological Medicine, 6*: 551–63.

Comstock, G.W., Tockman, M.S., Helsing, K.J. and Henesy, K.M. (1979). Standardised respiratory questionnaires: Comparison of the old with the new. *American Review of Respiratory Disease, 119*: 45–53.

Conn, V.S., Taylor, S.G. and Abele, P.B. (1991). Myocardial infarction survivors: Age and gender differences in physical health, psychosocial state and regimen adherence. *Journal of Advanced Nursing, 16*: 1026–34.

Conners, C.K. (1973). Rating scales for use in drug studies with children. *Psychopharmacology Bulletin, Special Issue: Pharmacotherapy of Children*, 24–84.

Convery, F.R., Minteer, M.A., Amiel, D. and Connett, K.L. (1977). Polyarticular disability: A functional assessment. *Archives of Physical Medicine and Rehabilitation, 58*: 494–9.

Cook, D.G., Shaper, A.G. and MacFarlane, P.W. (1989). Using the WHO (Rose angina) questionnaire in cardiovascular epidemiology. *International Journal of Epidemiology, 18*: 607–13.

Cooper, J.E. and Mackenzie, S. (1981). The rapid prediction of low scores on a standardised psychiatric interview (Present State Examination). In: J.K. Wing, P. Bebbington and L.N. Robins (eds), *What is a Case? The Problem of Definition in Psychiatric Community Surveys*. London: Grant McIntyre.

Cooper, J.E., Copeland, J.R.M., Brown, G.W. *et al.* (1977). Further studies on interview training and inter-rater reliability of the Present State Examination (PSE). *Psychological Medicine, 7*: 517–23.

Cooper, P., Osborn, M., Gath, D. and Fegetter, G. (1982). Evaluation of a modified self-report measure of social adjustment. *British Journal of Psychiatry, 141*: 68–75.

Cooperating Clinics Committee of the American Rheumatism Association (1965). A seven day variability study of 499 patients with peripheral rheumatoid arthritis. *Arthritis and Rheumatism, 8*: 302–34.

Coopersmith, S. (1975). *Developing Motivation in Young Children*. San Francisco, CA: Albion Publishing.

Coopersmith, S. (1981a). *The Antecedents of Self-esteem*. Palo Alto, CA: Consulting Psychologists Press.

Coopersmith, S. (1981b). *Self-esteem Inventories*. Palo Alto, CA: Consulting Psychologists Press.

Copeland, J.R.M. (1990). Suitable instruments for detecting dementia in community samples. *Age and Ageing, 19*: 81–3.

Copeland, J.R.M. and Gurland, B.J. (1978). Evaluation of diagnostic methods: An international comparison. In: A.D. Isaacs and F. Post (eds), *Studies in Geriatric Psychiatry*. Chichester: John Wiley.

Copeland, J.R.M. and Wilson, K.C.M. (1989). Rating scales in old age psychiatry. In: C. Thompson (ed.), *The Instruments of Psychiatric Research*. Chichester: John Wiley.

Copeland, J.R.M., Kelleher, M.H., Kellet, J.M. *et al.* (1976). A semi-structured clinical interview for the assessment of diagnosis and mental state in the elderly: The geriatric mental state. Schedule I: Development and reliability. *Psychological Medicine, 6*: 439–49.

Copeland, J.R.M., Dewey, M.E. and Griffiths Jones, H.M. (1986). A computerised psychiatric diagnostic system and case nomenclature for elderly subjects: GMS and AGECAT. *Psychological Medicine, 16*: 89–99.

Copeland, J.R.M., Gurland, B.J., Dewey, M.E. *et al.* (1987). The distribution of dementia, depression and neurosis in elderly men and women in an urban community: Assessed using the GMS-AGECAT package. *International Journal of Geriatric Psychiatry, 2*: 177–84.

Corney, R.H. (1988). Development and use of a short self-rating instrument to screen for psychosocial disorder. *Journal of the Royal College of General Practitioners, 38*: 263–6.

Corney, R.H. and Clare, A.W. (1985). The construction, development and testing of a self-report questionnaire to identify social problems. *Psychological Medicine, 15*: 637–49.

Cornoni-Huntley, J.C., Foley, D.J., White, L.R. *et al.* (1985). Epidemiology of disability in the oldest old: Methodologic issues and preliminary findings. *Milbank Memorial Fund Quarterly (Health and Society), 63*: 350–76.

Coronary Artery Surgery Study (CASS) (1983). Coronary Artery Surgery Study (CASS): A randomised trial of coronary artery bypass surgery. Quality of life in patients randomly assigned to treatment groups. *Circulation, 68*: 951–60.

Costa, P. and McCrae, R. (1985). *The NEO Personality Inventory Manual*. Odessa, FL: Psychological Assessment Resources.

Côté, R. and Hachinski, V. (1992). The Canadian Neurological Scale: Cerebrovascular diseases (abstract). *Second European Stroke Conference Issue, 2*: 243–4.

Côté, R., Hachinski, V., Shurvell, B.L. *et al.* (1986). The Canadian Neurological Scale: A preliminary study in acute stroke. *Stroke, 17*: 731–7.

Côté, R., Battista, R.N., Wolfson, C. and Hachinski, V. (1988). Stroke assessment scales: Guidelines for development, validation and reliability assessment. *Canadian Journal of Neurological Sciences, 15*: 261–5.

Côté, R., Battista, R.N., Wolfson, C. *et al.* (1989). The Canadian Neurological Scale: Validation and Reliability Assessment. *Neurology, 39*: 638–43.

Coulter, A. (1987). Lifestyles and social class: Implications for primary care. *Journal of the Royal College of General Practitioners, 37*: 533–6.

Coulton, C.J., Hyduk, C.M. and Chow, J.C. (1989). An assessment of the Arthritis Impact Measurement Scales in 3 ethnic groups. *Journal of Rheumatology, 16*: 1110–15.

Cousins, N. (1979). *Anatomy of an Illness*. New York: Norton.

Cox, B.D., Blaxter, M., Buckle, A.L.J. *et al.* (1987). *The Health and Lifestyle Survey*. London: Health Promotion Research Trust.

Cox, J.B., Brown, T.R., Peterson, P.D. and Row, M.M. (1978). *The Two-State Collaborative Mental Health Outcome Study: State of Washington (Vol. 1)*. Olympia, WA: Office of Research, Division of Analysis and Information Services and the Division of Mental Health, Department of Health and Social Services.

Crawford-Little, J. and McPhail, N.I. (1973). Measures of depressive mood at monthly intervals. *British Journal of Psychiatry, 122*: 447–52.

Creed, F. and Ash, G. (1992). Depression in rheumatoid arthritis: Aetiology and treatment. *International Review of Psychiatry, 4*: 23–34.

Creed, F., Murphy, S. and Jayson, M.V. (1989). Measurement of psychological disorders in RA. *Journal of Psychosomatic Research, 33*: 79–87.

Creer, C. and Wing, J.K. (1974). *Schizophrenia at Home*. London: National Schizophrenia Fellowship.

Creer, T.L. (1987). Living with asthma: Replications and extensions. *Health Education Quarterly, 14*: 319–31.

Creer, T.L., Wigal, J.S., Tobin, D.L. *et al.* (1986a). *Asthma Attitude Scale for Adults*. Athens, OH: Self Management Systems.

Creer, T.L., Tobin, D.L., Wigal, J.S. and Winder, J.A.

(1986b). *Revised Problem Behaviour Checklist*. Athens, OH: Self Management Systems.

Criteria Committee of the New York Heart Association (1964). *Nomenclature and Criteria for Diagnosis of Disease of the Heart and Blood Vessels*, 6th edn. Boston, MA: Little, Brown and Co.

Cronbach, L.J. (1951). Coefficient alpha and the internal structure of tests. *Psychometrika, 22*: 293–6.

Cronbach, L.J., Glaser, G., Nada, H. and Rajaratnam, R. (1972). The Dependability of Behavioral Measurements: Theory of generalisability for scores and profiles. New York: John Wiley.

Croog, S.H. and Levine, S. (1977). *The Heart Patient Recovers*. New York: Human Sciences Press.

Croog, S.H. and Levine, S. (1982). *Life after a Heart Attack: Social and Psychological Factors Eight Years Later*. New York: Human Sciences Press.

Croog, S.H., Levine, S., Testa, M.A. *et al.* (1986). The effects of antihypertensive therapy on quality of life. *New England Journal of Medicine, 314*: 1657–64.

Croog, S.H., Kong, W., Levine, S. *et al.* (1990). Hypertensive black men and women: Quality of life and effects of anti-hypertensive medications. *Archives of Internal Medicine, 150*: 1733–41.

Crosby, C. (1990). *Evaluation of the CLWYD Mental Health Community Service: Interim Report*. Bangor: Health Services Research Unit, University College of North Wales.

Crosby, C. (1991). *Evaluation of the CLWYD Mental Health Community Service: Community Care – Initial Findings – 6 Weeks After Discharge from North Wales Hospital*. Bangor: Health Services Research Unit, University College of North Wales.

Crosby, C., Barry, M., Fitzgerald Carter, M. and Lowe, C.F. (1993). Psychiatric rehabilitation and community care: Resettlement from a North Wales Hospital. *Health and Social Care, 1*: 355–63.

Crown, S. and Crown, J.M. (1973). Personality in early rheumatoid disease. *Journal of Psychosomatic Research, 17*: 189–97.

Crowne, D. and Marlowe, D. (1960). A new scale of social desirability independent of psycho-pathology. *Journal of Consulting Psychology, 24*: 349–54.

Curb, J.D., Borhani, N.O., Blaszkanski, T.P. *et al.* (1985). Long term surveillance for adverse effects of antihypertensive drugs. *Journal of the American Medical Association, 253*: 3263–8.

Curbow, B., Somerfield, M., Legro, M. and Sonnega, J. (1990). Self concept and cancer in adults: Theoretical and methodological issues. *Social Science and Medicine, 31*: 115–28.

Currer, C. and Stacey, M. (1986). *Concepts of Health, Illness and Disease*. Leamington Spa: Berg.

Dahlstrom, W.D. and Welsh, G.S. (1960). *An MMPI Handbook: A Guide to Use in Clinical Practice and*

Research. Minneapolis, MN: University of Minnesota Press.

Dahlstrom, W.D., Welsh, G.S. and Dahlstrom, L.E. (1972). *An MMPI handbook: Clinical Interpretation*, Vol. I, revised edn. Minneapolis, MN: University of Minnesota Press.

Dalkey, N.C. (1972). *Studies in the Quality of Life*. Lexington, MA: Lexington Books.

Danchin, N., Brengard, A., Ethevenot, G. *et al.* (1988). Ten year follow-up of patients with single vessel coronary artery disease that was suitable for percutaneous transluminal coronary angioplasty. *British Heart Journal, 59*: 275–9.

Davies, A.R. and Ware, J.E. (1981). *Measuring Health Perceptions in the Health Insurance Experiment*. Publication No. R-2711-HHS. Santa Monica, CA: Rand Corporation.

Davies, A.R. and Ware, J.E. (1991). *GHAA'S Consumer Satisfaction Survey and User's Manual*. Washington, DC: Group Health Association of America.

Davies, A.R., Sherbourne, C.D., Peterson, J.R. and Ware J.E. (1988). *Scoring Manual: Adult Health Status and Patient Satisfaction Measures Used in RAND's Health Insurance Experiment*. Publication No. N-2190-HHS. Santa Monica, CA: Rand Corporation.

Davies, B., Burrows, G. and Poynton, C.A. (1975). Comparative study of four depression rating scales. *Australian and New Zealand Journal of Psychiatry, 9*: 21–4.

Davis, F. (1963). *Passage Through Crisis: Polio Victims and Their Families*. Indianapolis, IN: Bobbs-Merrill.

Davis, M.Z. (1973). *Living with Multiple Sclerosis: A Social Psychological Analysis*. Springfield, IL: C.C. Thomas.

Day, A.T. (1991). *Remarkable Survivors: Insights into Successful Aging Among Women*. Washington, DC: Urban Institute Press.

Dayson, D., Durham, F., Oerton, J. and Wills, W. (1990). Assessing social behaviour – whose perspective? In: *Better Out Than In? Report of the 5th Annual Conference of the Team for the Assessment of Psychiatric Services*. London: North East Thames Regional Health Authority.

Dayson, D., Gooch, C. and Thornicroft, G. (1992). Difficult to place, long term psychiatric patients: Risk factors for failure to resettle long stay patients in community facilities. *British Medical Journal, 305*: 993–5.

de Bruin, A.F., Diederiks, J.P.M., de Witte, I.P. and Stevens, F.C.J. (1993). The first testing of the SIP-68, a short generic version of the Sickness Impact Profile. Paper presented to the *Fifth European Health Services Research Conference*, Maastricht, December.

de Haes, J.C.J.M. and van Knippenberg, F.C.E. (1985). The quality of life of cancer patients: A review of the literature. *Social Science and Medicine, 20*: 809–17.

de Haes, J.C.J.M. and van Knippenberg, F.C.E. (1987). Quality of life of cancer patients: Review of the literature. In: N.K. Aaronson and J.H. Beckmann (eds), *The Quality of Life of the Cancer Patient*. New York: Raven Press.

de Haes, J.C.J.M. and Welvaart, K. (1985). Quality of life after breast cancer surgery. *Journal of Surgery and Oncology, 28*: 123–5.

de Haes, J.C.J.M., Pruyn, J.F.A. and van Knippenberg, F.C.E. (1983). Klachtenlijst voor Kankerpatienten, eerste ervaringen. *Nederlands Tijdschrift Psychol. 38*: 403.

de Haes, J.C.J.M., van Ostrom, M.A. and Welvaart, K. (1986). The effect of radical and conserving surgery on the quality of life of early breast cancer patients. *European Journal of Surgical Oncology, 12*: 337–42.

de Haes, J.C.J.M., Pennink, B.J.W. and Welvaart, K. (1987a). The distinction between affect and cognition. *Social Indicators Research, 19*: 367–78.

de Haes, J.C.J.M., Raatgever, J.W., van der Burg, M.E.L. *et al.* (1987b). Evaluation of the quality of life of patients with advanced ovarian cancer treated with combination therapy. In: N.K. Aaronson and J. Beckman (eds), *The Quality of Life of Cancer Patients*. New York: Raven Press.

de Haes, J.C.J.M., van Knippenberg, F.C. and Neijt, J.P. (1990). Measuring psychological and physical distress in cancer patients: Structure and application of the Rotterdam Symptom Checklist. *British Journal of Cancer, 62*: 1034–8.

de Haes, J.C.J.M., de Ruiter, J.H., Tempelaar, R. and Pennink, B.J.W. (1992). The distinction between affect and cognition in the quality of life of cancer patients – sensitivity and stability. *Quality of Life Research, 1*: 315–22.

Demeurisse, G., Demol, O. and Robaye, E. (1980). Motor evaluation in vascular hemiplegia. *European Neurology, 19*: 382–9.

Deniston, O.L. and Jette, A.M. (1980). A functional status assessment instrument: Validation in an elderly population. *Health Services Research, 15*: 21–34.

Department of Health (1992). *Assessing the Effects of Health Technologies: Principles, Practice, Proposals*. Advisory Group on Health Technology Assessment. London: HMSO.

Department of Health and Social Security (1989). *Caring for People*. London: Department of Health and Social Security.

Derogatis, L.R. (1977). *Psychosocial Adjustment to Illness Scale (PAIS and PAIS-SR): Scoring, Procedures and Administration I*. Baltimore, MD: Clinical Psychometric Research.

Derogatis, L.R. (1986). The Psychological Adjustment to Illness Scale (PAIS). *Journal of Psychosomatic Research, 30*: 77–91.

Derogatis, L.R. (1993a). *BSI – Brief Symptom Inventory: Administration, Scoring and Procedures Manual.* Minneapolis, MN: National Computer Systems.

Derogatis, L.R. (1993b). *SCL-90-R: Bibliography.* Minneapolis, MN: National Computer Systems.

Derogatis, L.R. (1993c). *BSI Bibliography.* Minneapolis, MN: National Computer Systems.

Derogatis, L.R. and Cleary, P.A. (1977). Confirmation of the dimensional structure of the SCL-90-R: A study in construct validation. *Journal of Clinical Psychology, 33*: 981–9.

Derogatis, L.R. and Lopez, M. (1983). *PAIS and PAIS-SR: Administration, Scoring and Procedures Manual I.* Baltimore, MD: Clinical Psychometric Research.

Derogatis, L.R. and Spencer. P.M. (1982). *The Brief Symptom Inventory (BSI): Administration, Scoring and Procedures Manual I.* Baltimore, MD: Johns Hopkins University Press.

Derogatis, L.R. and Spencer, P.M. (1984). *Administration and Procedures: BSI Manual I.* Baltimore, MD: Johns Hopkins University Press.

Derogatis, L.R., Lipman, R.S., Covi, L. et al. (1971). Neurotic symptom dimensions. *Archives of General Psychiatry, 24*: 454–64.

Derogatis, L.R., Lipman, R.S., Rickels, K. et al. (1974a). The Hopkins Symptom Checklist (HSCL): A self report symptom inventory. *Behavioural Science, 19*: 1–15.

Derogatis, L.R., Lipman, R.S. and Covi, L. (1974b). SCL-90: An outpatient psychiatric rating scale – preliminary report. *Psychopharmacology Bulletin, 9*: 13–28.

Derogatis, L.R., Rickels, K. and Rock, A. (1976). The SCL-90 and the MMPI: A step in validation of a new self-report scale. *British Journal of Psychiatry, 128*: 280–9.

Derogatis, L.R., Rickels, K. and Rock, A. (1977). *The SCL-90-R: Administration, Scoring and Procedures Manual, I.* Baltimore, MD: Clinical Psychometric Research.

Derogatis, L.R., Akeloff, M.D. and Melisaratos, N. (1979). Psychological coping mechanisms and survival time in breast cancer. *Journal of the American Medical Association, 242*: 1504–9.

Devlen, J.L. (1987). The psychological and social consequences of Hodgkin's disease and its treatment. In: P. Selby and T.J. McElwain (eds), *Hodgkin's Disease.* Oxford: Blackwell Scientific.

Dewey, M.E. and Copeland, J.R.M. (1986). Computerised psychiatric diagnosis in the elderly: AGECAT. *Journal of Microcomputer Applications, 9*: 135–40.

Deyo, R.A. (1984a). Pitfalls in measuring the health status of Mexican Americans: Comparative validity of the English and Spanish Sickness Impact Profile. *American Journal of Public Health, 74*: 569–73.

Deyo, R.A. (1984b). Measuring functional outcomes in therapeutic trials for chronic disease. *Controlled Clinical Trials, 5*: 223–40.

Deyo, R.A. (1993). Measuring the quality of life of patients with rheumatoid arthritis. In: S.R. Walker and R.M. Rosser (eds), *Quality of Life Assessment: Key Issues in the 1990s.* Dordrecht: Kluwer Academic.

Deyo, R.A. and Diehl, A. (1983). Measuring physical and psychosocial function in patients with low back pain. *Spine, 8*: 635–42.

Deyo, R.A., Inui, T.S., Leininger, J.D. et al. (1982).' Physical and psychological functioning in rheumatoid arthritis: Clinical use of a self-administered instrument. *Archives of Internal Medicine, 142*: 879–82.

Deyo, R.A., Inui, T.S., Leininger, J.D. et al. (1983). Measuring functional outcomes in chronic disease: A comparison of traditional scales and a self-administered health status questionnaire in patients with rheumatoid arthritis. *Medical Care, 21*: 180–92.

Dhillon, R., Palmer, B., Pittam, B. and Shaw, H. (1982). Rehabilitation after major head and neck surgery – the patient's view. *Clinics in Orolaryngology, 7*: 319–24.

D'Houtard, A. and Field, M.G. (1984). The image of health: Variations in perception by social class in a French population. *Sociology of Health and Illness, 6*: 30–60.

D'Houtard, A., Field, M.G., Tax, B. and Gueguen, R. (1990). Representations of health in two Western European populations. *International Journal of Health Sciences, 1–4*: 243–55.

Diabetes Control and Complications Trial Research Group (1988). Reliability and validity of a diabetes quality of life measure for the diabetes control and complications trial (DCCT). *Diabetes Care, 11*: 725–32.

Dick, J.P.R., Guiloff, R.J., Stewart, A., Blackstock, J. et al. (1984). Mini-Mental State Examination in neurological patients. *Journal of Neurology, Neurosurgery and Psychiatry, 47*: 496–8.

Dickinson, E. (1993). Developing a consensus for the assessment of elderly people – the SAFE (Standardised Assessment for the Elderly) multi-centre project. *Journal of Interprofessional Care, 7*: 67–70.

Dickson, J.S. and Bird, H.A. (1981). Reproducibility along a 10 cm vertical visual analogue scale. *Annals of Rheumatic Diseases, 40*: 87–9.

Dodrill, C.B. (1978). A neuropsychological battery for epilepsy. *Epilepsia, 19*: 611–23.

Dodrill, C.B. and Wilensky, A.J. (1990). Intellectual impairment as an outcome of status epilepticus. *Neurology, 40*: 23–7.

Dodrill, C.B., Batzel, L.W., Queisser, H.R. and Temkin, N.R. (1980). An objective method for the assessment of psychological and social problems among epileptics. *Epilepsy, 21*; 123–35.

Dohrenwend, B.S., Krasnoff, L., Askenasy, A.R. and Dohrenwend, B.P. (1978). Exemplification of a method for scaling life events: The PERI life events scale. *Journal of Health and Social Behaviour, 19*: 205–29.

Dohrenwend, B.S., Cook, D. and Dohrenwend, B.P. (1981). Measurement of social functioning in community populations. In: J.K. Wing, P. Bebbington and L. Robbins (eds), *What is a Case? The Problem of Definition in Community Surveys*. London: Grant McIntyre.

Dolan, P., Gudex, C., Kind, P. and Williams, A. (1993). The valuation of health states: A comparison of methods. Paper presented at the *Fifth European Health Services Research Conference*, Maastricht, December.

Donabedian, A. (1985). *Explorations in Quality Assessment and Monitoring*, Vols 1–3. Ann Arbor, MI: Health Administration Press.

Donovan, K., Sanson-Fisher, R.W. and Redman, S. (1989). Measuring quality of life in cancer patients. *Journal of Clinical Oncology, 7*: 959–68.

Downing, R.W. and Rickels, K. (1972). Some properties of the Popoff Index. *Clinical Medicine, 79*: 11–18.

Drummond, N., Abdalla, M., Buckingham, J.K. *et al.* (1994). Integrated care for asthma: A clinical, social and economic evaluation. *British Medical Journal, 308*: 559–64.

Dubos, R. (1959). *Mirage of Health: Utopias, Progress and Biological Change*. New York: Harper.

Dubuisson, D. and Melzack, R. (1976). Classification of clinical pain descriptions by multiple group discriminant analysis. *Experimental Neurology, 51*: 480–7.

Dudley, D.L., Glaser, E.M., Jorgenson, B.N. and Logan, D.L. (1980). Psychosocial concomitants to rehabilitation in chronic obstructive pulmonary disease. Part 1: Psychosocial and psychological considerations. *Chest, 77*: 413–20.

Dunbar, G.C., Stoker, M.J., Hodges, T.C.P. and Beaumont, G. (1992). The development of SBQOL: A unique scale for measuring quality of life. *British Journal of Health Economics, 2*: 65–74.

Duncan, J.S. and Sander, J.W.A.S. (1991). The Chalfont Seizure Severity Scale. *Journal of Neurology, Neurosurgery and Psychiatry, 54*: 873–6.

Dunn, M., O'Driscoll, C., Dayson, D. *et al.* (1990). The TAPS project, 4: An observational study of the social life of long stay patients. *British Journal of Psychiatry, 157*: 842–8.

Dunnell, K. and Cartwright, A. (1972). *Medicine Takers, Prescribers and Hoarders*. London: Routledge and Kegan Paul.

Dupuy, H.J. (1973). *Developmental Rationale, Substantive, Derivatable, and Conceptual Relevance of the General Well-Being Schedule*. Fairfax, VA: National Center for Health Statistics.

Dupy, H.J. (1974) Utility of the National Center for Health Statistics' General Well-Being Schedule in the Assessment of Self-Representations of Subjective Well-Being and Distress. In *Report of The National Conference on Evaluation in Alcohol, Drug Abuse and Mental Health Programs*. Washington DC: ADA MHA.

Dupuy, H.J. (1978). Self representations of general psychological well-being of American adults. Paper presented to the *American Public Health Association Meeting*, Los Angeles. CA, October.

Dupuy, H.J. (1984). The Psychological General Well-being Index. In: N.K. Wenger, M.E. Mattson, C.P. Furberg and J. Elinson (eds), *Assessment of Quality of Life in Clinical Trials of Cardiovascular Therapies*. New York: Le Jacq.

Durnin, J.G.V.A. and Passmore, R. (1967). *Energy, Work and Leisure*. London: Heinemann.

Dworkin, R.J. (1992). *Researching Persons with Mental Illness*. Newbury Park, CA: Sage.

Dye, C.J. (1982). Intellectual functioning. In: D.A. Mangen and W.A. Peterson (eds), *Clinical and Social Psychology, Vol. I. Research Instruments in Social Gerontology*. Minneapolis, MN: University of Minnesota Press.

Eakin, E.G., Kaplan, R.M. and Ries, A.L. (1993). Measurement of dyspnoea in chronic obstructive pulmonary disease. *Quality of Life Research, 2*: 181–91.

Early Breast Cancer Trialists' Collaborative Group (1992). Systemic treatment of early breast cancer by hormonal, cytotoxic, or immune therapy: 133 trials involving 31,000 recurrences and 24,000 deaths among 75,000 women. *Lancet, 339*: 71–85.

Eaton, W.W. and Kessler, L.G. (1981). Rates of symptoms of depression in a national sample. *American Journal of Epidemiology, 114*: 528–38.

Ebbs, S.R., Fallowfield, L.J., Fraser, S.C.A. and Baum, M. (1989). Treatment outcomes and quality of life. *International Journal of Technology Assessment in Health Care, 5*: 391–400.

Ebel, R.L. (1951). Estimation of the reliability of ratings. *Psychmetrica, 16*: 407–24.

Ebmeier, K.P., Beson, J.A.O., Eagles, J.N. *et al.* (1988). Continuing care of the demented elderly in Inverurie. *Health Bulletin, 46*: 32–41.

Ebrahim, S., Nouri, F. and Barer, D. (1985). Measuring disability after stroke. *Journal of Epidemiology and Community Health, 39*: 86–9.

Ebrahim, S., Barer, D. and Nouri, F. (1986). Use of the Nottingham Health Profile with patients after stroke. *Journal of Epidemiology and Community Health, 40*: 166–9.

Edelstyn, G.A., MacRae, K.D. and MacDonald, F.M. (1979). Improvements of life quality in cancer patients undergoing chemotherapy. *Clinical Oncology, 5*: 43–9.

Edlund, M. and Tancredi, L.R. (1985). Quality of life:

An ideological critique. *Perspectives in Biological Medicine, 28*: 591–607.

Edwards, D.W., Yarvis, R.M., Mueller, D.P. *et al.* (1978). Test-taking and the stability of adjustment scales: Can we assess patient deterioration? *Evaluation Quarterly, 2*: 278–91.

Eisen, M., Donald, C.A., Ware, J.E. and Brook, R.A. (1980). Conceptual measurement of health for children in the Health Insurance Study. R-2313-HEW. Santa Monica, CA: Rand Corporation.

Elbert, J.C. and Holden, E.W. (1985). Wechsler Preschool and Primary Scale of Intelligence. In: D.J. Keyser and R.C. Sweetland (eds), *Test Critiques*, Vol. III. Kansas City, MO: Test Corporation of America.

Elliot, C.D. (1983). *The British Ability Scales: Introductory Handbook, Technical Handbook and Manual for Administration and Scoring*. Windsor: NFER-Nelson.

Elster, J. and Roemer, J.E. (eds) (1993). *International Comparisons of Well-being*. Cambridge: Cambridge University Press.

Endicott, J. (1984). Measurement of depression in patients with cancer. *Cancer, 53*: 2243–8.

Endicott, J. and Spitzer, R.L. (1978). A diagnostic interview: The Schedule for Affective Disorders and Schizophrenia. *Archives of General Psychiatry, 35*: 837–44.

Endicott, J., Spitzer, R.L., Fleiss, J.L. and Cohen, J. (1976). The global assessment scales: A procedure for measuring overall severity of psychiatric disturbance. *Archives of General Psychiatry, 33*: 766–71.

Endler, N.S. and Parker, J.D.A. (1990). Multidimensional assessment of coping: a critical examination. *Journal of Personality and Social Psychology, 58*: 844–54.

Endler, N.S. and Parker, J.D.A. (1992). Towards a reliable and valid method for the multidimensional assessment of coping. Paper presented to the *Annual Meeting of the Canadian Psychological Association*, Quebec City, June.

Engblom, E., Hamalainen, H., Lind, J. *et al.* (1992). Quality of life during rehabilitation after coronary artery bypass surgery. *Quality of Life Research, 1*: 167–75.

Engel, J. (1987). Outcome with respect to epileptic seizures. In: J. Engel (ed.), *Surgical Treatment of the Epilepsies*. New York: Raven Press.

Erdman, R.A.M., Lorstman, L., van Domburg *et al.* (1993). Compliance with the medical regimen and partner's quality of life after heart transplantation. *Quality of Life Research, 2*: 205–12.

Etzioni, A. (1968). *The Active Society*. New York: Free Press.

EURIDISS (1990). European research on incapacitating diseases and social support. *International Journal of Health Sciences, 1*: 217–28.

European Coronary Surgery Study Group (1982). Long term results of prospective randomised study of coronary artery bypass surgery in stable angina pectoris. *Lancet, 2*: 1173–80.

European Organization for Research on Treatment of Cancer (EORTC) (1983). Quality of life: Methods of measurement and related areas. Proceedings of the *4th Workshop EORTC Study Group on Quality of Life*. Odense, Denmark: Odense University Hospital.

Euroqol Group (1990). Euroqol: A new facility for the measurement of health related quality of life. *Health Policy, 16*: 199–208.

Evans, D. and Cope, W. (1993). *The Quality of Life Questionnaire-D (QLQ-D)*. Tonawanda, NY: Multi-Health Systems.

Evans, R.W., Manninen, D.L., Overcaste, T.D. *et al.* (1984). *The National Heart Transplantation Study: Final Report*. Washington: Battelle Human Affairs Research Center.

Evans, R.W., Manninen, D.L., Garrison, L.P. *et al.* (1985). The quality of life of patients with end stage renal disease. *New England Journal of Medicine, 312*: 553–9.

Eysenck, H.J. (1976). *The Measurement of Personality*. Baltimore, MD: University Park Press.

Eysenck, H.J. and Eysenck, S.B.G. (1985). *Manual for the Eysenck Personality Questionnaire*. London: Hodder and Stoughton.

Fairbank, J.C.T., Cooper, J., Davies, J.B. and O'Brien, J.P. (1980). The Oswestry low back pain disability questionnaire. *Physiotherapy, 66*: 271–3.

Fallowfield, L.J. (1990). *The Quality of Life: The Missing Measurement in Health Care*. London: Souvenir Press.

Fallowfield, L.J. (1993). Quality of life measurement in breast cancer. *Journal of the Royal Society of Medicine, 86*: 10–12.

Fallowfield, L.J. and Hall, A. (1991). Psychosocial and sexual impact of diagnosis and treatment of breast cancer. *British Medical Bulletin, 47*: 388–99.

Fallowfield, L.J., Baum, M. and Maguire, G.P. (1986). Effects of breast conservation on psychological morbidity associated with diagnosis and treatment of early breast cancer. *British Medical Journal, 293*: 1331–4.

Fallowfield, L.J., Baum, M. and Maguire, G.P. (1987). Do psychological studies upset patients? *Journal of the Royal Society of Medicine, 80*: 59.

Fallowfield, L.J., Hall, A., Maguire, G.P. and Baum, M. (1990). Psychological outcomes of different treatment policies in women with early breast cancer outside a clinical trial. *British Medical Journal, 301*: 575–80.

Falotico-Taylor, J., McClellan, M. and Mosteller, F. (1989). The use of quality of life measures in technology assessment. In: F. Mosteller and J. Falotico-Taylor (eds), *Quality of Life and Technology Assessment*.

Monograph of the Council on Health Care Technology. Washington, DC: National Academy Press.

Fanshel, S. and Bush, J.W. (1970). A Health Status Index and its applications to health services outcome. *Operational Research, 18*: 1021–66.

Faris, J.A. and Stotts, N.A. (1990). The effect of percutaneous transluminal coronary angioplasty on quality of life. *Progress in Cardiovascular Nursing, 5*: 132–40.

Farquhar, M. (1995). Elderly people's definitions of quality of life. *Social Science and Medicine, 10*: 1439–46.

Fava, G.A. and Freyberger, H. (eds) (1990) Quality of life in the medically ill: A psychosomatic approach. *Psychotherapy and Psychosomatics, 54*: 57–179.

Fava, G.A., Kellner, R., Munari, F. and Pavan, L. (1982). The Hamilton Depression Rating Scale in normals and depressives. *Acta Psychiatrica Scandinavica, 66*: 26–32.

Fayers, P.M. and Jones, D.R. (1983). Measuring and analysing quality of life in cancer clinical trials: A review. *Statistics in Medicine, 2*: 429–46.

Fays-Dunne, N. and Willner, A.E. (1989). Changes in psychometric test scores after cardiac surgery. In: A. Willner and G. Rodewald (eds), *Impact of Cardiac Surgery on Quality of Life: Neurological and Psychological Aspects*. New York: Plenum Press.

Fazio, A.F. (1977). *A Concurrent Validation Study of the NCHS General Well-Being Schedule*. Hyattsville, MD: US Department of Health, Education and Welfare, National Center for Health Statistics: Vital and Health Statistics Series 2, No. 73. DHEW Publication No. (HRA) 78–1347.

Feeny, D., Barr, R.D., Furlong, W. *et al.* (1991). Quality of life of the treatment process in pediatric oncology: An approach to measurement. In: D. Osoba (ed.), *Effect of Cancer on Quality of Life*. Boston, MA: CRC Press.

Feighner, J.P., Robins, E., Guze, S.B. *et al.* (1972). Diagnostic criteria for use in psychiatric research. *Archives of General Psychiatry, 26*: 57–63.

Feinstein, A.R., Josephy, B.R. and Carolyn, K. (1986). Scientific and clinical problems in indexes of functional disability. *Annals of Internal Medicine, 105*: 413–20.

Feinstein, A.R., Fisher, M.B. and Pigeon, J.G. (1989). Changes in dyspnoea–fatigue ratings as indicators of quality of life in the treatment of congestive heart failure. *American Journal of Cardiology, 64*: 50–5.

Felson, D.T., Anderson, J.J., Boers, M. *et al.* (1993). The American College of Rheumatology core set of disease activity measures for rheumatoid arthritis clinical trials. *Arthritis and Rheumatism, 36*: 729–39.

Felton, B.J. and Revenson, T.A. (1984). Coping with chronic illness: A study of illness controllability and the influence of coping strategies on psychological adjustment. *Journal of Consulting and Clinical Psychology, 52*: 343–53.

Felton, B.J., Revenson, J.A. and Hinrichsen, G.A. (1984). Stress and coping in the explanation of psychological adjustment among chronically ill adults. *Social Science and Medicine, 18*: 889–98.

Fendrich, M., Weissman, M.M. and Warner, V. (1990). Screening for depressive disorder in children and adolescents: Validating the Center for Epidemiologic Studies Depression Scale for Children. *American Journal of Epidemiology, 131*: 538–51.

Fentiman, I.S., Tirelli, U., Monfardini, S. *et al.* (1990). Cancer in the elderly: Why so badly treated? *Lancet, 335*: 1020–2.

Fergusson, R.J. and Cull, A. (1991). Quality of life measurements for patients undergoing treatment for lung cancer. *Thorax, 46*: 671–5.

Ferrans, C.E. and Ferrell, B.R. (1990). Development of a quality of life index for patients with cancer. *Oncology Nursing Forum, 17*: 15–19 (suppl.).

Ferrans, C.E. and Powers, M.J. (1985). Quality of Life Index: Development and psychometric properties. *Advances in Nursing Science, 8*: 15–24.

Ferrell, B. (1990). Development of a quality of life index for patients with cancer: Critique of the study. *Oncology Nursing Forum, 17*: 20–1 (suppl.).

Ferrell, B., Wisdom, C., Wenzl, C. and Brown, J. (1989). Effects of controlled-release morphine on quality of life for cancer pain. *Oncology Nursing Forum, 16*: 521–6.

Ferrell, B., Grant, M., Schmidt, G. *et al.* (1992a). The meaning of quality of life for bone marrow transplant survivors: Part I. The impact of BMT on QOL. *Cancer Nursing, 15*: 153–60.

Ferrell, B., Grant, M., Schmidt, G. *et al.* (1992b). The meaning of quality of life for bone marrow transplant survivors: Part II. Improving QOL for BMT survivors. *Cancer Nursing, 15*: 247–53.

Fillenbaum, G.G. (1978). *Multidimensional Functional Assessment: The OARS Methodology – A Manual*, 2nd edn. Durham, NC: Center for the Study of Aging and Human Development, Duke University.

Fillenbaum, G.G. (1980). Comparison of two brief tests of organic brain impairment: The MSQ and the Short Portable MSQ. *Journal of the American Geriatrics Society, 28*: 381–4.

Fillenbaum, G.G. and Smyer, M.A. (1981). The development, validity and reliability of the OARS Multidimensional Functional Assessment Questionnaire. *Journal of Gerontology, 36*: 428–34.

Findlay-Jones, R.A. and Murphy, E. (1979). Severity of psychiatric disorder and the 30-item General Health Questionnaire. *British Journal of Psychiatry, 134*: 609–16.

Finkelstein, D.M., Cassileth, B.R., Bonomi, P.D. *et al.*

(1988). A pilot study of the Functional Living Index–Cancer (FLIC) Scale for the assessment of quality of life for metastatic lung cancer patients. *American Journal of Clinical Oncology*, 11: 630–3.

Finlay, A.Y. and Kelly, S.E. (1987). Psoriasis: An index of disability. *Clinics in Experimental Dermatology*, 12: 8–11.

Fischl, M.A., Richmann, D.D., Grieco, M.H. *et al.* (1987). The efficacy of azidothymidine (AZT) in the treatment of patients with AIDS and AIDS related complex: A double blind, placebo controlled trial. *New England Journal of Medicine*, 317: 185–91.

Fischl, M.A., Richmann, D.D., Hansen, N. *et al.* (1990). The safety and efficacy of zidovudine (AZT) in the treatment of subjects with mildly symptomatic human immunodeficiency virus type 1 (HIV) infection. A double-blind placebo-controlled trial. The AIDS Clinical Trials Group. *Annals of Internal Medicine*, 112: 727–37.

Fishman, D.B. and Petty, T.L. (1971). Physical, symptomatic and psychological improvement in patients receiving comprehensive care for chronic airway obstruction. *Journal of Chronic Diseases*, 24: 775–85.

Fiske, D.W. (1974). The use of significant others in assessing the outcome of psychotherapy. In: I. Waskow and M. Parloff (eds), *Psychotherapy Change Measures*. Rockville, MD: National Institute of Mental Health.

Fitts, W. (1965). *Tennessee Self Concept Scale Manual*. Nashville, TN: Counselor Recordings and Tests.

Fitzgerald, J.M. and Hargreave, F.E. (1990). Acute asthma: Emergency department management and prospective evaluation of outcome. *Canadian Medical Association Journal*, 142: 591–5.

Fitzpatrick, R. (1990). Measurement of patient satisfaction: Measuring the outcomes of medical care. In: A. Hopkins and D. Costain (eds), *Measuring the Outcomes of Medical Care*. London: Royal College of Physicians.

Fitzpatrick, R., Newman, S., Lamb, R. and Shipley, M. (1988). Social relationships and psychological well-being in rheumatoid arthritis. *Social Science and Medicine*, 27: 399–403.

Fitzpatrick, R., Newman, S., Lamb, R. and Shipley, M. (1990). Helplessness and control in rheumatoid arthritis. *International Journal of Health Sciences*, 1: 17–23.

Fitzpatrick, R., Ziebland, S., Jenkinson, C. and Mowat, A. (1992). A generic health status instrument in the assessment of rheumatoid arthritis. *British Journal of Rheumatology*, 31: 87–90.

Flax, M.J. (1972). *A Study in Comparative Urban Indicators: Conditions in 18 Large Metropolitan Areas*. Washington, DC: The Urban Institute.

Fleiss, J.L. (1981a). *Statistical Methods for Rates and Proportions*, 2nd edn. New York: John Wiley.

Fleiss, J.L. (1981b). The measurement of inter-rater agreement. In: J.L. Fleiss, *Statistical Methods for Rates and Proportions*. New York: John Wiley.

Fleiss, J.L. (1986). *The Design and Analysis of Clinical Experiments*. New York: John Wiley.

Fletcher, A.E. and Bulpitt, C.J. (1989). Quality of life during antihypertensive treatment: Results from a randomised double-blind trial of pinacidil and nifedipine. *Journal of Hypertension*, 7: S364 (suppl. 6).

Fletcher, A.E. and Bulpitt, C.J. (1993). Measuring quality of life in hypertension. In: S.R. Walker and R.M. Rosser (eds), *Quality of Life Assessment: Key Issues in the 1990s*. Dordrecht: Kluwer Academic.

Fletcher, A.E., Hunt, B. and Bulpitt, C.J. (1987). Evaluation of quality of life in clinical trials of cardiovascular disease. *Journal of Chronic Diseases*, 40: 557–66.

Fletcher, A.E., Dickinson, E. and Philp, I. (1992a). Review: Audit measures – quality of life instruments for everyday use with elderly patients. *Age and Ageing*, 21: 142–50.

Fletcher, A.E., Gore, S., Jones, D. *et al.* (1992b). Quality of life measures in health care. II. Design, analysis, and interpretation. *British Medical Journal*, 305: 1145–8.

Fletcher, C.M. (1952). The clinical diagnosis of pulmonary emphysema – an experimental study. *Proceedings of the Royal Society of Medicine*, 45: 577–84.

Fletcher, C.M., Elmes, P.C., Fairbairn, A.S. and Wood, C.H. (1959). The significance of respiratory symptoms and the diagnosis of chronic bronchitis in a working population. *British Medical Journal*, 2: 257–66.

Fletcher, C.M., Peto, R., Tinker, C. and Speizer, F.E. (1976). *The Natural History of Chronic Bronchitis and Emphysema*. Oxford: Oxford University Press.

Fobair, P.A. (1987). The adaptation process in surviving cancer. In: *Proceedings of the Fifth National Conference on Human Values and Cancer*. American Cancer Society, San Francisco, March 19–21.

Fobair, P., Hoppe, R.T., Bloom, J. *et al.* (1986). Psychosocial problems among survivors of Hodgkin's disease. *Journal of Clinical Oncology*, 4: 805–14.

Folkman, S. and Lazarus, R.S. (1980). An analysis of coping in a middle aged community sample. *Journal of Health and Social Behaviour*, 21: 219–39.

Folkman, S. and Lazarus, R.S. (1985). If it changes it must be a process: Study of emotion and coping during three stages of college examination. *Journal of Personality and Social Psychology*, 48: 150–70.

Folkman, S. and Lazarus, R.S. (1986). Stress processes and depressive symptomatology. *Journal of Abnormal Psychology*, 95: 107–13.

Folkman, S. and Lazarus, R.S. (1988a). *Manual of the Ways of Coping Questionnaire*. Palo Alto, CA: Consulting Psychologists Press.

Folkman, S. and Lazarus, R.S. (1988b). Coping as a

mediator of emotion. *Journal of Personality and Social Psychology, 54*: 466–75.

Folkman, S., Lazarus, R.S., Gruen, R.J. and DeLongis, A. (1986a). Appraisal, coping, health status and psychological symptoms. *Journal of Personality and Social Psychology, 50*: 571–9.

Folkman, S., Lazarus, R.S., Dunkel-Schetter, C. *et al.* (1986b). Dynamics of a stressful encounter: Cognitive appraisal, coping and encounter outcomes. *Journal of Personality and Social Psychology, 50*: 992–1003.

Folks, D.G., Blake, D.J., Fleece, L. *et al.* (1986). Quality of life six months after coronary artery bypass surgery: A preliminary report. *Southern Medical Journal, 79*: 397–9.

Folsom, T. and Popkin, M. (1987). Current and future perspectives on psychiatric involvement in bone marrow transplantations. *Psychiatric Medicine, 4*: 319–28.

Folstein, M.F., Folstein, S.E. and McHugh, P.R. (1975). 'Mini-Mental State': A practical method for grading the cognitive state of patients for the clinician. *Journal of Psychiatric Research, 12*: 189–98.

Foltz, A.T. (1987). The influence of cancer on self-concept and life quality. *Seminars Oncology Nursing, 3*: 303–12.

Ford, D.E., Anthony, J.C., Nestadt, G.R. and Romanoski, A.J. (1989). The General Health Questionnaire by interview: Performance in relation to recent use of health services. *Medical Care, 27*: 367–75.

Forsberg, C. and Bjorvell, H. (1993). Swedish population norms for the GHRI, HI and STAI-state. *Quality of Life Research, 2*: 349–56.

Fortinsky, R.H., Granger, C.V. and Seltzer, G.B. (1981). The use of functional assessment in understanding home care needs. *Medical Care, 19*: 489–97.

Fowlie, M. and Berkeley, J. (1987). Quality of life – a review of the literature. *Family Practice, 4*: 226–34.

Frank, E. and Kupfer, D.J. (1976). In every marriage there are two marriages. *Journal of Sex Therapy, 2*: 137–43.

Frank, E. and Kupfer, D.J. (undated). The KDS-15: A marital questionnaire. Pittsburgh, PA: University of Pittsburgh, Pitts-Western Psychiatric Institute and Clinic.

Frank, J.D., Gliedman, L.H., Imber, S.D. *et al.* (1957). Why patients leave psychotherapy. *Archives of Neurology and Psychiatry, 77*: 283–99.

Frank, R.G., Beek, N.C., Parker, J.C. *et al.* (1988). Depression in rheumatoid arthritis. *Journal of Rheumatology, 15*: 920–5.

Fraser, S.C.A., Ebbs, S.R., Dobbs, H.J. *et al.* (1990). The design of advanced breast cancer trials. *Acta Oncology, 29*: 397–400.

Frater, A. (1992). Health outcomes: A challenge to the *status quo. Quality in Health Care, 1*: 87–8.

Frayn, M. (1991). *A Landing on the Sun*. London: Viking.

Fredriksson, T. and Pettersson, U. (1978). Severe psoriasis – oral therapy with a new retinoid. *Dermatologica, 157*: 238–44.

Freemantle, N., Pollock, T.A., Sheldon, T.A. *et al.* (1992). Formal rehabilitation after stroke. *Quality in Health Care, 1*: 134–7.

Freemantle, N., Long, A., Mason, J. *et al.* (1993). The treatment of depression in primary care. *Effective Health Care, 5* (whole issue).

Fridlund, B., Hogstedt, B., Lidell, E. and Larsson, P.A. (1991). Recovery after myocardial infarction: Effects of a caring rehabilitation programme. *Scandinavian Journal of Caring Science, 5*: 23–32.

Fries, J.F. (1983). The assessment of disability from first to future principles. Paper presented to the *Conference on Advances in Assessing Arthritis*. The London Hospital, March.

Fries, J.F., Hess, E.V. and Klinenberg, J. (1974). A standard database for rheumatic disease. *Arthritis and Rheumatism, 17*: 327–36.

Fries, J.F., Spitz, P.W., Kraines, R.G. and Holman, H.R. (1980). Measurement of patient outcome in arthritis. *Arthritis and Rheumatism, 23*: 137–45.

Fries, J.F., Spitz, P.W. and Young, D.Y. (1982). The dimensions of health outcomes: The Health Assessment Questionnaire, disability and pain scales. *Journal of Rheumatology, 9*: 789–93.

Furberg, C.D., Schuker, B., Chesney, M.A. *et al.* (1984). Report of the Working Group: Mild hypertension. In: N.K. Wenger, M.E. Mattson, C.P. Furberg and J. Elinson (eds), *Assessment of Quality of Life in Clinical Trials of Cardiovascular Therapies*. New York: Le Jacq.

Gallagher, D., Nies, G. and Thompson, L.W. (1982). Reliability of the Beck Depression Inventory with older adults. *Journal of Consulting and Clinical Psychology, 50*: 152–3.

Gallup, G.H. (1976). Human needs and satisfaction: A global survey. *Public Opinion Quarterly, 40*: 459–67.

Ganster, C.D. and Victor, B. (1988). The impact of social support on mental and physical health. *British Journal of Medical Psychology, 61*: 17–36.

Ganz, P.A., Rofessart, J., Polinsky, M.L., Schag, C.A.C. and Heinrich, R.L. (1986). A comprehensive approach to the assessment of cancer patients' rehabilitation needs: The Cancer Inventory of Problem Situations and a companion interview. *Journal of Psychosocial Oncology, 4*: 27–42.

Ganz, P.A., Schag, C.A.C., Polinsky, M.L. *et al.* (1988a). Rehabilitation needs and breast cancer: The first month after primary therapy. *Breast Cancer Research and Treatment, 10*: 243–53.

Ganz, P.A., Haskell, C.M., Figlin, R.A. *et al.* (1988b). Estimating the quality of life in a clinical trial of patients with metastatic lung cancer using the Karnofsky Performance Status and the Functional Living Index – Cancer. *Cancer, 61*: 849–56.

Ganz, P.A., Polinsky, M.L., Schag, C.A.C. and Heinrich, R.L. (1989). Rehabilitation of patients with primary breast cancer: Assessing the impact of adjuvant therapy. *Recent Results in Cancer Research, 115*: 244–54.

Ganz, P.A., Schag, C.A.C., Cheng, H.L. (1990). Assessing the quality of life – a study in newly diagnosed breast cancer patients. *Journal of Clinical Epidemiology, 43*: 75–86.

Ganz, P.A., Schag, C.A.C., Lee, J.J. and Sim, M.S. (1992). The CARES: A generic measure of health related quality of life for patients with cancer. *Quality of Life Research, 1*: 19–29.

Ganz, P.A., Schag, C.A.C., Kahn, B. *et al.* (1993). Describing the health related quality of life impact of HIV infection: Findings from a study using the HIV Overview of Problems–Evaluation System (HOPES). *Quality of Life Research, 2*: 109–19.

Garber, C.E., Carleton, R.A. and Heller, G.V. (1992). Comparison of the 'Rose Questionnaire Angina' to exercise thallium scintigraphy: Different findings in males and females. *Journal of Clinical Epidemiology, 45*: 715–20.

Garratt, A.M., Macdonald, L.M., Ruta, D.A. *et al.* (1993a). Towards measurement of outcome for patients with varicose veins. *Quality in Health Care, 2*: 5–10.

Garratt, A.M., Ruta, D.A., Abdalla, M.I. *et al.* (1993b). The SF-36 health survey questionnaire: An outcome measure suitable for routine use within the NHS? *British Medical Journal, 306*: 1440–4.

Geil, R. (1991). Transcultural psychiatry: A question of interpretation. In: P.E. Bebbington (ed.), *Social Psychiatry: Theory, Methodology and Practice*. London: Transaction Publishers.

Gelber, R.D. and Goldhirsh, A. (1986). A new endpoint for the assessment of adjuvant therapy in postmenopausal women with operable breast cancer. *Journal of Clinical Oncology, 4*: 1772–9.

Gelber, R.D., Richard, D. and Goldhirsh, A. (1989). Comparison of adjuvant therapies using quality of life considerations. *International Journal of Technology Assessment in Health Care, 5*: 401–13.

George, L.K. and Fillenbaum, G.G. (1985). OARS methodology: A decade of experience in geriatric assessment. *Journal of the American Geriatric Society, 33*: 607–15.

Gibbons, J.S., Horn, S.H ., Powell, J.M. and Gibbons, J.L. (1984). Schizophrenic patients and their families: A survey in a psychiatry service based on a DGH unit. *British Journal of Psychiatry, 144*: 70–7.

Gift, A.G. (1989). Validation of a vertical visual analogue scale as a measure of clinical dyspnoea. *Rehabilitation Nursing, 14*: 323–5.

Gift, A.G., Plaut, S.M. and Jacox, A. (1986). Psychological and physiological factors related to dyspnoea in subjects with chronic obstructive pulmonary disease. *Heart and Lung, 15*: 595–601.

Gijn, J. van and members of the Dutch TIA Trial Study Group (1991). A comparison of two doses of aspirin (30 mg *vs* 283 mg a day) in patients after a transient ischaemic attack or minor ischaemic stroke. *New England Journal of Medicine, 325*: 1261–6.

Gilson, B., Bergner, M., Bobbitt, R.A. *et al.* (1975). The Sickness Impact Profile: Development of an outcome measure of health care. *American Journal of Public Health, 65*: 1304–10.

Gilson, B.S., Bergner, M., Bobbitt, R.A. *et al.* (1979). *The Sickness Impact Profile; Final Development and Testing, 1975–1978*. Seattle, WA: University of Washington Press.

Glazer, W., Aaronson, H.S., Prusoff, B.A. *et al.* (1980). Assessment of social adjustment in chronic ambulatory schizophrenics. *Journal of Nervous Mental Disease, 168*: 493–7.

Gleser, G.C. and Ihilevich, D. (1969). An objective instrument for measuring defense mechanisms. *Journal of Consulting and Clinical Psychology, 35*: 51–60.

Goffman, E. (1961). *Asylums: Essays on the Social Situation of Mental Patients and Other Inmates*. New York: Doubleday.

Goldberg, D.P. (1972). *The Detection of Psychiatric Illness by Questionnaire*. Maudsley Monograph No. 21. Oxford: Oxford University Press.

Goldberg, D.P. (1978). *Manual of the General Health Questionnaire*. Windsor: NFER-Nelson.

Goldberg, D.P. and Huxley, P. (1980). *Mental Illness in the Community: The Pathway to Psychiatric Care*. London: Tavistock.

Goldberg, D.P. and Williams, P. (1988). *A User's Guide to the General Health Questionnaire*. Windsor: NFER-Nelson.

Goldberg, D.P., Cooper, B., Eastwood, M.R. *et al.* (1970). A standardised psychiatric interview for use in community surveys. *British Journal of Preventive and Social Medicine, 24*: 18–23.

Goldberg, D.P., Rickels, K., Downing, R. and Hesbacher, P. (1976). A comparison of two psychiatric screening tests. *British Journal of Psychiatry, 129*: 61–7.

Goldberg, D.P. and Hillier, V.F. (1979). A scaled version of the General Health Questionnaire. *Psychological Medicine, 9*: 139–45.

Goldfried, M.R. and D'Zurilla, T.J. (1969). A behavior-analytic model for assessing competence. In: C.D. Spielberger (ed.), *Current Topics in Clinical and Community Psychology*, Vol. 1. New York: Academic Press.

Goldhirsh, A., Gelber, R.D., Simes, J., Glasziou, P. and Coates, A.S. (1989). Costs and benefits of adjuvant therapy in breast cancer: A quality adjusted survival analysis. *Journal of Clinical Oncology*, 7: 36–44.

Goldman, H.H., Morrissey, J.P., Ridgely, M.S. *et al.* (1992). Lessons from the program on chronic mental illness. *Health Affairs*, Fall, pp. 51–68.

Goldman, L., Hashimoto, B., Cook, E.F.L. and Loscalzo, A. (1981). Comparative reproducibility and validity of systems for assessing cardiovascular functional class: Advantages of a new specific activity scale. *Circulation*, 64: 1227–34.

Goldman, L., Cook, E.F., Mitchell, N. *et al.* (1982). Pitfalls in the serial assessment of cardiac functional states: How a reduction of 'ordinary' activity may reduce the apparent degree of cardiac compromise and give a misleading impression of improvement. *Journal of Chronic Diseases*, 35: 763–71.

Goligher, J.C. (1987). Judging the quality of life after surgical operations. *Journal of Chronic Diseases*, 40: 631–3.

Gompertz, P., Pound, P. and Ebrahim, S. (1993a). The reliability of stroke outcome measurement. *Clinical Rehabilitation*, 7: 290–6.

Gompertz, P., Pound, P. and Ebrahim, S. (1993b). *Kudo: A Kit for Describing the Outcome of Stroke.* London: Department of Public Health, Royal Free Hospital Medical School.

Goodall, T.A. and Halford, W.K. (1991). Self-management of diabetes mellitus: A critical review. *Health Psychology*, 10: 1–8.

Goodchilld, M.E. and Duncan-Jones, P. (1985). Chronicity and the General Health Questionnaire. *British Journal of Psychiatry*, 146: 55–61.

Gortner, S.R., Gilliss, C.L., Moran, J.A. *et al.* (1985). Expected and realised benefits from coronary bypass surgery in relation to severity of illness. *Cardiovascular Nursing*, 21: 13–18.

Gotay, C.C. and Moore, T.D. (1992). Assessing quality of life in head and neck cancer. *Quality of Life Research*, 1: 5–17.

Gottschalk, L.A. (1983). Measurement of mood and affect in cancer patients. *Cancer*, 53: 2236–40 (suppl.).

Gough, I.R., Furnival, C.M., Schilder, L. and Grove, W. (1983). Assessment of the quality of life of patients with advanced cancer. *European Journal of Cancer and Clinical Oncology*, 19: 1161–5.

Granger, C.V. (1982). Health accounting – functional assessment of the long term patient. In: F.J. Kottke, G.K. Stillwell and J.F. Lehmann (eds), *Krusen's Handbook of Physical Medicine and Rehabilitation*, 3rd edn. Philadelphia, PA: W.B. Saunders.

Granger, C.V. and McNamara, M.A. (1984). Functional assessment utilisation: The Long Range Evaluation System (LRES). In: C.V. Granger and G.E. Gresham (eds), *Functional Assessment in Rehabilitation Medicine.* Baltimore, MD: Williams and Williams.

Granger, C.V., Albrecht, G.L. and Hamilton, B.B. (1979a). Outcome of comprehensive medical rehabilitation: Measurement by PULSES Profile and the Barthel Index. *Archives of Physical Medicine and Rehabilitation*, 60: 145–54.

Granger, C.V., Dewis, L.S., Peters, N.C. *et al.* (1979b). Stroke rehabilitation: Analysis of repeated Barthel Index measures. *Archives of Physical Medicine and Rehabilitation*, 60: 14–17.

Grant, I. and Heaton, R. (1985). Neuropsychiatric abnormalities. In: T.L. Petty (ed.), *Chronic Obstructive Pulmonary Disease.* New York: Dekker.

Grant, M., Padilla, G.V., Ferrell, B.R. and Rhiner, M. (1990). Assessment of quality of life with a single instrument. *Seminars in Oncology Nursing*, 6: 260–70.

Grant, M., Ferrell, B., Schmidt, G.M. *et al.* (1992). Measurement of quality of life in bone marrow transplantation survivors. *Quality of Life Research*, 1: 375–84.

Green, C.J. (1993). The use of psychodiagnostic questionnaires in predicting risk factors and health outcomes. In: P. Koroly (ed.), *Measurement Strategies in Health Psychology.* Chichester: John Wiley.

Greenfield, T.K. (1989). *Consumer Satisfaction with the Delaware Drinking Driver Program in 1987–1988.* Report to the Delaware Drinker Driver Program. San Francisco, CA: Department of Psychiatry, University of California.

Greenfield, T.K. and Attkisson, C.C. (1989). *Family Satisfaction with Services.* Report to Northwest Residential Services Inc. San Francisco, CA: Department of Psychiatry, University of California.

Greenough, C.G. and Fraser, R.D. (1992). Assessment of outcome in patients with low back pain. *Spine*, 17: 36–41.

Greenwald, A.G., Bellezza, F.S. and Banaji, M.R. (1988). Is self-esteem a central ingredient of the self-concept? *Personality and Social Psychology Bulletin*, 14: 34–45.

Greenwald, H.P. (1987). The specificity of quality of life measures among the seriously ill. *Medical Care*, 25: 642–51.

Greer, S. (1984). The psychological dimension in cancer treatment. *Social Science and Medicine*, 18: 345–9.

Greer, S., Moorey, S., Baruch, J. *et al.* (1992). Adjuvant psychological therapy for patients with cancer: A prospective randomised trial. *British Medical Journal*, 304: 675–80.

Grieco, A. and Long, C.J. (1984). Investigation of the Karnofsky Performance Status as a measure of quality of life. *Health Psychology*, 3: 129–42.

Griffiths, R. (1970). *The Abilities of Young Children: A Comprehensive System of Mental Measurement for the First*

Eight Years of Life. London: Child Development Research Centre.

Grimby, A., Milsom, I., Molander, U. *et al.* (1993). The influence of urinary incontinence on the quality of life of elderly women. *Age and Ageing, 22*; 82–9.

Grimley Evans, J. (1992). Quality of life assessments and elderly people. In: A. Hopkins (ed.), *Measures of the Quality of Life and the Uses to which such Measures May be Put.* London: Royal College of Physicians.

Grotevant, H.D. and Carlson, C.I. (1989). *Family Assessment: A Guide to Methods and Measures.* New York: Guilford Press.

Gruenberg, A.M., Kendler, K.S. and Tsuang, M.T. (1985). Reliability and concordance in the subtyping of schizophrenia. *American Journal of Psychiatry, 142*: 1355–8.

Grundy, E., Bowling, A. and Farquhar, M. (1992). *Differentials in Mortality: Results from a Follow-up Study.* Working Paper No. 5. London: Age Concern Institute of Gerontology and Joseph Rowntree Foundation.

Gulliford, M.C. (1992). Evaluating prognostic factors: Implications for measurement of health care outcome. *Journal of Epidemiology and Community Health, 46*: 323–6.

Gunderson, E. and Ronson, A. (1969). A brief mental health index. *Journal of Abnormal Psychology, 74*: 100–4.

Gurin, G., Verloff, J. and Field, S. (1960). *Americans View Their Mental Health.* New York: Basic Books.

Gurland, B.J. and Yorkston, N.Y. (1971). *The Structured and Scaled Interview to Assess Maladjustment: Training Manual.* Mimeographed.

Gurland, B.J., Yorkston, N.J., Stone, A.R. and Frank, J.D. (1972a). The Structured and Scaled Interview to Assess Maladjustment (SSIAM). I. Description, rationale and development. *Archives of General Psychiatry, 27*: 259–64.

Gurland, B.J., Yorkston, N.J., Goldberg, K. *et al.* (1972b). The Structured and Scaled Interview to Assess Maladjustment. II. Factor analysis, reliability and validity. *Archives of General Psychiatry, 27*: 264–7.

Gurland, B.J., Kuriansky, L., Sharpe, R. *et al.* (1977). The Comprehensive Assessment and Referral Evaluation (CARE) – rationale, development and reliability. Part II. A factor analysis. *International Journal of Aging and Human Development, 8*: 9–42.

Gurland, B.J., Copeland, J.R.M. and Kelleher, M.J. *et al.* (1983). *The Mind and Mood of Ageing: The mental Health Problems of the Community Elderly in New York and London.* London: Croom Helm.

Gurland, B.J., Golden, R.R., Teresi, J.A. and Challop, J. (1984). The SHORT-CARE: An efficient instrument for the assessment of depression, dementia and disability. *Journal of Gerontology, 39*: 166–9.

Gurtman, M.B. (1985). Self-rating Depression Scale. In: D.J. Keyser and R.C. Sweetland (eds), *Test Critiques,* Vol. III. Kansas City, MO: Test Corporation of America.

Guttman, L. (1944). A basis for scaling qualitative data. *American Sociological Review, 9*: 139–51.

Guyatt, G.H. (1993). The philosophy of health-related quality of life translation. *Quality of Life Research, 2*: 461–5.

Guyatt, G.H., Pugsley, S.O., Sullivan, M. *et al.* (1984). Effect of encouragement on walking test performance. *Thorax, 39*: 818–22.

Guyatt, G.H., Thompson, P.J., Berman, L.B. *et al.* (1985a). How should we measure function in patients with chronic lung disease? *Journal of Chronic Diseases, 38*: 517–24.

Guyatt, G.H., Sullivan, M.J., Fallen, E.L. *et al.* (1985b). The six minute walk: A new measure of exercise capacity in patients with chronic heart failure. *Canadian Medical Association Journal, 132*: 919–23.

Guyatt, G.H., Bombardier, C. and Tugwell, P. (1986). Measuring disease specific quality of life in clinical trials. *Canadian Medical Association Journal, 134*: 895–9.

Guyatt, G.H., Berman, L.B., Townsend, M. *et al.* (1987a). A measure of quality of life for clinical trials in chronic lung disease. *Thorax, 42*: 773–8.

Guyatt, G.H., Walter, S. and Geoff, N. (1987b). Measuring change over time: Assessing the usefulness of evaluative instruments. *Journal of Chronic Diseases, 40*: 171–8.

Guyatt, G.H., Townsend, M., Berman, L. and Pugsley, S.O. (1987c). Quality of life in patients with chronic airflow limitation. *British Journal of Diseases of the Chest, 81*: 45–54.

Guyatt, G.H., Sullivan, M.J.J., Fallen, E.L. *et al.* (1988). A controlled trial of digoxin in heart failure. *American Journal of Cardiology, 61*: 371–5.

Guyatt, G.H., Nogradi, S., Halcrow, S. *et al.* (1989a). Development and testing of a new measure of health status for clinical trials in heart failure. *Journal of General Internal Medicine, 4*: 101–7.

Guyatt, G.H., Van Zanten, S.J.O.V., Feeny, D.H. and Patrick, D.L. (1989b). Measuring quality of life in clinical trials: A taxonomy and review. *Canadian Medical Association Journal, 140*: 1441–8.

Guyatt, G.H., Deyo, R.A., Charlson, M. *et al.* (1989c). Responsiveness and validity in health status measurement: A clarification. *Journal of Clinical Epidemiology, 42*: 403–8.

Guyatt, G.H., Mitchell, A., Irvine, E.J. *et al.* (1989d). A new measure of health status for clinical trials in inflammatory bowel disease. *Gastronenterology, 96*: 804–10.

Guyatt, G.H., Townsend, M., Keller, J. *et al.* (1991). Measuring functional status in chronic lung disease: Conclusions from a randomised controlled trial. *Respiratory Medicine, 85*: 17–21 (suppl. B).

Haberman, M.R. (1988). Psychosocial aspects of bone marrow transplantation. *Seminars in Oncology Nursing, 4*: 55–9.

Hackett, T. and Cassem, N. (1974). Development of a quantitative rating scale to assess denial. *Journal of Psychosomatic Research, 18*: 93–100.

Hadhorn, D. and Hays, R.D. (1991). Multi-trait-multimethod analysis of health related quality of life preferences. *Medical Care, 29*: 829–40.

Hall, J. and Baker, R. (1983). *REHAB: A User's Manual.* Aberdeen: Vine Publishing.

Hamilton, M. (1960). Rating scale for depression. *Journal of Neurology, Neurosurgery and Psychiatry, 23*: 56–62.

Hamilton, M. (1967). Development of a rating scale for primary depressive illness. *British Journal of Social Clinical Psychiatry, 6*: 278–96.

Hamilton, M. (1969). Standardised assessment and recording of depressive symptoms. *Psychiatrica, Neurologia, Neurochirurgia, 72*: 201–5.

Hamilton, M. (1970). The Hamilton Depression Scale. In: W. Guy and R. Bonato (eds), *ECDFU Assessment Manual*. Rockville, MD: National Institutes of Mental Health.

Hamilton, M. (1976). Clinical evaluation of depression: Clinical criteria and rating scales, including a Guttman Scale. In: D.M. Gallant and G.M. Simpson (eds), *Depression: Behaviour, Biochemical Diagnosis and Treatment Concepts*. New York: Spectrum Publications.

Hammond, G.S. and Aoki, T.T. (1992). Measurement of health status in diabetic patients. *Diabetes Care, 15*: 469–77.

Hanestad, B.R. (1993). Quality of life as an outcome measure in a study of people with diabetes using Hörnquist's model. Paper presented to the *WONCA/ SIMG Congress*, Quality of Care in Family Medicine/ General Practice. The Hague, Netherlands, June 13–17.

Hanestad, B.R., Hörnquist, J.O. and Albrektsen, G. (1991). Self-assessed quality of life and metabolic control in persons with insulin–dependent diabetes mellitus (IDDM). *Scandinavian Journal of Social Medicine, 19*: 57–65.

Hargreaves, W.A., McIntyre, M.H. and Attkisson, C.C. (1979). Outcome measurement instruments for use in community mental health program evaluation. In: W.A. Hargreaves, C.C. Attkisson and J.E. Sorensen (eds), *Resource Materials for Community Mental Health Program Evaluation*, 2nd edn. Washington DC: US Department of Health, Education and Welfare.

Harris, B.A., Jette, A.M., Campion, E.W. and Cleary, P.D. (1986). Validity of self report measures of functional disability. *Topics in Geriatric Rehabilitation, 1*: 31–41.

Harris, W.H. (1969). Traumatic arthritis of the hip after dislocation and acetabular fractures: Treatment by mold arthroplasty. An end–result study using a new method of result evaluation. *Journal of Bone and Joint Surgery, 51A*: 737–55.

Harver, A. and Mahler, D.A. (1990). The symptom of dyspnea. In: D.A. Mahler (ed.), *Dyspnea*. New York: Futura.

Harvey, R.M., Doyle, E.F., Ellis, K. (1974). Major changes made by the Criteria Committee of the New York Heart Association. *Circulation, 49*: 390.

Harvey, V.J., Slevin, M.L., Cheek, S.P. *et al.* (1987). A randomised trial comparing vindesine and cisplatinum to vindesine and methotrexate in advanced non–small cell lung carcinoma. *European Journal of Cancer and Clinical Oncology, 23*: 1615–19.

Hasin, D.S. and Skodol, A.E. (1989). Standardised diagnostic interviews for psychiatric research. In: C. Thompson (ed.), *The Instruments of Psychiatric Research*. Chichester: John Wiley.

Hathaway, S.R. and McKinley, J.C. (1940a). A Multiphasic Personality Schedule (Minnesota). I. Construction of the schedule. *Journal of Psychology, 10*: 249–54.

Hathaway, S.R. and McKinley, J.C. (1940b). A Multiphasic Personality Schedule (Minnesota). II. A differential study of hypochondriasis. *Journal of Psychology, 10*: 255–68.

Hathaway, S.R. and McKinley, J.C. (1942a). A Multiphasic Personality Schedule (Minnesota). III. The measurement of symptomatic depression. *Journal of Psychology, 14*: 73–84.

Hathaway, S.R. and McKinley, J.C. (1942b). A Multiphasic Personality Schedule (Minnesota). IV. Psychasthenia. *Journal of Applied Psychology, 26*: 614–24.

Hathaway, S.R. and McKinley, J.C. (1951). *Manual for the Minnesota Multiphasic Personality Inventory*, revised. New York: Psychological Corporation.

Hathaway, S. and McKinley, J. (1990). *Minnesota Multiphasic Personality Inventory*, 2nd edn. Windsor: NFER-Nelson.

Hauser, A. (1987). Postscript: How should outcome be determined and reported? In: J. Engel (ed.), *Surgical Treatment of the Epilepsies*, 1st edn. New York: Raven Press.

Havighurst. R.J. (1963). Successful aging. In: R.H. Williams, C. Tibbits and W. Donahue (eds), *Processes of Aging*, Vol. I, New York: Atherton Press.

Hawkins, N.G., Davies, R. and Holmes, T.H. (1957). Evidence of psychosocial factors in the development of pulmonary tuberculosis. *American Review of Tuberculosis and Pulmonary Disease, 75*: 5.

Hays, R.D. and Hadhorn, D. (1992). Responsiveness to change: An aspect of validity, not a separate dimension. *Quality of Life Research, 1*: 73–5.

Hays, R.D. and Shapiro, M.F. (1992). An overview of

generic health related quality of life measures for HIV research. *Quality of Life Research, 1*: 91–7.

Hays, R.D., Vickrey, B.G. and Engel, J. (1993). Post-script: Epilepsy surgery outcome assessment. In: J. Engel (ed.), *Surgical Treatment of the Epilepsies*, 2nd edn. New York: Raven Press.

Headey, B., Holmstrom, E. and Wearing, A. (1984). The impact of life events and changes in domain satisfactions on well-being. *Social Indicators Research, 15*: 203–27.

Health Outcomes Institute (1990). *User's Manual: SF-36 Health Status Questionnaire.* Bloomington, MN: HOI.

Hedlund, J.L. and Vieweg, B.W. (1979). The Hamilton Rating Scale for Depression: A comprehensive review. *Journal of Operational Psychiatry, 10*: 149–65.

Hedlund, J.L. and Vieweg, B.W. (1980). The Brief Psychiatric Rating Scale (BPRS): A comprehensive review. *Journal of Operational Psychiatry, 11*: 48–65.

Heiby, E.M. (1984). Wechsler Memory Scale. In: D.J. Keyser and R.C. Sweetland (eds), *Test Critiques*, Vol. I. Kansas City, MO: Test Corporation of America.

Heinrich, R.L., Schag, C.A.C. and Ganz, P.A. (1984). Living with cancer: The cancer inventory of problem situations. *Journal of Clinical Psychology, 40*: 972–80.

Heinrichs, D.W., Hanlon, T.E. and Carpenter, W.T. (1984). The Quality of Life Scale: An instrument for rating the schizophrenic deficit syndrome. *Schizophrenia Bulletin, 10*: 388–97.

Heller, A., Wade, D.T., Wood, V.A. *et al.* (1987). Arm function after stroke: Measurement and recovery over the first three months. *Journal of Neurology, Neurosurgery and Psychiatry, 50*: 714–19.

Helmstater, G.C. (1964). *Principles of Psychological Measurement.* New York: Appleton-Century-Crofts.

Helzer, J.E., Robins, L.N., Croughan, J.L. and Weiner, A. (1981). Renard diagnosis interview: Its reliability and procedural validity with physicians and lay interviewers. *Archives of General Psychiatry, 38*: 393–8.

Helzer, J.E., Robins, L.N., McEvoy, L.T. *et al.* (1985). A comparison of Clinical and Diagnostic Interview Schedule diagnoses: Physician reexamination of lay-interviewed cases in a general population. *Archives of General Psychiatry, 42*: 657–66.

Henderson, A.A., Duncan-Jones, P. and Finlay-Jones, R.A. (1983). The reliability of the Geriatric Mental State Examination. *Acta Psychiatrica Scandinavica, 67*: 281–9.

Henderson, S.H., Byrne, D.G. and Duncan-Jones, P. (1981). *Neurosis and the Social Environment.* Sydney: Academic Press.

Herlitz, J., Hjalmarson, M., Lomsky, M. *et al.* (1988). The relationship between infarct size and mortality and morbidity during short term and long term

follow-up after acute myocardial infarction. *American Heart Journal, 5*: 1378–82.

Herrick, A.L., Walker, P.C., Berkin, K.E., Pringle, S.D., Callender, J.S., Robertson, M.P., Findlay, J.G. and Murray, G.D. (1989). Comparison of atenolol and enalapril in mild to moderate hypertension. *American Journal of Medicine, 86*: 421–6.

Herzlich, C. (1973). *Health and Illness.* A social psychological analysis. New York: Academic Press.

Heyrman, J. and van Hoeck, K. (1993). Measuring health outcome: Shouldn't we first define health? Paper presented to the *WONCA/SIMG Congress*, Quality of Care in Family Medicine/General Practice. The Hague, Netherlands, June 13–17.

Hibbs, P. (1989). *Achievable Standards of Care for the Elderly Patient Cared for in the Acute Assessment Wards, the Continuing Care Wards, Nursing Homes and Day Hospitals within the City and Hackney Health Authority.* London: St Bartholomew's Hospital.

Higginson, I.J. (1992). The development, validity, reliability and practicality of a new measure of palliative care: The Support Team Assessment Schedule. PhD thesis, University College, University of London.

Hill, S. and Harries, U. (1994). Assessing the outcome of health care for the older person in community settings: Should we use the SF-36? *Outcomes Briefing, UK Clearing House for the Assessment of Health Outcomes 4*: 26–7.

Hinterberger, W., Gadner, H., Hocker, P. *et al.* (1987). Survival and quality of life in 23 patients with severe aplastic anaemia treated with BMT. *BLUT, 54*: 137–46.

Hirsch, A.R., Platt, S.D., Knights, A.C. and Weyman, A. (1979). Shortening hospital stay for psychiatric care: Effect on patients and their families. *British Medical Journal, 1*: 442–6.

Hochberg, M.C., Chang, R., Dwosh, I. *et al.* (1990). Preliminary revised ACR criteria for functional status in rheumatoid arthritis (abstract). *Arthritis and Rheumatism, 33*: S15 (suppl. 9).

Hodkinson, H.M. (1972). Evaluation of a mental test score for assessment of mental impairment in the elderly. *Age and Ageing, 1*: 233–8.

Hoffmeister, J.K. (1976). Some information regarding the characteristics of the two measures developed from the Self-Esteem Questionnaire (SEQ-3). Boulder, CO: Test Analysis and Development Corporation.

Hogan, M.J., Wallin, J.D. and Baer, R.M. (1980). Antihypertensive therapy and male sexual dysfunction. *Psychosomatics, 21*: 234–7.

Hogarty, G.E. and Katz, M.M. (1971). Norms of adjustment and social behaviour. *Archives of General Pschiatry, 25*: 470–80.

Hogg, L.I. and Marshall, M. (1992). Can we measure need in the homeless mentally ill? Using the MRC

Needs for Care Assessment in hostels for the homeless. *Psychological Medicine, 22*: 1027–34.

Holahan, C.J. and Moos, R.H. (1981). Social support and psychological distress: A longitudinal analysis. *Journal of Abnormal Psychology, 90*: 365–70.

Holbrook, M. and Skilbeck, C.E. (1983). An activities index for use with stroke patients. *Age and Ageing, 12*: 166–70.

Holden, M.K., Gill, K.M., Magliozzi, M.R., Nathan, J. and Piehl-Baker, L. (1984). Clinical gait assessment in the neurologically impaired: Reliability and meaningfulness. *Physical Therapy, 64*: 35–40.

Holden, R.H. (1988). Wechsler Memory Scale – Revised. In D.J. Keyser and R.C. Sweetland (eds), *Test Critiques*, Vol. VII. Kansas City, MO: Test Corporation of America.

Holland, J.C., Silberfarb, P., Tron, S. and Cella, D. (1986). Psychosocial research in cancer: The Cancer and Leukemia Group B (CALGB) experience. In: V. Ventafridda, F.S.A.M. van Dam, R. Yancik and M. Tamburini (eds), *Assessment of Quality of Life and Cancer Treatment*. Amsterdam: Elsevier.

Hollandsworth, J.G. (1988). Evaluating the impact of medical treatment on the quality of life: A five year update. *Social Science and Medicine, 26*: 425–34.

Holmes, C.S. (1987). Cognitive functioning and diabetes: Broadening the paradigm for behavioural and health psychology? *Diabetes Care, 10*: 135–6.

Holmes, D.R., van Raden, M.J., Reeder, G.S. *et al.* (1984). Return to work after coronary angioplasty: A report from the National Heart, Lung and Blood Institute Percutaneous Transluminal Coronary Angioplasty Registry. *American Journal of Cardiology, 52*: 48–51.

Holmes, S. (1989). Use of a modified symptom distress scale in assessment of the cancer patient. *International Journal of Nursing Studies, 26*: 69–79.

Holmes, S. and Dickerson, J. (1987). The quality of life: Design and evaluation of a self assessment instrument for use with cancer patients. *International Journal of Nursing Studies, 1*: 15–24.

Holmes, T.H. and Rahe, R.H. (1967). The Social Readjustment Rating Scale. *Journal of Psychosomatic Research, 11*: 213–18.

Holzemer, S., Henry, S.B., Stewart, A. and Janson-Bjerklie, S. (1993). The HIV quality audit marker (HIV-QAM): An outcome measure for hospitalised AIDS patients. *Quality of Life Research, 2*: 99–107.

Hopkins, A. (ed.) (1992). *Measures of the Quality of Life and the Uses to which such Measures May be Put*. London: Royal College of Physicians.

Hopwood, P. (1984). Measurement of psychological morbidity in advanced breast cancer. In: M. Watson and S. Greer (eds), *Psychosocial Issues in Malignant Disease*. Oxford: Pergamon Press.

Hopwood, P. and Maguire, P. (1992). Priorities in the psychological care of cancer patients. *International Review of Psychiatry, 4*: 35–44.

Hopwood, P., Howell, A. and Maguire, P. (1991). Screening for psychiatric morbidity in patients with advanced breast cancer: Validation of two self-report questionnaires. *British Journal of Cancer, 64*: 353–6.

Hörnquist, J.O. (1982). The concept of quality of life. *Scandinavian Journal of Social Medicine, 10*: 57–61.

Hörnquist, J.O. (1989). Quality of life: Concept and assessment. *Scandinavian Journal of Social Medicine, 18*: 69–79.

Hörnquist, J.O. and Elton, M.A. (1983). A prospective longitudinal study of abusers of alcohol granted disability pension. *Scandinavian Journal of Social Medicine, 23*: 1171–95.

Hörnquist, J.O., Wikby, A., Andersson, P.O. and Dufva, A.M. (1990). Insulin-pen treatment, quality of life and metabolic control: Retrospective intra-group evaluations. *Diabetes Research and Clinical Practice, 10*: 221–30.

Hörnquist, J.O., Hansson, B., Akerlind, I. and Larsson, J. (1992). Severity of disease and quality of life: A comparison in patients with cancer and benign disease. *Quality of Life Research, 1*: 135–41.

Hörnquist, J.O., Wikby, A., Hansson, B. and Andersson, P.O. (1993). Quality of life: Status and change (QLSC): Reliability, validity and sensitivity of a generic assessment approach tailored for diabetes. *Quality of Life Research, 2*: 263–79.

Horowitz, M.J. and Cohen, F.M. (1968). Temporal lobe epilepsy: Effect of a lobectomy on psychosocial functioning. *Epilepsia, 9*: 23–41.

Horowitz, M.J., Schaefer, C., Hiroto, D. *et al.* (1977). Life events questionnaires for measuring presumptive stress. *Psychosomatic Medicine, 39*: 413–31.

Horowitz, M.J., Wilner, N. and Alvarez, W. (1979). Impact of Event Scale: A measure of subjective stress. *Psychomatic Medicine, 41*: 209–18.

Horowitz, M.J., Simon, N., Holden, N. *et al.* (1983). The stressful impact of news of risk for premature heart disease. *Psychosomatic Medicine, 45*: 31–7.

Horsley, J.R. (1985). *A Study to Determine the Prevalence of Respiratory Disease in the Elderly*. Southampton: Hampshire Health Authority, Department of Geriatric Medicine, Southampton General Hospital.

Horsley, J.R., Sterling, I.J.N., Waters, W.E. and Howell, J.B.L. (1991). Respiratory symptoms among elderly people in the New Forest area as assessed by postal questionnaire. *Age and Ageing, 20*: 325–31.

Horsley, J.R., Sterling, I.J.N., Waters, W.E. and Howell, J.B.L. (1993). How common is increased airway reactivity amongst the elderly? *Gerontology, 39*: 38–48.

House, J.S. (1981). *Work, Stress and Social Support*. Reading, MA: Addison-Wesley.

House, J.S., Landis, K.R. and Umberson, D. (1988). Social relationships and health. *Science*, July, pp. 540–45.

Hulicka, J., Morganti, J. and Cataldo, J. (1975). Perceived latitude of choice of institutionalized and non-institutionalized elderly women. *Experimental Aging Research*, 1: 27–39.

Hunt, S.M. (1984). Nottingham Health Profile. In: N.K. Wenger, M.E. Mattson, C.P. Furberg and J. Elinson (eds), *Assessment of Quality of Life in Clinical Trials of Cardiovascular Therapies*. New York: Le Jacq.

Hunt, S.M. (1988). Subjective health indicators and health promotion. *Health Promotion*, 3: 23–34.

Hunt, S.M. and McKenna, S.P. (1992). *Adaptation of the General Well-Being Index for Use in Britain*. Manchester: Galen Research and Consultancy.

Hunt, S.M. and McKenna, S.P. (1993). Measuring quality of life in psychiatry. In: S.R. Walker and R.M. Rosser (eds), *Quality of Life Assessment: Key Issues in the 1990s*. Dordrecht: Kluwer Academic.

Hunt, S.M., McEwan, J. and McKenna, S.P. (1986). *Measuring Health Status*. Beckenham: Croom Helm.

Hurny, C., Piasetsky, E., Bagin, R. and Holland, J. (1987). High social desirability in patients being treated for advanced colorectal or bladder cancer: Eventual impact on the assessment of quality of life. *Journal of Psychosocial Oncology*, 5: 19–29.

Hurry, J. (1989). Social factors and the use of psychiatric services. PhD thesis, Institute of Psychiatry, University of London.

Hurry, J. and Sturt, E. (1981). Social performance in a population sample: Relation to psychiatric symptoms. In: J.K. Wing, P.E. Bebbington and L. Robins (eds), *What is a case? The Problem of Definition in Psychiatric Community Surveys*. London: Grant MacIntyre.

Hurry, J., Sturt, E., Bebbington, P. and Tennant, C. (1983). Socio-demographic associations with social disablement in a community sample. *Social Psychiatry*, 18: 113–21.

Hurry, J., Bebbington, P.E. and Tennant, C. (1987). Psychiatric symptoms, social disablement and illness behaviour. *Australian and New Zealand Journal of Psychiatry*, 21: 68–73.

Husaini, B.A., Neff, J.A., Harrington, J.B. *et al.* (1979). *Depression in Rural Communities: Establishing CES-D Cutting Points*. Mental Health Project. Final Report, National Institute of Mental Health Contract 278-77-0044 (DBE).

Hutchinson, A. and Fowler, P. (1992). Outcome measures for primary health care: What are the research priorities? *British Journal of General Practice*, 42: 227–31.

Hutchinson, T.A., Boyd, N.F., Feinstein, A.R. *et al.* (1979). Scientific problems in clinical scales as demonstrated in the Karnofsky Index of Performance Status. *Journal of Chronic Diseases*, 32: 661–6.

Huxley, P.J. (1988). *The General Satisfaction Questionnaire Pilot Study: Technical Details*. Manchester: University of Manchester, Mental Health Social Work Research Unit.

Huxley, P.J. (1990). *The General Satisfaction Questionnaire (GSQ): Field Trial Results I. GSQ Subscales*. Manchester: University of Manchester, Mental Health Social Work Research Unit.

Huxley, P.J. and Warner, R. (1992). Case management, quality of life, and satisfaction with services of long-term psychiatric patients. *Hospital and Community Psychiatry*, 43: 799–802.

Hyde, L., Wolf, J., McCracken, S. and Yesner, R. (1973). Natural course of inoperable lung cancer. *Chest*, 64: 309–12.

Hyland, M.E. (1991). The Living with Asthma Questionnaire. *Respiratory Medicine*, 85: 13–16 (suppl. B).

Hyland, M.E. (1992a). Quality-of-life assessment in respiratory disease. An examination of the content and validity of four questionnaires. *PharmacoEconomics*, 2: 43–53.

Hyland, M.E. (1992b). Selection of items and avoidance of bias in quality of life scales. *PharmacoEconomics*, 1: 182–90.

Hyland, M.E. (1993). The validity of health assessments: Resolving some recent differences. *Journal of Clinical Epidemiology*, 46: 1019–23.

Hyland, M.E. and Kenyon, C.A.P. (1992). A measure of positive health-related quality of life: The satisfaction with illness scale. *Psychological Reports*, 71: 1137–8.

Hyland, M.E., Finnis, S. and Irvine, S.H. (1991). A scale for assessing quality of life in adult asthma sufferers. *Journal of Psychosomatic Research*, 35: 99–110.

Hyland, M.E., Kenyon, C.A.P. and Jacobs, P.A. (1994). Sensitivity to quality of life domains and constructs to longitudinal change in a clinical trial comparing salmeterol with placebo in asthmatics. *Quality of Life Research*, 3: 121–6.

Hyman, M.D. (1971). The stigma of stroke. *Geriatrics*, 5: 132–41.

Hypertension Detection and Follow-up Program Co-operative Group (1982). The effect of treatment on mortality in 'mild' hypertension: Results of the Hypertension Detection and Follow-up Program. *New England Journal of Medicine*, 307: 976–80.

Idler, E.L. (1992). Self-assessed health and mortality: A review of studies. In: S. Maes, H. Leventhal and M. Johnston (eds), *International Review of Health Psychology*, Vol. I. Chichester: John Wiley.

Isacson, J., Allander, E. and Brostrom, L.A. (1987). A seventeen-year follow-up of a population survey of rheumatoid arthritis. *Scandinavian Journal of Rheumatology*, 16: 145–52.

Izsak, F.C. and Medalie, J.H. (1971). Comprehensive follow-up of carcinoma patients. *Journal of Chronic Diseases, 24*: 179–91.

Jachuk, S.J., Brierly, H., Jachuck, S. and Wilcox, P.M. (1982). The effect of hypotensive drugs on the quality of life. *Journal of the Royal College of General Practitioners, 32*; 103–5.

Jacoby, A. (1992). Epilepsy and the quality of everyday life: Findings from a study of people with well controlled epilepsy. *Social Science and Medicine, 34*: 657–66.

Jacoby, A., Baker, G., Smith, D. *et al.* (1993). Measuring the impact of epilepsy: The development of a novel scale. *Epilepsy Research, 16*: 83–8.

Jagger, C., Clarke, M., Anderson, J. and Battock, T. (1992). Dementia in Melton Mowbray – a validation of earlier findings. *Age and Ageing, 21*: 205–10.

Jahoda, M. (1958). *Current Concepts in Positive Mental Health*. New York: Basic Books.

Jaivenois, M.F., Delvaux, N., Badii, N. *et al.* (1993). A preparation and rehabilitation programme (PRP) for patients undergoing bone marrow transplantation (BMT): Development of an intervention module (abstract). *Quality of Life Research, 2*: 69.

Jalowiec, A., Murphy, S.P. and Powers, M.J. (1984). Psychometric assessment of the Jalowiec Coping Scale. *Nursing Research, 33*: 157–61.

Jellinek, M.S. and Murphy, J.M. (1988). Screening for psychosocial disorders in pediatric practice. *American Journal of Diseases of Childhood, 142*: 1153–7.

Jenkins, C.D., Rosenman, R.H. and Friedman, M. (1967). Development of an objective psychological test for the determination of the coronary-prone behaviour pattern in employed men. *Journal of Chronic Diseases, 20*: 371–9.

Jenkins, C.D., Stanton, B.A., Savageau, J.A. *et al.* (1983a). Physical, psychological, social and economic outcomes after cardiac valve surgery. *Archives of Internal Medicine, 143*: 2107–13.

Jenkins, C.D., Stanton, B.A., Savageau, J.A. *et al.* (1983b). Coronary artery bypass surgery: Physical, psychological, and economic outcomes six months later. *Journal of the American Medical Association, 250*: 782–8.

Jenkinson, C., Wright, L. and Coulter, A. (1993a). *Quality of Life Measurement in Health Care: A Review of Measures and Population Norms for the UK SF-36*. Oxford: University of Oxford, Health Services Research Unit, Department of Public Health and Primary Care.

Jenkinson, C., Coulter, A. and Wright, L. (1993b). Short Form-36 (SF-36) health survey questionnaire: Normative data for adults of working age. *British Medical Journal, 306*: 1437–40.

Jennett, B. (1976). Resource allocation for the severely brain damaged. *Archives of Neurology, 33*: 595–7.

Jennett, B. (1984). The measurement of outcome. In: N. Brooks (ed.), *Closed Head Injury: Psychological, Social and Family Consequences*. Oxford: Oxford University press.

Jennett, B. and Bond, M. (1975). Assessment of outcome after severe brain damage: A practical scale. *Lancet, 1*: 480–4.

Jensen, I. and Larsen, K. (1979). Mental aspects of temporal lobe epilepsy. *Journal of Neurology, Neurosurgery and Psychiatry, 42*: 256–65.

Jette, A.M. (1980a). The Functional Status Index: Reliability of a chronic disease evaluation instrument. *Archives of Physical Medicine and Rehabilitation, 61*: 395–401.

Jette, A.M. (1980b). Functional capacity evaluation: An empirical approach. *Archives of Physical Medicine and Rehabilitation, 61*: 85–9.

Jette, A.M. (1987). The Functional Status Index: Reliability and validity of a self-report functional disability measure. *Journal of Rheumatology, 14*: 15–21 (suppl.).

Jette, A.M. and Cleary, P.D. (1987). Functional disability assessment. *Physical Therapy, 67*: 1854–9.

Jette, A.M. and Deniston, O.L. (1978). Inter-observer reliability of a functional status assessment instrument. *Journal of Chronic Diseases, 31*: 573–80.

Jette, A.M., Davies, A.R., Cleary, P.D. *et al.* (1986). The Functional Status Questionnaire: Reliability and validity when used in primary care. *Journal of General and Internal Medicine, 1*: 143–9.

Jitapunkul, S., Pillay, I. and Ebrahim, S. (1991). The Abbreviated Mental Test. *Age and Ageing, 20*: 332–6.

Johnson, A.N., Cooper, D.F. and Edwards, R.H.T. (1977). Exertion of stair climbing in normal subjects and in patients with chronic obstructive bronchitis. *Thorax, 32*: 711–16.

Johnson, J.R. and Temple, R. (1985). Food and Drug Administration requirements for approval of new anticancer drugs. *Cancer Treatment Reviews, 69*: 1155–7.

Jollife, I.T. and Morgan, B.J.T. (1992). Principal component analysis and exploratory factor analysis. *Statistical Methods in Medical Research, 1*: 69–95.

Jones, E., Lund, V.J., Howard, D.J. *et al.* (1992). Quality of life of patients treated surgically for head and neck cancer. *Journal of Laryngology and Ontology, 106*: 238–42.

Jones, P.W. (1991a). Quality of life measurement for patients with diseases of the airways. *Thorax, 46*: 676–82.

Jones, P.W. (1991b). Symptoms and 'quality of life' in asthma – a one year placebo controlled trial with nedocromil sodium (abstract). *Thorax, 46*: 759.

Jones, P.W. (1993). Measurement of health related quality of life in asthma and chronic obstructive airways disease. In: S.R. Walker and R.M. Rosser (eds), *Quality of Life Assessment: Key Issues in the 1990s*. Dordrecht: Kluwer Academic.

Jones, P.W. (with the Nedocromil Sodium Quality of Life Study Group) (1994). Quality of life, symptoms, and pulmonary function in asthma. Long term treatment with nedocromil sodium examined in a controlled multicentre trial. *European Respiratory Journal*, 7: 55–62.

Jones, P.W., Baveystock, C.M. and Littlejohns, P. (1989). Relationships between general health measured with the Sickness Impact Profile and respiratory symptoms, physiological measures and mood in patients with chronic airflow limitation. *American Review of Respiratory Diseases, 140*: 1538–43.

Jones, P.W., Quirk, F.H. and Baveystock, C.M. (1991). The St. George's Respiratory Questionnaire. *Respiratory Medicine, 85*: 25–31 (suppl. B).

Jones, P.W., Quirk, F.H., Baveystock, C.M. and Littlejohns, P. (1992). A self-complete measure of health status for chronic airflow limitation: The St. George's Respiratory Questionnaire. *American Review of Respiratory Diseases, 145*: 1321–7.

Jones, W.G., Akaza, H., van Oosterom, A.T *et al.* (1988). Objective response criteria in phase II and phase III studies. *Progress in Clinical and Biological Research, 269*: 243–60.

Jorm, A.F. (1990). *The Epidemiology of Alzheimer's Disease and Related Disorders*. London: Chapman and Hall.

Jorm, A.F., Scott, R., Henderson, A.S. *et al.* (1988). Educational differences on the Mini-Mental state: The role of test bias. *Psychological Medicine, 18*: 727–33.

Julian, D.G. (1987). Quality of life after myocardial infarction. *American Heart Journal, 5*: 1378–82.

Juniper, E.F., Guyatt, G.H., Epstein, R.S. *et al.* (1992). Evaluation of impairment of health related quality of life in asthma: Development of a questionnaire for use in clinical trials. *Thorax, 47*: 76–83.

Juniper, E.F., Guyatt, G.H., Ferrie, P.J. and Griffith, L.E. (1993a). Measuring quality of life in asthma. *American Review of Respiratory Disease, 147*: 832–8.

Juniper, E.F., Johnston, P., Borkhoff, C. *et al.* (1993b). Effect of salmeterol on asthma quality of life. *American Review of Respiratory Disease, 147*: A60.

Juniper, E.F., Guyatt, G.H., Willan, A. and Griffith, L.E. (1994). Determining a minimal important change in a disease specific quality of life questionnaire. *Journal of Clinical Epidemiology, 47*: 81–7.

Kahn, R.L., Goldfarb, A.I., Pollack, M. *et al.* (1960a). The relationship of mental and physical status in institutionalized aged persons. *American Journal of Psychiatry, 117*: 120–4.

Kahn, R.L., Goldfarb, A.I., Pollack, M. *et al.* (1960b). Brief objective measures for the determination of mental status in the aged. *American Journal of Psychiatry, 117*: 326–8.

Kahneman, D. and Tversky, A. (1983). Choices, values and frames. *American Psychologist, 39*: 341–50.

Kalra, L. and Crome, P. (1993). The role of prognostic scores in targeting stroke rehabilitation in elderly patients. *Journal of the American Geriatrics Society, 41*: 396–400.

Kammann, R. and Flett, R. (1983). Affectometer 2: A scale to measure current level of general happiness. *Australian Journal of Psychology, 35*: 259–65.

Kane, R.A. and Kane, R.L. (1988). *Assessing the Elderly*. Lexington, MA: Lexington Books.

Kantz, M.E., Harris, W.J., Levitsky, K. *et al.* (1992). Methods for assessing condition-specific and generic functional status outcomes after total knee replacement. *Medical Care, 30*: MS240–MS252 (suppl.).

Kaplan, R.M. (1985). Quality of life measurement. In: P. Karoly (ed.), *Measurement Strategies in Health Psychology*. New York: John Wiley.

Kaplan, R.M. and Anderson, J.P. (1990). The general health policy model: An integrated approach. In: B. Spilker (ed.), *Quality of Life Assessments in Clinical Trials*. New York: Raven Press.

Kaplan, R.M. and Bush, J.W. (1982). Health related quality of life measurement for evaluation research and policy analysis. *Health Psychology, 1*: 61–80.

Kaplan, R.M., Bush, J.W. and Berry, C.C. (1976). Health status: Types of validity and the Index of Well-being. *Health Services Research, 11*: 478–507.

Kaplan, R.M., Bush, J.W. and Berry C.C. (1978). The reliability, stability and generalisability of a health status index. *Proceedings of the American Statistical Association, Social Statistics Section*: 704–9. Washington, DC: American Statistical Association.

Kaplan, R.M., Bush, J.W. and Berry, C.C. (1979). Health status index: Category rating versus magnitude estimation for measuring levels of well-being. *Medical Care, 17*: 501–23.

Kaplan, R.M., Atkins, C.J., Times, R. *et al.* (1984). Validity of quality of well-being scale as an outcome measure in chronic obstructive pulmonary disease. *Journal of Chronic Diseases, 37*: 85–95.

Kaplan, R.M., Feeny, D. and Revicki, D.A. (1993a). Methods for assessing relative importance in preference based outcome measures. *Quality of Life Research, 2*: 467–75.

Kaplan, R.M., Anderson, J.P. and Ganiats, T.G. (1993b). The Quality of Well-being Scale: Rationale for a single quality of life index. In: S.R. Walker and R.M. Rosser (eds), *Quality of Life Assessment: Key Issues in the 1990s*. Dordrecht: Kluwer Academic.

Kaplan-DeNour, N. (1982). Psychosocial Adjustment to Illness Scale (PAIS): A study of chronic hemodialysis patients. *Journal of Psychosomatic Research, 26*: 11–26.

Karnofsky, D.A. and Burchenal, J.H. (1949). The clinical evaluation of chemotherapeutic agents against cancer. In: C.M. McLeod (ed.), *Evaluation of Chemotherapeutic Agents*. New York: Columbia University Press.

Karnofsky, D.A., Abelmann, W.H., Craver, L.F. *et al.* (1948). The use of nitrogen mustards in the palliative treatment of carcinoma. *Cancer, I*: 634–56.

Kasl, S.V. and Cooper, C.L. (1987). *Stress and Health Issues in Research Methodology*. Chichester: John Wiley.

Kaszniak, A.W. and Allender, J. (1985). Psychological assessment of depression in older adults. In: G.M. Chaisson-Stewart (ed.), *Depression in the Elderly: An Interdisciplinary Approach*. New York: John Wiley.

Katz, M.M. and Lyerly, S.S. (1963). Methods for measuring adjustment and social behaviour in the community: I. Rationale, description, discriminative validity and scale development. *Psychological Reports, Monograph, 13*: 503–35 (suppl.).

Katz, M.M., Secunda, S.K., Hirschfeld, R.M.A. and Koslow, S.H. (1979). NIMH Clinical Research Branch: Collaborative program on the psychobiology of depression. *Archives of General Psychiatry, 36*: 765–71.

Katz, S. and Akpom, C.A. (1976a). A measure of primary sociobiological functions. *International Journal of Health Services, 6*: 493–508.

Katz, S. and Akpom, C.A. (1976b). Index of ADL. *Medical Care, 14*: 116–18.

Katz, S., Ford, A.B., Moskowitz, R.W. *et al.* (1963). Studies of illness in the aged: The index of ADL – a standardized measure of biological and psychosocial function. *Journal of the American Medical Association, 185*: 914–19.

Katz, S., Ford, A.B., Chinn, A.B. *et al.* (1966). Prognosis after strokes. Long term course of 159 patients with stroke. *Medicine, 45*: 236–46.

Katz, S., Vignos, P.J., Moskowitz, R.W. *et al.* (1968). Comprehensive out-patient care in rheumatoid arthritis: A controlled study. *Journal of the American Medical Association, 206*: 1249–54.

Katz, S., Akpom, C.A., Papsidero, J.A. *et al.* (1973). Measuring the health status of populations. In: R.L. Berg (ed.), *Health Status of Populations*. Chicago, IL: Hospital Research and Educational Trust.

Kazis, L.E., Meenan, R.F. and Anderson, J.J. (1983). Pain in the rheumatic diseases: Investigation of a key health status component. *Arthritis and Rheumatism, 26*: 1017–22.

Kazis, L.E., Anderson, J.J. and Meenan, R.F. (1988). Health status information in clinical practice: The development and testing of patient profile reports. *Journal of Rheumatology, 15*: 338–44.

Kearns, N.P., Cruickshank, C.A., McGuigan, K.J. *et al.* (1982). A comparison of depression rating scales. *British Journal of Psychiatry, 141*: 45–9.

Kellerman, A.L. and Hackman, B.B. (1988). Emergency department 'dumping'. *American Journal of Public Health, 78*: 1287–92.

Kellner, R. (1983). *Abridged Manual of the Symptom Rating Test*. Albuquerque, NM: University of New Mexico.

Kellner, R. and Sheffield, B.F. (1973). A self-rating scale of distress. *Psychological Medicine, 3*: 88–100.

Kemm, J.R. and Booth, D. (1992). *Promotion of Healthy Eating: How to Collect and Use Information for Planning, Monitoring and Evaluation*. London: HMSO.

Kendell, R.E., Everitt, B., Cooper, J.E. *et al.* (1968). Reliability of the Present State Examination. *Social Psychiatry, 3*: 123–9.

Kertesz, A. and Poole, E. (1974). The aphasia quotient: The taxonomic approach to measurement of aphasic disability. *Canadian Journal of Neurological Sciences, 1*: 7–16.

Keyser, D.J. and Sweetland, R.C. (eds) (1984). *Test Critiques*, Vol. I. Kansas City, MO: Test Corporation of America.

Keyser, D.J. and Sweetland, R.C. (eds) (1985a). *Test Critiques*, Vol. II. Kansas City, MO: Test Corporation of America.

Keyser, D.J. and Sweetland, R.C. (eds) (1985b). *Test Critiques*, Vol. III. Kansas City, MO: Test Corporation of America.

Keyser, D.J. and Sweetland, R.C. (eds) (1986). *Test Critiques*, Vol. V. Kansas City, MO: Test Corporation of America.

Keyser, D.J. and Sweetland, R.C. (eds) (1988). *Test Critiques*, Vol. VII. Kansas City, MO: Test Corporation of America.

Kiébert, G.M., de Haes, J.C.J.M. and van de Velde, C.J.H. (1991). The impact of breast conserving treatment and mastectomy on the quality of life of early-stage breast cancer patients: A review. *Journal of Clinical Oncology, 9*: 1059–70.

Kind, P. and Carr-Hill, R. (1987). The Nottingham Health Profile: A useful tool for epidemiologists? *Social Science and Medicine, 25*: 905–10.

Kind, P. and Gudex, C. (1991). *The HMQ: Measuring Health Status in the Community*. York: University of York, Centre for Health Economics.

Kind, P., Rosser, R. and Williams, A. (1982). Valuation of quality of life: Some psychometric evidence. In: M.W. Jones-Lee (ed.), *The Value of Life and Safety*. Amsterdam: Elsevier.

Kinsman, R.A., Luparello, T., O'Banion, K. and Spector, S. (1973). Multidimensional analysis of the subjective symptomatology of asthma. *Psychosomatic Medicine, 35*: 250–67.

Kinsman, R.A., Dahlem, N.W., Spector, S. and Staudenmayer, H. (1977). Observations on subjective symptomatology, coping behaviour, and medical decisions in asthma. *Psychosomatic Medicine, 39*: 102–19.

Kinsman, R.A., Yaroush, R.A., Fernandez, E. *et al.* (1983). Symptoms and experiences in chronic bronchitis and emphysema. *Chest, 83*: 755–61.

Kirwan, R.J. and Reeback, J.S. (1983). Using a modified Stanford Health Assessment Questionnaire to assess disability in UK patients with rheumatoid arthritis. *Annals of Rheumatic Diseases, 42*: 219–20.

Kitsuse, J. and Cicourel, A.B. (1963). A note on the official use of statistics. *Social Problems, 11*: 131–9.

Klassen, D., Hornstra, R.K. and Anderson, P.B. (1975). Influence of social desirability on symptom and mood reporting in a community survey. *Journal of Consulting and Clinical Psychology, 45*: 448–52.

Klein, D.C. (1970). The community and mental health: An attempt at a conceptual framework. In: P.E. Cook (ed.), *Community Psychology and Community Mental Health: Introductory Readings.* San Francisco, CA: Holden Day.

Kleinman, A. (1986). Culture, the quality of life and cancer pain: Anthropological and cross-cultural perspectives. In: V. Ventifridda, F.S.A.M. van Dam, R. Yancik and M. Tamburini (eds), *Assessment of Quality of Life and Cancer Treatment: Proceedings of the International Workshop on Quality of Life Assessment and Cancer Treatment,* Milan, December 1985. Amsterdam: Excerpta Medica.

Kline, P. (1986). *A Handbook of Test Construction.* London: Methuen.

Klonoff, H., Clark, C., Kavanagh-Gray, D. *et al.* (1989). Two-year follow-up study of coronary bypass surgery. *Journal of Thoracic and Cardiovascular Surgery, 97*: 78–85.

Knesevich, J.W., Biggs, J.T., Clayton, P.J. and Ziegler, V.E. (1977). Validity of the Hamilton rating scale for depression. *British Journal of Psychiatry, 131*: 49–52.

Knight, R.G., Waal-Manning, H.J. and Spears, G.F. (1983). Some norms and reliability data for the State–Trait Anxiety Inventory and the Zung Self-Rating Depression Scale. *British Journal of Clinical Psychology, 22*: 245–9.

Kobasa, S.O. (1979). Stressful life events, personality and health: An enquiry into hardiness. *Journal of Personality and Social Psychology, 39*: 1–11.

Kober, B., Kuchler, Th., Broelsch, B. *et al.* (1990). A psychological support concept and quality of life research in a liver transplantation program: An interdisciplinary multicenter study. *Psychotherapy and Psychosomatics, 54*: 117–31.

Koch, U. and Muthny, F.A. (1990). Quality of life in patients with end-stage renal disease in relation to the method of treatment. *Psychotherapy and Psychosomatics, 54*: 161–71.

Koos, E. (1954). *The Health of Regionville: What People Thought and Did About It.* New York: Columbia University Press.

Kornfeld, D.S., Heller, S.S., Frank, K.A., Wilson, S.N. and Malm, J.R. (1984). Psychologic and behavioural responses after coronary artery bypass graft surgery. In: N.K. Wenger, M.E. Mattson, C.P. Furberg and J. Elinson (eds), *Assessment of Quality of Life in Clinical Trials of Cardiovascular Therapies.* New York: Le Jacq.

Kovacs, M. and Beck, A.T. (1977). An empirical–clinical approach toward a definition of childhood depression. In: J.G. Schulterbrandt and A. Raskin (eds), *Depression in Childhood: Diagnosis, Treatment and Conceptual Models.* New York: Raven Press.

Kranth, J. (1981). Objective measurements of the quality of life. In: M. Baum, R. Kay and H. Scheurlen (eds), *Clinical Trials in Early Breast Cancer.* Second Heidelberg Symposium. Basel: Birkhauser Verlag.

Krauskopf, C.J. (1984). Wechsler Adult Intelligence Scale. In: D.J. Keyser and R.C. Sweetland (eds), *Test Critiques,* Vol. I. Kansas City, MO: Test Corporation of America.

Krischer, J.P. (1979). Indexes of severity: Conceptual development. *Health Services Research, 14*: 56–67.

Kronenberg, Y., Blumensohn, R. and Apter, A. (1988). A comparison of different diagnostic tools for childhood depression. *Acta Psychiatrica Scandinavica, 77*: 194–8.

Krupinski, J. (1980). Health and quality of life. *Social Science and Medicine, 14A*: 203–11.

Kuhn, W.F., Davis, M.H. and Lippman, S.B. (1988). Emotional adjustment to cardiac transplantation. *General Hospital Psychiatry, 10*: 108–13.

Kuhn, W.F., Brennan, A.F., Lacefield, P.K. *et al.* (1990). Psychiatric distress during stages of heart transplant protocol. *Journal of Heart Transplantation, 9*: 25–9.

Kunsebeck, H.W., Korber, J. and Freyberger, H. (1990). Quality of life in patients with inflammatory bowel disease. *Psychotherapy and Psychosomatics, 54*: 110–16.

Kurtin, P.S., Davies, A.R., Meyer, K.B. *et al.* (1992). Patient-based health status measurements in outpatient dialysis: Early experiences in developing an outcomes assessment program. *Medical Care, 30*: MS136–MS149 (suppl. 5).

Kutner, N.G., Fair, P.L. and Kutner, M.H. (1985). Assessing depression and anxiety in chronic dialysis patients. *Journal of Psychosomatic Research, 29*: 23–31.

Laerum, E., Johnsen, N., Smith, P. and Arnesen, H. (1991). Positive psychological and life style changes after myocardial infarction: A follow-up study after 2–4 years. *Family Practice, 8*: 229–33.

Langley, G.B. and Sheppard, H. (1984). Problems associated with pain measurement in arthritis: Comparison of the visual analogue and verbal rating scales. *Clinics in Experimental Rheumatology, 2*: 231–4.

Langner, T.S. (1962). Twenty-two item screening scale of psychiatric symptoms indicating impairment. *Journal of Health and Human Behaviour, 3*: 269–76.

Larsen, D.L., Attkisson, C.C., Hargreaves, W.A. and Nguyen, T.D. (1979). Assessment of client/patient satisfaction: Development of a general scale. *Evaluation and Program Planning, 2*: 197–207.

Larsson, G. and Setterlind, S. (1990). Work load/work control and health: Moderating effects of heredity, self-image, coping and health behaviour. *International Journal of Health Sciences, 1*: 79–88.

Lasry, J.C. (1991). Women's sexuality following breast cancer. In: D. Osoba (ed.), *Effect of Cancer on Quality of Life*. Boston, MA: CRC Press.

Lasry, J.C., Margolese, R.G., Poisson, R., Shibata, H. *et al.* (1987). Depression and body image following mastectomy and lumpectomy. *Journal of Chronic Diseases, 40*: 529–34.

Laszlo, J. (1983). Nausea and vomiting as major complications of cancer chemotherapy. *Drugs, 25*: 1–7.

Lawrence, K., McWhinnie, D., Coulter, A. *et al.* (1993). Quality of life assessment in a randomised controlled trial of laparoscopic versus open inguinal hernia repair. Paper presented to the *Fifth European Health Services Research Conference*, Maastricht, December.

Lawton, M.P. (1972). The dimensions of morale. In: D. Kent, R. Kastenbaum and S. Sherwood (eds), *Research, Planning and Action for the Elderly*. New York: Behavioural Publications.

Lawton, M.P. (1975). The Philadelphia Geriatric Center Morale Scale: A revision. *Journal of Gerontology, 30*: 85–9.

Lawton, M.P. (1983). Environment and other determinants of well-being in older people. *The Gerontologist, 23*: 349–57.

Lawton, M.P. (1991). Functional status and aging well. *Generations, 15*: 31–4.

Lawton, M.P. and Brody, E.M. (1969). Assessment of older people: Self maintaining and instrumental activities of daily living. *The Gerontologist, 9*: 179–86.

Lawton, M.P., Moss, M. and Glicksman, A. (1990). The quality of the last year of life of older persons. *The Milbank Quarterly, 68*: 1–28.

Lazarus, R.S. (ed.) (1966). *Psychological Stress and the Coping Process*. New York: McGraw-Hill.

Lazarus, R.S. (1980). The stress and coping paradigm. In: C. Eisdorfer, D. Cohen, A. Kleinman and P. Maxim (eds), *Theoretical Bases for Psychopathology*. New York: Spectrum.

Lazarus, R.S. and Cohen, J.B. (1977). Environmental stress. In: I. Altman and J.F. Wohlwill (eds), *Human Behavior and Environment*, Vol. 2. New York: Plenum Press.

Lazarus, R.S. and Folkman, S. (1984). *Stress, Appraisal and Coping*. New York: Springer Verlag.

Lazarus, R.S., Averill, J.R. and Opton, E.M. (1974). The psychology of coping: Issues of research and assessment. In: G.V. Coelho, D.A. Hamburg and J.E. Adams (eds), *Coping and Adaptation*. New York: Basic Books.

Lebowitz, M.D. and Burrows, B. (1976). Comparison of questionnaires: The BMRC and NHLI respiratory questionnaires and new self-completion questionnaire. *American Review of Respiratory Disease, 113*: 627–35.

Lee, T.H., Shammash, J.B., Ribeiro, J.P. *et al.* (1988). Estimation of maximum oxygen uptake from clinical data: Performance of the Specific Activity Scale. *American Heart Journal, 115*: 203–4.

Lefcourt, H.M. (1991). Locus of control. In: J.P. Robinson, P.R. Shaver and L.S. Wrightsman (eds), *Measures of Personality and Social Psychological Attitudes*, Vol. 1. San Diego, CA: Academic Press.

Leff, J. (1988). *Team for the Assessment of Psychiatric Services: Preliminary Report on Baseline Data from Friern and Claybury Hospitals*. London: North East Thames Regional Health Authority.

Leff, J. (1991a). The relevance of psychosocial risk factors for treatment and prevention. In: P.E. Bebbington (ed.), *Social Psychiatry: Theory, Methodology and Practice*. London: Transaction Publishers.

Leff, J. (1991b). The evaluation of reprovision for psychiatric hospitals. In: P.E. Bebbington (ed.), *Social Psychiatry: Theory, Methodology and Practice*. London: Transaction Publishers.

Leff, J. (ed.) (1993). The TAPS project: Evaluating community placement of long stay psychiatric patients. *British Journal of Psychiatry, 162*: 1–56 (suppl. 19).

Leff, J. and Vaughan, C. (1985). *Expressed Emotion in Families*. New York: Guilford Press.

Leff, J., O'Driscoll, C., Dayson, D. *et al.* (1990). The TAPS project. 5: The structure of social-network data obtained from long stay patients. *British Journal of Psychiatry, 157*: 848–52.

Lehman, A.F. (1983). The well-being of chronic mental patients: Assessing their quality of life. *Archives of General Psychiatry, 40*: 369–73.

Lehman, A.F. (1988). A quality of life interview for the chronically mentally ill. *Evaluation and Program Planning, 11*: 51–62.

Lehman, A.F., Ward, N.C. and Lynn, L.S. (1982). Chronic mental patients: The quality of life issue. *American Journal of Psychiatry, 139*: 1271–6.

Lehman, A.F., Possidente, S. and Hawker, F. (1986). The well-being of chronic mental patients in a state hospital and community residences. *Hospital and Community Psychiatry, 37*: 901–7.

Lehman, A.F., Postrado, L.T. and Rachuba, L.T. (1993). Convergent validation of quality of life assessments for persons with severe mental illnesses. *Quality of Life Research, 2*: 327–33.

Lehman, A.F., Postrado, L.T., Roth, D. *et al.* (1994).

Continuity of care and client outcomes in the Robert Wood Johnson Foundation Program on chronic mental illness. *The Milbank Quarterly, 72*: 105–22.

Leighton, D.C., Harding, J.S., Macklin, D., Hughes, C. and Leighton, A. (1963). Psychiatric findings of the Sterling County Study. *American Journal of Psychiatry, 119*: 1021–6.

Leiner, G.C., Abramowitz, S., Lewis, W.A. and Small, M.J. (1965). Dyspnoea and pulmonary function tests. *American Review of Respiratory Disease, 92*: 822–3.

Lerner, M. (1973). Conceptualisation of health and social welfare. In: R.L. Berg (ed.), *Health Status Indexes*. Chicago, IL: Hospital Research and Educational Trust.

Lesko, L. and Hawkins, D. (1983). *Psychological Aspects of Transplantation Medicine*. New York: Aronson.

Lester, D.M. (1973). The psychological impact of chronic obstructive pulmonary disease. In: R.F. Johnson (ed.), *Pulmonary Care*. New York: Grune and Stratton.

Levin, G., Wilder, J.F. and Gilbert, J. (1978). Identifying and meeting clients' needs in six community mental health centers. *Hospital and Community Psychiatry, 29*: 185–8.

Levine, S. and Croog, S.H. (1984). What constitutes quality of life? A conceptualisation of the dimensions of life quality in healthy populations and patients with cardiovascular disease. In: N.K. Wenger, M.E. Mattson, C.D. Furberg and J. Elinson (eds), *Assessment of Quality of Life in Clinical Trials of Cardiovascular Therapies*. New York: Le Jacq.

Levine, S. and Croog, S.H. (1989). Quality of life measures used to study antihypertensive medications. In: F. Mosteller and J. Falotico-Taylor (eds), *Quality of Life and Technology Assessment*. Monograph of the Council on Health Care Technology. Washington, DC: National Academy Press.

Levine, M.N., Guyatt, G.H., Gent, M. *et al.* (1988). Quality of life in stage II breast cancer: An instrument for clinical trials. *Journal of Clinical Oncology, 6*: 1798–1810.

Levinson, H. (1974). Activism and powerful others: Distinctions within the concept of internal–external control. *Journal of Personality Assessment, 38*: 377–83.

Levinson, H. (1975). Multidimensional locus of control in prison inmates. *Journal of Applied Social Psychology, 5*: 342–7.

Levy, S.M., Heberman, R.B., Lee, J.R., Lippman, M.E. and d'Angelo, T. (1989). Breast conservation *v.* mastectomy: Distress sequelae as a function of choice. *Journal of Clinical Oncology, 7*: 367–75.

Lewin, K., Dembo, T., Festinger, L. and Sears, P. (1944). *Level of Aspirations*. New York: Ronald Press.

Lewis, F.M. (1982). Experienced personal control and quality of life in late stage cancer patients. *Nursing Research, 31*: 113–19.

Lewis, F.M. (1989). Attributions of control, experienced meaning and psychosocial well-being in patients with advanced cancer. *Journal of Psychosocial Oncology, 7*: 105–19.

Lewis, G. and Wessely, S. (1990). Comparison of the General Health Questionnaire and the Hospital Anxiety and Depression Scale. *British Journal of Psychiatry, 157*: 860–4.

Lezak, M.D. (1989). *Assessment of the Behavioural Consequences of Head Trauma*. New York: Alan L. Liss.

Liang, J., Levin, J.S. and Krause, N.M. (1989). Dimensions of the OARS mental health measures. *Journal of Gerontology (Psychological Sciences), 44*: 127–38.

Liang, M.H. and Jette, A. M. (1981). Measuring functional ability in chronic arthritis: A critical review. *Arthritis and Rheumatism, 24*: 80–6,

Liang, M.H. and Katz, J.N. (1992). Measurement of outcome in rheumatoid arthritis. In D.L. Scott (ed.), *The Course and Outcome of Rheumatoid Arthritis: Bailliere's Clinical Rheumatology*, Vol. 6 No. 1. London Bailliere Tindall.

Liang, M.H., Cullen, K. and Larson, M. (1982). In search of a more perfect mousetrap (health status or quality of life instrument). *Journal of Rheumatology, 9*: 775–9.

Liang, M.H., Larson, M., Cullen, K. and Schwartz, J. (1985). Comparative measurement efficiency and sensitivity of five health status instruments for arthritis research. *Arthritis and Rheumatism, 28*: 524–47.

Liang, M.H., Fossel, A.H. and Larson, M.G. (1990). Comparisons of five health status instruments for orthopedic evaluation. *Medical Care, 28*: 632–42.

Liddle, J., Gilleard, C. and Neil, A. (1993). Elderly patients' and their relatives' views on CPR (letter). *Lancet, 342*: 1055.

Likert, R. (1952). A technique for the development of attitude scales. *Educational and Psychological Measurement, 12*: 313–15.

Lindal, E. (1990). Post-operative depression and coronary bypass surgery. *International Disability Studies, 12*: 70–4.

Lindenstrom, E. Boysen, G., Christiansen, L.W., Rogvi-Hansen, B. and Nielsen, P.W. (1991). Reliability of Scandinavian Neurological Stroke Scale. *Cerebrovascular Disease, 1*: 103–7.

Lindley, C.M. (1992). Quality of life measurements in oncology. *Pharmacotherapy, 12*: 346–52.

Lindley, C.M., Hirsch, J.D., O'Neill, C.V. *et al.* (1992). Quality of life consequences of chemotherapy-induced emesis. *Quality of Life Research, 1*: 331–40,

Lindsay, R.M., Burton, H.J. and Kline, S.A. (1985). Quality of life and psychosocial aspects of chronic peritoneal dialysis. In: K.D. Nolph (ed.), *Peritoneal Dialysis*, 2nd edn. Boston, MA: Martinus Nijoff.

Linn, B.S., Linn, M.W. and Gurel, L. (1968). Cumulative Illness Rating Scale. *Journal of the American Geriatrics Society, 16*: 622–6.

Linn, M.W. (1976). Studies in rating the physical, mental and social dysfunction of the chronically ill aged. *Medical Care, 14*: 119–25 (suppl. 5).

Linn, M.W. (1979). Assessing community adjustment in the elderly. In: A. Raskin and L.F. Jervik (eds), *Assessment of Psychiatric Symptoms and Cognitive Loss in the Elderly*. Washington, DC: Hemisphere Press.

Linn, M.W., Sculthorpe, W.B., Evje, M. *et al.* (1969). A Social Dysfunction Rating Scale. *Journal of Psychiatric Research, 6*: 299–306.

Lipman, R.S., Rickles, K., Covi, L. *et al.* (1969). Factors of symptom distress. *Archives of General Psychiatry, 24*: 454–64.

Little, A., Hemsley, D., Bergmann, K. *et al.* (1987). Comparison of the sensitivity of three instruments for the detection of cognitive decline in the elderly living at home. *British Journal of Psychiatry, 150*: 808–14.

Littlewood, R. and Lipsedge, M. (1982). *Aliens and Alienists*. Harmondsworth: Penguin.

Liu, B.C. (1974). Quality of life indicators: A preliminary investigation. *Social Indicators Research, 1*: 187–208.

Llewellyn-Thomas, H.A., Sutherland, H.J., Hogg, S.A. *et al.* (1984). Linear analogue self-assessment of voice quality in laryngeal cancer. *Journal of Chronic Diseases, 37*: 917–24.

Lohr, K.N. and Ware, J.E. (eds) (1987). Proceedings of the Advances in Health Assessment Conference, Palm Springs, CA, February 1986. *Journal of Chronic Diseases, 40*: S1–S193 (suppl.).

Long, A.F., Bate, L. and Sheldon, T.A. (1992). Establishment of UK clearing house for assessing health services outcomes. *Quality in Health Care, 1*: 131–3.

Loo, R. (1983). Caveat on sample sizes in factor analysis. *Perceptual and Motor Skills, 56*: 371–4.

Lorr, M., McNair, D. and Fisher, S. (1982). Evidence for bipolar mood states. *Journal of Personality Assessment, 46*: 432–6.

Lough, M.E., Lindsey, A.M., Shinn, J.A. *et al.* (1987). Impact of symptom frequency and symptom distress on self-reported quality of life in heart transplant recipients. *Heart and Lung, 16*: 193–200.

Louks. J., Hayne, C. and Smith, J. (1989). Replicated factor structure of the Beck Depression Inventory. *Journal of Nervous Mental Disease, 177*: 473–9.

Lubeck, D.P. and Fries, J.F. (1992). Changes in quality of life among persons with HIV infection. *Quality of Life Research, 1*: 359–66.

Lubeck, D.P., Patrick, D.P., McNulty, P. *et al.* (1993). Quality of life with persons with onychomycosis. *Quality of Life Research, 2*: 341–8.

Luborsky, L. (1962). Clinician's judgements of mental health. *Archives of General Psychiatry, 7*: 407–17.

Luce, B.R., Wechsler, J.M. and Underwood, C. (1989). The uses of quality of life measures in the private sector. In: F. Mosteller and J. Falotico-Taylor (eds), *Quality of Life and Technology Assessment*. Washington, DC: National Academy Press.

Luria, R.E. and Berry, R. (1979). Reliability and descriptive validity of PSE syndromes. *Archives of General Psychiatry, 36*: 1187–95.

Lustig, F.M., Haas, A. and Castillo, R. (1972). Clinical and rehabilitation regime in patients with COPD. *Archives of Physical Medical Rehabilitation, 53*: 315–22.

MacCarthy, B., Benson, J. and Brewin, C.R. (1986). Task motivation and problem appraisal in long term psychiatric patients. *Psychological Medicine, 16*: 431–8.

MacCarthy, B., Lesage, A., Brewin, C.R. *et al.* (1989). Needs for care among the relatives of long term users of day care. *Psychological Medicine, 19*: 725–36.

MacDonald, A.P. (1973). Internal–external locus of control. In: J.P. Robinson and P. Shaver (eds), *Measures of Social Psychological Attitudes*. Ann Arbor, MI: Institute for Social Research, University of Michigan.

Mackenzie, R., Charlson, M., DiGioia, D. and Kelley, K. (1986). Can the Sickness Impact Profile measure change? An example of scale assessment. *Journal of Chronic Diseases, 39*: 429–38.

Mackillop, W.J., Ward, G.K. and O'Sullivan, B. (1986). The use of expert surrogates to evaluate clinical trials in non-small cell lung cancer. *British Journal of Cancer, 54*: 661–7.

Mackillop, W.J., Palmer, M.J., O'Sullivan, B. *et al.* (1988). Clinical trials in cancer: The role of surrogate patients in defining what constitutes an ethically acceptable clinical experiment. *British Journal of Cancer, 59*: 388–95.

Mackillop, W.J., Palmer, M.J., O'Sullivan, B. and Quirt, C.F. (1992). The expert surrogate system. In: C.J. Williams (ed.), *Introducing New Treatments for Cancer: Practical, Ethical and Legal Problems*. Chichester: John Wiley.

Magni, G., Unger, H.P., Valfe, C. *et al.* (1987). Psychosocial outcome one year after heart surgery. *Archives of Internal Medicine, 147*: 473–7.

Maguire, G.P., Tait, A., Brooke, M., Howat, J.M. and Sellwood, R.A. (1980). Psychiatric morbidity and physical toxicity associated with adjuvant chemotherapy after mastectomy. *British Medical Journal, 14*: 61–5.

Maguire, P. and Selby, P. (1989). Assessing the quality of life in cancer patients. *British Journal of Cancer, 60*: 437–40.

Mahler, D.A. and Harver, A. (1990). Clinical measurement of dyspnea. In: D.A. Mahler (ed.), *Dyspnea*. New York: Future Publishing.

Mahler, D.A. and Wells, C.K. (1988). Evaluation of

clinical methods for rating dyspnoea. *Chest, 93*: 580–6.

Mahler, D.A., Weinberg, D.H., Wells, C.K. and Feinstein, A.R. (1984). The measurement of dyspnea: Contents, interobserver agreement, and physiologic correlates of two new clinical indexes. *Chest, 85*: 751–8.

Mahler, D.A., Rosiello, R.A., Harver, A. *et al.* (1987). Comparison of clinical dyspnea ratings and psychophysical measurements of respiratory sensation in obstructive airway disease. *American Review of Respiratory Disease, 135*: 1229–33.

Mahoney, F.I. and Barthel, D.W. (1965). Functional evaluation: The Barthel Index. *Maryland State Medical Journal, 14*: 61–5.

Mai, F.M. (1993). Psychiatric aspects of heart transplantation. *British Journal of Psychiatry, 163*: 285–92.

Mallya, R. and Mace, B. (1981). The assessment of disease activity in rheumatoid arthritis using a multivariate analysis. *Rheumatology and Rehabilitation, 20*: 14–17.

Malm, U., May, P., Dencker, S. (1981). Evaluation of the quality of life of the schizophrenic outpatient: A checklist. *Schizophrenia Bulletin, 7*: 477–87.

Manchanda, R., Hirsch, S.R. and Barnes, T.R.E. (1989). A review of rating scales for measuring symptom changes in schizophrenic research. In: C. Thompson (ed.), *The Instruments of Psychiatric Research*. Chichester: John Wiley.

Mangen, D.J. and Peterson, W.A. (1982). *Clinical and Social Psychology*. Minneapolis, MN: University of Minnesota Press.

Mangen, S. and Brewin, C.R. (1991). The measurement of need. In: P.E. Bebbington (ed.). *Social Psychiatry: Theory, Methodology and Practice*. London: Transaction Publishers.

Mangione, C.M., Marcantonio, E.R., Goldman, L. *et al.* (1993). Influence of age on measurement of health status in patients undergoing elective surgery. *Journal of the American Geriatrics Society, 41*: 377–83.

Mann, A.H. (1977). The psychological effects of a screening programme and clinical trial for hypertension upon the participants. *Psychological Medicine, 7*: 431–8.

Mann, A.H. (1984). Hypertension: Psychological aspects and diagnostic impact in a clinical trial. *Psychological Medicine Monograph*, suppl. 5.

Manning, W.G., Newhouse, J.P. and Ware, J.E. (1982). The status of health in demand estimation. In: V.R. Fuchs (ed.), *Economic Aspects of Health*. Chicago, IL: University of Chicago Press.

Martin, J., Meltzer, H. and Elliot, D. (1988). *The Prevalence of Disability Among Adults*. OPCS Surveys of Disability in Great Britain, Report No. 1. London: HMSO.

Mashberg, D., Ostroff, J. and Lesko, L. (1989). Psychosexual sequelae among adult leukemia survivors. *Proceed ASCO, 8*: 311.

Maslow, A. (1954). *Motivation and Personality*. New York: Harper Row.

Maslow, A. (1962a). *Towards a Psychology of Being*. Princeton, NJ: Van Nostrand.

Maslow, A. (1962b). *The Farther Reaches of Human Nature*. New York: Viking Press.

Mason, J.H., Anderson, J.J. and Meenan, R.F. (1988). A model for health status for rheumatoid arthritis: A factor analysis of the Arthritis Impact Measurement Scales. *Arthritis and Rheumatism, 31*: 714–20.

Mason, R. and Faulkenberry, G.D. (1978). Aspirations, achievement and life satisfaction. *Social Indicators Research, 5*: 133–50.

Matazzo, J.D. (1972). *Wechsler's Measurement and Appraisal of Intelligence*. Baltimore, MD: Williams and Wilkins.

Mathiowetz, V., Volland, G., Kashman, N. and Weber, K. (1985). Adult norms for the nine-hole peg test of finger dexterity. *Occupational Therapy Journal of Research, 5*: 24–37.

Matthews, J.L., Bush, B.A. and Ewall, F.W. (1989). Exercise responses during incremental and high intensity and low intensity steady state exercise in patients with obstructive lung disease and normal control subjects. *Chest, 96*: 11–17.

Mattison, P.G., Aitken, R.C.B. and Prescot, R.J. (1991). Rehabilitation status – the relationship between the Edinburgh Rehabilitation Status Scale (ERSS), Barthel Index and PULSES Profile. *International Disability Studies, 13*: 9–11.

Maylath, N.S. (1990). Development of the Children's Health Rating Scale. *Health Education Quarterly, 17*: 89–97.

Mayou, R. (1990). Quality of life in cardiovascular disease. *Psychotherapy and Psychosomatics, 54*: 99–109.

Mayou, R., Williamson, B. and Foster, A. (1976). Attitudes and advice after myocardial infarction. *British Medical Journal, i*: 1577–9.

McArdle, C.S., Calman, K.C., Cooper, A.F., Hughson, A.W.M., Russell, A.R. and Smith, D.C. (1981). The social, emotional and financial implications of adjuvant chemotherapy in breast cancer. *British Journal of Surgery, 68*: 261–6.

McCarthy, P.R. (1985). Self-esteem Questionnaire. In: D.J. Keyser and R.C. Sweetland (eds), *Test Critiques*, Vol. II. Kansas City, MO: Test Corporation of America.

McColl, E., Meadows, K.A., Hutchison, A. *et al.* (1993). Outcome measures in ambulatory care: Developing measures for asthma and diabetes. A summary. Paper presented to the *Society for Social Medicine, Health Related Quality of Life Workshop*, Sheffield, May.

McColl, E., Steen, I.N., Meadows, K. *et al.* (1995). Developing outcome measures for ambulatory care: An application to asthma and diabetes. *Social Science and Medicine, 10*: 1339–48.

McCorkle, R. (1987). The measurement of symptom distress. *Seminars Oncology Nursing, 3*: 248–56.

McCorkle, R. and Quint-Benoliel, J. (1981). *Cancer Patient Responses to Psychosocial Variables*. Final Report of Project Supported by Grant NU 00730, DHHS. Seattle, WA: University of Washington.

McCorkle, R. and Quint-Benoliel, J. (1983). Symptom distress, current concerns and mood disturbances after diagnosis of life threatening disease. *Social Science and Medicine, 17*: 431–8.

McCorkle, R. and Young, K. (1978). Development of a symptom distress scale. *Cancer Nursing, 1*: 373–8.

McCorkle, R., Quint-Benoliel, J., Donaldson, G. *et al.* (1986). *Evaluation of Cancer Management*. Final Report. PHS grant NU01001. Seattle, WA: University of Washington, Division of Nursing, Bureau of Health Professions, Health Resources and Services Administration.

McCorkle, R., Quint-Benoliel, J., Donaldson, G. *et al.* (1989). A randomised clinical trial of home nursing care for lung cancer patients. *Cancer, 64*: 1375–82.

McCrae, P.R. (1984). Situational determinants of coping responses: Loss, threat and challenge. *Journal of Personality and Social Psychology, 46*: 919–28.

McDonald, B.W., Pugh, W.M., Gunderson, E.K.E. and Rahe, R.H. (1972). Reliability of life change cluster scores. *British Journal of Social and Clinical Psychology, 11*: 407–9.

McDowell, I. and Newell, I. (1987). *Measuring Health: A Guide to Rating Scales and Questionnaires*. New York: Oxford University Press.

McGavin, C.R., Gupta, G.P. and McHardy, G.J.R. (1976). Twelve minute walking test for assessing disability in chronic bronchitis. *British Medical Journal, i*: 822–3.

McGavin, C.R., Artvinli, M., Naoe, H. and McHardy, G.J.R. (1978). Dyspnoea, disability and distance walked: A comparison of estimates of exercise performance in respiratory disease. *British Medical Journal, 2*: 241–3.

McGee, H.M., O'Boyle, C.A., Hickey, A. *et al.* (1991). Assessing the quality of life of the individual: The SEIQoL with a healthy and a gastroenterology unit population. *Psychological Medicine, 21*: 749–59.

McGee, H.M. and Bradley, C. (1994). *Quality of Life Following Renal Failure*. Reading: Harwood Academic.

McHorney, C.A., Ware, J.E., Rogers, W. *et al.* (1992). The validity and relative precision of the MOS Short- and Long-form health status scales and Dartmouth Coop Charts. *Medical Care 30*: MS253–MS265.

McHorney, C.A., Ware, J.E. and Raczek, A.E. (1993). The MOS 36-Item Short Form Health Survey (SF-36): II. Psychometric and clinical tests of validity in measuring physical and mental health constructs. *Medical Care, 31*: 247–63.

McKenna, S.P. (1993). The Nottingham Health Profile. Paper presented to the *Fifth European Health Services Research Conference*, Maastricht, December.

McKenna, S.P. and Hunt, S.M. (1992a). The General Well-being Index: Adapting and retesting an American measure for use in the United Kingdom. *British Journal of Medical Economics, 4*: 41–50.

McKenna, S.P. and Hunt, S.M. (1992b). A new measure of quality of life in depression: Testing the reliability and construct validity of the QLDS. *Health Policy, 22*: 321–30.

McKennell, A.C. and Andrews, F.M. (1980). Models of cognition and affect in perceptions of well-being. *Social Indicators Research, 8*: 257–98.

McMurdo, M.E.T. and Rennie, L. (1993). A controlled trial of exercise by residents of old people's homes. *Age and Ageing, 22*: 11–15.

McNair, D.M., Lorr, M. and Droppleman, L.F. (1971). *Manual for the Profile of Mood States*. San Diego, CA: Educational and Industrial Testing Services.

McNair, D.M., Lorr, M. and Droppleman, L.F. (1992). *EdITS Manual for the Profile of Mood States (POMS)*. San Diego, CA: EdITS/Educational and Industrial Testing Service.

McNeil, B.J., Weichselbaum, R. and Pauker, S.G. (1978). Fallacy of the five year survival in lung cancer. *New England Journal of Medicine, 299*: 1397–1401.

McNeil, B.J., Weichselbaum, R. and Pauker, S.G. (1981). Speech and survival, trade-offs between quality and quantity of life in laryngeal cancer. *New England Journal of Medicine, 305*: 982–7.

McPhee, C.B., Zusman, J. and Joss, R.H. (1975). Measurement of patient satisfaction: A survey of practices in community mental health centres. *Comprehensive Psychiatry, 16*: 399–404.

McQuay, H.J. (1990). Assessment of pain, and effectiveness of treatment. In: A. Hopkins and D. Costain (eds), *Measuring the Outcomes of Medical Care*. London: Royal College of Physicians.

McSweeny, A.J. (1984). Assessing the quality of life in patients with chronic obstructive pulmonary disease. In: N.K. Wenger, M.E. Mattson, C.P. Furberg and J. Elinson (eds), *Assessment of Quality of Life in Clinical Trials of Cardiovascular Therapies*. New York: Le Jacq.

McSweeny, A.J., Heaton, R.K., Grant, I. *et al.* (1980). Chronic obstructive pulmonary disease: Socio-emotional adjustment and life quality. *Chest, 77*: 309–11 (suppl.).

McSweeny, A.J., Grant, I., Heaton, R.K. *et al.* (1982). Life quality of patients with chronic obstructive pulmonary disease. *Archives of Internal Medicine, 142*: 473–8.

McSweeny, A.J. and Labuhn, K.T. (1990). Chronic obstructive pulmonary disease. In: B. Spilker (ed.), *Quality of Life Assessment in Clinical Trials*. New York: Raven Press.

Meadows, K.A. (1991). Assessing quality of life. In: C. Bradley, P. Home and M. Christie (eds), *The Technology of Diabetes Care: Converging Medical and Psychosocial Perspectives*. Reading: Harwood Academic.

Meadows, K.A., Brown, K., Thompson, C. *et al.* (1988). An instrument for screening psychosocial problems in IDDM. *Diabetes Research Clinical Practice, 5* (suppl. 1): ORA/005/003 (abstract).

Meadows, K.A., Brown, K.G., Thompson, C. and Wise, P.H. (1989). The Diabetes Health Questionnaire (DHQ): Preliminary validation of a new instrument. *Diabetic Medicine, 6*: 78 (suppl. 2).

Mechanic, D. (1962). The concept of illness behaviour. *Journal of Chronic Diseases, 17*: 189–94.

Mechanic, D. and Angel, R.J. (1987). Some factors associated with the report and evaluation of back pain. *Journal of Health and Social Behaviour, 28*: 131–9.

Mechanic, M. (1991). Researching the idea of health. In: P.E. Bebbington (ed.), *Social Psychiatry: Theory, Methodology and Practice*. London: Transaction Publishers.

Medical Outcomes Institute (1990). *Report on a Survey of Elderly Rural Residents: Health Status, Use of Health Care Services, and Satisfaction with Quality of Care*. Bloomington, MN: HOI.

Medical Outcomes Trust (1993a). SF-36 responses of end-stage renal patients. *Medical Outcomes Trust Bulletin, 1*: 3. Boston, MA: MOT.

Medical Outcomes Trust (1993b). Medical Outcomes Trust instruments. *Medical Outcomes Trust Bulletin, 1*: 1. Boston, MA: MOT.

Medical Outcomes Trust (1994). Confidence intervals for individual scores. *Medical Outcomes Trust Bulletin, 2*: 3. Boston, MA: MOT.

Medical Research Council (1960). Committee on the Aetiology of Chronic Bronchitis: Standardised questionnaires on respiratory symptoms. *British Medical Journal, ii*: 1665.

Medical Research Council (1965). Committee on the Aetiology of Chronic Bronchitis: Definitions and classification of chronic bronchitis for clinical and epidemiological purposes. *Lancet, 1*: 775.

Medical Research Council (1966). *Committee on Research into Chronic Bronchitis: Instructions for the Use of the Questionnaire on Respiratory Symptoms*. Devon: W.J. Holman.

Medical Research Council (1981). Working Party on Mild to Moderate Hypertension: Adverse reactions to bendrofluazide and propanolol for the treatment of mild hypertension. *Lancet, 2*: 539–43.

Medical Research Council (1986). *Questionnaire on Respiratory Symptoms: Instructions to Interviewers*. MRC Committee on Environmental and Occupational Health. London: MRC.

Meenan, R.F. (1982). The AIMS approach to health status measurement: Conceptual background and measurement properties. *Journal of Rheumatology, 9*: 785–8.

Meenan, R.F. (1985). New approaches to outcome assessment: The AIMS questionnaire for arthritis. In: G.H. Stollerman (ed.), *Advances in Internal Medicine*, Vol. 31. New York: Year Book Medical.

Meenan, R.F. and Mason, J.H. (1990). *AIMS2 Users' Guide*. Boston, MA: Boston University School of Medicine, Department of Public Health.

Meenan, R.F., Gertman, P.M. and Mason, J.H. (1980). Measuring health status in arthritis: The arthritis impact measurement scales. *Arthritis and Rheumatism, 23*: 146–52.

Meenan, R.F., Gertman, P.M., Mason, J.H. *et al.* (1982). The arthritis impact measurement scales: Further investigations of a health status measure. *Arthritis and Rheumatism, 25*: 1048–53.

Meenan, R.F., Anderson, J.J., Kazis, L.E. *et al.* (1984). Outcome assessment in clinical trials: Evidence for the sensitivity of a health service measure. *Arthritis and Rheumatism, 27*: 1344–52.

Melzack, R. (1975). The McGill Pain Questionnaire: Major properties and scoring methods. *Pain, 1*: 277–99.

Melzack, R. (1980). Psychological aspects of pain. In: J.J. Bonica (ed.), *Pain*. New York: Raven Press.

Melzack, R. (1983). *Pain Measurement and Assessment*. New York: Raven Press.

Melzack, R. (1987). The Short-Form McGill Pain Questionnaire. *Pain, 30*: 191–7.

Melzack, R. and Torgerson, W.S. (1971). On the language of pain. *Anaesthesiology, 34*: 50–9.

Melzer, D., Hale, A.S. and Malik, S.J. (1991). Community care for patients with schizophrenia one year after hospital discharge. *British Medical Journal, 303*: 1023–6.

Mercier, M., Schraub, S., Bransfield, D.D. and Barthod, L. (1992a). Measurement of quality of life: Application to the screening of psychological distress in cancer patients. *Bulletin du Cancer (Paris), 79*: 193–204.

Mercier, M., Schraub, S., Bransfield, D.D. and Fournier, J. (1992b). Patient acceptance and differential perceptions of quality of life measures in a French oncology setting. *Quality of Life Research, 1*: 53–61.

Metcalfe, M. and Goldman, E. (1965). Validation of an inventory for measuring depression. *British Journal of Psychiatry, 111*: 240–2.

Meyer, A. (1919). The life chart and the obligation of specifying positive data in psycho–pathological diagnosis. In: *Contributions to Medical and Biological Research*, Vol. II. New York: Paul B. Hoeber.

Meyerowitz, B.E., Vasterling, J., Muirhead, J. and Frist, W. (1989). Quality of life and coping in heart transplant patients. In: A. Willner and G. Rodewald (eds), *Impact of Cardiac Surgery on Quality of Life: Neurological and Psychological Aspects*. New York: Plenum Press.

Miklowitz, D.J., Goldstein, M.J., Falloon, I.R.H. and Doane, J.A. (1984). Interactional correlates of expressed emotion in the families of schizophrenics. *British Journal of Psychiatry, 144*: 482–7.

Miller, A.B., Hoogstraten, B., Staquet, N. *et al*. (1981). Reporting results of cancer treatment. *Cancer, 47*: 207–14.

Miller, I.W., Bishop, S., Norman, W.H. and Maddever, H. (1985). The modified Hamilton Rating Scale for Depression: Reliability and validity. *Psychiatric Research, 14*: 131–42.

Minet, P., Bartsch, P., Chevalier, P. *et al*. (1987). Quality of life of inoperable non-small cell lung carcinoma: A randomised phase II clinical study comparing radiotherapy alone and combined radio-chemotherapy. *Radiotherapy and Oncology, 8*: 217–30.

Moinpour, C.M., Feigel, P., Metch, B. *et al*. (1989). Quality of life end points in cancer clinical trials: Review and recommendations. *Journal of the National Cancer Institute, 81*: 486–95.

Moinpour, C.M., Hayden, K.A., Thompson, I.M. *et al*. (1990). Quality of life assessment in Southwest Oncology Group trials. *Oncology, 4*: 79–89.

Monk, M. (1981). Blood pressure awareness and psychological well-being in the Health and Nutrition Examination Survey. *Clinical Investigative Medicine, 4*: 183–9.

Monroe, S.M. (1982). Assessment of life events: Retrospective *vs* concurrent strategies. *Archives of General Psychiatry, 39*: 606–10.

Montgomery, S.A. and Asberg, M. (1979). A new depression scale designed to be sensitive to change. *British Journal of Psychiatry, 134*: 382–9.

Montgomery, S.A., Asberg, M., Traskman, L. and Montgomery, D. (1978). Cross cultural studies on the use of the CPRS in English and Swedish depressed patients. *Acta Psychiatrica Scandinavica, 271*: 3–37 (suppl.).

Moody, L. (1988). *Psychophysiologic Responses of Adults with Chronic Lung Disease*. Gainesville, FL: Division of Sponsored Research, University of Florida.

Moody, L. (1990). Measurement of psychophysiological response variables in chronic bronchitis and emphysema. *Applied Nursing Research, 3*: 36–8.

Moody, L., McCormick, K.M. and Williams, A.R. (1990). Disease and symptom severity, functional status, and quality of life in chronic bronchitis and emphysema (CBE). *Journal of Behavioural Medicine, 13*: 297–306.

Moody, L., McCormick, K.M. and Williams, A.R. (1991). Psychophysiologic correlates of quality of life in chronic bronchitis and emphysema. *Western Journal of Nursing Research, 13*: 336–52.

Moos, R.H. and Tsu, V.D. (1977). The crisis of physical illness: An overview. In: R. Moos (ed.), *Coping with Physical Illness*. New York: Plenum Press.

Moos, R.H., Cronkite, R.C., Billings, A.G. and Finney, J.W. (1982). *Health and Daily Living Form Manual*. Stanford, CA: Stanford University School of Medicine.

Moos, R.H., Cronkite, R.C., Billings, A.G. and Finney, J.W. (1986). *Health and Daily Living Form*, revised version. Palo Alto, CA: Veterans Administration and Stanford University Medical Centres.

Moos, R.H., Cronkite, R.C. and Finney, J.W. (1990). Health and Daily Living Form Manual (revised), 2nd edn. Palo Alto: MIND GARDEN.

Mor, V. (1987). Cancer patients' quality of life over the disease course: Lessons from the real world. *Journal of Chronic Diseases, 40*: 535–44.

Mor, V., Laliberte, L., Morris, J.N. and Wiemann, M. (1984). The Karnofsky performance status scale: An examination of its reliability and validity in a research setting. *Cancer, 53*: 2002–7.

Morgan, A.E. (1934). An attempt to measure happiness. *International Journal of Ethics, 44*: 271–4.

Morgan, M.D.L. (1991). Experience of using the CRQ (Chronic Respiratory Questionnaire). *Respiratory Medicine, 85*: 23–4 (suppl. B).

Morris, J.N. (1990). *The Quality of Life of Head and Neck Cancer Patients: A Review of the Literature*. Discussion Paper No. 72. York: Centre for Health Economics, Health Economics Consortium.

Morris, J.N. and Royle, G.T. (1988). Offering patients a choice of surgery for early breast cancer: A reduction in anxiety and depression in patients and their husbands. *Social Science and Medicine, 26*: 583–5.

Morris, J.N. and Sherwood, S. (1987). Quality of life of cancer patients at different stages in the disease trajectory. *Journal of Chronic Diseases, 40*: 545–53.

Morris, J.N., Wolf, R.S. and Klerman, L.V. (1975). Common themes among morale and depression scales. *Journal of Gerontology, 30*: 209–15.

Morris, J.N., Suissa, S., Sherwood, S. *et al*. (1986). Last days: A study of terminally ill cancer patients. *Journal of Chronic Diseases, 39*: 47–62.

Morrissey, J.P., Calloway, J., Bartko, T.W. *et al*. (1994). Local mental health authorities and service system changes: Evidence from the Robert Wood Johnson Foundation Program on chronic mental illness. *The Milbank Quarterly, 72*: 49–80.

Morrissey, T., Mauschkin, C. and Franks, D. *et al.* (1990). *Client Needs, Service System Characteristics, and Mental Health Authority Performance: Interim Report from the Site Level Evaluation of the Robert Wood Johnson Foundation Program on Chronic Mental Illness.* Chapel Hill, NC: University of North Carolina, Sheps Center for Health Services Research.

Morrow, G.R. (1984). The assessment of nausea and vomiting: Past problems, current issues and suggestions for future research. *Cancer, 53*: 2267–78.

Morrow, G.R. and Morrell, C. (1982). Behavioral treatment for anticipatory nausea and vomiting induced by cancer chemotherapy. *New England Journal of Medicine, 307*: 1476–80.

Morrow, G.R., Chiarello, R.J. and Derogatis, L.R. (1978). A new scale for assessing patients' psychosocial adjustment to medical illness. *Psychological Medicine, 8*: 605–10.

Morrow, G.R., Feldstein, M., Adler, L.M. *et al.* (1981). Development of brief measures of psychosocial adjustment to medical illness applied to cancer patients. *General Hospital Psychiatry, 3*: 79–81.

Morrow, G.R., Lindke, J. and Black, P. (1992). Measurement of quality of life in patients: Psychometric analysis of the Functional Living Index – Cancer (FLIC). *Quality of Life Research, 1*: 287–96.

Morton, R., Davies, A., Baker, J., Baker, G. and Stell, P. (1984). Quality of life in treated head and neck cancer patients: A preliminary report. *Clinics in Otolaryngology, 9*: 181–5.

Moser, C.A. and Kalton, G. (1971). *Survey Methods in Social Investigation.* London: Heinemann.

Mosteller, F., Gilbert, J.P. and McPeek, B. (1980). Reporting standards and research strategies for controlled trials: Agenda for the editor. *Controlled Clinical Trials, 1*: 37–58.

Motley, R.J. and Finlay, A.Y. (1989). How much disability is caused by acne? *Clinics in Experimental Dermatology, 14*: 194–8.

Moum, T., Naess, S., Sorensen, T. *et al.* (1990). Coping processes and quality of life changes among previously unaware hypertensives. *International Journal of Health Sciences, 1*: 157–70.

Mowbray, R.M. (1972). The Hamilton Rating Scale for Depression: A factor analysis. *Psychological Medicine, 2*: 272.

Mulder, P.H. and Sluijs, E.M. (1993). *Dependent Elderly: Quality of Life Indicators.* Bibliography No. 48. Utrecht: Netherlands Institute for Primary Health Care (NIVEL).

Murphy, F.E., Donald, F.J. and Molla, A.C. (1976). A single blind comparative clinical trial of lymecycline and amoxycillin in the treatment of acute bronchitis in general practice. *Journal of International Medical Research, 4*: 65–8.

Murphy, S., Creed, F. and Jayson, M.I.V. (1988). Psychiatric disorder and illness behaviour in rheumatoid arthritis. *British Journal of Rheumatology, 27*: 357–63.

Myers, J.K. and Weissman, M.M. (1980). Use of a self-report symptom scale to detect depression in a community sample. *American Journal of Psychiatry, 137*: 1081–4.

Najman, J.M. and Levine, S. (1981). Evaluating the impact of medical care and technologies on the quality of life: A review and critique. *Social Science and Medicine, 15*: 107–15.

National Center for Health Statistics (1971). *Chronic Conditions and Limitations of Activity and Mobility: US, July 1965–June 1967.* PHS Publication No. 1000, Series 10, No. 61. Rockville, MD: US Department of Health, Education and Welfare.

National Center for Health Statistics (1974). *Prevalence of Chronic Circulatory Conditions, United States, 1972.* DHEW Publication No. (HRA) 75–1521, Series 10, No. 94. Rockville, MD: US Department of Health, Education and Welfare.

National Center for Health Statistics (1978). *Plan and Operation of the HANES I: Augmentation of Adults 25–74 years. Vital and Health Statistics.* PHS Publication No. 78–1314, Series 1, No. 14. Washington, DC: US Department of Health, Education and Welfare.

National Clearing House on Health Indexes (1993). Research Roundtable. *Bibliography on Health Indexes, 3*: 31–3. Washington DC: National Center for Health Statistics.

National Heart and Lung Institute (1971). *Proceedings, First NHLI Epidemiology Workshop.* Washington DC: US Department of Health, Education and Welfare.

National Heart, Lung and Blood Institute (1978). *Epidemiology Standardization project.* Washington DC: US Department of Health and Human Services.

Naughton M.J. and Wiklund, I. (1993). A critical review of dimension-specific measures of health-related quality of life in cross-cultural research. *Quality of Life Research, 2*: 397–432.

Nayfield, S.G., Ganz, P.A., Moinpour, C.M., Cella, D.F. and Hailey, B.J. (1992). Report from a National Cancer Institute (USA) workshop on quality of life assessment in cancer clinical trials. *Quality of Life Research, 1*: 203–10.

Nelson, A., Fogal, B.S. and Faust, D. (1986). Bedside cognitive screening instruments: A critical assessment. *Journal of Nervous and Mental Diseases, 174*: 73–83.

Nelson, E.C., Wasson, J., Kirk, J. *et al.* (1987). Assessment of function in routine clinical practice: Description of the Coop chart method and preliminary findings. *Journal of Chronic Diseases, 40*: 55S–63S (suppl.).

Nelson, E.C., Landgraf, J.M., Hays, R.D. *et al.* (1990).

The Coop Function Charts: A system to measure patient function in physicians' offices. In: M. Lipkin (ed.), *Functional Status Measurement in Primary Care: Wonca Classification Committee*. New York: Springer-Verlag.

Neugarten, B.L., Havighurst, R.J. and Tobin, S.S. (1961). The measurement of life satisfaction. *Journal of Gerontology, 16*: 134–43.

Neuhauser, D.B. and Studer, J. (1989). Who is to decide: Functional disability screening as an example. *Annals of Internal Medicine, 111*: 775–6.

Newark, C.S. and Faschingbauer, T.R. (1978). Bibliography of short forms of the MMPI. *Journal of Personality Assessment, 42*: 496–502.

Newson-Smith, J. and Hirsch, S. (1979). Psychiatric symptoms in self poisoning patients. *Psychological Medicine, 9*: 493–500.

Nguyen, T.D., Attkisson, C.C. and Stegner, B.L. (1983). Assessment of patient satisfaction: Development and refinement of a service evaluation questionnaire. *Evaluation and Program Planning, 6*: 299–314.

Nicassio, M., Wallston, A., Callahan, L. *et al.* (1985). The measurement of helplessness in rheumatoid arthritis: The development of the Arthritis Helplessness Index. *Journal of Rheumatology, 12*: 462–7.

Niezgoda, H.E. and Pater, J.L. (1993). A validation study of the domains of the core EORTC Quality of Life Questionnaire. *Quality of Life Research, 2*: 319–25.

Nocon, A. and Booth, T. (1989). *The Social Impact of Asthma*. Report to the Sheffield Asthma Society. Sheffield: University of Sheffield, Joint Unit for Social Services Research.

Nocon, A. and Booth, T. (1991). The social impact of asthma. *Family Practice, 8*: 37–41.

Nocturnal Oxygen Therapy Trial (NOTT) Group (1980). Continuous or nocturnal oxygen therapy in hypoxemic chronic obstructive lung disease. *Annals of Internal Medicine, 93*: 391–8.

Norcross, J.C., Guadagnoli, E. and Prochaska, J.O. (1984). Factor structure of the Profile of Mood States (POMS): Two partial replications. *Journal of Clinical Psychology, 40*: 77.

Normand, C. and Bowling, A. (in press). Cost–benefit analysis. In: M. Swash and J. Wilden (eds), *Outcomes in Neurological and Neurosurgical Disorders*. Cambridge: Cambridge University Press.

Nou, E. and Aberg, T. (1980). Quality of survival in patients with surgically treated bronchial carcinoma. *Thorax, 35*: 255–63.

Nou, E. and Eklund, G. (1979). Bronchial carcinoma IV: A methodological evaluation of the vitagram index for measurement of quality of survival. *Scandinavian Journal of Respiratory Disease, 104*: 131–72 (suppl.).

Nouri, F.M. and Lincoln, N.B. (1987). An extended activities of daily living scale for stroke patients. *Clinical Rehabilitation, 1*: 301–5.

Nunnally, J. (1978). *Psychometric Theory*, 2nd edn. New York: McGraw Hill.

O'Boyle, C.A., McGee, H., Hickey, A. *et al.* (1989). Reliability and validity of judgement analysis as a method for assessing quality of life. *British Journal of Clinical Pharmacology, 27*: 155.

O'Boyle, C.A., McGee, H., Hickey, A. *et al.* (1992). Individual quality of life in patients undergoing hip replacement. *Lancet, 339*: 1088–91.

O'Boyle, C.A., McGee, H., Hickey, A. *et al.* (1993). *The Schedule for the Evaluation of Individual Quality of Life (SEIQoL): Administration Manual*. Dublin: Department of Psychology, Royal College of Surgeons in Ireland.

O'Brien, B.J. (1988). Assessment of treatment in heart disease. In: G. Teeling Smith (ed.), *Measuring Health: A Practical Approach*. Chichester: John Wiley.

O'Brien, B., Buxton, M.J. and Ferguson, B.A. (1987). Measuring the effectiveness of heart transplant programmes: Quality of life data and their relationship to survival analysis. *Journal of Chronic Diseases, 40*: 137S–153S (suppl. 1).

O'Connor, P. and Brown, G.W. (1984). Supportive relationships: Fact or fancy? *Journal of Social and Personal Relationships, 1*: 159–75.

O'Driscoll, C., Marshall, J. and Reed, J. (1990). Chronically ill psychiatric patients in a district general hospital unit: A survey and two year follow-up in an inner London health district. *British Journal of Psychiatry, 157*: 694–702.

O'Reilly, J.F., Shaylor, J.M., Fromings, K.M. and Harrison, B.D.W. (1982). The use of the 12 minute walking test in assessing the effect of oral steroid therapy in patients with chronic airways obstruction. *British Journal of Diseases of the Chest, 76*: 374–82.

O'Riordan, T.G., Haynes, J.P. and O'Neil, D. (1990). The effect of mild to moderate dementia on the Geriatric Depression Scale and on the General Health Questionnaire. *Age and Ageing, 19*: 57–61.

O'Young, J. and McPeek, B. (1987). Quality of life variables in surgical trials. *Journal of Chronic Diseases, 40*: 513–22.

Oberman, A., Mattson, M.E., Alderman, E. (1984). Report of the working group: Coronary artery bypass graft surgery. In: N.K. Wenger, M.E. Mattson, C.P. Furberg and J. Elinson (eds), *Assessment of Quality of Life in Clinical Trials of Cardiovascular Therapies*. New York: Le Jacq.

Office of Health Economics (1977). *Preventing Bronchitis*. London: OHE.

Office of Health Economics (1985). *Back Pain*. London: OHE.

Office of Health Economics (1989). *Measurement and Management in the NHS*. London: OHE.

Oliver, J.P.J. (1991a). The quality of life in community care: A consideration of hostel wards prompted by a survey of residential facilities. In: R. Young (ed.), *Residential Needs for Severely Disabled Psychiatric Patients: The Case for Hospital Hostels*. London: HMSO.

Oliver, J.P.J. (1991b). The social care directive: Development of a quality of life profile for use in community services for the mentally ill. *Social Work and Social Sciences Review, 3*: 5–45.

Oliver, J.P.J. and Mohamad, H. (1992). The quality of life of the chronically mentally ill: A comparison of public, private and voluntary residential provision. *British Journal of Social Work, 22*: 391–404.

Oliver, J.P.J., Huxley, P.J., Bridges, K. *et al.* (in press). *Quality of Life and Mental Health Service Evaluation*. London: Routledge.

Olson, M., Smoyer, S., Stevens, L. and Bigelow, D. (1991). *Program Impact Monitoring System*. Portland, OR: Department of Psychiatry, Oregon Health Sciences University.

Olsson, G., Lubsen, J., van Es, G.A. and Rehnqvist, N. (1986). Quality of life after myocardial infarction: Effect of long term metoprolol on mortality and morbidity. *British Medical Journal, 292*: 1491–3.

Oppenheim, A.N. (1968). *Questionnaire Design and Attitude Measurement*. London: Heinemann Educational.

Ormel, J., Koeter, M.W. and van den Brink, W. (1989). Measuring change with the General Health Questionnaire (GHQ): The problem of retest effects. *Social Psychiatry and Psychiatric Epidemiology, 24*: 227–32.

Orth-Gomer, K., Britton, M. and Rehnqvist, N. (1979). Quality of care in an out-patient department: The patient's view. *Social Science and Medicine, 13A*: 347–57.

Osberg, T.M. (1985). Social Behaviour Assessment Schedule. In: D.J. Keyser and R.C. Sweetland (eds), *Test Critiques*, Vol. III. Kansas City, MO: Test Corporation of America.

Osgood, C.E., Suci, G.J. and Tannenbaum. P.H. (1957). *The Measurement of Meaning*. Urbana, IL: University of Illinois Press.

Osoba, D. (1992). The Quality of Life Committee of the Clinical Trials Group of the National Cancer Institute of Canada: Organization and functions. *Quality of Life Research, 1*: 211–18.

Ott, C.R., Sivarajan, E.S., Newton, K.M. *et al.* (1983). A controlled randomised study of early cardiac rehabilitation: The Sickness Impact Profile as an assessment tool. *Heart and Lung, 12*: 162–70.

Overall, J.E. (1974). The brief psychiatric rating scale in psychopharmacology research. *Modern Problems in Pharmacopsychiatry, 7*: 67–78.

Overall, J.E. and Gorham, D.R. (1962). The Brief Psychiatric Rating Scale. *Psychological Reports, 10*: 799–812.

Overall, J.E. and Hollister, L.E. (1986). Assessment of depression using the Brief Psychiatric Rating Scale. In: N. Sartorius and T.A. Ban (eds), *Assessment of Depression*. Heidelberg: Springer-Verlag.

Øvretveit, J. (1993). Purchasing for health gain: The problems and prospects for purchasing for health gain in the 'managed markets' of the NHS and other European health systems. *European Journal of Public Health, 3*: 77–84.

Paci, E. (1992). Assessment of validity and clinical application of an Italian version of the Rotterdam Symptom Checklist. *Quality of Life Research, 1*: 129–34.

Packa, D.R. (1989). Quality of life of adults after a heart transplant. *Journal of Cardiovascular Nursing, 3*: 12–22.

Padilla, G.V. (1990). Gastrointestinal side effects and quality of life in patients receiving radiation therapy. *Nutrition, 6*: 367–70.

Padilla, G.V. (1992). Validity of health-related quality of life subscales. *Progress in Cardiovascular Nursing, 7*: 13–20.

Padilla, G.V. and Grant, M.M. (1985). Quality of life as a cancer nursing outcome variable. *Advances in Nursing Science, 8*: 45–60.

Padilla, G.V., Presant, C.A., Grant, M.M. *et al.* (1981). Assessment of quality of life in cancer patients. *Proceedings of the American Association of Cancer Research, 22*: 397.

Padilla, G.V., Presant, C.A., Grant, M.M. *et al.* (1983). Quality of life index for patients with cancer. *Research in Nursing and Health, 6*: 117–26.

Padilla, G.V., Ferrell, B., Grant, M.M. and Rhiner, M. (1990). Defining the content domain of quality of life for cancer patients with pain. *Cancer Nursing, 13*: 108–15.

Padilla, G.V., Mishel, M.H. and Grant, M.M. (1992a). Uncertainty, appraisal and quality of life. *Quality of Life Research, 1*: 155–65.

Padilla, G.V., Grant, M.M. and Ferrell, B. (1992b). Nursing research into quality of life. *Quality of Life Research, 1*: 341–8.

Palmer, A.J., Fletcher, A.E. and Rudge, P.J. (1992). Quality of life in hypertensives treated with atenolol or captopril: A double blind crossover trial. *Journal of Hypertension, 10*: 1409–16.

Palmer, B.V., Walsh, G.A., McKinnae, J.A. and Greening, W.P. (1980). Adjuvant chemotherapy for breast cancer: Side effects and quality of life. *British Medical Journal, 281*: 1594–7.

Palmer, M.J., O'Sullivan, B., Steele, R. and Mackillop, W.J. (1990). Controversies in the management of non-small cell lung cancer: The results of an expert surrogate study. *Radiation Oncology, 19*: 17–28.

Palmore, E. (1979). Predictors of successful ageing. *The Gerontologist, 19*: 427–31.

Pantell, R.H. and Lewis, C.C. (1987). Measuring the impact of medical care on children. *Journal of Chronic Diseases, 40*: 99S–108S (suppl. 1).

Papageorgiou, A.C. and Badley, E.M. (1989). The quality of pain in arthritis: The words patients use to describe overall pain and pain in individual joints at rest and on movement. *Journal of Rheumatology, 16*: 106–12.

Parducci, A. (1984). Value judgement: Toward a relational theory of happiness. In: J.B. Eiser (ed.), *Attitudinal Judgement*. New York: Springer Verlag.

Parfrey, P.S., Vavasour, H., Bullock, M. *et al.* (1989). Development of a health questionnaire specific for end-stage renal disease. *Nephron, 52*: 20–8.

Parker, D.F., Levinson, W., Mullooly, J.P. and Frymark, S.L. (1989). Using the quality of life index in a cancer rehabilitation program. *Journal of Psychosocial Oncology, 7*: 47–61.

Parker, J.D.A. and Endler, N.S. (1992). Coping with coping assessment: A critical review. *European Journal of Personality, 6*: 321–44.

Parkerson, G.R., Broadhead, W.E. and Tse, C.K.J. (1990). The Duke Health Profile: A 17 item measure of health and dysfunction. *Medical Care, 28*: 1056–72.

Parkerson, G.R., Broadhead, W.E. and Tse, C.K.J. (1993a). The Duke Severity of Illness checklist (DUSOI) for measurement of severity and comorbidity. *Journal of Clinical Epidemiology, 46*: 379–93.

Parkerson, G.R., Connis, R.T., Broadhead, W.E. *et al.*, (1993b). Disease-specific versus generic measurement of health related quality of life in insulin dependent diabetic patients. *Medical Care, 31*: 629–39.

Parkes, K.R. (1984). Locus of control, cognitive appraisal and coping in stressful episodes. *Journal of Personality and Social Psychology, 46*: 655–68.

Parloff, M.B., Kelman, H.C. and Frank, J.D. (1954). Comfort, effectiveness and self-awareness as criteria of improvement in psychotherapy. *American Journal of Psychiatry, 111*: 343–51.

Parsons, T. (1958). Definitions of health and illness in the light of American values and social structure. In: E.G. Jaco (ed.), *Patients, Physicians and Illness*. New York: Free Press.

Partridge, C.J., Johnson, M. and Morris, L. (1991). *Disability and Health Services: Perceptions, Beliefs and Experiences of Elderly People*. London: Centre for Physiotherapy Research, King's College, University of London.

Patrick, D.L. (ed.) (1982a) *Health and Care of the Physically Disabled in Lambeth: Phase I Report*. London: Department of Community Medicine, St Thomas' Hospital Medical School.

Patrick, D.L. (ed.) (1982b). *Health and Care of the Physically Disabled in Lambeth: Report of Phase II of the Longitudinal Disability Interview Survey*. London: Department of Community Medicine, St Thomas' Hospital Medical School.

Patrick, D.L., Bush, J.W. and Chen, M.M. (1973). Methods for measuring levels of well-being for a health status index. *Health Services Research, 8*: 228–45.

Patrick, D.L., Danis, M., Southerland, L. and Hong, G. (1988). Quality of life following intensive care. *Journal of General Internal Medicine, 3*: 218–23.

Pattie, A.H. and Gilleard, C.J. (1979). *Manual of the Clifton Assessment Procedures for the elderly (CAPE)*. Sevenoaks: Hodder and Stoughton Educational.

Paulhus, D.L. (1991). Measurement and control of response bias. In: J.P. Robinson, P.R. Shaver and L.S. Wrightsman (eds), *Measures of Personality and Social Psychological Attitudes*, Vol. 1. New York: Academic Press.

Paykel, E.S. (1974). Recent life events and clinical depression. In: E.K.E. Gunderson and R.H. Rahe (eds), *Life Stress and Illness*. Springfield, IL: Charles C. Thomas.

Paykel, E.S. (1983). Methodological aspects of life events research. *Journal of Psychosomatic Research, 27*: 341–52.

Paykel, E.S. (1985). Clinical interview for depression, development, reliability and validity. *Journal of Affective Disorders, 9*: 85–96.

Paykel, E.S. and Dowlatshahi, D. (1988). Life events and mental disorder. In: S. Fisher and J. Reason (eds), *Handbook of Life Stress, Cognition and Health*. Chichester: John Wiley.

Paykel, E.S., Myers, J.K., Dienelt, M.N. *et al.* (1969). Life events and depression: A controlled study. *Archives of General Psychiatry, 21*: 753–60.

Paykel, E.S., Prusoff, B.A. and Uhlenhuth, E.H. (1971a). Scaling of life events. *Archives of General Psychiatry, 25*: 340–7.

Paykel, E.S., Weissman, M., Prusoff, B.A. and Tonks, C.M. (1971b). Dimensions of social adjustment in depressed women. *Journal of Nervous and Mental Diseases, 152*: 158–72.

Paykel, E.S., Klerman, G.L. and Di Mascio, A. (1973). Maintenance antidepressants, psychotherapy, symptoms and social function. In: J.O. Cole, A. Friedhogg and A. Freeman (eds), *Psychopathology and Psychopharmacology*. Baltimore, MD: Johns Hopkins University Press.

Payne, R.L. and Graham-Jones, J. (1987). Measurement and methodological issues in social support. In: S.V. Kasl and C.L. Cooper (eds), *Stress and Health: Issues in Research Methodology*. Chichester: John Wiley.

Peace, S., Hall., J.F. and Hamblin, J.R. (1979). *The Quality of Life of the Elderly in Residental Care*. Survey Research Centre Report No. 1. London: Department of Applied Social Studies, University of North London.

Pearlin, L.I. (1989). The sociological study of stress. *Journal of Health and Social Behaviour, 30*: 241–56.

Pearlin, L.I. and Lieberman, M.A. (1978). Social sources of emotional distress. In R. Simmons (ed.) *Research in Community and Mental Health*. Greenwich, CT: JAI.

Pearlin, L.I. and Schooler, C. (1978). The structure of coping. *Journal of Health and Social Behaviour, 19*: 2–21.

Pearlin, L.I., Menaghan, E.G., Lieberman, M.A. and Mullen, J.Y.T. (1981). The stress process. *Journal of Health and Social Behaviour, 22*: 337–56.

Pearlman, R.A. (1987). Development of a functional assessment questionnaire for geriatric patients: The Comprehensive Older Persons Evaluation (COPE). *Journal of Chronic Diseases, 40*: 85S–94S (suppl.).

Pearlman, R.A., Cain, K.C. and Patrick, D.L. (1993). Insights pertaining to patient assessments of states worse than death. *Journal of Clinical Ethics, 4*: 33–41.

Peduzzi, P., Hultgren, H., Thomsen, J. *et al.* (1987). Ten year effect of medical and surgical therapy on quality of life: Veterans Administration Cooperative Study of coronary artery surgery. *American Journal of Cardiology, 59*: 1017–23.

Percy-Smith, J. and Sanderson, I. (1992). *Understanding Local Needs*. London: Institute for Public Policy Research.

Permanyer-Miralda, G., Alonso, J., Anto, J.M. *et al.* (1991). Comparison of perceived health status and conventional functional evaluation in stable patients with coronary artery disease. *Journal of Clinical Epidemiology, 44*: 779–86.

Peterson, R.A. and Headen, S.W. (1985). Profile of Mood States. In: D.J. Keyser and R.C. Sweetland (eds), *Test Critiques*, Vol. I. Kansas City, MO: Test Corporation of America.

Pfeiffer, E. (1975a). A short portable mental status questionnaire for the assessment of organic brain deficit in elderly patients. *Journal of the American Geriatric Society, 23*: 433–41.

Pfeiffer, E. (1975b). A short psychiatric evaluation schedule: A new 15 item monotonic scale indicative of functional psychiatric disorder (abstract). *The Gerontologist, 15*: 34.

Pill, R. and Stott, N.C.H. (1985). Choice or chance: Further evidence on ideas of illness and responsibility for health. *Social Science and Medicine, 20*: 981–91.

Pill, R. and Stott, N.C.H. (1988). Invitation to attend a health screening in a general practice setting: The views of a cohort of non-attenders. *Journal of the Royal College of General Practitioners, 38*: 57–60.

Pilowsky, I., Spence, N.D. and Waddy, J.L. (1979). Illness behaviours and coronary artery bypass surgery. *Journal of Psychosomatic Research, 23*: 39–44.

Pim, J.B. and Jude, J.R. (1989). Beck Depression Inventory scores of coronary bypass patients with or without psychological intervention. In: A. Willner and G. Rodewald (eds), *Impact of Cardiac Surgery on Quality of Life: Neurological and Psychological Aspects*. New York: Plenum Press.

Pincus, T. and Callahan, L.F. (1992). Quantitative measures to assess, monitor and predict morbidity and mortality in rheumatoid arthritis. In: D.L. Scott (ed.), *The Course and Outcome of Rheumatoid Arthritis*. Bailliere's Clinical Rheumatology, Vol. 6, No. 1. London: Bailliere Tindall.

Pincus, T., Callahan, L.F., Bradley, L.A. *et al.* (1986). Elevated MMPI scores for hypochondriasis, depression and hysteria in patients with rheumatoid arthritis reflect disease rather than psychological status. *Arthritis and Rheumatism, 29*: 1456–66.

Place, M., Kolvin, I. and Morton, S.M. (1987). The Newcastle Adolescent Behaviour Screening Questionnaire. *British Journal of Psychiatry, 151*: 45–51.

Platt, S. and Hirsch, S.R. (1981). The effects of brief hospitalisation upon the psychiatric patient's household. *Acta Psychiatrica Scandinavica, 64*: 199–216.

Platt, S.D., Weyman, A.J., Hirsch, S.R. and Hewett, S. (1980). The Social Behaviour Assessment Schedule (SBAS): Rationale, contents, scoring and reliability of a new interview schedule. *Social Psychiatry, 15*: 43–55.

Platt, S.D., Hirsch, S.R. and Knights, A.C. (1981). Effects of brief hospitalisation on psychiatric patients' behaviour and social functioning. *Acta Psychiatrica Scandinavica, 63*: 117–28.

Platt, S., Hirsch, S. and Weyman, A. (1983). *Training Manual and Rating Guide: Social Behaviour Assessment Schedule*, 3rd edn. Windsor: NFER-Nelson.

Pocock, S.J. (1983). *Clinical Trials: A Practical Approach*. Chichester: John Wiley.

Poon, M.A., O'Connell, M.J., Moertel, C.G. *et al.* (1989). Biochemical modulation of Fluorouracil: Evidence of significant improvement of survival and quality of life in patients with advanced colorectal carcinoma. *Journal of Clinical Oncology, 7*: 1407–18.

Portenoy, R. (1992). Cancer pain: Pathophysiology and syndromes. *Lancet, 339*: 1026–31.

Potts, M.K., Daniels, M., Burnam, A. and Wells, K.B. (1990). A structured interview version of the Hamilton Depression Rating Scale: Evidence of reliability and versatility of administration. *Journal of Psychiatric Research, 24*: 335–50.

Pound, P., Gompertz, P. and Ebrahim, S. (1993). Development and results of a questionnaire to measure carer satisfaction after stroke. *Journal of Epidemiology and Community Health, 47*: 500–5.

Pound, P., Gompertz, P. and Ebrahim, S. (1994). Patients' satisfaction with stroke services. *Clinical Rehabilitation, 8*: 7–17.

Presant, C.A. (1984). Quality of life in cancer patients:

Who measures what? *American Journal of Clinical Oncology*, 7: 571–3.

Priestman, T.J. (1984). Quality of life after cytotoxic chemotherapy: Discussion paper. *Journal of the Royal Society of Medicine*, 77: 494–5.

Priestman, T. and Baum, M. (1976). Evaluation of quality of life in patients receiving treatment for advanced breast cancer. *Lancet, i*: 899–901.

Priestman, T., Baum, M., Jones, V. and Forbes, J. (1977). Comparative trial of endocrine versus cytotoxic treatment in advanced breast cancer, *British Medical Journal*, 1: 1248–50.

Prieto, E.J. and Geisinger, K.F. (1983). Factor-analytic studies of the McGill Pain Questionnaire. In: R. Melzack (ed.), *Pain Measurement and Assessment*. New York: Raven Press.

Prigatano, G.P., Parsons, O., Wright, E. *et al.* (1983). Neuropsychological test performance in mildly hypoxemic patients with chronic obstructive pulmonary disease. *Journal of Consulting and Clinical Psychology*, 51: 108–16.

Pruyn, J.F.A., van den Heuval, W.J.A. and Jonkers, R. (1980). *Verantwoording van de klachtenlijst voor kankerpatienten*. Rotterdam: Studiecentrum Sociale Oncologie.

Pruyn, J.F.A., Maguire, P. and de Haes, J.C.J.M. (1981). Two methods of measuring some aspects of quality of life: A comparison of subjective versus objective methods in monitoring the quality of life in cancer patients. In: *Quality of Life. Methods of Measurement and Related Areas: Proceedings of the Second EORTC Quality of Life Workshop*, Copenhagen, November 13–14.

Quality of Life Research (1994). Proceedings of the Inaugural Meeting of the International Health-related Quality of Life Society, Brussels, February. *Quality of Life Research*, 3(1): 41–102.

Quirk, F.H. and Jones, P.W. (1990). Patients' perceptions of distress due to symptoms and effects of asthma on daily living and an investigation of possible influential factors. *Clinical Science*, 79: 17–21.

Quirk, F.H., Baveystock, C.M., Wilson, R.C. and Jones, P.W. (1991). Influence of demographic and disease related factors on the degree of distress associated with symptoms and restrictions on daily living due to asthma in six countries. *European Respiratory Journal*, 4: 167–71.

Qureshi, K.N. and Hodkinson, H.M. (1974). Evaluation of a 10 question mental test in the institutionalized elderly. *Age and Ageing*, 3: 152–7.

Rabins, P. and Brooks, B. (1981). Emotional disturbance in multiple sclerosis patients: Validity of the General Health Questionnaire. *Psychological Medicine*, 11: 425–7.

Radley, A. (1988). *Prospects of Heart Surgery: Psychological Adjustment to Coronary Bypass Grafting*. Heidelberg: Springer-Verlag.

Radloff, L.S. (1975). Sex differences in depression: The effects of occupation and marital status. *Sex Roles*, 1: 249–65.

Radloff, L.S. (1977). The CES-D scale: A self report depression scale for research in the general population. *Applied Psychological Measurement*, 1: 385–401.

Radloff, L.S. and Locke, B.Z. (1986). The community mental health assessment survey and the CES-D scale. In: M.M. Weissman, J.K. Myers and C.E. Ross (eds), *Community Surveys of Psychiatric Disorders*. New Brunswick, NJ: Rutgers University Press.

Raft, D., McKee, D.D., Popio, K.A. *et al.* (1985). Life adaptation after percutaneous transluminal coronary angioplasty and coronary artery bypass grafting. *American Journal of Cardiology*, 56: 395–8.

Rahe, R.H. (1969). Life crisis and health change. In: R.A. Philip and J.R. Wittenborn (eds), *Psychotropic Drug Response: Advances in Prediction*. Springfield, IL: Charles C. Thomas.

Rahe, R.H. (1974). Life change and subsequent illness reports. In: E.K.E. Gunderson and R.H. Rahe (eds), *Life Stress and Illness*. Springfield, IL: Charles C. Thomas.

Rahe, R.H. (1988). Recent life changes and coronary heart disease: 10 years' research. In: S. Fisher and J. Reason (eds), *Handbook of Life Stress, Cognition and Health*. Chichester: John Wiley.

Rahe, R.H., Meyer, M., Smith, M. *et al.* (1964). Social stress and illness onset. *Journal of Psychosomatic Research*, 8: 35–44.

Rand (1992). *Rand 36-Item Health Survey, 1.0*. Rand Health Sciences Program. Santa Monica, CA, Rand Corporation.

Rand (1993). *Epilepsy Surgery Inventory (ESI)-55: Scoring Manual*. Rand Health Sciences Program. Santa Monica, CA: Rand Corporation.

Ranhoff, A.H. and Laake, K. (1993). The Barthel ADL Index: Scoring by the physician from patient interview is not reliable. *Age and Ageing*, 22: 171–4.

Rankin, J. (1957). Cerebral vascular accidents in people over the age of 60. II. Prognosis. *Scottish Medical Journal*, 2: 200–15.

Rankin, S.H. (1990). Differences in recovery from cardiac surgery: A profile of male and female patients. *Heart and Lung*, 19: 481–5.

Rapp, E., Pater, J.L., Willan, A. *et al.* (1988). Chemotherapy can prolong survival in patients with advanced non-small-cell lung cancer: Report of a Canadian multi-center randomised trial. *Journal of Clinical Oncology*, 6: 633–41.

Rausch, R. and Crandall, P.H. (1982). Psychological status related to surgical control of temporal lobe seizures. *Epilepsia*, 23: 191–202.

Reading, A.E. (1983). The McGill Pain Questionnaire: An Appraisal. In: R. Melzack (ed.), *Pain Measurement and Assessment*. New York: Raven Press.

Rector, T.S., Kubo, S.H. and Cohn, J.N. (1993). Validity of the Minnesota Living with Heart Failure Questionnaire as a measure of therapeutic response: Effects of enalapril and placebo. *American Journal of Cardiology, 71*: 1006–7.

Redd, W.H. and Andrykowski, M.A. (1982). Behavioural interventions in cancer treatment: Controlling aversion reactions to chemotherapy. *Journal of Consulting and Clinical Psychology, 50*: 1018–29.

Reddon, J.R., Marceau, R. and Holden, R.R. (1985). A confirmatory evaluation of the Profile of Mood States: Convergent and discriminant item validity. *Journal of Psychopathology and Behavioral Assessment, 7*: 243–59.

Redeker, N.S. (1992). A description of the nature and dynamics of coping following coronary artery bypass surgery. *Scholarly Inquiry for Nursing Practice, 6*: 63–75.

Regier, D.A., Myers, J.K., Kramer, M. *et al.* (1984). The NIMH epidemiological catchment area program. *Archives of General Psychiatry, 41*: 934–41.

Rehm, L.P. (1981). *Behaviour Therapy for Depression*. New York: Academic Press.

Reisine, S.T., Goodenow, C. and Grady, K.E. (1987). The impact of rheumatoid arthritis on the homemaker. *Social Science and Medicine, 25*: 89–95.

Reitan, R.M. (1955). The relation of the Trail-making Test to organic brain damage. *Journal of Consulting Psychology, 19*: 393–4.

Reitan, R.M. (1958). *Trail-making Manual for Administration, Scoring and Interpretation*. Indianapolis, IN: Indiana University Medical Center.

Reitan, R.M. and Tarsches, E.T. (1959). Differential effects of lateralised brain lesions. *Journal of Nervous and Mental Diseases, 129*: 257–62.

Remington, M. and Tyrer, P. (1979). The social functioning schedule – a brief semi-structured interview. *Social Psychiatry, 14*: 151–7.

Remington, M., Tyrer, P.J., Newsom-Smith, J. and Cichetti, D.V. (1979). Comparative reliability of categorical and analogue scales in the assessment of psychiatric symptomatology. *Psychological Medicine, 9*: 765–70.

Renfroe, K.L. (1988). Effect on progressive relaxation on dyspnoea and state anxiety in patients with chronic obstructive pulmonary disease. *Heart and Lung, 17*: 403–13.

Revenson, T.A. (1981). Coping with loneliness: The impact of causal attributions. *Personality and Social Psychology Bulletin, 7*: 565–71.

Revill, S.I., Robinson, J.O., Rosen, M. and Hogg, I.J. (1976). The reliability of a linear analogue for evaluating pain. *Anaesthesia, 31*: 1191–8.

Reynolds, W.M. and Gould, J.W. (1981). A psychometric investigation of the standard and short form Beck Depression Inventory. *Journal of Consulting and Clinical Psychology, 49*: 306–7.

Rhoads, G.G., Kagan, A. and Yano, K. (1975). Usefulness of community surveillance for the ascertainment of coronary heart disease and stroke. *International Journal of Epidemiology, 4*: 265–70.

Rhoades, H.M. and Overall, J.E. (1988). The semistructured BPRS Interview and Rating Guide. *Psychopharmacology Bulletin, 24*: 101–4.

Richman, N. and Graham, P.J. (1971). A behavioural screening questionnaire for use with 3-year-old children: Preliminary findings. *Journal of Child Psychology and Psychiatry, 12*: 5–33.

Ridgely, M.S., Goldman, H.H. and Morrissey, J.P. (1992). Assessing systems of care for the long-term mentally ill in urban settings. In: G. Thornicroft, C.R. Brewin and J. Wing (eds), *Measuring Mental Health Needs*. London: Royal College of Psychiatrists.

Rieker, P.P., Clark, E.J. and Fogelberg, P.R. (1992). Perceptions of quality of life and quality of care for patients with cancer receiving biological therapy. *Oncology Nursing Forum, 19*: 433–40.

Ries, A.L. (1990). Scientific basis of pulmonary rehabilitation: Position paper of the American Association of Cardiovascular and Pulmonary Rehabilitation. *Journal of Cardiopulmonary Rehabilitation, 10*: 418–41.

Ringdal, G.I. and Ringdal, K. (1993). Testing the EORTC quality of life questionnaire on cancer patients with heterogeneous diagnoses. *Quality of Life Research, 2*: 129–40.

Ritchie, D., Boyle, J. and McInnes, J. *et al.* (1968). Clinical studies with an articular index for the assessment of joint tenderness in patients with rheumatoid arthritis. *Quarterly Journal of Medicine, 147*: 393–406.

Robb, B. (1967). *Sans Everything*. London: Nelson.

Roberts, J.G. and Tugwell, P. (1987). Comparison of questionnaires determining patient satisfaction with medical care. *Health Services Research, 22*: 637–54.

Roberts, M.S. (1989). Quality of life measures in liver transplantation. In: F. Mosteller and J. Falotico-Taylor (eds), *Quality of Life and Technology Assessment*. Washington, DC: National Academy Press.

Robin, A., Currey, S.H. and Whelpton, R. (1974). Clinical and biochemical comparison of chlorazepate and diazepam. *Psychological Medicine, 4*: 338–92.

Robine, J.M., Blanchet, M. and Dowd, J.E. (eds) (1992). *Health Expectancy: First Workshop of the International Healthy Life Expectancy Network (REVES)*. OPCS Studies on Medical and Population Subjects, No. 54. London: HMSO.

Robins, L.N., Helzer, J.E., Croughan, J.L. *et al.* (1979). *The National Institute of Mental Health Diagnostic*

Interview Schedule. Rockville, MD: National Institute of Mental Health.

Robins, L.N., Helzer, J.E., Croughan, J.L. and Ratcliff, K. (1981). The NIMH diagnostic interview schedule: Its history, characteristics and validity. In: J.K. Wing, P. Bebbington and L.N. Robins (eds), *What is a Case? The Problem of Definition in Psychiatric Community Surveys*. London: Grant MacIntyre.

Robins, L.N., Helzer, J.E., Ratcliff, K.S. and Seyfried, W. (1982). Validity of the Diagnostic Interview Schedule, version II: DSM-III diagnoses. *Psychological Medicine, 12*: 855–70.

Robins, L.N., Helzer, J.E., Orvaschel, H. *et al*. (1985). The Diagnostic Interview Schedule. In: W.W. Eaton and L.G. Kessler (eds), *Epidemiological Field Methods in Psychiatry: The NIMH Epidemiological Catchment Area Program*. Orlando, FL: Academic Press.

Robinson, R. and Price, T. (1981). Post-stroke depressive disorders: A follow-up study of 103 patients. *Stroke, 13*: 635–41.

Rodgers, H., Curless, R. and James, O.F.W. (1993). Standardized functional assessment scales for elderly patients. *Age and Ageing, 22*: 161–3.

Rodin, G. (1990). Quality of life in adults with insulin-dependent diabetes mellitus. *Psychotherapy and Psychosomatics, 54*: 132–9.

Rogerson, R.J., Findlay, A.M. and Morris, A.S. (1989). Indicators of quality of life: Some methodological issues. *Environment and Planning, 21*: 1655–66.

Roila, F., Lupattelli, M., Sassi, M. *et al*. (1991). Intra- and interobserver variability in cancer patients' performance status assessed according to Karnofsky and ECOG scales. *Annals of Oncology, 2*: 437–9.

Rokeach, M. (1973). *The Nature of Human Values*. New York: Free Press.

Ropes, M.W.G., Bennett, G.A., Cobb, S. *et al*. (1958). 1958 revision of diagnostic criteria for rheumatoid arthritis. *Bulletin on Rheumatic Diseases, 9*: 175–6.

Rose, G.A. (1962). The diagnosis of ischaemic heart pain and intermittent claudication in field surveys. *Bulletin of the World Health Organization, 27*: 645.

Rose, G.A. (1965). Chest pain questionnaire. *Milbank Memorial Fund Quarterly, 43*: 32–9.

Rose, G.A. (1968). Variability of angina: Some implications for epidemiology. *British Journal of Preventive and Social Medicine, 22*: 12–15.

Rose, G.A. (1971). Predicting coronary heart disease from minor symptoms and electrocardiographic findings. *British Journal of Preventive and Social Medicine, 25*: 94–6.

Rose, G.A. and Blackburn, H. (1968). *Cardiovascular Survey Methods*. World Health Organization Monograph Series No. 56. Geneva: WHO.

Rose, G., McCartney, P. and Reid, D.D. (1977). Self-administration of a questionnaire on chest pain:

Intermittent claudication. *British Journal of Preventive and Social Medicine, 31*: 42–8.

Rose, G.A., Blackburn, H., Gillum, R.F. *et al*. (1982). *Cardiovascular Survey Methods*, 2nd edn. WHO Monograph No. 56. Geneva: WHO.

Rose, R.M., Jenkins, C.D. and Hurst, M.W. (1978). *Air Traffic Controller Health Change Study*. Report to Federal Aviation Administration, August, 1978. Boston, MA; Boston University School of Medicine.

Rosen, A., Hadzi-Pavlovic, D. and Parker, G. (1989). The life skills profile: A measure assessing function and disability in schizophrenia. *Schizophrenia Bulletin, 15*: 325–37.

Rosen, B.M., Lawrence, L., Goldsmith, H.F., Windle, C.D. and Shambaugh, J.P. (1975). *Mental Health Demographic Profile System Description: Purpose, Contents and Sampler of Uses*. NIMH Series C, No. 11. DEHW Publication ADM 76–263. Washington, DC: US Government Printing Office.

Rosenberg, M. (1965). *Society and the Adolescent Self Image*. Princeton, NJ: Princeton University Press.

Rosenberg, M. (1986). *Conceiving the Self*, 2nd edn. Malabar, FL: Krieger.

Rosenberg, R. (1992). Quality of life, ethics, and philosophy of science. *Nordic Journal of Psychiatry, 46*: 75–7.

Rosenhan, D.L. (1973). On being sane in insane places. *Science, 179*: 250–8.

Rosenthal, M., Lohr, K.N., Rubenstein, R.S. *et al*. (1981). *Conceptualisation and Measurement of Physiologic Health in Adults, Vol. 5: Congestive Heart Failure*. R-2262/5-HHS. Santa Monica, CA: Rand Corporation.

Rosser, R.M. (1992). Index of health-related quality of life. In: A. Hopkins (ed.), *Measures of the Quality of Life and the Uses to which Such Measures may be Put*. London: Royal College of Physicians.

Rosser, R., Denford, J., Heslop, A. *et al*. (1983). Breathlessness and psychiatric morbidity in chronic bronchitis and emphysema: A study of psychotherapeutic management. *Psychological Medicine, 13*: 93–110.

Rosser, R.M. and Watts, V.C. (1972). The measurement of hospital output. *International Journal of Epidemiology, 1*: 361–8.

Rosser, R.M. and Watts, V.C. (1978). The measurement of illness. *Journal of the Operational Research Society, 29*: 529–40.

Rosser, R.M., Cottee, M., Rabin, R. and Selai, C. (1992). Index of health related quality of life. In: A. Hopkins (ed.), *Measures of the Quality of Life and the Uses to which Such Measures may be Put*. London: Royal College of Physicians.

Rosser, R.M., Allison, R., Butler, C. *et al*. (1993). The Index of Health Related Quality of Life (IHRQL): A new tool for audit and cost-per-QALY analysis. In:

S.R. Walker and R.M. Rosser (eds), *Quality of Life Assessment: Key Issues in the 1990s*. Dordrecht: Kluwer Academic.

Rossi, P.H. (1972). Community social indicators. In: A. Campbell and P. Converse (eds), *The Human Meaning of Social Change*. New York: Russell Sage Foundation.

Roth, M. (1986). Differential diagnoses of psychiatric disorders in old age. *Hospital Practice, 15*: 111–25.

Roth, M., Tyme, E., Mountjoy, C.Q. *et al.* (1986). CAMDEX: A standardised instrument for the diagnosis of mental disorder in the elderly with special reference to the early detection of dementia. *British Journal of Psychiatry, 149*: 698–709.

Roth, M., Huppert, F.A., Tym, E. and Mountjoy, C.Q. (1988) *CAMDEX: The Cambridge Examination for Mental Disorders of the Elderly*. Cambridge: Cambridge University Press.

Rotter, J.B. (1966). Generalised expectancies for internal versus external control of reinforcement. *Psychological Monographs, 80*: 1–23.

Rowe, B.H. (1991). Steroid treatment of asthma exacerbations: A meta analysis, evaluation of a quality of life instrument and design of a randomised factorial trial. MSc thesis, McMaster University, Hamilton, Canada.

Royal College of General Practitioners, Office of Population Censuses and Surveys and Department of Health and Social Security (1986). *1981–82 Morbidity Statistics from General Practice*. London: HMSO.

Royal College of Physicians (1981). *Disabling Chest Disease: Prevention and Care*. London: RCP.

Rubeck, M.F. (1971). *Social and Emotional Effects of Chronic Bronchitis*. London: The Chest and Heart Association.

Rubenstein, L.V., Calkins, D.R., Greenfield, S. *et al.* (1989a). Health status assessment for elderly patients: Report of the Society of General Internal Medicine Task Force on Health Assessment. *Journal of the American Geriatrics Society, 37*: 562–9.

Rubenstein, L.V., Calkins, D.R., Young, R.T. *et al.* (1989b). Improving patient function: A randomised trial of functional disability screening. *Annals of Internal Medicine, 111*: 836–42.

Rubenstein, R.S., Lohr, K.N., Brook, R.H. and Goldberg, G.A. (1982). *Conceptualisation and Measurement of Health for Adults. Vol. 12. Vision Impairments*. Santa Monica, CA: Rand Corporation.

Rubenstein, R.S., Beck, S., Lohr, K.N. *et al.* (1983). *Conceptualisation and Measurement of Health for Adults. Vol. 15. Surgical Conditions*. Santa Monica, CA: Rand Corporation.

Ruberman, W., Weinblatt, E., Goldberg, J.D. *et al.* (1984). Psychosocial influences on mortality after myocardial infarction. *New England Journal of Medicine, 311*: 552–9.

Russell, D., Peplau, L.A. and Cutrona, C.E. (1980). The revised UCLA Loneliness Scale: Concurrent and discriminant validity evidence. *Journal of Personality and Social Psychology, 39*: 472–80.

Russell, E. (1982). Factor analysis of the revised Wechsler Memory Scale Tests in a neuropsychological battery. *Perceptual and Motor Skills, 54*: 971–4.

Ruta, D.A. (1992). A new approach to the measurement of quality of life. The patient generated index. Paper presented to the *Workshop on Quality of Life, Society for Social Medicine 36th Annual Conference*, Nottingham, September.

Ruta, D.A., Garratt, A.M., Wardlaw, D. and Russell, I.T. (1994a). Developing a valid and reliable measure of health outcome for patients with low back pain. *Spine, 19*: 1887–96.

Ruta, D.A., Garratt, A.M., Leng, M. *et al.* (1994b). A new approach to the measurement of quality of life: The patient generated index (PGI). *Medical Care, 32*: 1109–26.

Rutter, B.M. (1977). Some psychological concomitants of chronic bronchitis. *Psychological Medicine, 7*: 459–64.

Rutter, M., Tizard, J. and Whitmore, K. (1970). *Education, Health and Behaviour*. London: Longman.

Sackett, D.L., MacDonald, L., Haynes, R.B. *et al.* (1983). Labelling of hypertensive patients. *New England Journal of Medicine, 309*: 1253.

Sadura, A., Pater, J., Osoba, D. *et al.* (1992) Quality-of-life assessment: Patient compliance with questionnaire completion. *Journal of the National Cancer Institute, 84*: 1023–6.

Salek, M.S. (1993). Measuring the quality of life of patients with skin disease. In: S.R. Walker and R.M. Rosser (eds), *Quality of Life Assessment: Key Issues in the 1990s*. Dordrecht: Kluwer Academic.

Santanello, N.O., Epstein, R.S., Demuro-Mercon, C. and Hartmaier, S.L. (1994). Development of a 24 hour disease specific questionnaire to assess the impact of migraine headache on the quality of life (abstract). *Quality of Life Research, 3*: 62.

Sarason, I.G., Johnson, J.G. and Siegel, J.M. (1978). Assessing the impact of life changes: Development of the Life Experiences Survey. *Journal of Consulting and Clinical Psychology, 46*: 932–46.

Sarna, L. (1993). Women with lung cancer: Impact on quality of life. *Quality of Life Research, 2*: 13–22.

Sartorius, N. (1993). A WHO method for the assessment of health related quality of life (WHOQOL). In: S.R. Walker and R.M. Rosser (eds), *Quality of Life Assessment: Key Issues in the 1990s*. Dordrecht: Kluwer Academic.

Sartorius, N., Brooke, E. and Lin, T.Y. (1970). Reliability of psychiatric assessment in international research. In: E.H. Hare and J.K. Wing (eds), *Psychiatric Epidemiology*. Oxford: Oxford University Press.

Sattler, J. (1982). *Assessment of Children's Intelligence and Special Abilities*. Boston, MA; Allyn and Bacon.

Sauer, W.J. and Warland, R. (1982). Morale and life satisfaction. In: D.J. Mangen and W.A. Peterson (eds), *Research Instruments in Social Gerontology. Vol. 1. Clinical and Social Psychology*. Minneapolis, MN: University of Minnesota Press.

Saunders, C.M. and Baum, M. (1992). Quality of life during treatment for cancer. *British Journal of Hospital Medicine, 48*: 119–23.

Scandinavian Stroke Study Group (1985). Multicentre trial of hemodilution in ischemic stroke. Background and study protocol. *Stroke, 16*: 885–90.

Scandinavian Stroke Study Group (1987). Multicentre trial of hemodilution in ischemic stroke. *Stroke, 18*: 691–9.

Scanlon, T. (1993). Value, desire and quality of life. In: M. Nussbaum and A. Sen (eds), *The Quality of Life*. Oxford: Clarendon Press.

Schaefer, C., Coyne, J.C. and Lazarus, R.S. (1982). The health related functions of social support. *Journal of Behavioural Medicine, 4*: 381–406.

Schag, C.A.C. and Heinrich, R.L. (1988). *Cancer Rehabilitation Evaluation System (CARES): Manual*, 1st edn. Los Angeles, CA: Cares Consultants.

Schag, C.A.C. and Heinrich, R.L. (1990). Development of a comprehensive quality of life measurement tool: CARES. *Oncology, 4*: 135–8.

Schag, C.A.C., Heinrich, R.L. and Ganz, P.A. (1983). Cancer Inventory of Problem Situations: An instrument for assessing cancer patients' rehabilitation needs. *Journal of Psychosocial Oncology, 1*: 11–24.

Schag, C.A.C., Heinrich, R.L. and Ganz, P.A. (1984). Karnofsky Performance Status Revisited: Reliability, validity and guidelines. *Journal of Clinical Oncology, 2*: 187–93.

Schag, C.A.C., Coscarelli, C.A., Heinrich, R.L. *et al.* (1990). Assessing problems of cancer patients: Psychometric properties of the cancer inventory of problem situations. *Health Psychology, 9*: 83–102.

Schag, C.A.C., Ganz, P.A., and Heinrich, R.L. (1991). Cancer Rehabilitation Evaluation System – short form (CARES-SF): A cancer-specific rehabilitation and quality of life instrument. *Cancer, 68*: 1406–13.

Schag, C.A.C., Ganz, P.A., Kahn, B. and Petersen, L. (1992). Assessing the needs and quality of life of patients with HIV infection: Development of the HIV Overview of Problem Situations Evaluation System (HOPES). *Quality of Life Research, 1*: 397–413.

Schag, C.A.C., Ganz, P.A., Polinksy, M.L. *et al.* (1993). Characteristics of women at risk for psychosocial distress in the year after breast cancer. *Journal of Clinical Oncology, 4*: 783–93.

Schag, C.A.C., Ganz, P.A., Wing, D.J. *et al.* (1994). Quality of life in adult survivors of lung, colon and prostate cancer. *Quality of Life Research, 3*: 127–41.

Schain, W. (1980). Sexual functioning, self-esteem and cancer care. *Frontiers Radiation Therapy and Oncology, 14*: 12–29.

Scheff, T. (1961). *Becoming Mentally Ill*. Chicago, IL: Aldine.

Scheidt, S. (1987). Ischaemic heart disease: A patient specific therapeutic approach with emphasis on quality of life considerations. *American Heart Journal, 114*: 251–7.

Scheier, M.F. and Carver, C.S. (1985). Optimism, coping and health: Assessment and implications of generalised outcome expectancies. *Health Psychology, 4*: 219–47.

Schennel, F.J. and Schonell, F.E. (1949). *Diagnostic and Attainment Testing*. Edinburgh: Oliver and Boyd.

Scherwitz, L.W., Perkins, L.L., Chesney, M.A. *et al.* (1992). Hostility and health behaviours in young adults: The CARDIA Study. Coronary Artery Risk Development in Young Adults Study. *American Journal of Epidemiology, 136*: 136–45.

Schipper, H. (1983). Why measure quality of life? *Journal of the Canadian Medical Association, 128*: 1367–70.

Schipper, H. and Levitt, M. (1985). Measuring quality of life: Risks and benefits. *Cancer Treatment Reports, 69*: 1115–23.

Schipper, H. and Levitt, M. (1986). Quality of life in cancer trials: What is it? Why measure it? In: V. Ventafridda, F.S.A.M. van Dam, R. Yancik and M. Tamburini (eds), *Assessment of Quality of Life and Cancer Treatment*. Amsterdam: Elsevier.

Schipper, H., Clinch, J., McMurray, A. and Levitt, M. (1984). Measuring the quality of life of cancer patients: The functional living index – cancer: Development and validation. *Journal of Clinical Oncology, 2*: 472–83.

Schneider, M. (1976). The 'quality of life' and social indicators research. *Public Administration Review, 36*: 297–305.

Schneiderman, L.J., Kaplan, R.M., Pearlman, R.A. *et al.* (1993). Do physicians' own preferences for life-sustaining treatment influence their perceptions of patients' preferences? *Journal of Clinical Ethics, 4*: 28–33.

Schooler, N., Hogarty, G. and Weissman, M.M. (1979). Social Adjustment Scale (SAS-II). In: W.A. Hargreaves, C.C. Attkisson and J.E. Sorenson (eds), *Resource Materials for Community Mental Health Programme Evaluators*. Publication No. (ADM) 79–328. Washington, DC: US Department of Health, Education and Welfare.

Schrier, A.C., Dekker, F.W., Kaptein, A.A. and Dijkman, J.H. (1990). Quality of life in elderly patients with chronic non-specific lung disease seen in family practice. *Chest, 90*: 894–9.

Schwab, J.J., Brolow, M.R. and Holser, C.E. (1967). A comparison of two rating scales for depression. *Journal of Clinical Psychology, 23*: 94–6.

Schwartz, C., Myers, J. and Astrachan, B. (1974). Psychiatric labelling and the rehabilitation of the mental patient: implications of research findings for mental health policy. *Archives of General Psychiatry, 31*: 329–34.

Scott, B., Goldberg, G., Brook, R.H. and Lohr, K.N. (1980). *Conceptualisation and Measurement of Health for Adults. Vol. 6: Anemia*. Santa Monica, CA: Rand Corporation.

Scott, B., Brook, R.H., Lohr, K.N. and Goldberg, G.A. (1981) *Conceptualisation and Measurement of Physiologic Health for Adults. Vol. 10: Joint Disorders*. Santa Monica, CA: Rand Corporation.

Scott, J. and Huskisson, E.C. (1976). Graphic representation of pain. *Pain, 2*: 175–87.

Scott, P.J., Ansell, B.M. and Huskisson, E.C. (1977). The measurement of pain in juvenile chronic polyarthritis. *Annals of Rheumatic Diseases, 36*: 186–7.

Secretaries of State for Health, Wales, Northern Ireland and Scotland (1989a). *Contracts for Services and Role of District Health Authorities*. London: HMSO.

Secretaries of State for Health, Wales, Northern Ireland and Scotland (1989b). *Working for Patients*. London: HMSO.

Seeman, M. and Seeman, T.E. (1983). Health behaviour and personal autonomy: A longitudinal study of the sense of control in illness. *Journal of Health and Social Behaviour, 24*: 144–60.

Selby, P. (1992). Measurement of the quality of life: The particular problems of cancer patients. In: A. Hopkins (ed.), *Measures of the Quality of Life*. London: Royal College of Physicians.

Selby, P. (1993). Measuring the quality of life of patients with cancer. In: S.R. Walker and R.M. Rosser (eds), *Quality of Life Assessment: Key Issues in the 1990s*. Dordrecht: Kluwer Academic.

Selby, P., Chapman, J.A.W., Etazadi-Amoli, J. *et al.* (1984). The development of a method for assessing the quality of life of cancer patients. *British Journal of Cancer, 50*: 13–22.

Selby, P. and Robertson, B. (1987). Measurement of quality of life in patients with cancer. *Cancer Surveys, 6*: 521–43.

Sengupta, R.P., Chiu, J.S.P. and Brierley, H. (1975). Quality of survival following direct surgery for anterior communicating artery aneurysms. *Journal of Neurosurgery, 43*: 58–63.

Serban, G. (1979). Mental status, functioning, and stress in chronic schizophrenic patients in community care. *American Journal of Psychiatry, 136*: 948–52.

Serban, G. and Gidynski, C.B. (1979). Relationship between cognitive defect, affect response and community adjustment in chronic schizophrenics. *British Journal of Psychiatry, 134*: 602–8.

Sergeant, P., Lasaffre, E., Flameng, W. *et al.* (1986). How predictable is the postoperative work resumption after aortocoronary bypass surgery? *Acta Cardiologica, 41*: 41–52.

Shaffer, D., Gould, M.S., Brasic, J. *et al.* (1983). Children's Global Assessment Scale (CGAS). *Archives of General Psychiatry, 40*: 1228–31.

Shah, S., Frank, V. and Cooper, B. (1989). Improving the sensitivity of the Barthel Index for stroke rehabilitation. *Journal of Clinical Epidemiology, 42*: 703–9.

Shah, S., Vanclay, F. and Cooper, B. (1991). Stroke rehabilitation: Australian patient profile and functional outcome. *Journal of Clinical Epidemiology, 44*: 21–8.

Shahtahmasebi, S., Davies, R. and Wenger, G.C. (1992). A longitudinal analysis of factors related to survival in old age. *The Gerontologist, 32*: 404–13.

Shandu, H. (1986). Psychosocial issues in chronic obstructive pulmonary disease. *Clinics in Chest Medicine, 7*: 629–42.

Shaver, P.R. and Brennan, K.A. (1991). Measures of depression and loneliness. In: J.P. Robinson, P.R. Shaver and L.S. Wrightsman (eds), *Measures of Personality and Social Psychological Attitudes*. San Diego, CA: Academic Press.

Shaw, A. (1977). Defining the quality of life. *Hastings Center Report*, 11 October.

Shaw, P.J. (1986). Neurological dysfunction following coronary artery bypass graft surgery. *Journal of the Royal Society of Medicine, 79*: 130–1.

Shaw, R.E., Cohen, F., Fishman-Rosen, J. *et al.* (1986). Psychological predictors of psychosocial and medical outcomes in patients undergoing coronary angioplasty. *Psychosomatic Medicine, 48*: 582–97.

Shepherd, G. (1988). Evaluation and service planning. In: A. Lavender and F. Holloway (eds), *Community Care in Practice*. Chichester: John Wiley.

Shepherd, M. and Watt, D. (1975). Impact of long-term neuroleptics on the community: Advantages and disadvantages. In: J.R. Boissier *et al.* (eds), *Neuropsychopharmacology*. New York: Elsevier.

Sherbourne, C.D. (1988). The role of social support and life stress events in use of mental health services. *Social Science and Medicine, 27*: 1393–400.

Sherbourne, C.D. and Hays, R.D. (1990). Marital status, social support, and health transitions in chronic disease patients. *Journal of Health and Social Behaviour, 31*: 328–43.

Sherbourne, C.D. and Stewart, A.L. (1991). The MOS social support survey. *Social Science and Medicine, 32*: 705–14.

Sherbourne, C.D., Meredith, L.S., Rogers, W. and Ware, J.E. (1992). Social support and stressful life events: Age differences in their effects on health related quality of life among the chronically ill. *Quality of Life Research, 1*: 235–46.

Sherwood, S.J., Morris, J., Mor, V. and Gutkin, C. (1977). *Compendium of Measures for Describing and Assessing Long Term Care Populations*. Boston, MA: Hebrew Rehabilitation Center for the Aged.

Shindler, J.S., Brown, R., Welburn, P. and Parkes, J.D. (1993). Measuring the quality of life of patients with Parkinson's disease. In: S.R. Walker and R.M. Rosser (eds), *Quality of Life Assessment: Key Issues in the 1990s*. Dordrecht: Kluwer Academic.

Shrout, P.E. and Fleiss, J.L. (1979). Intraclass correlations: Uses in assessing rater reliability. *Psychological Bulletin, 86*: 420–8.

Shumaker, S.A., Schron, E. and Ockene, J. (eds) (1990). *The Handbook of Health Behavior Change*. New York: Springer-Verlag.

Sibbald, B. (1989). Patient self care in acute asthma. *Thorax, 44*: 97–101.

Sibbald, B., Collier, J. and D'Souza, M. (1986). Questionnaire assessment of patients' attitudes and beliefs about asthma. *Family Practice, 3*: 37–41.

Sibbald, B., White, P., Pharoah, C. *et al.* (1988). Relationship between psychosocial factors and asthma morbidity. *Family Practice, 5*: 12–17.

Siegler, I.C., Peterson, B.L., Barefott, J.C. and Williams, R.B. (1992). Hostility during late adolescence predicts coronary risk factors at mid life. *American Journal of Epidemiology, 136*: 146–54.

Siegrist, J. and Junge, A. (1990). Measuring the social dimension of subjective health in chronic illness. *Psychotherapy and Psychosomatics, 54*: 90–8.

Siegrist, J., Broer, M. and Junge, A. (1993). *Profil der Lebensqualitat bei Chronischkranken*. Dusseldorf: Institut für Medizinische Soziologie, Universität Dusseldorf.

Sigurdardottir, V., Bolund, C., Brandberg, Y. and Sullivan, M. (1993). The impact of generalised malignant melanoma on quality of life evaluated by the EORTC questionnaire technique. *Quality of Life Research, 2*: 193–203.

Silberfarb, P.L., Maurer, H.L. and Crouthamel, C.S. (1980). Psychological aspects of neoplastic disease: Functional status of breast cancer patients during different treatment regimens. *American Journal of Psychiatry, 137*: 450–5.

Simmons, R.G. and Abress, L. (1990). Quality of life issues for end-stage renal disease patients. *American Journal of Kidney Diseases, XV*: 201–8.

Simmons, S. (1994). Quality of life in community mental health care – a review. *International Journal of Nursing Studies, 2*: 183–93.

Sinclair, I. (1988) *Residential Care: The Research Reviewed*. London: HMSO.

Sinclair, I. and Clarke, R.V. (1991). Studies of residential

environments: Lessons from the past and pointers to the future. In: P.E. Bebbington (ed.), *Social Psychiatry: Theory, Methodology and Practice*. London: Transaction Publishers.

Skeel, R.T. (1989). Quality of life assessment in cancer clinical trials – it's time to catch up. *Journal of the National Cancer Institute, 81*: 472–3.

Skilbeck, C.E. and Woods, R.T. (1980). The factorial structure of the Wechsler Memory Scale: Samples of neurological and psychogeriatric patients. *Journal of Clinical Neuropsychology, 2*: 293–300.

Slevin, M.L. (1984). Quality of life in cancer patients. *Clinics in Oncology, 3*: 371–90.

Slevin, M.L. (1992). Quality of life: Philosophical question or clinical reality? *British Medical Journal, 305*: 466–9.

Slevin, M.L., Plant, H., Lynch, D. *et al.* (1988). Who should measure quality of life, the doctor or the patient? *British Journal of Cancer, 57*: 109–12.

Slevin, M.L., Stubbs, L., Plant, H.J., Wilson, P., Gregory, W.M., Armes, P.J. *et al.* (1990). Attitudes to chemotherapy: Comparing views of patients with cancer with those of doctors, nurses and the general public. *British Medical Journal, 300*: 1458–60.

Smart, C.R. and Yates, J.W. (1987). Quality of life. *Cancer, 60*: 620–2.

Smith, D.F., Baker, G.A., Dewey, M. *et al.* (1991). Seizure frequency, patient perceived seizure severity and the psychosocial consequences of intractable epilepsy. *Epilepsy Research, 9*: 231–41.

Smith, D., Baker, G., Davies, G. *et al.* (1993). Outcomes of add-on treatment with lamotrigine in partial epilepsy. *Epilepsia, 34*: 312–22.

Smith, H.C.L., Frye, R.L. and Piehler, J.M. (1983). Does coronary bypass surgery have a favourable influence on the quality of life? *Cardiovascular Clinics, 13*: 253–64.

Smith, R. (1990). Crisis in American health care. *British Medical Journal, 300*: 765.

Smith, W.C., Kenicer, M.B., Tunstall-Pedoe, H. *et al.* (1990). Prevalence of coronary heart disease in Scotland: Scottish Heart Health Survey. *British Heart Journal, 64*: 295–8.

Snaith, R.P. (1985). A mood chart for use in clinical practice. *British Journal of Clinical and Social Psychiatry, 3*: 16–18.

Snaith, R.P. (1987). The concepts of mild depression. *British Journal of Psychiatry, 150*: 387–93.

Snaith, R.P. (1993). What do depression rating scales measure? *British Journal of Psychiatry, 163*: 293–8.

Snaith, R.P. and Taylor, C.M. (1985). Rating scales for depression and anxiety: A current perspective. *British Journal of Clinical Pharmacology, 19*: 17S–20S (suppl.).

Sommerville, S. (1982). The Functional Limitations Profile: Comparison with the Harris self-care measure. In: D.L. Patrick (ed.) Health and care of the physically disabled in Lambeth. Report of Phase III of the Longitudinal Disability Interview Survey. London: St Thomas' Hospital Medical School, Department of Community Medicine.

Spanier, G.B. (1976). Measuring dyadic adjustment: New scales for assessing the quality of marriage and similar dyads. *Journal of Marriage and the Family*, *38*: 15–28.

Sparrow, S., Balla, D. and Ciccetti, D. (1984a). *Vineland Adaptive Behaviour Scales (Survey Form)*. Circle Pines, MN: American Guidance Service.

Sparrow, S., Balla, D. and Ciccetti, D. (1984b). *Vineland Adaptive Behaviour Scales (Expanded Form)*. Circle Pines, MN: American Guidance Service.

Sparrow, S., Balla, D. and Ciccetti, D. (1985). *Vineland Adaptive Behaviour Scales (Classroom Edition)*. Circle Pines, MN: American Guidance Service.

Spector, T.D. and Hochberg, M.C. (1992). An epidemiological approach to the study of outcome in rheumatoid arthritis. In: D. Scott (ed.), *The Course and Outcome of Rheumatoid Arthritis*. Baillière's Clinical Rheumatology, Vol. 6, No. 1. London: Bailliere Tindall.

Spector, T.D. and Thompson, S.J. (1991). The potential and limitations of meta-analysis. *Journal of Epidemiology and Community Health*, *45*: 89–92.

Spector, W.D., Katz, S., Murphy, J.B. *et al.* (1987). The hierarchical relationship between activities of daily living and instrumental activities of daily living. *Journal of Chronic Diseases*, *40*: 481–9.

Spencer, S.S. and Spencer, D.D. (1991). Dogma, data and directions. In: S.S. Spencer and D.D. Spencer, *Surgery for Epilepsy*. Oxford: Blackwell Scientific.

Spielberger, C.D., Gorsuch, R.L., Luchene, R.E. (1970). *Manual for the State–Trait Anxiety Inventory*. Palo Alto, CA: Consulting Psychologists Press.

Spielberger, C.D., Davidson, K., Lighthall, F. *et al.* (1973). *STAI Preliminary Manual*. Palo Alto, CA: Consulting Psychologists Press.

Spielberger, C.D., Gorsuch, R.L., Luchene, R.E. *et al.* (1983). *Manual for the State–Trait Anxiety Inventory* (revised edition). Palo Alto, CA: Consulting Psychologists Press.

Spilker, B., Molinek, F.R., Johnston, K.A. *et al.* (eds) (1990). Quality of life bibliography and indexes. *Medical Care*, *28*: DS1–DS77.

Spitzer, R.L. (ed.) (1987). *Diagnostic and Statistical Manual of Mental Disorders*, 3rd edn, revised. Washington, DC: American Psychiatric Association.

Spitzer, R.L. and Williams, J.B.W. (1988). Revised diagnostic criteria and a new structured interview for diagnosing anxiety disorders. *Journal of Psychiatric Research*, *22*: 55–85 (suppl. 1).

Spitzer, R.L., Endicott, J., Fliess, J.L. *et al.* (1970).

Psychiatric status schedule: A technique for evaluating psychopathology and impairment in role functioning. *Archives of General Psychiatry*, *23*: 41–55.

Spitzer, R.L., Endicott, J. and Robins, E. (1975a). Clinical criteria for psychiatric diagnosis and DSM-III. *American Journal of Psychiatry*, *132*: 1187–92.

Spitzer, R.L., Endicott, J. and Robins, E. (1975b). Research Diagnostic Criteria (RDC). *Psychopharmacology Bulletin*, *11*: 22–4.

Spitzer, R.L., Endicott, J. and Robins, E. (1978). Research Diagnostic Criteria: Rationale and reliability. *Archives of General Psychiatry*, *35*: 773–82.

Spitzer, W.O., Dobson, A.J., Hall, J. *et al.* (1981). Measuring quality of life of cancer patients: A concise QL-index for use by physicians. *Journal of Chronic Diseases*, *34*: 585–97.

Splinter, T.A.W. (1990). Chemotherapy in advanced non-small cell lung cancer. *European Journal of Cancer*, *26*: 1093–9.

Sprangers, M.A.G., Cull, A., Bjordal, K. *et al.* (1993). The European Organisation for Research and Treatment of Cancer approach to quality of life assessment: Guidelines for developing questionnaire modules. *Quality of Life Research*, *2*: 287–95.

Spruill, J. (1984). Wechsler Adult Intelligence Scale – Revised. In: D.J. Keyser and R.C. Sweetland (eds), *Test Critiques*, Vol. I. Kansas City, MO: Test Corporation of America.

Stanley, K.E. (1980). Prognostic factors for survival in patients with inoperable lung cancer. *Journal of the National Cancer Institute*, *65*: 25–32.

Stark, R.D., Gambles, S.A. and Lewis, J.A. (1981). Methods to assess breathlessness in healthy subjects: A critical evaluation and application to analyse the acute effects of diazepam and promethazine on breathlessness induced by exercise or by exposure to raised levels of carbon dioxide. *Clinical Science*, *61*: 429–39.

Stark, R.D., Gambles, S.A. and Chattergee, S.S. (1982). An exercise test to assess clinical dyspnoea: Estimation of reproducibility and sensitivity. *British Journal of Diseases of the Chest*, *76*: 269–78.

Steer, R.A., Beck, A.T. and Garrison, B. (1986). Applications of the Beck Depression Inventory. In: N. Sartorius and T.A. Ban (eds), *Assessment of Depression*. Berlin: Springer-Verlag.

Stein, M., Wallston, K. and Nicassio, P. (1988). Factor structure of the Arthritis Helplessness Index. *Journal of Rheumatology*, *15*: 427–32.

Steinberg, M.D., Juliano, M.A. and Wise, L. (1985). Psychological outcome of lumpectomy versus mastectomy in the treatment of breast cancer. *American Journal of Psychiatry*, *142*: 34–9.

Steinbrocker, O., Traeger, C.H. and Batterman, R.C. (1949). Therapeutic criteria in rheumatoid arthritis. *Journal of the American Medical Association*, *140*: 659–62.

Stern, M.J., Pascale, L. and Ackerman, A. (1977). Life adjustment post-myocardial infarction. *Archives of Internal Medicine, 137*: 1680–5.

Stevens, B. (1972). Dependence of schizophrenic patients on elderly relations. *Psychological Medicine, 2*: 17–32.

Stewart, A.L. and Ware, J.E. (eds) (1992). *Measuring Functioning and Well-being: The Medical Outcomes Study Approach*. Durham, NC: Duke University Press.

Stewart, A.L., Ware, J.E., Brooke, R.H. *et al.* (1978). *Conceptualisation and Measurement of Health for Adults in the Health Insurance Study. Vol. 2. Physical Health in Terms of Functioning*. Santa Monica, CA: Rand Corporation.

Stewart, A.L., Ware, J.E., Brook, R.H. *et al.* (1981). Advances in the measurement of functional status: Construction of aggregate indexes. *Medical Care, 19*: 473–88.

Stewart, A.L., Hays, R.D. and Ware, J.E. (1988). The MOS short form general health survey: Reliability and validity in a patient population. *Medical Care, 26*: 724–35.

Stewart, A.L., Greenfield, S., Hays, R.D. *et al.* (1989). Functional status and well-being of patients with chronic conditions: Results from the Medical Outcomes Study. *Journal of the American Medical Association, 262*: 907–13.

Stewart, A.L., Sherbourne, C., Hays, R.D. *et al.* (1992a). Summary and discussion of MOS measures. In: A.L. Stewart and J.E. Ware (eds), *Measuring Functioning and Well-being: The Medical Outcomes Study Approach*. Durham, NC: Duke University Press.

Stewart, A.L., Ware, J.E., Sherbourne, C.D. and Wells, K.B. (1992b). Psychological distress/well-being and cognitive functioning measures. In: A.L. Stewart and J.E. Ware (eds), *Measuring Functioning and Well-being: The Medical Outcomes Study Approach*. Durham, NC: Duke University Press.

Stewart, D.A., Burns, J.M.A., Dunn, S.G. and Roberts, M.A. (1990). The two-minute walking test: A sensitive index of mobility in the rehabilitation of elderly patients. *Clinical Rehabilitation, 4*: 273–6.

Stewart, R. and Poaster, L. (1975). Methods of assessing mental and physical health needs from social statistics. *Evaluation, 2*: 67–70.

Stiff, J.E. and Silver, D.L. (1990). *The City of Pasadena Quality of Life Index: California Healthy Cities Project*. Pasadena, CA: City of Pasadena Health Department.

Stineman, M.G., Escarce, J.J., Goin, J.E. *et al.* (1994). A case mix classification system for medical rehabilitation. *Medical Care, 32*: 366–79.

Stocksmeier, U. (1979) *Questionnaire Used in the Rehabilitation of Myocardial Infarction Patients*. Tutzing, Germany: Institute for Preventive and Social Medicine.

Stoker, M.J., Dunbar, G.C. and Beaumont, G. (1992).

The SmithKline Beecham 'quality of life' scale: A validation and reliability study in patients with affective disorder. *Quality of Life Research, 1*: 385–95.

Stoller, J.K., Ferranti, R. and Feinstein, A.R. (1986). Further specification and evaluation of a new clinical index for dyspnoea. *American Review of Respiratory Diseases, 34*: 1129–34.

Stone, A.A. and Neale, J.M. (1984). New measures of daily coping: Development and preliminary results. *Journal of Personality and Social Psychology, 46*: 892–906.

Stone, A.A., Greenberg, M.A., Kenney-Moore, E. and Newman, M.G. (1991). Self-report, situation specific coping questionnaires: What are they measuring? *Journal of Personality and Social Psychology, 61*: 648–58.

Strachan, A.M., Leff, J.P., Goldstein, M.J. *et al.* (1986). Emotional attitudes and direct communication in the families of schizophrenics: A cross-national replication. *British Journal of Psychiatry, 149*: 279–87.

Strahan, R. and Gerbasi, K. (1972). Short, homogeneous version of the Marlowe–Crowne social desirability scale. *Journal of Clinical Psychology, 28*: 191–3.

Strauss, A.L. (ed.) (1975). *Chronic Illness and the Quality of Life*. St Louis, MO: C.V. Mosby.

Strauss, B., Thormann, T., Strenge, E.B., Foerst, U., Stauch, C., Torp, U., Bernhard, A. and Speidel, H. (1992). Psychosocial, neuropsychological and neurological status in a sample of heart transplant recipients. *Quality of Life Research, 1*: 119–28.

Strauss, J.S. and Carpenter, W.T. (1974). The prediction of outcome in schizophrenia: II. Relationships between predictor and outcome variables. A report from the WHO International Pilot Study of Schizophrenia. *Archives of General Psychiatry, 31*: 37–42.

Streiner, G.L. and Norman, D.R. (1990). *Health Measurement Scales: A Practical Guide to Their Development and Use*. Oxford: Oxford University Press.

Strunk, R.C., Fukuhara, J.T., Labrecque, J.F. *et al.* (1989). Outcome of long-term hospitalisation for asthma in children. *Journal of Allergy and Clinical Immunology, 83*: 17–25.

Sturt, E. and Wykes, T. (1987) Assessment schedules for chronic psychiatric patients. *Psychological Medicine, 17*: 485–93.

Sudman, S. and Bradburn, N.M. (1983). *Asking Questions*. New York: Jossey Bass.

Sugarbaker, P.H., Barofsky, I., Rosenberg, S.A. and Gianola, P.J. (1982). Quality of life assessment of patients in extremity sarcoma clinical trials. *Surgery, 91*: 17–23.

Sullivan, G. (1989). *Rehospitalization of the Seriously Mentally Ill in Mississippi: Conceptual Models, Study Design, and Implementation*. N–2996–RWJ/NIMH/HCFA. Santa Monica, CA: Rand Corporation.

Sullivan, M. (1992). Quality of life assessment in medicine: Concepts, definitions, purposes and basic tools. *Nordic Journal of Psychiatry, 46*: 79–83.

Sullivan, M., Ahlmen, M., Archenholt, B. *et al.* (1986). Measuring health in rheumatic disorders by means of a Swedish version of the Sickness Impact Profile. *Scandinavian Journal of Rheumatology, 15*: 193–200.

Sullivan, M., Ahlmen, M. and Bjelle, A. (1990). Health status assessment in rheumatoid arthritis. I. Further work on the validity of the Sickness Impact Profile. *Journal of Rheumatology, 17*: 439–47.

Sunderland, A., Harris, J.E. and Baddeley, A.D. (1983). Do laboratory tests predict everyday memory? A neuropsychological study. *Journal of Verbal Learning and Verbal Behaviour, 22*: 341–57.

Sunderland, T., Hill, J.L., Mellow, A.M. *et al.* (1989). Clock drawing in Alzheimer's disease: A novel measure of dementia severity. *Journal of the American Geriatrics Society, 37*: 725–9.

Sutherland, H.J., Llewellyn-Thomas, H., Hogg, S.A. *et al.* (1984). Do patients and physicians agree on the assessment of voice quality in laryngeal cancer? *Journal of Otolaryngology, 13*: 325–30.

Suurmeijer, Th. P.B.M. and Kempen, G.I.J.M. (1990). Behavioural change as an outcome of disease: The development of an instrument. *International Journal of Health Sciences, 1*: 189–94.

Swieten, J.C., Koudstaal. P.J., Visser, M.C. *et al.* (1988). Interobserver agreement for the assessment of handicap in stroke patients. *Stroke, 19*: 604–7.

Swinburn, C.R., Wakefield, J.M. and Jones, P.W. (1985). Performance, ventilation and oxygen consumption in three different types of exercise test in patients with chronic obstructive lung disease. *Thorax, 40*: 581–6.

Swinburn, C.R., Wakefield, J.M., Newman, S.P. *et al.* (1988). Evidence of prednisolone induced mood change ('steroid euphoria') in patients with chronic obstructive airways disease. *British Journal of Clinical Pharmacology, 26*: 709–13.

Syme, S.L. (1986). Social networks in relation to morbidity and mortality. In: S.O. Isacsson and L. Janzon (eds), *Social Support, Health and Disease*. Sixth International Berzelius Symposium sponsored by the Delegation for Social Research. Stockholm: Almqvist and Wiksell International.

Szasz, T. (1971). *The Manufacture of Madness*. London: Routledge and Kegan Paul.

Szmuckler, G.I., Berkowitz, R., Eisler, I. *et al.* (1987). Expressed emotion in individual and family settings: A comparative study. *British Journal of Psychiatry, 151*: 174–8.

Tamburini, M., Rosso, S., Gamba, A., Mecanglia, E., De Conno, F. and Ventafridda, V. (1992). A therapy impact questionnaire for quality of life assessment in advanced cancer research. *Annals of Oncology, 3*: 565–70.

Tartar, R.E., Hegedus, A.M., Gavaler, J.S.J. *et al.* (1983). Acute effects of liver transplantation on neuropsychological capacity as determined by studies performed pre-transplantation and four to six weeks following surgery (abstract). *Hepatology, 3*: 830.

Tartar, R.E., van Thiel, D.H., Hegedus, A.M. *et al.* (1984). Neuropsychiatric status after liver transplantation. *Journal of Laboratory and Clinical Medicine, 103*: 776–82.

Tartar, R.E., Erb, S., Biller, P.A. *et al.* (1988). The quality of life following liver transplantation: A preliminary report. *Gastroenterology Clinics of North America, 17*: 207–17.

Task Force on Health Risk Assessment (US Department of Health and Human Services) (1986). *Determining Risks to Health*. Dover, MA: Aubern House.

Tatarkiewicz, W. (1975). *Analysis of Happiness*. The Hague: Martinus Nijhoff.

Taylor, D.C. (1987). Psychiatric and social issues in measuring the input and outcome of epilepsy surgery. In: J. Engel (ed.), *Surgical Treatment of the Epilepsies*. New York: Raven Press.

Taylor, D.C. and Falconer, M.A. (1968). Clinical, socio-economic and psychological changes after temporal lobectomy for epilepsy. *British Journal of Psychiatry, 114*: 1247–61.

Taylor, S.H. (1987). Drug therapy and quality of life in angina pectoris. *American Heart Journal, 114*: 234–40.

Tchekmedyian, N.S. and Cella, D.F. (1990). Quality of life in current oncology practice and research: Appendix 1. *Oncology, 4*: 215.

Team for the Assessment of Psychiatric Services (TAPS) (1986–). *Annual Conferences of the Team for the Assessment of Psychiatric Services*. Conference reports from 1986 onwards (annual). Purchasable from the TAPS Research Unit, Hampstead Road Group Practice Building, 69 Fleet Road, London NW3 2QU, UK.

Team for the Assessment of Psychiatric Services (TAPS) (1990). *Better Out Than In*. London: North East Thames Regional Health Authority.

Tebbi, C.K., Bromberg, C., Sills, I. *et al.* (1990). Vocational adjustment and general well-being of adults with IDDM. *Diabetes Care, 13*: 98–113.

Tennen, H. and Herzberger, S. (1985a). Ways of Coping Scale. In: D.J. Keyser and R.C. Sweetland (eds), *Test Critiques*, Vol. III. Kansas City, MO: Test Corporation of America.

Tennen, H. and Herzberger, S. (1985b). Impact of Event Scale. In: D.J. Keyser and R.C. Sweetland (eds), *Test Critiques*, Vol. III. Kansas City, MO: Test Corporation of America.

Tennen, H., Affleck, G. and Herzberger, S. (1985). Schedule of Recent Experience. In: D.K. Keyser and R.C. Sweetland (eds), *Test Critiques*, Vol. III. Kansas City, MO: Test Corporation of America.

Thomas, M., Goddard, E., Hickman, M. and Hunter, P. (1994). *General Household Survey 1992*. Compiled for Office of Population Censuses and Surveys. London: HMSO.

Thomas, M.R. and Lyttle, D. (1980). Patient expectations about success of treatment and reported relief from low back pain. *Journal of Psychosomatic Research, 24*: 297–301.

Thompson, P. (1989a). Affective disorders. In: P. Thompson (ed.), *The Instruments of Psychiatric Research*. Chichester: John Wiley.

Thompson, P. (1989b). Anxiety. In: P. Thompson (ed.), *The Instruments of Psychiatric Research*. Chichester: John Wiley.

Thompson, P. (ed.) (1989c). *The Instruments of Psychiatric Research*. Chichester: John Wiley.

Thompson, P. and Blessed, G. (1987). Correlation between the 37-item Mental Test Score and Abbreviated 10-item Mental Test Score by psychogeriatric day patients. *British Journal of Psychiatry, 151*: 206–9.

Thornicroft, G., Gooch, C. and Dayson, D. (1992). Readmission to hospital for long term psychiatric patients after discharge to the community. *British Medical Journal, 305*: 994–8.

Thornicroft, G., Gooch, C., O'Driscoll, D. and Reda, S. (1993). The TAPS Project. 9: The reliability of the Patient Attitude Questionnaire. *British Journal of Psychiatry, 162*: 25–9 (suppl. 19).

Thurstone, L.L. (1927a). Psychophysical analysis. *American Journal of Psychology, 38*: 368–89.

Thurstone, L.L. (1927b). A law of comparative judgement. *Psychology Review, 34*: 273–86.

Till, J.R., Sutherland, H.J. and Meslin, E.M. (1992). Is there a role for preference assessments in research on quality of life in oncology? *Quality of Life Research, 1*: 31–40.

Tilson, H. and Spilker, B. (1990). Guest editorial. *Medical Care, 28*: 1 (suppl. 12).

Tobin, D.L., Wigal, J.K., Winder, J.A. *et al.* (1987). The Asthma Self Efficacy Scale. *Annals of Allergy, 59*: 273–7.

Todd, C.J., Williams, D.R.R, Pryor, G. *et al.* (1991). Early discharge to 'hospital at home' after fracture of neck of femur: Psychosocial factors. In: G. Brenner and I. Weber (eds), *Health Services Research and Primary Health Care*. Cologne: Deutscher Artze Verlag.

Toner, J., Gurland, B. and Teresi, J. (1988). Comparison of self-administered and rater-administered methods of assessing levels of severity of depression in elderly patients. *Journal of Gerontology, 43*: 136–40.

Torrance, G.W. (1986). Measurement of health state utilities for economic appraisal: A review. *Journal of Health Economics, 3*: 1–30.

Torrance, G.W. (1987). Utility approach to measuring health related quality of life. *Journal of Chronic Diseases, 40*: 593–600.

Torrance, G.W., Thomas, W.H. and Sackett, D.L. (1972). A utility maximization model for the evaluation of health care programmes. *Health Services Research, 7*: 118–33.

Torrance, G.W., Boyle, M.H. and Horwood, S.P. (1982). Application of multiattribute utility theory to measure social preferences for health states. *Operations Research, 30*: 1043–69.

Townsend, P. (1962). *The Last Refuge*. London: Routledge and Kegan Paul.

Treanton, J.R. (1962). Some sociological considerations on the problem of adjustment in older people. In: C. Tibbits and W. Donahue (eds), *Social and Psychological Aspects of Aging. Proceedings of the Fifth Congress of the International Association of Gerontology*, Vol. I. New York: Columbia University Press.

Tugwell, P., Sackett, D.L., Goldsmith, C.H. *et al.* (1983). *Quality of Care in Acute Myocardial Infarction: Final Report*. US National Center for Health Service Research Grant No. R01 HS 03239.

Tugwell, P., Bombardier, C., Buchanan, W.W. *et al.* (1987). The MACTAR Patient Preference Disability Questionnaire. *Journal of Rheumatology, 14*: 446–51.

Tugwell, P., Bombardier, C., Buchanan, W.W. *et al.* (1990). Methotrexate in rheumatoid arthritis: Impact on quality of life assessed by traditional standard-item and individualised patient preference health status questionnaire. *Archives of Internal Medicine, 150*: 59–62.

Turk, D.C. (1979). Factors influencing the adaptive process with chronic illness. In: I.G. Sarason and C.D. Spielberger (eds), *Stress and Anxiety*, Vol. 6. Washington, DC: Hemisphere.

Twaddle, A.C. (1969). Health decisions and sick role variations: An exploration. *Journal of Health and Social Behavior, 10*: 105–15.

Tyrer, P. (1990). Personality disorder and social functioning. In D.F. Peck and C.M. Shapiro (eds) *Measuring Human Problems*. Chichester: John Wiley.

Tyrer, P., Merson, S., Harrison-Read, P. *et al.* (1990). A pilot study of the effects of early intervention on clinical symptoms and social functioning in psychiatric emergencies. *Irish Journal of Psychological Medicine, 7*: 132–4.

Tyroler, H.A., Cutler, J.A., Cohen, F. *et al.* (1984). Report of the working group: Congestive heart failure. In: N.K. Wenger, M.E. Mattson, C.P. Furberg and J. Elinson (eds), *Assessment of Quality of Life in Clinical Trials of Cardiovascular Therapies*. New York: Le Jacq.

UK-TIA Study Group (1988). The UK-TIA aspirin trial: Interim results. *British Medical Journal, 296*: 316–20.

Unden, A.L., Schenck-Gustafsson, K., Axelsson, P.O., Karlsson, I., Orth-Gomer, K. and Ydrefors, A.M.

(1993). Positive effects of increased nurse support for male patients after acute myocardial infarction. *Quality of Life Research, 2*: 121–7.

Van Agt, H.M.E., Essink-Bot, M.L., van der Meer, J.B.W. and Bonsel, G.J. (1993). The NHP (Dutch version) in general and specified populations. Paper presented to the *Fifth European Health Services Research Conference*, Maastricht, December.

Van Campen, C., Friele, R.D. and Kerssens, J.J. (1992). *Methods for Assessing Patient Satisfaction with Primary Care: Review and Annotated Bibliography*. Utrecht: Netherlands Institute of Primary Care (NIVEL).

Van Dam, F.S.A.M., Linssen, C.A.G. and Couzijn, A.L. (1984). Evaluating 'quality of life' in cancer clinical trials. In: M.E. Buyse *et al.* (eds), *Cancer Clinical Trials: Methods and Practice*. New York: Oxford University Press.

Vandenburg, M.J. (1993). Measuring quality of life of patients with angina. In: S.R. Walker and R.M. Rosser (eds), *Quality of Life Assessment: Key Issues in the 1990s*. Dordrecht: Kluwer Academic.

Van Knippenberg, F.C.E. and de Haes, J.C.J.M. (1988). Measuring the quality of life of cancer patients. Psychometric properties of instruments. *Journal of Clinical Epidemiology, 11*: 1043–53.

Van Swieten, J.C., Koudstaal, P.J., Visser, M.C. *et al.* (1988). Interobserver agreement for the assessment of handicap in stroke patients. *Stroke, 19*: 604–7.

Vardon, V.M. and Blessed, G. (1986). Confusion ratings and abbreviated mental test performance: A comparison. *Age and Ageing, 15*: 139–44.

Vaughan, C.E. and Leff, J.P. (1976). The measurement of expressed emotion in the families of psychiatric patients. *British Journal of Clinical and Social Psychology, 15*: 157–65.

Veenhoven, R. (1984). *Conditions of Happiness*. Dordrecht: Reidel.

Veenhoven, R. (1988). The utility of happiness. *Social Indicators Research, 20*: 333–54.

Veenhoven, R. (1989). National economic prosperity and individual happiness. In: K.G. Grunert and T. Olander (eds), *Understanding Economic Behaviour*. London: Kluwer Academic.

Veenhoven, R. (1991). Is happiness relative? *Social Indicators Research, 24*: 1–34.

Veit, C.T. and Ware, J.E. (1983). The structure of psychological distress and well-being in general populations. *Journal of Consulting and Clinical Psychology, 51*: 730–42.

Ventafridda, V., van Dam, F.S.A.M., Yancik, R. and Tamburini, M. (eds) (1986). *Assessment of Quality of Life and Cancer Treatment: Proceedings of the International Workshop on Quality of Life Assessment and Cancer Treatment*, Milan, December 1985. Amsterdam: Elsevier.

Vera, M.I. (1981). Quality of life following pelvic exenteration. *Gynecologic Oncology, 12*: 355–66.

Verbrugge, L.M. (1992). Disability transitions for older persons with arthritis. *Journal of Aging and Health, 4*: 212–43.

Verger, E., Salamero, M. and Conill, C. (1992). Can Karnofsky performance status be transformed to the Eastern Cooperative Oncology Group scoring scale and vice versa? *European Journal of Cancer, 28A*: 1328–30.

Vernon, P.A. (1984). Wechsler Intelligence Scale for Children – Revised. In: D.J. Keyser and R.C. Sweetland (eds), *Test Critiques*, Vol. I. Kansas City, MO: Test Corporation of America.

Vetter, N., Smith, A., Sastry, D. and Tinker, G. (1989). *Day Hospital – Pilot Study Report*. Research Team for the Care of Elderly People. Cardiff: Department of Geriatrics, St David's Hospital.

Vickrey, B.G. (1993). A procedure for developing a quality of life measure for epilepsy surgery patients. *Epilepsia, 34*: (supplement 4) S22–7.

Vickrey, B.G., Hays, R.D., Brooks, R.H. and Rausch, R. (1992a). Reliability and validity of the Katz Adjustment Scales in an epilepsy sample. *Quality of Life Research, 1*: 63–72.

Vickrey, B.G., Hays, R.D., Graber, J. *et al.* (1992b). A health related quality of life instrument for patients evaluated for epilepsy surgery. *Medical Care, 30*: 299–319.

Vickrey, B.G., Hays, R.D., Hermann, B., Bladin, P.F. *et al.* (1993). Quality of life outcomes. In: J. Engel (ed.), *Surgical Treatment of the Epilepsies*, 2nd edn. New York: Raven Press.

Vieweg, B.W. and Hedlund, J.L. (1983). The General Health Questionnaire: A comprehensive review. *Journal of Operational Psychiatry, 14*: 74–81.

Vingerhoets, A.J.J.M. and Flohr, P.J.M,. (1984). Type A behaviour and self-reports of coping preferences. *British Journal of Medical Psychology, 57*: 15–21.

Vinokur, A.D., Threat, B.A., Caplan, R.D. and Zimmerman, B.L. (1989). Physical and psychosocial functioning and adjustment to breast cancer. *Cancer, 63*: 394–405.

Vinokur, A.D., Threat, B.A., Vinokur-Kaplan, D. and Satariano, W.A. (1990). The process of recovery from breast cancer for younger and older patients: Changes during the first year. *Cancer, 65*: 1242–54.

Visser, M.C., Fletcher, A.E., Parr, G. *et al.* (1994). A comparison of three quality of life instruments in subjects with angina pectoris: The Sickness Impact Profile, the Nottingham Health Profile, and the Quality of Well-Being Scale. *Journal of Clinical Epidemiology, 47*: 157–63.

Vitaliano, P.P. (1987). *Manual for Revised Ways of Coping Checklist (WCCL): The Stress and Coping Project*. Seattle, WA: University of Washington.

Vitaliano, P.P., Russo, J., Carr, J.E. *et al.* (1985). The Ways of Coping Checklist: Revision and psychometric properties. *Multivariate Behavioral Research, 20*: 3–26.

Volkmar, F.R., Sparrow, S.S., Goudreau, D. *et al.* (1987). Social deficit in autism: An operational approach using the Vineland Adaptive Behaviour Scales. *Journal of the American Academy of Child and Adolescent Psychiatry, 26*: 156–61.

Wachtel, T., Piette, J., Mor, V. *et al.* (1992). Quality of life in persons with human immunodeficiency virus infection: Measurement by the Medical Outcomes Study Instrument. *Annals of Internal Medicine, 116*: 129–37.

Waddell, G. and Main, C.J. (1984). Assessment of severity in low back-pain disorders. *Spine, 9*: 204–8.

Wade, D.T. (1988). Measurement in rehabilitation. *Age and Ageing, 17*: 289–92.

Wade, D.T. (1992). *Measurement in Neurological Rehabilitation*. Oxford: Oxford University Press.

Wade, D.T. and Collin, C. (1988). The Barthel ADL Index: A standard measure of physical disability? *International Disability Studies, 10*: 64–7.

Wade, D.T. and Langton-Hewer, R. (1987). Functional abilities after stroke: Measurement, natural history and prognosis. *Journal of Neurology, Neurosurgery and Psychiatry, 50*: 177–82.

Wade, D.T., Legh-Smith, G.L. and Langton-Hewer, R. (1985). Social activities after stroke: Measurement and natural history using the Frenchay Activities Index. *International Rehabilitation Medicine, 7*: 176–81.

Wade, D.T., Collen, F.M., Robb, G.F. and Warlow, C.P. (1992). Physiotherapy intervention late after stroke and mobility. *British Medical Journal, 304*: 609–13.

Wagner, E.H., La Croix, A.Z., Grothaus, L.C. and Hecht, J.A. (1993). Responsiveness of health status measures to change among older adults. *Journal of the American Geriatrics Society, 41*: 241–8.

Wainwright, T., Holloway, F. and Brugha, T.S. (1988). Day care in an inner city. In: A. Lavendar and F. Holloway (eds), *Community Care in Practice: Services for the Continuing Care Client*. Chichester: John Wiley.

Walker, C.E. and Kaufman, K. (1984). State–Trait Anxiety Inventory for Children. In: D.J. Keyser and R.C. Sweetland (eds), *Test Critiques*, Vol. I. Kansas City, MO: Test Corporation of America.

Wallace, P. (1994). Health checks for people aged 75 and over in general practice: An international package for assessment (abstract). *Family Practice, 10*: 477.

Wallston, B.S., Wallston, K.A., Kaplan, G.D. and Maides, S.A. (1976). Development and validation of the Health Locus of Control (HLC) Scale. *Journal of Consulting and Clinical Psychology, 44*: 580–5.

Wallston, K.A., Wallston, B.S. and de Vellis, R. (1978). Development of the Multidimensional Health Locus of Control (MHLC) Scales. *Health Education Monographs, 6*: 160–71.

Wallston, K.A., Brown, G.K., Stein, M.J. and Dobbins, C.J. (1989). Comparing the short and long versions of the Arthritis Impact Measurement Scales. *Journal of Rheumatology, 16*: 1105–9.

Wallwork, J. and Caine, N. (1985). A comparison of the quality of life of cardiac transplant patients and coronary artery bypass graft patients before and after surgery. *Quality of Life and Cardiovascular Care, 1*: 317–31.

Walter, J.J. and Shannon, T.A. (1990). Foreword: An overview of 'quality of life'. In: J.J. Walter and T.A. Shannon (eds), *Quality of Life: The New Medical Dilemma*. Mahwah, NJ: Paulist Press.

Walter, P.J. and Mohan, R. (1994). Health related quality of life in octogenarians 5 years after coronary bypass surgery (abstract). *Quality of Life Research, 3*: 63.

Walter, P.J., Mohan, R. and Dahan-Mizrahl, S. (1992). Quality of life after open heart surgery, 16–18 May 1991. Conference report. *Quality of Life Research, 1*: 77–83.

Waltz, C., Strickland, O. and Lenz, E. (1984). *Measurement in Nursing Research*. Philadelphia, PA: F.A. Davis.

Wan, T.T.H. and Livieratos, B. (1977). A validation of the General Well-being Index: A two-stage multivariate approach. Paper presented to the *American Public Health Association Meeting*. Washington, DC, October/November.

Ward, T., Dawe, B., Procter, A. *et al.* (1993). Assessment in severe dementia: The Guy's Advanced Dementia Schedule. *Age and Ageing, 22*: 183–9.

Warde, P., Sturgeon, J.F., Fine, S. *et al.* (1984). Quality of life assessment in patients with carcinoma of the ovary. *Proceedings of the American Society of Clinical Oncology*, ASCO abstracts of the 26th annual meetings of the American Society of Clinical Oncology, May 6–8, 3: 68. Toronto: Canada.

Ware, J.E. (1976). Scales for measuring general health perceptions. *Health Services Research, 11*: 394–415.

Ware, J.E. (1984a). General Health Rating Index. In: N.K. Wenger, M.E. Mattson, C.P. Furberg and J. Elinson (eds), *Assessment of Quality of Life in Clinical Trials of Cardiovascular Therapies*. New York: Le Jacq.

Ware, J.E. (1984b). Methodological considerations in the selection of health status assessment procedures. In: N.K. Wenger, M.E. Mattson, C.D. Furberg and J. Elinson (eds), *Assessment of Quality of Life in Clinical Trials of Cardiovascular Therapies*. New York: Le Jacq.

Ware, J.E. (1987). Standards for validating health measures: Definition and content. *Journal of Chronic Diseases, 40*: 473–80.

Ware, J.E. (1992). Measures for a new era of health

assessment. In: A.L. Stewart and J.E. Ware (eds), *Measuring Functioning and Well-being: The Medical Outcomes Study Approach*. Durham, NC: Duke University Press.

Ware, J.E. (1993). Measuring patients' views: The optimum outcome measure. *British Medical Journal, 306*: 1429–30.

Ware, J.E. and Hays, R.D. (1988). Methods for measuring patient satisfaction with specific medical encounters. *Medical Care, 26*: 393–402.

Ware, J.E. and Karmos, A.H. (1976). *Development and Validation of Scales to Measure Perceived Health and Patient Role Propensity*. Vol. 2 of a Final Report, No. PB288–331. Springfield, VA: National Technical Information Services.

Ware, J.E. and Sherbourne, C.D. (1992). The MOS 36-item short form health survey (SF-36): I. Conceptual framework and item selection. *Medical Care, 30*: 473–83.

Ware, J.E., Davies-Avery, A. and Donald, C.A. (1978). *Conceptualisation and Measurement of Health for Adults in the Health Insurance Study, Vol. V*. Santa Monica, CA: Rand Corporation.

Ware, J.E., Johnson, S.A., Davies-Avery, A. and Brook, R.H. (1979) *Conceptualisation and Measurement of Health for Adults in the Health Insurance Study, Vol. 3. Mental Health*. Santa Monica. CA: Rand Corporation.

Ware, J.E., Brook, R.H., Davies-Avery, A.R. *et al.* (1980). *Conceptualisation and Measurement of Health for Adults in the Health Insurance Study. Vol.VI. Analysis of Relationships among Health Status Measures*. Santa Monica, CA: Rand Corporation.

Ware, J.E., Brook, R.H., Rogers, W.H. *et al.* (1987). *Health Outcomes for Adults in Prepaid and Fee-for-Service Systems of Care: Results from the Health Insurance Experiment*. Santa Monica, CA: Rand Corporation.

Ware, J.E., Sherbourne, C.D. and Davies, A.R. (1992). Developing and testing the MOS 20-item Short Form Health Survey: A general population application. In: A.L. Stewart and J.E. Ware (eds), *Measuring Functioning and Well-being: The Medical Outcomes Study Approach*. Durham, NC: Duke University Press.

Ware, J.E., Snow, K.K., Kosinski, M. and Gandek, B. (1993). *SF-36 Health Survey: Manual and Interpretation Guide*. Boston, MA: The Health Institute, New England Medical Center.

Watchel, T., Piette, J., Mor, V. *et al.* (1992). Quality of life in persons with human immunodeficiency virus infection: Measurement by the medical outcomes study instrument. *Annals of Internal Medicine, 116*: 129–37.

Waters, W.E., Heikkinen, E. and Dontas, A.S. (eds) (1989). *Health, Lifestyles and Services for the Elderly*. Report from the World Health Organization Regional Office for Europe. Public Health in Europe No. 29. Copenhagen: WHO.

Watts, D., Freeman, A.M., McGriffin, D.K. *et al.* (1984). Psychiatric aspects of cardiac transplantation. *General Hospital Psychiatry, 10*: 108–13.

Webb, E.J., Campbell, D.T., Schwartz, R.D. and Sechrest, L. (1966). *Unobtrusive Measures: Non-reactive Research in the Social Sciences*. Chicago, IL: Rand McNally College Publishing.

Wechsler, D. (1945). A standardized memory scale for clinical use. *Journal of Psychology, 19*: 87–95.

Wechsler, D. (1948). *The Measurement and Appraisal of Adult Intelligence*. Baltimore, MD: Williams and Wilkins.

Wechsler, D. (1958). *The Measurement and Appraisal of Adult Intelligence*, 4th edn. Baltimore, MD: Williams and Wilkins.

Wechsler, D. (1967). *Wechsler Pre-school and Primary Scale of Intelligence*. Cleveland, OH: Psychological Corporation.

Wechsler, D. (1974). *Manual for the Wechsler Intelligence Scale for Children – Revised*. New York: Psychological Corporation.

Wechsler, D. (1981a). The psychometric tradition: Developing the Wechsler Adult Intelligence Scale. *Contemporary Educational Psychology, 6*: 82–5.

Wechsler, D. (1981b). *WAIS-R Manual: Wechsler Adult Intelligence Scale – Revised*. New York: Psychological Corporation.

Wechsler, D. (1986). *Wechsler Adult Intelligence Scale: Revised UK Edition (WAIS-R UK)*. Sidcup: Psychological Corporation.

Wechsler, D. (1987). *A Manual for the Wechsler Memory Scale – Revised*. San Antonio, TX: Psychological Corporation.

Wechsler, D. (1988). *Wechsler Memory Scale – Revised (WMS-R)*. Sidcup: Psychological Corporation.

Wechsler, D. and Stone, C.P. (1973). *Instruction Manual for the Wechsler Memory Scale*. New York: Psychological Corporation.

Wechsler, H., Grosser, G.H. and Busfield, B. (1963). The depression rating scale. *Archives of General Psychiatry, 9*: 334–43.

Weckowicz, T.E. (1978). Profile of Mood States. In: O.K. Buros (ed.), *The Eighth Mental Measurements Yearbook*, Vol. I. Highland Park, NJ: Gryphon Press.

Weckowicz, T.E., Muir, W. and Cropley, A. (1967). A factor analysis of the Beck Inventory of Depression. *Journal of Consulting Psychology, 31*: 23–8.

Weinberger, M., Hiner, S.L. and Tierney, W.M. (1987). Assessing social support in elderly adults. *Social Science and Medicine, 25*: 1049–55.

Weinberger, M., Tierney, W.M., Booher, P. and Hiner, S.L. (1990). Social support, stress and functional status in patients with osteoarthritis. *Social Science and Medicine, 30*: 503–8.

Weiner, C. (1975). The burden of rheumatoid arthritis: Tolerating the uncertainty. *Social Science and Medicine, 9*: 97–104.

Weinert, C. and Brandt, P. (1987). Measuring social support with the personal resource questionnaire. *Nursing Research, 9*: 589–602.

Weinstein, M.C. and Stason, W.B. (1976). *Hypertension: A Policy Perspective*. Cambridge, MA: Harvard University Press.

Weinstein, M.C., Fineberg, H.V., Elstein, A.S. *et al.* (1980). *Clinical Decision Analysis*. Philadelphia, PA: W.B. Saunders.

Weisman, A.D. (1979). *Coping with Cancer*. New York: McGraw Hill.

Weissman, M.M. and Bothwell, S. (1976). The assessment of social adjustment by self report. *Archives of General Psychiatry, 33*: 1111–15.

Weissman, M.M. and Paykel, E. (1974). *The Depressed Woman: A Study of Social Relations*. Chicago, IL: University of Chicago Press.

Weissman, M.M., Paykel, E., Siegel, R. and Klerman, G. (1971). The social role of depressed women: Comparisons with a normal group. *American Journal of Orthopsychiatry, 41*: 390–405.

Weissman, M.M., Klerman, G.L., Paykel, E.S. *et al.* (1974). Treatment effects on the social adjustment of depressed out-patients. *Archives of General Psychiatry, 30*: 771–8.

Weissman, M.M., Prusoff, B. and Newberry, P.B. (1975). *Comparisons of CES-D, Zung and Beck Self-Report Depression Scales*. Technical Report ADM 42–47–83. Rockville, MD: Center for Epidemiologic Studies, National Institute of Mental Health.

Weissman, M.M., Sholamskas, D., Pottenger, M. *et al.* (1977). Assessing depressive symptoms in five psychiatric populations: A validation study. *American Journal of Epidemiology, 106*: 203–14.

Weissman, M.M., Prusoff, B.A., Thompson, W.D. *et al.* (1978). Social adjustment by self report in a community sample and in psychiatric out-patients. *Journal of Nervous and Mental Disorders, 166*: 317–26.

Weissman, M.M., Sholomskas, D. and John, K. (1981). The assessment of social adjustment: An update. *Archives of General Psychiatry, 38*: 1250–8.

Wellisch, D.K. (1987). Surviving and its effects on the family. In: *Proceedings of the Fifth National Conference on Human Values and Cancer*, San Francisco, California, March 19–21. American Cancer Society.

Wellisch, D.K., Landsverk, J., Guidera, K. *et al.* (1983a). Evaluation of psychosocial problems of the home bound cancer patient: I. Methodology and problem frequencies. *Journal of Psychosomatic Medicine, 45*: 11–21.

Wellisch, D.K., Fawzy, F.I., Landsverk, J. *et al.* (1983b). Evaluation of psychosocial problems for the home-bound cancer patient: The relationship of disease and the socio-demographic variables of patients to family problems. *Journal of Psychosocial Oncology, 1*: 1–15.

Welsh, G.S. and Dahlstrom, W.D. (1956). *Basic Readings on the MMPI in Psychology and Medicine*. Minneapolis, MN: University of Minnesota Press.

Wenger, N.K., Mattson, M.E., Furberg, C.D. and Elinson, J. (eds) (1984). *Assessment of Quality of Life in Clinical Trials of Cardiovascular Therapies*. New York: Le Jacq.

Wennberg, J.E., Mulley, A.G., Hanley, D. *et al.* (1988). An assessment of prostatectomy for benign urinary tract obstruction: Geographic variations and the evaluation of medical care outcomes. *Journal of the American Medical Association, 259*: 3027–30.

Westaby, S., Sapsford, R.N. and Bentall, H.H. (1979). Return to work and quality of life after surgery for coronary artery disease. *British Medical Journal, 2*: 1028–31.

White, A., Nicolaas, G., Foster, K. *et al.* (1993). *Health Survey for England 1991*. London: HMSO.

WHOQOL Group (1991). *Assessment of Quality of Life in Health Care*. Geneva: WHO.

WHOQOL Group (1993a) Study protocol for the World Health Organization project to develop a Quality of Life assessment instrument (WHOQOL). *Quality of Life Research, 2*: 153–9.

WHOQOL Group (1993b). *Measuring Quality of Life: The Development of the World Health Organization Quality of Life Instrument (WHOQOL)*. Geneva: WHO.

WHOQOL Group (1993c). *WHOQOL Study Protocol*. MNH/PSF/93.9, Division of Mental Health. Geneva: WHO.

WHOQOL Group (1994a). The development of the WHO Quality of Life assessment instrument (the WHOQOL). In: J. Orley and W. Kuyken (eds), *International Quality of Life Assessment in Health Care Settings*. Heidelberg: Springer-Verlag.

WHOQOL Group (1994b). Quality of life assessment: An annotated bibliography (compiled by L. Hubanks and W. Kuyken). Geneva: WHO.

Wigton, R.S. (1988). Medical applications. In: B. Brehmer and C.R.B. Joyce (eds), *Human Judgement: The SJT View*. Advances in Psychology Vol. 54. Amsterdam: North-Holland.

Wikby, A., Hörnquist, J.O., Stenstrom, U. and Andersson, P.O. (1993). Background factors, long-term complications, quality of life and metabolic control in insulin dependent diabetes. *Quality of Life Research, 2*: 281–6.

Wiklund, I., Lindvall, K., Swedberg, K. *et al.* (1987). Self-assessment of quality of life in severe heart failure:

An instrument for clinical use. *Scandinavian Journal of Psychology, 28*: 220–5.

Wiklund, I., Gorkin, L., Pawitan, Y. *et al.* (1992). Methods for assessing quality of life in the cardiac arrhythmia suppression trial (CAST). *Quality of Life Research, 1*: 187–201.

Wilkin, D. and Jolley, D.J. (1979). *Behavioural Problems Among Old People in Geriatric Wards, Psychogeriatric Wards and Residential Homes, 1976–1978*. Research Report No. 1, Research Section, Psychiatric Unit. Manchester: University Hospital of South Manchester.

Wilkin, D., Hallam, L. and Doggett, A.M. (1992). *Measures of Need and Outcome for Primary Health Care*. Oxford: Oxford University Press.

Wilkinson, G., Borsey, D.Q., Leslie, P. *et al.* (1988). Psychiatric morbidity and social problems in patients with insulin-dependent diabetes mellitus. *British Journal of Psychiatry, 153*: 38–43.

Wilkinson, M.J.B. and Barczak, P. (1988). Psychiatric screening in general practice: Comparison of the General Health Questionnaire and the Hospital Anxiety and Depression Scale. *Journal of the Royal College of General Practitioners, 38*: 311–13.

Willer, B. and Biggin, P. (1974). *Self-assessment Guide: Rationale, Development, Evaluation*. Toronto: Lakeshore Psychiatric Hospital.

Williams, A. (1985a). The value of QALYS. *Health and Social Services Journal, 95*: 3–5.

Williams, A. (1985b). Economics of coronary artery bypass grafting. *British Medical Journal, 291*: 326–9.

Williams, A. and Kind, P. (1992). The present state of play about QALYs. In: A. Hopkins (ed.), *Measures of the Quality of Life and the Uses to which such Measures may be Put*. London: Royal College of Physicians.

Williams, D.R.R. (1989). Outcome indicators for diabetes services – what do we have and what do we need? *Community Medicine, 11*: 57–64.

Williams, G. (1987). Disablement and the social context of daily activity. *International Disability Studies, 9*: 97–102.

Williams, G. and Wood, P. (1988). Coming to terms with chronic illness: The negotiation of autonomy in rheumatoid arthritis. *International Disability Studies, 10*: 1228–37.

Williams, I.P. and McGavin, C.R. (1980). Corticosteroids in chronic airways obstruction: Can the patient's assessment be ignored? *British Journal of Diseases of the Chest, 74*: 142–8.

Williams, J.G., Barlow, D.H. and Agras, W.S. (1972). Behavioural measurement of severe depression. *Archives of General Psychiatry, 27*: 330–3.

Williams, J.I. and Wood-Dauphinee, S. (1989). Assessing quality of life: Measures and utility. In: F. Mosteller and J. Falotico-Taylor (eds), *Quality of Life and Technology Assessment*. Washington, DC: National Academy Press.

Williams, J.M.G. (1984). *The Psychology of Depression*. Beckenham: Croom Helm.

Williams, O.D., Kelner-Schron, E., Barofsky, I. *et al.* (1984). Report of the working group: Acute myocardial infarction. In: N.K. Wenger, M.E. Mattson, C.D. Furberg and J. Elinson, *Assessment of Quality of Life in Clinical Trials of Cardiovascular Therapies*. New York: Le Jacq.

Williams, P. (1987). Depressive thinking in general practice patients. In: P. Freeling, L.J. Downey and J.C. Malkin (eds), *The Presentation of the Depression: Current Approaches*. Occasional Paper No. 36, pp. 17–20. London: Royal College of General Practitioners.

Williams, R.H. and Wirths, C.G. (1965). *Lives Through the Years: Styles of Life and Successful Aging*. New York: Atherton Press.

Williams, S.J. (1989). Chronic respiratory illness and disability: A critical review of the psychosocial literature. *Social Science and Medicine, 28*: 791–803.

Williams, S.J. and Bury, M.R. (1989). Impairment, disability and handicap in chronic respiratory illness. *Social Science and Medicine, 29*: 609–16.

Willner, A.E. (1989). The use of cognitive tests to assess cognitive impairment in cardiac surgery patients: With emphasis on the CLAT Analogy Test. In: A. Willner and G. Rodewald (eds), *Impact of Cardiac Surgery on Quality of Life: Neurological and Psychological Aspects*. New York: Plenum Press.

Willner, A.E. and Rodewald, G. (1990). *The Impact of Cardiac Surgery on the Quality of Life*. New York: Plenum Press.

Wilson, B.A., Cockburn, J. and Baddeley, A.D. (1985). *The Rivermead Behavioural Memory Test*. Titchfield, Hants: Thames Valley Test Company.

Wilson, B.A., Cockburn, J., Baddeley, A.D. and Hierns, R.W. (1989). The development and validation of a test battery for detecting and monitoring everyday memory problems. *Journal of Clinical and Experimental Neuropsychology, 11*: 855–70.

Wilson, J.H., Taylor, P.J. and Robertson, G. (1985). The validity of the SCL-90 in a sample of British men remanded to prison for psychiatric reports. *Psychological Medicine, 10*: 101–14.

Wilson, L.A. and Brass, W. (1973). Brief assessment of the mental state in geriatric domiciliary practice: The usefulness of the mental status questionnaire. *Age and Ageing, 2*: 92–101.

Wilson, L.A., Roy, S.K. and Bursill, A.E. (1973). The reliability of the mental status questionnaire in geriatric practice. Unpublished manuscript. (Referred to in Wilson and Brass, 1973.)

Wilson, R.C. and Jones, P.W. (1989). A comparison of the visual analogue scale and modified Borg scale for the measurement of dyspnoea during exercise. *Clinical Science*, 76: 277–82.

Wilson, R.C. and Jones, P.W. (1991). Differentiation between the intensity of breathlessness and the distress it evokes in normal subjects during exercise. *Clinical Science*, 80: 65–70.

Wilson, R.G., Hart, A. and Dawes, P.J.D.K. (1988). Mastectomy or conservation: The patient's choice. *British Medical Journal*, 297: 1167–9.

Wilson-Barnett, J. (1981). Assessment of recovery: With special reference to a study with post-operative cardiac patients. *Journal of Advanced Nursing*, 6: 435–45.

Winefield, H.R. (1982). Reliability and validity of the health locus of control scale. *Journal of Personality Assessment*, 46: 614–19.

Wing, J.K. (1989). The measurement of 'social disablement': The MRC social behaviour and social performance schedules. *Social Psychiatry and Psychiatric Epidemiology*, 24: 173–8.

Wing, J.K. (1991). Measuring and classifying clinical disorders: Learning from the PSE. In: P.E. Bebbington (ed.), *Social Psychiatry: Theory, Methodology and Practice*. London: Transaction Publishers.

Wing, J.K. (1992). *SCAN: Schedules for Clinical Assessment in Neuropsychiatry*. Geneva: WHO.

Wing, J.K. (1993). *Trials of a Set of Brief Outcomes Scales to Measure the First Target of Mental Health of the Nation: Report on the Start-up Phase*. London: Royal College of Psychiatrists.

Wing, J.K. and Brown, G.W. (1970). *Institutionalism and Schizophrenia*. Cambridge: Cambridge University Press.

Wing, J.K. and Sturt, E. (1978). *The PSE-ID-Catego System: A Supplementary Manual*. London: Institute of Psychiatry.

Wing, J.K., Birley, J.L.T., Cooper, J.E. *et al.* (1967). Reliability of a procedure for measuring and classifying 'present psychiatric state'. *British Journal of Psychiatry, 113:*, 499–515.

Wing, J.K., Cooper, J.E. and Sartorius, N. (1974). *The measurement and classification of psychiatric symptoms: An Instruction Manual for the PSE and Catego Program*. Cambridge: Cambridge University Press.

Wing, J.K., Nixon, J.M., Mann, S.A. and Leff, J.P. (1977a). Reliability of the PSE (ninth edition) used in a population survey. *Psychological Medicine*, 7: 505–16.

Wing, J.K., Henderson, A.S. and Winckle, M. (1977b). The rating of symptoms by a psychiatrist and a non-psychiatrist: A study of patients referred from general practice. *Psychological Medicine*, 7: 713–15.

Wing, J.K., Babor, T., Brugha, T. *et al.* (1990). SCAN: Schedules for Clinical Assessment in Neuropsychiatry. *Archives of General Psychiatry*, 47: 589–93.

Wing, J.K., Brewin, C.R. and Thornicroft, G. (1992).

Defining mental health needs. In: G. Thornicroft, C.R. Brewin and J.K. Wing (eds), *Measuring Mental Health Needs*. London: Royal College of Psychiatrists.

Wing, J.K., Sartorius, N. and Ustun, T.B. (eds) (in press). *Diagnosis and Clinical Management in Psychiatry: An Instruction Manual for the SCAN System*. Cambridge: Cambridge University Press.

Wing, L., Wing, J.K., Griffith, D. and Stevens, B. (1972). An epidemiological and experimental evaluation of industrial rehabilitation for chronic psychotic patients in the community. In: J.K. Wing and A.M. Hailey (eds), *Evaluating a Community Psychiatric Service*. Oxford: Oxford University Press.

Wingard, J.R., Curbow, B., Baker, F. *et al.* (1991). Health, functional status and employment of adult survivors of bone marrow transplantation. *Annals of Internal Medicine*, 144: 113–18.

Wingo, L. and Evans, A. (1978). *Public Economics and the Quality of Life*. Baltimore, MD: Johns Hopkins University Press.

Winslow, C.M., Soloman, D.H., Chassin, M.R. *et al.* (1988). The appropriateness of carotid endarterectomy. *New England Journal of Medicine*, 318: 721–7.

Wolberg, W.H. (1991). Surgical options in 424 patients with primary breast cancer without systemic metastases. *Archives of Surgery*, 126: 817–20.

Wolberg, W.H., Tanner, M.A., Romsaas, E.P. *et al.* (1987). Factors influencing options in primary breast cancer treatment. *Journal of Clinical Oncology*, 5: 68–74.

Wolcott, D.L., Wellisch, D.K. and Fawzy, F.I. (1986). Adaptation of adult bone marrow transplant recipient long term survivors. *Transplantation*, 41: 478–84.

Wolcott, D.L., Fawzy, F.I. and Wellisch, D.K. (1987). Psychiatric aspects of BMT: A review and current issues. *Psychiatric Medicine*, 4: 299–317.

Wolkove, N., Dajozman, E., Colacone, A. and Kreisman, H. (1989). The relationship between pulmonary function and dyspnoea in obstructive lung disease. *Chest*, 96: 1247–51.

Wood-Dauphinee, S. and Williams, J.I. (1987). Reintegration to normal living as a proxy to quality of life. *Journal of Chronic Diseases*, 40: 491–9.

Wood-Dauphinee, S. and Williams, J.I. (1991). The Spitzer Quality of Life Index: Its performance as a measure. In: D. Osoba (ed.), *Effect of Cancer on Quality of Life*. Boston, MA: CRC Press.

Woodworth, R. S. (1918). *Personal Data Sheet*. Chicago, IL: Stoelting.

Woody, G.R., McLellan, A.T., Luborsky, L. and O'Brien, C.P. (1985). Sociopathy and psychotherapy outcome. *Archives of General Psychiatry*, 42: 1081–6.

World Health Organization (1947). *Constitution of the World Health Organization*. Geneva: WHO.

World Health Organization (1948). *Official Records of the*

World Health Organization, No. 2, p. 100. Geneva: WHO.

World Health Organization (1958). *The First Ten Years of the World Health Organization*. Geneva: WHO.

World Health Organization (1977). *International Classification of Diseases*, 9th edn. Geneva: WHO.

World Health Organization (1978). *Mental Disorders: Glossary and Guide to Their Classification in Accordance with the Ninth Edition of the International Classification of Diseases (ICD-9)*. Geneva: WHO.

World Health Organization (1979). *Handbook for Reporting Results of Cancer Treatments*. WHO Offset Publication No. 48. Geneva: WHO.

World Health Organization (1980). *International Classification of Impairments, Disabilities and Handicaps*. Geneva: WHO.

World Health Organization (1984). *Uses of Epidemiology in Aging: Report of a Scientific Group, 1983*. Technical Report Series, No. 706. Geneva: WHO.

World Health Organization (1988). *Psychiatric Disability Assessment Schedule*. Geneva: WHO.

World Health Organization (1990). *DCR ICD 10*. Geneva: WHO.

World Health Organization (1991). *Assessment of Quality of Life in Health Care: A Working Party Report*. Geneva: WHO.

World Health Organization (1992). *International Classification of Diseases*, 10th edn. Geneva: WHO.

World Health Organization (1993). *Rehabilitation after Cardiovascular Diseases, with Special Emphasis on Developing Countries: Report of a WHO Expert Committee*. WHO Technical Report Series 831. Geneva: WHO.

Wray, J., Radley-Smith, R. and Yacoub, M. (1992). Effect of cardiac or heart–lung transplantation on the quality of life of the paediatric patient. *Quality of Life Research, 1*: 41–6.

Wright, S.J. (1987). Self-ratings of health: The influence of age and smoking status and the role of different explanatory models. *Psychology and Health, 1*: 379–97.

Wright, S.J. (1990). Conceptions and dimensions of health. In: R. Shute and G. Penny (eds), *Psychology and Health Promotion: Proceedings of the Welsh Branch of the British Psychological Society Conference on 'Psychology and Health Promotion'*. Cardiff: British Psychological Society (Welsh Branch).

Wright, S.J. (in press). Health status assessment. In: A. Baum, C. McManus, S. Newman *et al.* (eds), *Cambridge Handbook of Psychology, Health and Medicine*. Cambridge: Cambridge University Press.

Wright, S.J., Stein, A., Boyle, H. *et al.* (1994). Health-related quality of life in end-stage renal failure (abstract). *Quality of Life Research: 3*: 63.

Wright, S.J., Johnston, M. and Weinman, J. (in press). *Measures in Health Psychology: A User's Resource Pack*. Windsor: NFER-Nelson.

Wu, A.W., Mathews, W.C., Brysk, L.T. *et al.* (1990). Quality of life in a placebo-controlled trial of zidovudine patients with AIDS and AIDS related complex. *Acquired Immune Deficiency Syndrome, 3*: 683–90.

Wu, A.W., Rubin, H.R., Mathews, W.C. *et al.* (1991). A health status questionnaire using 30 items from the Medical Outcomes Study: preliminary validation in persons with early HIV infection. *Medical Care, 29*: 786–98.

Wykes, T. (1982). A hostel-ward for 'new' long stay patients: An evaluative study of 'a ward in a house' (Part II, Appendix). In: J.K. Wing (ed.), Long term community care: Experience in a London borough. *Psychological Medicine*, monograph supplement 2: 96.

Wykes, T. and Hurry, J. (1991). Social behaviour and psychiatric disorders. In: P.E. Bebbington (ed.), *Social Psychiatry: Theory, Methodology and Practice*. London: Transaction Publishers.

Wykes, T. and Sturt, E. (1986). The measurement of social behaviour in psychiatric patients: An assessment of the reliability and validity of the SBS schedule. *British Journal of Psychiatry, 148*: 1–11.

Wykes, T., Sturt, E. and Creer, C. (1982). Practices of day and residential units in relation to the social behaviour of attenders. In: J.K. Wing (ed.), Long term community care: Experience in a London borough. Part II. *Psychological Medicine*, monograph supplement 2: 15–27.

Wykes, T., Sturt, E. and Creer, C. (1985). The assessment of patients' needs for community care. *Social Psychiatry, 20*: 76–85.

Wylie, C.M. and White, B.K. (1964). A measure of disability. *Archives of Environmental Health, 8*: 834–9.

Yates, J.W., Chalmer, B. and McKegney, F.P. (1980). Evaluation of patients with advanced cancer using the Karnofsky Performance Status. *Cancer, 45*: 2220–4.

Yesavage, J.A., Brink, T.L., Rose, T.L. *et al.* (1983). Development and validation of a geriatric depression screening scale – a preliminary report. *Journal of Psychiatric Research, 17*: 37–49.

Yorkston, N.J., Zaki, S.A., Malik, M.K.U. *et al.* (1974). Propanolol in the control of schizophrenic symptoms. *British Medical Journal, iv*: 633–5.

Yorkston, N.J., Zaki, S.A., Weller, M.P. *et al.* (1981). DL-propanolol and chlorpromazine following admission for schizophrenia: A controlled comparison. *Acta Psychiatrica Scandinavica, 63*: 13–27.

Young, K.J. and Longman, A.J. (1983). Quality of life and persons with melanoma: A pilot study. *Cancer Nursing, 6*: 219–25.

Young, N., Williams, J.I., Wright, J.G. and Piexto, G. (1994). Rating difficulty in functioning in patients undergoing hip or knee replacements: Comparing the WOMAC and Physical Functioning (SF-36) Scales (abstract). *Quality of Life Research, 3*: 100.

Zautra, A. and Goodhart, D. (1979). Quality of life indicators: A review of the literature. *Community Mental Health Review, 4*: 1–10.

Zautra, A. and Simons, L.S. (1978). An assessment of a community's mental health needs. *American Journal of Community Psychology, 6*: 351–62.

Zeiner-Henriksen, T. (1972). The repeatability at interview of symptoms of angina and possible infarction. *Journal of Chronic Diseases, 25*: 407–14.

Zeller, R.A. and Carmines, E.G. (1980). *Measurement in the Social Sciences.* Cambridge: Cambridge University Press.

Ziebland, S. and Fitzpatrick, R. (1992). Assessing short term outcome (letter). *Quality in Health Care, 1*: 141–2.

Zielske, J.V., Lohr, K., Goldberg, G.A. *et al.* (1982). *Conceptualisation and Measurement of Health for Adults. Vol. 17. Peptic Ulcer Disease.* Santa Monica, CA: Rand Corporation.

Zigmond, A.S. and Snaith, R.P. (1983). The Hospital Anxiety and Depression Scale. *Acta Psychiatrica Scandinavica, 67*: 361–70.

Ziller, R.C. (1974). Self–other orientation and quality of life. *Social Indicators Research, 1*: 301–27.

Zonderman, A.B., Costa, P.T. and McCrae, R.R. (1989). Depression as a risk for cancer morbidity and mortality in a nationally representative sample. *Journal of the American Medical Association, 262*: 1191–5.

Zubrod, C.G., Schneiderman, M., Frei, E. *et al.* (1960).

Appraisal of methods for the study of chemotherapy of cancer in man: Comparative therapeutic trial of nitrogen mustard and triethylene thiophosphoramide. *Journal of Chronic Diseases, 11*: 7–33.

Zung, W.W.K. (1965). A self-rating depression scale. *Archives of General Psychiatry, 12*: 63–70.

Zung, W.W.K. (1967a). Factors influencing the Self-Rating Depression Scale. *Archives of General Psychiatry, 16*: 543–7.

Zung, W.W.K. (1967b). Depression in the normal aged. *Psychosomatics, 8*: 287–92.

Zung, W.W.K. (1972). The Depression Status Inventory: An adjunct to the self-rating depression scale. *Journal of Clinical Psychology, 28*: 539–43.

Zung, W.W.K. (1986). Zung Self-Rating Depression Scale and Depression Status Inventory. In: N. Sartorius and T.A. Ban (eds), *Assessment of Depression.* Heidelberg: Springer-Verlag.

Zung, W.W.K., Richards, C.B. and Short, M.J. (1965). Self-rating depression scale in an out-patient clinic: Further validation of the ZDS. *Archives of General Psychiatry, 13*: 508–15.

Zwick, R.J. (1982). The effect of pre-therapy orientation on client knowledge about therapy, improvement in therapy, attendance patterns, and satisfaction with services. *Masters Abstracts, 20*: 307 (Masters thesis, University of California, Berkeley).

INDEX

Visual Analogue Scale for Bone Marrow
    Transplant Patients, 55–6

Waddell Disability Score, 276
Wade, D. T., 177, 180, 182, 185, 186, 259
walking tests (dyspnoea), 154, 160
Wallston, K. A., 146–8
Ware, J. E., 15, 16, 21, 22, 23, 35, 59, 60, 177, 212, 229,
    260, 281–5, 291, 296
    see also Short Form-36
Washington Psychosocial Inventory, 190, 194–5, 208
Ways of Coping Scale, 25, 139–41, 148
Wechsler Memory and Intelligence Scales, 25, 178, 192,
    198–200, 206–7, 208, 240, 253

Western Ontario and McMaster Universities Arthritis
    Index (WOMAC), 222–4
Wing, J. K., 24, 61, 62, 66, 67–8, 69, 88, 102–3, 118,
    120, 121, 122, 123
Wood-Dauphinee, S., 25, 137, 292
Work Performance and Satisfaction Scale, 237
World Health Organization
    criteria on rehabilitation of mentally-ill patients, 252

definition of health, 2–3, 8, 9
definition of impairment, disability, handicap, 210,
    223
dyspnoea and cardiovascular questionnaires, 245–7
Functional Scale, 30
International Classification of Diseases, 67
Psychiatric Disability Assessment Schedule, 126–7
Quality of Life Assessment Instrument, 3, 58–9
Symptom Checklist, 33
WHOQoL Group, 3, 58–9, 61
Wright, S. J., 268–9
Wu, A. W., 272
Wykes, T., 62, 88, 103, 113, 119, 120, 121, 122, 123
    see also Social Behaviour Schedule, Assessment of
    Need Questionnaire

Yesavage, J. A., 189

Zigmond, A. S., 23, 24, 25, 34–5, 39, 47, 59, 76, 88,
    152, 165, 213
Zubrod Scale, 30–1
Zung Self-Rating Depression Scale, 82–4, 88, 238

MEASURING HEALTH
A REVIEW OF QUALITY OF LIFE MEASURE-MENT SCALES

Ann Bowling

Increasing attention is being paid to the consequences of health and ill-health and to the outcomes of health care provision. Indices of health status in current usage focus on ill-health and are based on negative conceptualizations of health (e.g. mortality and morbidity rates, the self-reporting of symptoms, illness and functional ability). More attention is now being given to the development of positive measures of health, a term which encompasses concepts of 'social health', 'social well-being' and 'quality of life'. This volume reviews a wide range of popular measures of functional disability and health status, as well as broader measures of health such as those concerned with psychological well-being (e.g. anxiety and depression), emotional well-being (e.g. life satisfaction, morale and happiness), and social networks, support and loneliness. The book will be an essential source book for social scientists and all health care professionals involved in the measurement of 'health'.

> This is a useful contribution to the literature on health measurement, presenting material which could be dull in an economical and lively fashion.
> (*Sociology of Health and Illness*)

> . . . Ann Bowling's review of quality-of-life measurement scales is timely and ought to be of value to a wide range of readers.
> (*The Health Service Journal*)

Contents
Preface – The conceptualization of functioning, health and quality of life – Theory of measurement – The measurement of functional ability – Broader measures of health status – Measures of psychological well-being – Measuring social networks and social support – Measures of life satisfaction and morale – References.

208pp   0 335 15435 2 (Paperback)